MEDICAL
ABBREVIATIONS
&
EPONYMS

2nd Edition

MEDICAL ABBREVIATIONS & EPONYMS

2nd Edition

SHEILA B. SLOANE

Formerly President, Medi-Phone, Inc.
Author, The Medical Word Book, 3rd Edition;
A Word Book in Radiology; and
A Word Book in Laboratory Medicine, 2nd Edition

W.B. SAUNDERS COMPANY
A Division of Harcourt Brace & Company
Philadelphia   London   Toronto   Montreal   Sydney   Tokyo

W.B. SAUNDERS COMPANY
A Division of Harcourt Brace & Company

The Curtis Center
Independence Square West
Philadelphia, Pennsylvania 19106

Library of Congress Cataloging-in-Publication Data

Sloane, Sheila B.

Medical abbreviations & eponyms / Sheila B. Sloane—2nd ed.

p.   cm.

ISBN 0–7216–7088–1

1. Medicine—Abbreviations.   2. Eponyms—Dictionaries.   I. Title.

R123.S569 1997
610′.148—DC20   96–28595

ESKIND BIOMEDICAL LIBRARY

SEP 1 6 1997

VANDERBILT UNIVERSITY
NASHVILLE, TN 37232-8340

MEDICAL ABBREVIATIONS & EPONYMS, 2nd Edition   ISBN 0–7216–7088–1

Copyright © 1997, 1985 by W.B. Saunders Company.

All rights reserved. No part of this publication may be reproduced or transmitted in any form or by any means, electronic or mechanical, including photocopy, recording, or any information storage and retrieval system, without permission in writing from the publisher.

Printed in the United States of America.

Last digit is the print number: 9   8   7   6   5   4   3   2   1

Dedicated
to
John,
my friend, mentor, and supporter

Preface to the Second Edition

Don't never look back:
something may be gaining on you.
Satchel Paige

Writing a preface is, however ill-advisedly, simply looking back. The reader will want to know what was done and why; the writer will wonder whether deletion has been wise, addition precise, and purpose fulfilled.

In the eighteenth century linguistic purists frowned on use of abbreviations and even eponyms. They regarded both as inelegant shortcuts in the art of discourse; but now stark necessity in science—especially in bioscience and its sister art, clinical medicine—has brought new and extensive use to the abbreviation. The immense proliferation of polysyllabic terms and mind-bending phrases enforces its need. Flesch, in his *The ABC of Style*, put the matter to rest: "It's a superstition that abbreviations shouldn't be used in serious writing. Nonsense: use abbreviations wherever they are customary and needed." They are needed especially in the research report that frequently reuses a customary phrase. Why repeat "superconducting quantum interference device" when SQUID will do, even though it may be confused with a ten-armed cephalopod?

So, too, eponyms have come into favor. Like the computer they save time and space, but they also evoke the names of physicians, patients, and places that have played a role in the ongoing development of medicine. The very name Addison's disease brings to mind the whole complex field of diseases of the ductless glands and the fact that Addison's pioneering work on their elucidation was regarded in its day as a medical curiosity. Similarly, O'nyong-nyong fever evokes the mosquito-infested African scene where this disease brings lymphadenitis, aching joints, and painful skin rash to thousands of people.

The section on eponyms, which are often a source of misspelling and confusion to the transcriptionist, medical secretary, record librarian, nurse, and physician, includes diseases, syndromes, operations, positions, instruments, stains, tests, signs, and pathological conditions named after the discoverer, the patient, or even mythological characters. Definitions have been given for the more common diseases, syndromes, and operations, but for those which are rarely seen only the eponymic names have been listed. No effort has been made to include all possible instruments under an eponymic entry; rather, emphasis has been placed on completeness of the eponyms themselves for the purpose of correct spelling and identification.

The abbreviation poses a problem in spelling. That Thoreau said, "I distrust a man who can spell a word only one way" is a pleasantry, not a license to misuse words. To write "compliment" instead of "complement" is to defeat the purpose of language. There are indeed canons of correctness in orthography but none in the formation of abbreviations. Every dictionary, journal, or word book consulted will afford examples of difference. The same abbreviation will appear in both capital and lower-case letters and with or without closing periods. The attempt here is not to state which usage is favored, but only which is more prevalent. The aim is to be inclusive—not arbitrary—so that in this second edition more than 10,000 new entries appear, including chemical formulas and symbols, physical and biochemical terms, and new elements, acronyms, and names of organizations.

The eponym poses the curious problem of proper use of the apostrophe—a useful device that for no discernible reason has come under attack. In an amusing essay (Its Academic, Or Is It?), Professor Charles Larson deplores both its misuse and its coming demise. Nevertheless, it still seems useful as a possessive, so Smith's disease and Sjogren's syndrome and Adams' disease and Bruns' syndrome appear here in their traditional forms.

Now that the weary pen is put away, the kitchen light dimmed, and the thousands of jigsaw notes and ideas consigned to oblivion, perhaps I may speak for myself.

I have enjoyed doing this revision, for writing is ever a pleasure, and renewed acquaintanceship with the miracle of modern medicine is always stimulating. All books call for decisions, and whether these have been properly made only the reader may decide. Whatever that decision, corrections and suggestions from readers will be deeply appreciated and acted upon.

In making these decisions I have consulted many books and journals in which the advance of medicine is chronicled, and I have made use of the abundant reference sources of the American Association for Medical Transcription. I have consulted too with colleagues and with my publisher. I owe a great debt of appreciation to Margaret Biblis and the staff of the W.B. Saunders Company for their dexterous help and counsel, to Wynette Kommer for her expert guidance and assistance, and to Donna Ciccotelli for her skillful typing. For his support and constant encouragement, I offer my deepest gratitude to my dear John Dusseau.

To the many readers of the first edition of *Medical Abbreviations and Eponyms* it is my hope that this second edition will continue to answer the needs of transcriptionists and health-care personnel in their search for the correct spelling of the often-enigmatic medical term.

SHEILA B. SLOANE

Preface to the First Edition

....

Since publication in 1973 of the first edition of The Medical Word Book, medical-record keeping has changed to a remarkable degree, becoming more sophisticated and expert than ever before. There are few more impressive success stories than that of the spectacular growth and professionalism achieved by the medical transcriptionist over these past years. A dramatic advancement in the practice of medicine, phenomenal progress in research, and the division of medicine into highly specialized fields have given birth to a vitally important new profession—that of the professional transcriptionist. It extends to all aspects of medicine, and two of its more difficult areas are in the use of medical abbreviations and eponyms.

It is, therefore, the purpose of this book to offer a comprehensive listing of medical abbreviations—in which are included chemical formulas, chemical symbols, many new biochemical terms, elements, acronyms, medical organizations, and some appropriate computer terms—and a complete listing of eponyms, which have long been a source of confusion to medical secretaries, transcriptionists, record librarians, physicians, nurses, and anyone involved directly or indirectly with medical terminology. Abbreviations are time-saving and space-saving as well as efficient, and therefore the attempt of the book is to be inclusive rather than selective. Often the same abbreviation has multiple meanings, and no attempt has been made to state which is the favored usage, all forms being listed. If there is any possibility of confusion in the significance of the abbreviation, its meaning should be spelled out in full.

Eponyms, too, are an ancient device for the storage and retrieval of information—a forerunner of the computer but considerably more handy. The very name Addison's disease brings to mind the whole complex field of diseases of the ductless glands and that Addison's great work on the subject was regarded in his day as merely a medical curiosity. The section on eponyms includes diseases, syndromes, positions, operations, instruments, stains, tests, signs, and any medical procedure or pathological condition named after the discoverer, the patient, or even mythological characters. In the case of diseases, syndromes and operations, a brief definition is given, whereas all other eponymic entries are simply listed alphabetically and characterized. No effort has been made to include under each eponymic entry all of its possible instruments; but rather, emphasis has been placed on completeness of the eponyms themselves for the purpose of correct spelling and identification. Occasionally the word "eponym" has been given a broad meaning to include difficult and obscure place names when they refer to diseases, viruses, and so on—for instance, O'nyong-nyong fever.

Every effort has been made to see that these listings are both accurate and current; thus many reference sources have been used to reach this goal. Nowhere was the question of proper usage more troublesome than in the use of upper and lower case letters and periods in listing the abbreviations. Since there are great differences in form from one reference to another, compilation of the book called for judgment and guidance. For their assistance I owe the Saunders editorial staff, particularly Wynette Kommer and Baxter Venable, my sincere thanks.

It is my hope that this book will provide a simple method of locating the sought-after abbreviation or eponym with ease and speed and eliminate the need to search through many reference books to achieve this end.

SHEILA B. SLOANE

Contents

Medical Abbreviations

Medical Abbreviations

A—
abnormal
abortion
absolute temperature
absorbance
acceptor
accommodation
acetone
acetum [vinegar]
acid
acidophil
acidophilic
acromion
actin
activity [radiation]
adenine
adenoma
adenosine
admittance
adrenaline
adult
age
akinetic
alanine
albino [guinea pig]
albumin
alive
allergologist
allergy
alpha [cell]
alpha (first letter of the
   Greek alphabet), uppercase
alveolar gas
ambulatory
ampere
amphetamine
ampicillin
amyloid
anaphylaxis

A — (continued)
androsterone
anesthesia
anesthetic
angioplasty
angle
angstrom
Ångstrom unit
anisotropic
annum (Lat.) year
anode
antagonism
ante (Lat.) before
anterior
antrectomy
apical
aqua (Lat.) water
aqueous
area
argon
arteria
assessment
atomic weight
atrium
atropine
auricle
auris
auscultation
axial
axilla
axillary
blood group
mass number
start of anesthesia
subspinale
total acidity
A. —
   Actinomyces
   Anopheles

1

A [band] — the dark-staining zone
    of a striated muscle
Å — Ångstrom unit
Ā —
    cumulated activity
    antinuclear antibody
A₁ —
    aortic first sound
    first auditory area
AI — angiotensin I
A₂ —
    aortic second sound
    second auditory area
A₂₋os — aortic second sound, open-
    ing snap
AII — angiotensin II
AIII — angiotensin III
A250 — 5% albumin, 250 ml
A1000 — 5% albumin, 1000 ml
a —
    absorptivity
    acceleration
    accommodation
    acid
    acidity
    agar
    ampere
    annum (Lat.) year
    anode
    anterior
    aqua (Lat.) water
    area
    arteria
    arterial blood
    artery
    asymmetric
    atto-
    axial
    thermodynamic activity
    total acidity
ā — *ante* (Lat.) before
α —
    acceleration
    activity
    alpha (first letter of the
        Greek alphabet), lowercase
    angular acceleration
    chain of hemoglobin
    constituent of plasma protein
        fraction

α — (*continued*)
    first in a series or group
    heavy chain of immunoglobu-
        lin A
    optical rotation [chemistry]
    probability of type I error
    [Bunsen's] solubility coeffi-
        cient
    specific absorptivity
α₁ — antichymotrypsin
α/A — α to A ratio
α₂-AP — alpha₂-antiplasmin
α-GLUC — alpha-glucosidase
α-KG — alpha-ketoglutarate
α-LP — alpha-lipoprotein
α₂M — alpha₂-macroglobulin
AA —
    acetic acid
    achievement age
    active alcoholic
    active assistive [range of mo-
        tion]
    active avoidance
    acupuncture analgesia
    acute asthma
    Addicts Anonymous
    adenine arabinoside
    adenylic acid
    adjuvant arthritis
    adrenal androgen
    adrenocortical autoantibody
    aggregated albumin
    agranulocytic angina
    alcohol abuse
    Alcoholics Anonymous
    allergic alveolitis
    alopecia areata
    alveolar-arterial
    aminoacetone
    amino acid
    aminoacyl
    amyloid-associated
    ana (Gr.) so much of each
    anaplastic astrocytoma
    anesthesiologist's assistant
    antiarrhythmic agent
    anticipatory avoidance
    antigen aerosol

AA — (continued)
    antiprotein accumulator
    aortic amplitude
    aortic aneurysm
    aortic arch
    aplastic anemia
    arachidonic acid
    arm-ankle
    arteries
    ascaris antigen
    ascending aorta
    Association of Anesthetists
    atlantoaxial
    atomic absorption
    audiologic assessment
    Australia antigen
    authorized absence
    autoanalyzer
    automobile accident
    axonal arborization

$\overline{AA}$ — ana (Gr.) so much of each

A&A — aid and attendance
    arthroscopy and arthrotomy
    awake and aware

A-a —
    alveolar-arterial [gradient]
    aortic artery

aA —
    abampere
    arterial to alveolar [oxygen ratio]
    azure A

aa — ana (Gr.) so much of each

aa. — arteriae (Lat.) arteries

AAA —
    abdominal aortic aneurysm
    abdominal aortic aneurysmectomy
    acne-associated arthritis
    acquired aplastic anemia
    acute anxiety attack
    addiction, autoimmune diseases, and aging
    amalgam
    American Academy of Allergy
    American Association of Anatomists

AAA — (continued)
    androgenic anabolic agent
    aneurysm of ascending aorta
    Area Agency on Aging
    aromatic amino acid

AAAA — American Academy of Anesthesiologist's Assistants

AAAAA — aphasia, agnosia, apraxia, agraphia, and alexia

AAAD — aromatic amino acid decarboxylase

AAAE — amino acid–activating enzymes

AAAF — albumin autoagglutinating factor

AAAHE — American Association for the Advancement of Health Education

AAAI — American Academy of Allergy and Immunology

AAALAC — American Association for Accreditation of Laboratory Animal Care

AA-AMP — amino acid adenylate [adenomonophosphate]

AAAS — American Association for the Advancement of Science

AAB —
    action against burns
    American Association of Bioanalysts
    aminoazobenzene

AABB — American Association of Blood Banks

AABCC — alertness (consciousness), airway, breathing, circulation, and cervical spine

AABS — automobile accident, broadside

AAC —
    antibiotic-associated colitis
    antimicrobial agent–induced colitis
    antimicrobial agents and chemotherapy
    augmentative and alternative communication

AACA — acylaminocephalosporanic acid

AACC — American Association for Clinical Chemistry

AACCN — American Association of Critical Care Nurses

AACE — antigen-antibody–crossed electrophoresis

AACG — acute angle closure glaucoma

AACHP — American Association for Comprehensive Health Planning

AACIA — American Association for Clinical Immunology and Allergy

AACN — American Association of Colleges of Nursing

AACO — American Association of Certified Orthoptists

AACP —
American Academy of Cerebral Palsy
American Academy of Child Psychiatry
American Association of Colleges of Pharmacy

AACPDM — American Academy for Cerebral Palsy and Developmental Medicine

AACSH — adrenal androgen corticotropin–stimulating hormone

AAD —
acid-ash diet
acute agitated delirium
alloxazine adenine dinucleotide
alpha$_2$-antitrypsin deficiency
American Academy of Dermatology
antibiotic-associated diarrhea
aromatic acid decarboxylase

AADC — amino acid decarboxylase

AAdC — anterior adductor of the coxa

AADE —
American Association of Dental Editors

AADE — (continued)
American Association of Dental Examiners

AADGP — American Academy of Dental Group Practice

$(A-a)D_{N_2}$ — alveolar-arterial nitrogen tension difference

aAD_{O_2}, $(a-A)D_{O_2}$ — arterio-alveolar oxygen tension difference

AADP —
American Academy of Dental Prosthetics
amyloid A–degrading protease

AADPA — American Academy of Dental Practice Administration

AADR — American Academy of Dental Radiology

AADS — American Academy of Dental Schools

AAE —
active assistive exercise
acute allergic encephalitis
American Association of Endodontists
annuloaortic ectasia

AAEE — American Association of Electromyography and Electrodiagnosis

AAEH — Association to Advance Ethical Hypnosis

AAEM — American Academy of Environmental Medicine

A/AEX, AAex — active assistive exercise

AAF —
acetic acid–alcohol–formalin [fixative]
acetylaminofluorine
ascorbic acid factor

AAFP — American Academy of Family Physicians

AAG —
allergic angiitis and granulomatosis
alpha$_1$-acid glycoprotein
alveolar-arterial gradient
autoantigen

AaG — alveolar-arterial gradient

AAGP —

American Academy of General Practice

American Association for Geriatric Psychiatry

AAGS — adult adrenogenital syndrome

A:AGT — blood group A antiglobulin test

AAHA — American Academy of Health Administration

AAHD — American Association of Hospital Dentists

AAHE — Association for the Advancement of Health Education

AAHPER — American Association for Health, Physical Education, and Recreation

AAHS — American Association for Hand Surgery

AAI —

acute alveolar injury

Adolescent Alienation Index

American Association of Immunologists

arm-ankle indices

AAIA — acquired artery immune augmentation

AAIB — alpha$_1$-aminoisobutyrate

AAID — American Academy of Implant Dentures

AAIN —

acute allergic intestinal nephritis

American Association of Industrial Nurses

AAK — allo-activated killer

AAL — anterior axillary line

AALAS — American Association of Laboratory Animal Science

AALL — American Association for Labor Legislation

AAM —

acute aseptic meningitis

American Academy of Microbiology

AAM — (continued)

amino acid mixture

AAMA —

American Academy of Medical Administrators

American Association of Medical Assistants

AAMC —

American Association of Medical Clinics

Association of American Medical Colleges

AAMD — American Association on Mental Deficiency

AAME — acetylarginine methyl ester

AAMFT — American Association for Marriage and Family Therapy

AAMI — Association for the Advancement of Medical Instrumentation

AAMIH — American Association for Maternal and Infant Health

AAMMC — American Association of Medical Milk Commissioners

AAMP —

American Academy of Maxillofacial Prosthetics

American Academy of Medical Prevention

AAMR —

American Academy of Mental Retardation

AAMRA — American Association of Medical Record Administrators

AAMRL — American Association of Medical Record Librarians

AAMRS — automated ambulatory medical record system

AAMS — acute aseptic meningitis syndrome

AAMSI — American Association for Medical Systems and Informatics

AAMT—
American Association for Medical Transcription
American Association for Music Therapy

AAN—
AIDS-associated nephropathy
alpha-amino nitrogen
American Academy of Neurology
American Academy of Nursing
American Academy of Nutrition
American Association of Neuropathologists
amino acid nitrogen
analgesic abuse nephropathy
analgesic-associated nephropathy
attending's admission notes

AANA—American Association of Nurse Anesthetists

AANM—American Association of Nurse-Midwives

AANPI—American Association of Nurses Practicing Independently

AANS—American Association of Neurological Surgeons

AAO—
American Academy of Ophthalmology
American Academy of Optometry
American Academy of Osteopathy
American Academy of Otolaryngology
American Association of Ophthalmologists
American Association of Orthodontists
amino acid oxidase
awake, alert, and oriented

A-aO$_2$—alveolar-arterial oxygen gradient

AAO×3—awake, alert, and oriented to time, place, and person

AAOC—antacid of choice

AAofA—Ambulance Association of America

AAOHN—American Association of Occupational Health Nurses

AAOM—American Academy of Oral Medicine

AAOO—American Academy of Ophthalmology and Otolaryngology

AAOP—
American Academy of Oral Pathology
American Academy of Orthotists and Prosthetists

AAOS—American Academy of Orthopaedic Surgeons

AAP—
air at atmospheric pressure
alpha$_1$-antiprotease
American Academy of Pediatrics
American Academy of Pedodontics
American Academy of Periodontology
American Academy of Psychoanalysts
American Academy of Psychotherapists
American Association of Pathologists
assessment adjustment pass
Association for the Advancement of Psychoanalysis
Association for the Advancement of Psychotherapy
Association of American Physicians

AAPA—
American Academy of Physicians Assistants
American Association of Pathologist Assistants

AAPB — American Association of Pathologists and Bacteriologists

AAPC — antibiotic-associated pseudomembranous colitis

AaP_{CO_2} — alveolar-arterial carbon dioxide tension difference

AAPF — anti-arteriosclerosis polysaccharide factor

AAPHD — American Association of Public Health Dentists

AAPHP — American Association of Public Health Physicians

AAPL — American Academy of Psychiatry and Law

AAPMC — antibiotic-associated pseudomembranous colitis

AAPMR — American Academy of Physical Medicine and Rehabilitation

AaP_{O_2} — alveolar-arterial oxygen tension difference

AAPS —
American Association of Plastic Surgeons
Arizona Articulation Proficiency Scale
Association of American Physicians and Surgeons

AAPSC — American Association of Psychiatric Services for Children

AAR —
active avoidance reaction
acute articular rheumatism
antigen-antiglobulin reaction
Australia antigen radioimmunoassay

aar — against all risks

AARC — American Association for Respiratory Care

AARE — automobile accident, rear end

AAROM — active-assistive range of motion

AART —
American Association for Rehabilitation Therapy

AART — (continued)
American Association for Respiratory Therapy

AAS —
acid aspiration syndrome
acute abdominal series
alcoholic abstinence syndrome
American Academy of Sanitarians
American Analgesia Society
aneurysm of atrial septum
anthrax antiserum
atlantoaxial subluxation
aortic arch syndrome
atomic absorption spectrophotometry
atypical absence seizure

AASCRN — amino acid screen

AASD — American Academy of Stress Disorders

Aase — asparaginase

aa seq — amino acid sequence

AASH — adrenal androgen–stimulating hormone

AASP —
acute atrophic spinal paralysis
American Association of Senior Physicians
ascending aorta synchronized pulsation

AASS — American Association for Social Security

AAT —
Aachen aphasia test
academic aptitude test
acute abdominal tympany
alanine aminotransferase
alkylating agent therapy
$alpha_1$-antitrypsin
amino-azotoluene
atrial-triggered [pacemaker]
auditory apperception test
automatic atrial tachycardia

A1AT — $alpha_1$-antitrypsin

AATA — American Art Therapy Association

AATS — American Association for Thoracic Surgery

AAU — acute anterior uveitis
AAV — adeno-associated virus
AAVMC — Association of American Veterinary Medical Colleges
AAVP — American Association of Veterinary Parasitologists
AAVV — accumulated alveolar ventilatory volume
AAW — anterior aortic wall
AB —
  abdominal
  abnormal
  aborta, abortus (Lat.) abortion
  Ace bandage
  active bilaterally
  Aid to the Blind
  air bleed
  alcian blue
  antibiotic
  antibody
  antigen binding
  apex beat
  apnea-bradycardia
  Artium Baccalaureus (Lat.) Bachelor of Arts
  asbestos body
  asthmatic bronchitis
  axiobuccal
  blood group in ABO system
A/B — acid-base ratio
A&B — apnea and bradycardia
A>B — air greater than bone [conduction]
3AB — 3-aminobenzamide
Ab —
  abortion
  antibody
aB — azure B
ab —
  abortion
  about
  antibody
  axiobuccal
a-b — air-bone
ABA —
  abscissic acid
  allergic bronchopulmonary aspergillosis

ABA — *(continued)*
  American Board of Anesthesiologists
  antibacterial activity
ABB —
  Albright-Butler-Bloomberg [syndrome]
  American Board of Bioanalysis
ABBQ — Acquired Immunodeficiency Syndrome Beliefs and Behavior Questionnaire
abbrev —
  abbreviated
  abbreviation
ABC —
  absolute band count
  abbreviated blood count
  absolute band count
  absolute basophil count
  absolute bone conduction
  acalculous biliary colic
  acid balance control
  aconite-belladonna-chloroform
  airway, breathing, and circulation
  alternative birth center
  alum, blood, and charcoal [purification and deodorizing method]
  alum, blood, and clay [sludge deodorizing method]
  American Blood Commission
  aneurysmal bone cyst
  antigen-binding capacity
  apnea, bradycardia, cyanosis
  applesauce, bananas, and cereal [diet]
  artificial beta cells
  aspiration biopsy cytology
  assessment of basic competency
  atomic, biological, chemical [warfare]
  avidin-biotin complex
  axiobuccocervical
A&BC — air and bone conduction

ABCC — Atomic Bomb Casualty Commission

ABCD — asymmetry, border, color, and diameter [of melanoma]

ABCDE — botulism toxin, pentavalent

ABCIL — antibody-mediated cell-dependent immunolympholysis

ABCN — American Board of Clinical Neuropsychology

ABCP — American Board of Cardiovascular Perfusion

ABD —
abdomen
after bronchodilator
aged, blind, and disabled
aggressive behavioral disturbance
average body dose

ABd — [type of] plain gauze dressing

abd —
abdomen
abdominal
abduction
abductor

ABDCT — atrial bolus dynamic computed tomography

Abd hyst — abdominal hysterectomy

Abdom —
abdomen
abdominal

ABDPH — American Board of Dental Public Health

abd poll — abductor pollicis

abduc — abduction

ABE —
acute bacterial endocarditis
adult basic education
American Board of Endodontics
botulism equine trivalent antitoxin

ABEP — auditory brainstem evoked potential

ABEPP — American Board of Examiners in Professional Psychology

aber — aberrant

ABF — aortobifemoral

ABFP — American Board of Forensic Psychiatry

ABG —
aortic bypass graft
arterial blood gases
axiobuccogingival

abg — addictive behavior group

ABI —
ankle/brachial index
atherothrombotic brain infarction

ABIC — Adaptive Behavior Inventory for Children

ABID — antibody identification

ABIG — absence of immunoglobulin G

ABIM — American Board of Internal Medicine

ABIMCE — American Board of Internal Medicine certifying examination

ABK — aphakic bullous keratopathy

ABL —
abetalipoproteinemia
African Burkitt's lymphoma
allograft-bound lymphocyte
angioblastic lymphadenopathy
antigen-binding lymphocyte
Army Biological Laboratory
Automated Biological Laboratory
axiobuccolingual

ABLB — alternate binaural loudness balance

ABM —
adjusted body mass
alveolar basement membrane
artificial basement membrane
autologous bone marrow

ABMA — anti-basement membrane antibody

ABMS—
    Advisory Board of Medical
      Specialties
    autologous bone marrow sup-
      port
ABMT—autologous bone marrow
    transplantation
ABN—
    abnormal
    abnormality
AbN—antibody nitrogen
ABNC—abnormal curve
ABN F%—abnormal forms per-
    cent [sperm count]
ABNG—AB-negative
ABNM—American Board of Nu-
    clear Medicine
ABNMP—alpha-benzyl-*N*-
    methyl phenethylamine
ABO—
    abortion
    absent bed occupancy
    American Board of Orthodon-
      tists
    blood group system of groups
      A, AB, B, and O
ABO-HD—ABO hemolytic dis-
    ease
ABOHN—American Board for
    Occupational Health Nurses
ABOMS—American Board of
    Oral and Maxillofacial Sur-
    gery
ABOP—American Board of Oral
    Pathology
Abor—abortion
ABOS—American Board of Or-
    thopaedic Surgery
ABP—
    ambulatory blood pressure
    American Board of Pedodon-
      tics
    American Board of Periodon-
      tology
    American Board of Prostho-
      dontists
    androgen-binding protein
    antigen-binding protein

ABP—(*continued*)
    arterial blood pressure
    avidin-biotin peroxidase
ABPA—
    acute bronchopulmonary
      asthma
    allergic bronchopulmonary as-
      pergillosis
ABPC—antibody-producing cell
ABPE—acute bovine pulmonary
    edema
ABPN—American Board of Psy-
    chiatry and Neurology
ABR—
    abortus Bang ring [test]
    absolute bed rest
    auditory brainstem response
ABr—agglutination [test for] bru-
    cellosis
Abr—abrasion
ABRET—American Board of Reg-
    istration of Electroencephalo-
    graphic Technicians
ABS—
    abdominal surgery
    abnormal brainstem
    absent
    absorbed
    absorption
    acrylonitrile-butadiene-styrene
    acute brain syndrome
    Adaptive Behavior Scale
    admitting blood sugar
    adult bovine serum
    aging brain syndrome
    alkylbenzene sulfonate
    aloin, belladonna, strychnine
    American Board of Surgery
    amniotic band sequence
    amniotic band syndrome
    anti-B serum
    Antley-Bixler syndrome
    arterial blood sample
    at bedside
1:5 ABS—1:5 Absorption-Reiter-
    Strain [cerebrospinal fluid
    test]
Abs—absorption

abs —
 absent
 absolute
 absorbance
absc —
 abscess
 abscissa
abs conf — absolute configuration
ABSe — ascending bladder septum
abs. feb. — *absente febre* (Lat.)
 while fever is absent
absorp — absorption
AbSR — abnormal skin reflex
A/B ss — apnea/bradycardia self-
 stimulation
abst —
 absent
 abstract
abstr — abstract
ABT — aminopyrine breath test
abt — about
ABTA — American Brain Tumor
 Association
ABTX — alpha-bungarotoxin
ABU —
 aminobutyrate
 asymptomatic bacteriuria
ABV — arthropod-borne virus
ABW — actual body weight
ABx — antibiotics
ABY — acid bismuth yeast [me-
 dium]
AC —
 abdominal circumference
 abdominal compression
 absorption coefficient
 abuse case
 acetate
 acetylcholine
 acetylcysteine
 acidified complement
 Acinetobacter calcoaceticus
 aconitine
 acromioclavicular
 activated charcoal
 acupuncture clinic
 acute
 acute cholecystitis
 adenocarcinoma

AC — *(continued)*
 adenylate cyclase
 adherent cell
 adrenal cortex
 adrenocorticoid
 air chamber
 air changes
 air conditioning
 air conduction
 alcoholic cirrhosis
 all culture (broth)
 alternating current
 alveolar crest
 ambulatory care
 ambulatory controls
 anchored catheter
 anesthesia circuit
 angiocellular
 anodal closure
 ante cibum (Lat.) before meals
 antecubital
 anterior chamber
 anterior column
 anterior commissure
 anterior cruciate
 antibiotic concentrate
 anticoagulant
 anticomplementary
 anti-inflammatory corticoid
 antiphlogistic corticoid
 aortic closure
 aortocoronary
 arm circumference
 arterial capillary
 ascending colon
 atriocarotid
 auriculocarotid
 axiocervical
A-C —
 adult-versus-child
 aortocoronary [bypass]
A/C —
 albumin to coagulin ratio
 anterior chamber of eye
 assist/control [ventilation]
5-AC —
 5-azacitidine
 5-azacytidine

A2C — apical two-chamber
Ac —
>accelerator [globulin]
>acetate
>acetyl
>actinium
>arabinosyl cytosine

aC —
>abcoulomb
>arabinosyl cytosine
>azure C

ac —
>acceleration
>acetyl
>acid
>acute
>alternating current
>antecubital
>anterior chamber
>assisted control
>axiocervical

a.c. — *ante cibum* (Lat.) before meals

ACA —
>abnormal coronary artery
>acrodermatitis chronica atrophicans
>acute cerebellar ataxia
>adenine-cytosine-adenine
>adenocarcinoma
>adenylate cyclase activity
>adult child of an alcoholic
>American Chiropractic Association
>American College of Allergists
>American College of Anesthesiologists
>American College of Angiology
>American College of Apothecaries
>American Council on Alcoholism
>aminocaproic acid
>aminocephalosporanic acid
>ammonia, copper, and arsenic
>amyotrophic choreo-acanthocytosis

ACA — (*continued*)
>anomalous coronary artery
>anterior cerebral artery
>anterior communicating aneurysm [or artery]
>anticardiolipin antibody
>anticentromere antibody
>anticollagen antibody
>anticomplement activity
>anticytoplasmic antibody
>Automatic Clinical Analyzer

AC/A — accommodative convergence/accommodation [ratio]

ACAC — activated charcoal artificial cell

ACACN — American Council of Applied Clinical Nutrition

AcAcOH — acetoacetic acid

ACAD — asymptomatic coronary artery disease

Acad — academy

A-CAH — autoimmune chronic active hepatitis

ACAN — acanthocyte

ACAO — acyl coenzyme A oxidase

ACAS — Asymptomatic Carotid Atherosclerosis Study

ACAT —
>acylcholesterol acyltransferase
>automated computerized axial tomography

ACB —
>alveolar-capillary block
>antibody-coated bacteria
>aortocoronary bypass
>arterialized capillary blood
>asymptomatic carotid bruit

AC/BC — air conduction/bone conduction [time ratio]

ACBE — air contrast barium enema

ACBG — aortocoronary bypass graft

ACC —
>accident
>accommodation

ACC — *(continued)*
    acetyl coenzyme A carboxylase
    acinic or acinar cell carcinoma
    acute care center
    adenoid cystic carcinoma
    administrative control center
    adrenocortical carcinoma
    alveolar cell carcinoma
    ambulatory care center
    American College of Cardiology
    amylase creatinine clearance
    anodal closure contraction
    antitoxin-containing cell
    aplasia cutis congenita
    articular chondrocalcinosis

Acc —
    acceleration
    accident
    adenoid cystic carcinoma

acc —
    acceleration
    accelerator
    accident
    accommodation
    according

accel — acceleration

ACCESS —
    Ambulatory Care Clinic Effectiveness Systems Study
    American College of Cardiology Extended Study Services

ACCH — Association for the Care of Children's Health

AcCh — acetylcholine

AcChR — acetylcholine receptor

AcCHS — acetylcholinesterase

accid. —
    accident
    accidental

acc insuff — accommodation insufficiency

ACCL — anodal closure clonus or contraction

Accl — anodal closure clonus

ACCME — Accreditation Council for Continuing Medical Education

AcCoA — acetyl coenzyme A

accom — accommodation

ACCP —
    American College of Chest Physicians
    American College of Clinical Pharmacology

accum —
    accumulated
    accumulation

accur. — *accuratissime* (Lat.) accurately

ACD —
    absolute cardiac dullness
    absolute claudication distance
    acid-citrate-dextrose
    actinomycin D
    adult celiac disease
    advanced care directive
    allergic contact dermatitis
    alpha-chain disease
    American College of Dentists
    angiokeratoma corporis diffusum
    anterior chamber diameter
    anterior chest diameter
    anticoagulant citrate dextrose
    anticonvulsant drug
    area of cardiac disease or dullness

AcD — alive with disease

AC-DC — alternating current–direct current

ACDF —
    adult child of dysfunctional family
    anterior cervical diskectomy and fusion

ACE —
    acetonitrile
    actinium emanation
    acute cerebral encephalopathy
    acute coronary event
    adrenocortical extract
    aerobic chair exercises

ACE — (*continued*)
  alcohol, chloroform, and ether
  angiotensin-converting enzyme
AICE — angiotensin I–converting enzyme
ace —
  acentric
  acetone
ACED — anhydrotic congenital ectodermal dysplasia
ACEDS — angiotensin-converting enzyme dysfunction syndrome
ACEH — acid cholesterol ester hydrolase
ACEI — angiotensin-converting enzyme inhibitor
ACEP — American College of Emergency Physicians
AcEst — acetyl esterase
ACET — acetone
acet. — *acetum* (Lat.) vinegar
acetyl-CoA — acetyl coenzyme A
ACF —
  accessory clinical findings
  acute care facility
  advanced communications function
  anterior cervical fusion
  area correction factor
ACFn — additional cost of false negatives
ACFO — American College of Foot Orthopedists
ACFp — additional cost of false positives
ACFS — American College of Foot Surgeons
ACG —
  accelerator globulin
  American College of Gastroenterology
  angiocardiogram
  angiocardiography
  aortocoronary graft
  apexcardiogram
AcG — accelerator globulin [coagulation factor V]

ACGIH — American Conference of Governmental Industrial Hygienists
ACGME — Accreditation Council for Graduate Medical Education
ACGP — American College of General Practitioners
ACGPOMS — American College of General Practitioners in Osteopathic Medicine and Surgery
ACGT — antibody-coated grid technique
ACH —
  acetylcholine
  achalasia
  active chronic hepatitis
  adrenal-cortical hormone
  aftercoming head
  amyotrophic cerebellar hypoplasia
  arm, chest, height
  arm girth, chest depth, and hip width [nutritional index]
ACh — acetylcholine
ACHA — American College of Hospital Administrators
AChA — anterior choroidal artery
ACHE — American Council for Headache Education
AChE — acetylcholinesterase
ACHOO — autosomal dominant compelling helio-ophthalmic outburst [syndrome]
AChR — acetylcholine receptor
AChRAb — acetylcholine receptor antibody
AChRP — acetylcholine receptor protein
AC&HS — *ante cibum & hora somni* (Lat.) before meals and at bedtime
AChS — Association of the Society of Chiropodists
ACI —
  acoustic comfort index

ACI — (continued)
  acute coronary infarction
  acute coronary insufficiency
  adenylate cyclase inhibitor
  adrenal-cortical insufficiency
  aftercare instructions
  anticlonus index
  average cost of illness
ACID — Arithmetic, Coding, Information, and Digit Span
ACIDS — acquired cellular immunodeficiency syndrome
ACIF — anticomplement immunofluorescence
ACIP —
  acute canine idiopathic polyneuropathy
  Advisory Committee on Immunization Practices
ACIR — Automotive Crash Injury Research
ACJ — acromioclavicular joint
AcK — francium [actinium K]
ACL —
  Achievement Check List
  acromegaloid features, cutis verticis gyrata, corneal leukoma [syndrome]
  acromioclavicular line
  anterior cruciate ligament
ACl — aspiryl chloride
ACLA — American Clinical Laboratory Association
ACLC — Assessment of Children's Language Comprehension
ACLD — Association for Children with Learning Disabilities
ACLI — American Council on Life Insurance
ACLM — American College of Legal Medicine
ACLPS — Academy of Clinical Laboratory Physicians and Scientists
ACLR — anterior cruciate ligament repair
ACLS — advanced cardiac life support

AcLV — (avian) acute leukemia virus
ACM —
  acute cerebrospinal meningitis
  albumin-calcium-magnesium
  alveolar capillary membrane
  anticardiac myosin
  Arnold-Chiari malformation
ACMA — American Occupational Medicine Association
ACME —
  Advisory Council on Medical Education
  aphakic cystoid macular edema
  Automatic Classification of Medical Entities
ACMF — arachnoid cyst of the middle fossa
ACML — atypical chronic myeloid leukemia
ACMP — alveolar-capillary membrane permeability
ACMR — Advisory Committee on Medical Research
ACMS — American-Chinese Medical Society
ACMT — artificial circus movement tachycardia
ACMV — assist-controlled mechanical ventilation
ACN —
  acute conditioned neurosis
  American College of Neuropsychiatrists
  American College of Nutrition
ACNM —
  American College of Nuclear Medicine
  American College of Nurse-Midwives
ACNP — American College of Nuclear Physicians
ACO —
  acute coronary occlusion
  alert, cooperative, and oriented

ACO — (continued)
  American College of Oto-
    laryngologists
  anodal closure odor
ACOA — adult child of alcoholic
ACoA — anterior communicating
  artery
ACOG — American College of
  Obstetricians and Gynecolo-
  gists
ACOHA — American College of
  Osteopathic Hospital Admin-
  istrators
ACO-HNS — American Council
  of Otolaryngology–Head and
  Neck Surgery
ACOI — American College of Os-
  teopathic Internists
ACOM — American College of
  Occupational Medicine
A-comm — anterior communicat-
  ing [artery]
ACOMS — American College of
  Oral and Maxillofacial Sur-
  geons
ACOOG — American College of
  Osteopathic Obstetricians and
  Gynecologists
ACOP — American College of Os-
  teopathic Pediatricians
ACORDE — A Consortium on Re-
  storative Dentistry Education
ACOS — American College of Os-
  teopathic Surgeons
acous —
  acoustical
  acoustics
ACP —
  accessory conduction pathway
  acid phosphatase
  acyl-carrier protein
  American College of Patholo-
    gists
  American College of Pharma-
    cists
  American College of Physi-
    cians
  American College of Prostho-
    dontists

ACP — (continued)
  American College of Psychia-
    trists
  Animal Care Panel
  anodal-closing picture
  aspirin-caffeine-phenacetin
  Association for Child Psychia-
    trists
  Association of Clinical Pa-
    thologists
  Association of Correctional
    Psychologists
AcP — acid phosphatase
ACPA —
  American Cleft Palate Associ-
    ation
  anticytoplasmic antibodies
ACPC — aminocyclopentane car-
  boxylic [acid]
AC-PH — acid phosphatase
ACPM — American College of
  Preventive Medicine
ACPP — adrenocortical polypep-
  tide
ACPP-PF — acid phosphatase prostatic fluid
ACPS — acrocephalopolysyndac-
  tyly
acq —
  acquired
  acquisition
ACR —
  abnormally contracting region
  absolute catabolic rate
  acriflavine
  adenomatosis of colon and
    rectum
  American College of Radiol-
    ogy
  anticonstipation regimen
  axillary count rate
Acr —
  acriflavine
  acrylic
ACRF — ambulatory care research
  facility
ACRM — American Congress of
  Rehabilitation Medicine

ACS—
    acetyl strophanthidin
    acrocallosal syndrome
    acrocephalosyndactyly
    acute chest syndrome
    acute confusional state
    Alcon Closure System
    ambulatory care services
    American Cancer Society
    American Chemical Society
    American College of Sur-
      geons
    American Society of Cytology
    anodal-closing sound
    antireticular cytotoxic serum
    aperture current setting
    arterial cannulation support
    Association of Clinical Scien-
      tists
ACSA — adenylate cyclase–
    stimulating activity
ACSM — American College of
    Sports Medicine
ACSP—
    adenylate cyclase–stimulating
      protein
    Advisory Council on Scien-
      tific Policy
ACSV — aortocoronary saphenous
    vein [graft]
ACSVBG — aortocoronary saphe-
    nous vein bypass graft
ACT—
    achievement through counsel-
      ing and treatment
    actinomycin
    activated clotting time
    activated coagulation time
    advanced coronary treatment
    allergen challenge test
    American Council on Trans-
      plantation
    anterocolic transposition
    antichymotrypsin
    anticoagulant therapy
    anxiety control training
    asthma care training
    atropine coma therapy

ACT — (continued)
    automated computed tomogra-
      phy
act —
    actinomycin
    active
    activity
ACTA —
    American Cardiovascular
      Technologists Association
    automatic computed trans-
      verse axial [scanning]
Act-C — actinomycin C
Act-D — actinomycin D
ACTe — anodal-closure tetanus
Act Ex — active exercise
ACTG —
    AIDS Clinical Treatment
      Group
    AIDS Clinical Trials Group
ACTH — adrenocorticotropic hor-
    mone
ACTH-LI — adrenocorticotropic
    hormone–like immunoreac-
    tivity
ACTH-RF — adrenocorticotropic
    hormone–releasing factor
ACTN — adrenocorticotropin
ACTP — adrenocorticotropic poly-
    peptide
ACTS —
    acute cervical traumatic
      sprain or syndrome
    Auditory Comprehension Test
      for Sentences
ACTSEB — anterior chamber tube
    shunt encircling band
ACU —
    acquired cold urticaria
    acute care unit
    agar colony-forming unit
    ambulatory care unit
ACUTENS — acupuncture and
    transcutaneous electrical
    nerve stimulation
ACV —
    acute cardiovascular [disease]
    acyclovir

ACV — (continued)
   atrial/carotid/ventricular
ACVB — aortocoronary venous bypass
ACVD —
   acute cardiovascular disease
   atherosclerotic cardiovascular
      disease
ACVRD — arteriosclerotic cardiovascular renal disease
AC/W — acetone in water
acyl-CoA — acyl coenzyme A
AD —
   abdominal diameter
   accident dispensary
   acetate dialysis
   achievement drive
   active disease
   acute dermatomyositis
   addict
   addiction
   adenoid degeneration
   adjuvant disease
   admitting diagnosis
   adult disease
   advanced directive
   aerosol deposition
   affective disorder
   after discharge
   alcohol dehydrogenase
   Aleutian disease
   alveolar diffusion
   alveolar duct
   Alzheimer's dementia
   Alzheimer's disease
   analgesic dose
   anodal duration
   anterior division
   antigenic determinant
   appropriate disability
   arthritic dose
   Associate Degree
   atopic dermatitis
   atrium dextrum (Lat.) right
      atrium
   attentional disturbance
   autonomic dysreflexia
   autosomal dominant

AD — (continued)
   average day
   average deviation
   axiodistal
   axis deviation
A.D. — auris dextra (Lat.) right ear
A/D — analog-to-digital [con-
   verter]
A&D —
   admission and discharge
   alcohol and drugs
   ascending and descending
   vitamins A and D
Ad —
   adenovirus
   adipocyte
   adrenal
   anisotropic disk
ad — axiodistal
ad. —
   adde (Lat.) add
   addetur (Lat.) let there be
      added [up to a specified
      amount]
a.d. — alternis diebus (Lat.) alternating days [every other day]
ADA —
   adenosine deaminase activity
   American Dental Association
   American Dermatological As-
      sociation
   American Diabetes Associa-
      tion
   American Dietetic Associa-
      tion
   Americans with Disabilities
      Act
   anterior descending artery
   antideoxyribonucleic acid an-
      tibody
   approved dietary allowance
ADAA — American Dental Assis-
   tants Association
ADAM — amniotic deformity, ad-
   hesion mutilation [syndrome]
ADAMHA — Alcohol, Drug
   Abuse, and Mental Health
   Administration

ADAP—
   American Dental Assistants'
      Program
   Assistant Director of Army
      Psychiatry
ADAS—Alzheimer's Disease Assessment Scale
ADAS-COG—cognitive portion
   of the Alzheimer's Disease Assessment Scale
ADase—adenosine deaminase
ADAU—adolescent drug abuse
   unit
ADB—accidental death benefit
ADC—
   affective disorders clinic
   Aid to Dependent Children
   AIDS-dementia complex
   albumin, dextrose, and cata-
      lase [medium]
   ambulance design criteria
   analog-to-digital converter
   anodal duration contraction
   antral diverticulum of the co-
      lon
   anxiety disorder clinic
   average daily census
   axiodistocervical
AdC—
   adenylate cyclase
   adrenal cortex
ADCC—
   acute disorder of cerebral cir-
      culation
   antibody-dependent cell-me-
      diated cytotoxicity
   antibody-dependent cellular
      cytotoxicity
ADCP—adenosine deaminase
   complexing protein
ADCS—Argonz del Castillo syndrome
ADD—
   adduction
   adenosine deaminase
   alcohol and drug dependency
   attention deficit disorder
   average daily dose

add—
   addition
   adduction
   adductor
add.—
   adde (Lat.) add
   addetur (Lat.) let there be
      added
add. c. trit.—*adde cum tritu* (Lat.)
   add with trituration
ad def. an.—*ad defectionem animi*
   (Lat.) to the point of fainting
ad deliq.—*ad deliquium* (Lat.) to
   the point of failure
addend.—*addendus* (Lat.) to be
   added
ADDH—attention deficit disorder
   with hyperactivity
ADD/HA—attention deficit
   disorder/hyperactivity
addict—
   addiction
   addictive
addn—addition
add poll—adductor pollicis [mus-
   cle]
ADDS—American Digestive Disease Society
ADDU—alcohol and drug dependence unit
ADE—
   acute disseminated encephali-
      tis
   antibody-dependent enhance-
      ment
   apparent digestible energy
Ade—adenine
AdeCbl—adenosyl cobalamin
ADEE—age-dependent epileptic
   encephalopathy
ad effect.—*ad effectum* (Lat.) until
   effective
ADEM—
   acute disseminated encephalo-
      myelitis
   acute disseminating encepha-
      lomyelitis
adeq—adequate

ad. feb. — *adstante febre* (Lat.) fever being present

ADFN — albinism-deafness [syndrome]

ADFu — agar diffusion for fungus

ADG —
    atrial diastolic gallop
    axiodistogingival

ADGMS — Assistant Director General of Medical Services

ad grat. acid. — *ad gratum aciditatem* (Lat.) to an agreeable acidity

ad grat. gust. — *ad gratum gustum* (Lat.) to an agreeable taste

ADH —
    Academy of Dentistry for the Handicapped
    adhesion
    alcohol dehydrogenase
    antidiuretic hormone
    arginine dihydrolase

adh —
    adhesion
    adhesive

ADHA — American Dental Hygienists Association

ADHD — attention deficit hyperactivity disorder

adhib. — *adhibendus* (Lat.) to be administered

ADI —
    Academy of Dentistry International
    acceptable daily intake
    allowable daily intake
    antral diverticulum of the ileum
    artificial diverticulum of the ileum
    atlas-dens interval
    autosomal-dominant ichthyosis
    axiodistoincisal

ad int. — *ad interim* (Lat.) meanwhile

adj —
    adjacent

adj — (*continued*)
    adjoining
    adjunct
    adjuvant

ADK — adenosine kinase

ADKC — atopic dermatitis with keratoconjunctivitis

ADL —
    activities of daily living
    Amsterdam Depression List

ADLC — antibody-dependent lymphocyte-mediated cytotoxicity

ad lib. — *ad libitum* (Lat.) as desired

ADM —
    abductor digiti minimi [muscles]
    administrative medicine
    administrator
    admission
    admit
    Adriamycin
    apparent distribution mass

AdM — adrenal medulla

adm —
    administration
    admission
    admove (Lat.) apply

Adm Dr — admitting doctor

ADME — absorption, distribution, metabolism, and excretion

Admin —
    administer
    administration

admov. — *admove, admoveatur* (Lat.) let there be applied

Adm Ph — admitting physician

ADMR — average daily metabolic rate

ADMX — adrenal medullectomy

ADN —
    antideoxyribonuclease
    aortic depressor nerve
    Associate Degree in Nursing

adn —
    adenoid
    adenoidectomy

ADNase — antideoxyribonuclease

ad naus. — *ad nauseam* (Lat.) to the point of producing nausea

ADN-B — antideoxyribonuclease B

ad neut. — *ad neutralizandum* (Lat.) to neutralization

ADO —
adolescent medicine
axiodisto-occlusal

Ado — adenosine

ADOD — arthrodento-osteodys-plasia

AdoDABA — adenosyldiamino-butyric acid

ADODM — adult-onset diabetes mellitus

AdoHcy — S-adenosylhomo-cysteine

adol — adolescent

AdoMet — S-adenosylmethionine

Adox — oxidized adenosine

ADP —
Academy of Dental Prosthet-ics
acute dermatomyositis and polymyositis
adenopathy
adenosine diphosphate
administrative psychiatry
advanced pancreatitis
ammonium dihydrogen phos-phate
approved drug product
area diastolic pressure
arterial demand pacing
automatic data processing

ADP/ATP — adenosine diphosphate/adenosine tri-phosphate [ratio]

AdP — adductor pollicis

ad part. dolent. — *ad partes dolentes* (Lat.) to the painful parts

ADPase — adenosine diphospha-tase

ADPKD — autosomal dominant polycystic kidney disease

ADPL — average daily patient load

ad pond. om. — *ad pondus omnium* (Lat.) to the weight of the whole

ADPR — adenosine diphosphate ribose

ADQ —
abductor digiti quinti [mus-cle]
adequate

ADR —
acceptable dental remedies
acute dystonic reaction
adrenodoxin reductase
Adriamycin
adverse drug reaction
airway dilation reflex
Alzheimer's disease research
ataxia-deafness-retardation [syndrome]

Adr —
adrenaline
Adriamycin

adr —
adrenal
adrenalectomy

ad rat. — *ad rationem* (Lat.) as rea-sonable

ADRBR — adrenergic beta-recep-tor

ADRDA — Alzheimer's Disease and Related Disorders Associ-ation

ADS —
acute death syndrome
acute diarrheal syndrome
Alcohol Dependence Scale
alternative delivery system
American Denture Society
anatomical dead space
anonymous donor's sperm
anterior drawer sign
antibody deficiency syndrome
antidiuretic substance
Army Dental Service

ad sat. — *ad saturandum* (Lat.) to saturation

adst. feb. — *adstante febre* (Lat.) while fever is present

ADT —
    accepted dental therapeutics
    adenosine triphosphate
    admission, discharge, transfer
    agar gel diffusion test
    alternate-day therapy
    anticipate discharge tomorrow
    any desired thing [a placebo]
    auditory discrimination test
    automated dithionite test
ADTA — American Dental Trade
    Association
ADTe — anodal duration tetanus
ADTP —
    adolescent day treatment pro-
      gram
    alcohol dependence treatment
      program
ADU — acute duodenal ulcer
ad us. — *ad usum* (Lat.) according
    to custom
ad us. ext. — *ad usum externum*
    (Lat.) for external application
ADV —
    adenovirus
    adventitia
    Aleutian disease virus
A/DV — arterio/deep venous
A-DV — arterial–deep venous dif-
    ference
adv —
    advanced
    advice
    advise
adv. — *adversum* (Lat.) against
ad 2 vic. — *ad duas vices* (Lat.) at
    two times, for two doses
ADVIRC — autosomal dominant
    vitreoretinochoroidopathy
ADW — assault with deadly
    weapon
A5D5W — alcohol 5%, dextrose
    5%, in water
ADX — adrenalectomized
AE —
    above elbow [amputation]
    accident and emergency
      [department]

AE — *(continued)*
    acrodermatitis enteropathica
    activation energy
    adrenal epinephrine
    adult erythrocyte
    after-effect
    agarose electrophoresis
    air embolism
    air entry
    alcoholic embryopathy
    anoxic encephalopathy
    antiepileptic
    Antitoxineinheit (Ger.) anti-
      toxin unit
    apoenzyme
    aryepiglottic
    atherosclerotic encephalopa-
      thy
    avian encephalomyelitis
A&E —
    accident and emergency
      [department]
    analysis and evaluation
AEA —
    above-elbow amputation
    alcohol, ether, and acetone
      [solution]
AEB —
    acute erythroblastopenia
    as evidenced by
    avian erythroblastosis
AEC —
    ankyloblepharon-ectodermal
      dysplasia-clefting
    aortic ejection click
    at earliest convenience
    Atomic Energy Commission
AECD — allergic eczematous con-
    tact dermatitis
AED —
    antiepileptic drug
    antihidrotic ectodermal dys-
      plasia
    automated external defibrilla-
      tor
AEDP — automated external defi-
    brillator pacemaker
AEE — Atomic Energy Establish-
    ment

AEEU — admission, entrance, and evaluation unit
AEF —
allogeneic effect factor
amyloid-enhancing factor
aryepiglottic fold
AEG —
air encephalogram
air encephalography
atrial electrogram
aeg. — *aeger, aegra* (Lat.) the patient
AEGIS — Aid for the Elderly in Government Institutions
AEI —
acrylic eye illustrator
arbitrary evolution index
atrial emptying index
AEL — acute erythroleukemia
AEM —
ambulatory electrocardiographic monitoring
analytical electron microscopy
avian encephalomyelitis
AEMC — Albert Einstein Medical Center
AEMIS — Aerospace and Environmental Medicine Information System
AEN — aseptic epiphyseal necrosis
AEP —
acute edematous pancreatitis
appropriateness evaluation protocol
artificial endocrine pancreas
auditory evoked potential
average evoked potential
AEq — age equivalent
aeq. — *aequalis* (Lat.) equal
AER —
abduction/external rotation
acoustic evoked response
acute exertional rhabdomyolysis
agranular endoplasmic reticulum
aided equalization response
albumin excretion rate

AER — *(continued)*
aldosterone excretion rate
apical ectodermal ridge
auditory evoked response
average electroencephalic response
average evoked response
aer — aerosol
AERA — average evoked response audiometry
AERE — Atomic Energy Research Establishment
Aer M — aerosol mask
Aero — *Aerobacter*
AERP —
antegrade effective refractory period
atrial effective refractory period
AERPAP — antegrade effective refractory period accessory pathway
Aer T — aerosol tent
AES —
acetone-extracted serum
American Electroencephalographic Society
American Encephalographic Society
American Endocrine Society
American Endodontic Society
American Epidemiological Society
American Equilibration Society
anterior esophageal sensor
antiembolic stockings
antieosinophilic sera
antral ethmoidal sphenoidectomy
aortic ejection sound
Auger's electron spectroscopy
autoerythrocyte sensitization
AESP — applied extrasensory projection
AEST — aeromedical evacuation support team

AET —
   absorption-equivalent thickness
   atrial ectopic tachycardia
aet. — *aetas* (Lat.) age
aetat. — *aetatis* (Lat.) aged
aetiol — *aetiology* (British) etiology
AEV — avian erythroblastosis virus
AEVS — automated eligibility verification system
AF —
   abnormal frequency
   acid-fast
   adult female
   afebrile
   aflatoxin
   albumin-free
   albumose-free
   aldehyde fuchsin
   alleged father
   amaurosis fugax
   amnionic fluid
   amniotic fluid
   anchoring fibril
   angiogenesis factor
   anteflexion
   anterior fontanelle
   anterofrontal
   antibody-forming
   antifibrinogen
   anti-fog
   aortic flow
   aortofemoral
   Arthritis Foundation
   artificial feeding
   ascitic fluid
   atrial fibrillation
   atrial flutter
   atrial fusion
   attenuation factor
   attributable fraction
   audiofrequency
   auricular fibrillation
A-F —
   ankle-foot [orthosis]
   antifibrinogen
A/F — air/fluid [level]
aF — abfarad

af — audiofrequency
AFA —
   advanced first aid
   alcohol-formaldehyde-acetic acid [fixative]
AFAFP — amniotic fluid alpha-fetoprotein
AFAR — American Foundation for Aging Research
AFB —
   acid-fast bacillus(i)
   aflatoxin B
   air-fluidized bed
   American Foundation for the Blind
   aortofemoral bypass
   aspirated foreign body
AFBG — aortofemoral bypass graft
AFC —
   acid-fast culture
   adult foster care
   air-filled cushion
   antibody-forming cells
AFCI — acute focal cerebral ischemia
AFCR — American Federation for Clinical Research
AFD — accelerated freeze drying
AFDC — Aid to Families with Dependent Children
AFDH — American Fund for Dental Health
AFDW — ash-free dry weight
AFE — amniotic fluid embolism
afeb — afebrile
AFF — atrial filling fraction
AF/F — atrial fibrillation and/or flutter
aff — afferent
aff. — *affinis* (Lat.) having an affinity with but not identical to
AFG —
   aflatoxin G
   alpha fetal globulin
   amniotic fluid glucose
   auditory figure-ground
AFH —
   angiofollicular hyperplasia

AFH — *(continued)*
anterior facial height
AFI —
amaurotic familial idiocy
amniotic fluid index
AFib — atrial fibrillation
AFIP — Armed Forces Institute of
Pathology
AFIS — amniotic fluid infection
syndrome
AFL —
air/fluid level
antifatty liver
antifibrinolysin
artificial limb
AFl — atrial flutter
AFLNH — angiofollicular lymph
node hyperplasia
AFLP — acute fatty liver of preg-
nancy
AFM — aflatoxin M
AFML — Armed Forces Medical
Library
AFN — afunctional neutrophil
AFNC — Air Force Nurse Corps
AFND — acute febrile neutrophilic
dermatosis
AFO — ankle-foot orthosis
AFP —
adiabatic fast passage
alpha-fetoprotein
anterior faucial pillar
atrial filling pressure
atypical facial pain
AfP — affiliate physician
aFP — alpha-fetoprotein
AfPh — affiliate physician
AFPP — acute fibropurulent pneu-
monia
AFQ — aflatoxin Q
AFQT — Armed Forces Qualifica-
tion Test
AFR —
aqueous flare response
ascorbic free radical
AFRAX — autism—fragile X [syn-
drome]
AFRD — acute febrile respiratory
disease

AFRI — acute febrile respiratory illness
AFS —
acid-fast smear
acquired or adult Fanconi syndrome
acromegaloid facial syndrome
American Fertility Society
antifibroblast serum
AFSAM — Air Force School of
Aviation Medicine
AFSP — acute fibroserous pneumonia
AFT —
aflatoxin
agglutination-flocculation test
AFT_3 — absolute free triiodothyronine
AFT_4 — absolute free thyroxine
AFTA — American Family Therapy Association
AFTC — apparent free testosterone concentration
AFTN — autonomously functioning thyroid nodule
AFV — amniotic fluid volume
AFVSS — afebrile, vital signs stable
AFX —
air-fluid exchange
atypical fibroxanthoma
AG —
abdominal girth
agarose
albumin-globulin [ratio]
aminoglutethimide
aminoglycoside
analytical grade
anion gap
antigen
antiglobulin
antigravity
atrial gallop
attached gingiva
axiogingival
azurophilic granule
A/G — albumin/globulin [ratio]
Ag —
antigen

Ag — (*continued*)
  silver (Lat., *argentum*)
ag —
  antigen
  atrial gallop
AGA —
  accelerated growth area
  acetylglutamate
  acute gonococcal arthritis
  allergic granulomatosis and
    angiitis
  American Gastroenterological
    Association
  American Genetics Association
  American Geriatrics Association
  American Goiter Association
  antiglomerular antibody
  anti-IgG autoantibody
  appropriate for gestational age
  average for gestational age
Ag-Ab — antigen-antibody complex
AGAG — acidic glycosaminoglycans
AGAS — acetylglutamate synthetase
AGBAD — Alexander Graham Bell Association for the Deaf
AGC —
  absolute granulocyte count
  automatic gain control
AGCT —
  antiglobulin consumption test
  Army General Classification Test
AGD —
  agar gel diffusion
  agarose gel diffusion
AGDD —
  agar gel double diffusion
  agarose gel double diffusion
AGE —
  acrylamide gel electrophoresis
  acute gastroenteritis
  agarose gel electrophoresis
  angle of greatest extension

AGED — automated general experimental device
AGEPC — acetyl glyceryl ether phosphoryl-choline
AGF —
  adrenal growth factor
  angle of greatest flexion
ag. feb. — *aggrediente febre* (Lat.) when the fever is coming on
AGG — agammaglobulinemia
agg —
  agglutinate
  agglutination
  aggravation
  aggregation
agglut — agglutination
aggrav —
  aggravated
  aggravation
aggred. feb. — *aggrediente febre* (Lat.) while the fever is coming on
aggreg —
  aggregated
  aggregation
AGGS — anti-gas gangrene serum
AgI — silver iodide
agit —
  agitated
  agitation
agit. — *agita* (Lat.) shake
agit. ante sum. — *agita ante sumendum* (Lat.) shake before taking
agit. ante us. — *agita ante usum* (Lat.) shake before using
agit. bene — *agita bene* (Lat.) shake well
agit. vas. — *agitato vase* (Lat.) the vial being shaken
AGL —
  acute granulocytic leukemia
  agglutination
  aminoglutethimide
A-GLACTO-LK — alpha-galactoside leukocytes
AGLMe — N-alpha-acetylglycyl-L-lysine methyl ester

AGMK — African green monkey
  kidney [cell]
AGMkK — African green monkey
  kidney [cell]
AGML — acute gastric mucosal
  lesion
AGN —
    acute glomerulonephritis
    agnosia
    antigen
VIII$_{AGN}$ — factor VIII antigen
agn — agnosia
AgNO$_3$ — silver nitrate
AgNOR — argyrophilic nucleolar
  organizer region
Ag$_2$O — silver oxide
AGOS — American Gynecological
  and Obstetrical Society
AGP —
    agar gel precipitation
    alpha$_1$-acid glycoprotein
AGPA —
    American Group Practice As-
      sociation
    American Group Psychother-
      apy Association
AGPI — agar gel precipitin inhibi-
  tion
AGPT — agar gel precipitin test
AGR —
    aniridia, genitourinary malfor-
      mations, and mental retar-
      dation [complex]
    anticipatory goal response
A/G ratio — albumin-globulin
  ratio
AGS —
    adrenogenital syndrome
    American Geriatrics Society
    American Gynecological Soci-
      ety
    audiogenic seizures
Ag$_2$SO$_4$ — silver sulfate
AGT —
    abnormal glucose tolerance
    activity group therapy
    acute generalized tuberculosis
    adrenoglomerulotropin

AGT — (continued)
    antiglobulin test
agt — agent
AGTH — adrenoglomerulotropic
  hormone
AGTr — adrenoglomerulotropin
AGTT — abnormal glucose toler-
  ance test
AGU — aspartylglucosaminuria
AGV — aniline gentian violet
AH —
    abdominal hysterectomy
    absorptive hypercalciuria
    accidental hypothermia
    acetohexamide
    acid hydrolysis
    acute hepatitis
    adrenal hypoplasia
    after-hyperpolarization
    agnathia-holoprosencephaly
    alcoholic hepatitis
    amenorrhea and hirsutism
    amenorrhea and hyperprolac-
      tinemia
    aminohippurate
    anterior hypothalamus
    antihyaluronidase
    arcuate hypothalamus
    Army Hospital
    arterial hypertension
    artificial heart
    ascites hepatoma
    astigmatic hypermetropia
    ataxic hemiparesis
    autonomic hyperreflexia
    axillary hair
A/H — amenorrhea-
  hyperprolactinemia
A&H — accident & health [pol-
  icy]
A·H — ampere hour
Ah — hypermetropic astigmatism
aH — abhenry
ah — hyperopic astigmatism
AHA —
    acetohydroxamic acid
    acquired hemolytic anemia
    acute hemolytic anemia

AHA — *(continued)*
  American Heart Association
  American Hospital Association
  anterior hypothalamic area
  anti-heart antibody
  antihistone antibody
  area health authority
  arthritis-hives-angioedema [syndrome]
  aspartyl-hydroxamic acid
  Associate, Institute of Hospital Administrators
  Australian hepatitis antigen
  autoimmune hemolytic anemia
AHB — alpha-hydroxybutyric [acid]
AHBC — hepatitis B core antibody
AHC —
  academic health care
  acute hemorrhagic conjunctivitis
  acute hemorrhagic cystitis
  antihemophilic factor C
AHCA — American Health Care Association
AHCPR — Agency for Health Care Policy and Research
AHCy — adenosyl homocysteine
AHD —
  acquired hepatocerebral degeneration
  acute heart disease
  antihyaluronidase
  antihypertensive drug
  arteriohepatic dysplasia
  arteriosclerotic heart disease
  atherosclerotic heart disease
  autoimmune hemolytic disease
AHDMS — automated hospital data management system
AHDP — azacycloheptane diphosphonate
AHE — acute hemorrhagic encephalomyelitis

AHEA — area health education activity
AHEC — area health education center
AHES — artificial heart energy system
AHF —
  acute heart failure
  American Health Foundation
  American Hepatic Foundation
  American Hospital Formulary
  antihemolytic factor
  antihemophilic factor [blood coagulation factor VIII]
  Argentinian hemorrhagic fever
  Associated Health Foundation
AHFS — American Hospital Formulary Service
AHFS-DI — American Hospital Formulary Service–Drug Information
AHG —
  aggregated human globulin
  antihemolytic globulin
  antihemophilic globulin [blood coagulation factor VIII]
  antihuman globulin
AHGG —
  aggregated human gamma globulin
  antihuman gamma globulin
AHGS — acute herpetic gingival stomatitis
AHH —
  alpha-hydrazine analog of histidine
  anosmia and hypogonadotropic hypogonadism [syndrome]
  arylhydrocarbon hydroxylase
  Association for Holistic Health
AHI —
  active hostility index

AHI — (continued)
Animal Health Institute
apnea-plus-hypopnea index
AHIP — Assisted Health Insurance Plan
AHIS — Automated Hospital Information System
AHJ — artificial hip joint
AHL — apparent half-life
AHLE — acute hemorrhagic leukoencephalitis
AHLG — antihuman lymphocyte globulin
AHLS — antihuman lymphocyte serum
AHM —
allied health manpower
ambulatory Holter monitor
AHMA —
American Holistic Medicine Association
antiheart muscle autoantibody
AHMC — Association of Hospital Management Committees
AHN —
adenomatous hyperplastic nodule
Army Head Nurse
assistant head nurse
AHO — Albright's hereditary osteodystrophy
AHP —
acute hemorrhagic pancreatitis
after-hyperpolarization
air at high pressure
American Health Professionals
Assistant House Physician
AHPA — American Health Planning Association
AHPI — American Health Professions Institute
AHPO — anterior hypothalamic preoptic [area]
AHR —
antihyaluronidase reaction
Association for Health Records

AHR — (continued)
autonomic hyperreflexia
AHRA — American Hospital Radiology Administration
AHRF —
acute hypoxemic respiratory failure
American Hearing Research Foundation
AHS —
Academy of Health Sciences
adaptive hand skills
African horse sickness
alveolar hypoventilation syndrome
American Hearing Society
American Hospital Society
Assistant House Surgeon
AHSDF — area health service development fund
AHSN — Assembly of Hospital Schools of Nursing
AHSR — Association for Health Services Research
AHT —
aggregation half-time
antihyaluronidase titer
augmented histamine test
autoantibodies to human thyroglobulin
autogenous hamster tumor
AHTG — antihuman thymocytic globulin
AHTP — antihuman thymocytic plasma
AHTS — antihuman thymus serum
AHU —
acute hemolytic-uremic [syndrome]
arginine, hypoxanthine, and uracil
AHuG — aggregated human IgG
AHV — avian herpesvirus
AI —
accidental injury
accidentally incurred
adiposity index

AI — *(continued)*
    aggregation index
    allergy and immunology
    allergy index
    anaphylatoxin inhibitor
    angiogenesis inhibitor
    angiotensin I
    anxiety index
    aortic incompetence
    aortic insufficiency
    apical impulse
    articulation index
    artificial insemination
    artificial intelligence
    atherogenic index
    atrial insufficiency
    autoimmune
    autoimmunity
    axioincisal
A-I — aortoiliac
A&I — allergy and immunology
aI — active ingredient
AIA —
    acquired artery immune augmentation
    allylisopropylacetamide
    amylase inhibitor activity
    anti-immunoglobulin antibody
    anti-insulin antibody
    aspirin-induced asthma
    automated image analysis
AI-Ab — anti-insulin antibody
AIB —
    aminoisobutyrate
    avian infectious bronchitis
AIBA — aminoisobutyric acid
AIBF — anterior interbody fusion
AIBS — American Institute of Biological Sciences
AIC —
    aminoimidazole carboxamide
    Association des Infirmières Canadiennes
A-IC — average integrated concentration
AICA —
    anterior inferior cerebellar artery

AICA — *(continued)*
    anterior inferior communicating artery
    anterior internal cerebral artery
AI-CAH — autoimmune-type chronic active hepatitis
AICAR — aminoimidazole carboxamide ribonucleotide
AICC — anti-inhibitor coagulant complex
AICD —
    automatic implantable cardioverter-defibrillator
    automatic implantable cardiovascular defibrillator
AICE — angiotensin I–converting enzyme
AICF — autoimmune complement fixation
AID —
    acquired immunodeficiency disease
    acute infectious disease
    acute ionization detector
    Agency for International Development
    anti-inflammatory drug
    argon ionization detector
    artificial insemination donor
    autoimmune deficiency
    autoimmune disease
    automatic implantable defibrillator
    average interocular difference
AIDH — artificial insemination donor, husband
AIDP — acute inflammatory demyelinating polyradiculopathy
AIDS —
    acquired immune deficiency syndrome
    acquired immunodeficiency syndrome
    acute infectious disease series
    adult immunodeficiency syndrome
    Assessment of Intelligibility of Dysarthric Speech

AIDSDRUGS — clinical trials of acquired immunodeficiency drugs [MEDLARS data base]

AIDS-KS — acquired immune deficiency syndrome with Kaposi's sarcoma

AIDSLINE — on-line information on acquired immunodeficiency syndrome [MEDLARS data base]

AIDSTRIALS — clinical trials of acquired immunodeficiency syndrome drugs [MEDLARS data base]

AIE —
acute inclusion body encephalitis
acute infectious encephalitis
acute infective endocarditis

AIEP — amount of insulin extractable from pancreas

AIF —
anemia-inducing factor
anti-inflammatory
anti-invasion factor
aortic-iliac-femoral

AIFD — acute intrapartum fetal distress

AIG — anti-immunoglobulin

AIGA — absence of immunoglobulin A

AIGM — absence of immunoglobulin M

A-IGP — activity-interview group psychotherapy

AIH —
American Institute of Homeopathy
artificial insemination, homologous
artificial insemination by husband

AIHA —
American Industrial Hygiene Association
autoimmune hemolytic anemia

AIHC — American Industrial Health Conference

AIHD — acquired immune hemolytic disease

AII —
acute intestinal infection
angiotensin II

AIII — angiotensin III

AIIS — anterior inferior iliac spine

AIIT — amiodarone-iodine–induced thyrotoxicosis

AIL —
acute infectious lymphocytosis
angiocentric immunoproliferative lesion
angioimmunoblastic lymphadenopathy

AILD —
alveolar interstitial lung disease
angioimmunoblastic lymphadenopathy with dysproteinemia

AILT — amiloride-inhibitable lithium transport

AIM —
Abridged Index Medicus
Amputees in Motion
artificial intelligence in medicine

AIMD — abnormal involuntary movement disorder

AIMS —
abnormal involuntary movement scale
arthritis impact measurement scale

AIN —
acute interstitial nephritides
acute interstitial nephritis
American Institute of Nutrition
anal intraepithelial neoplasia
anterior interosseous nerve

AINA — automated immunonephelometric assay

AINS — anti-inflammatory nonsteroidal

A Insuf — aortic insufficiency

AIO — amyloid of immunoglobulin origin

AION — anterior ischemic optic neuropathy

AIP —
  acute idiopathic pericarditis
  acute infectious polyneuritis
  acute inflammatory polyneuropathy
  acute intermittent porphyria
  aldosterone-induced protein
  annual implementation plan
  automated immunoprecipitation
  average intravascular pressure integral anatuberculin, Petragnani

AIPE — acute interstitial pulmonary emphysema

AIPFP — acute idiopathic peripheral facial nerve palsy

AIPS — American Institute of Pathologic Science

AIR —
  accelerated idioventricular rhythm
  amino-imidazole ribonucleotide
  average impairment rating

AIRA — anti-insulin receptor antibody

AIRF — alteration in respiratory function

AIRS — Amphetamine Interview Rating Scale

AIS —
  Abbreviated Injury Score
  amniotic infection syndrome
  androgen insensitivity syndrome
  anterior interosseous nerve syndrome
  anti-insulin serum

AISA — acquired idiopathic sideroblastic anemia

AIS/ISS — Abbreviated Injury Score/Injury Severity Score

AIS/MR — Alternative Intermediate Services for the Mentally Retarded

AIT —
  acute intensive treatment
  administrator-in-training

AITP — autoimmune idiopathic thrombocytopenic purpura

AITT —
  arginine insulin tolerance test
  augmented insulin tolerance test

AIU —
  absolute iodine uptake
  antigen-inducing unit

AIUM — American Institute of Ultrasound in Medicine

AIVR — accelerated idioventricular rhythm

AIVV — anterior internal vertebral vein

A/J — ankle jerk

AJCCS — American Joint Committee on Cancer Staging

AJR — abnormal jugular reflex

AJS — acute joint syndrome

AK —
  above knee
  acetate kinase
  actinic keratosis
  adenosine kinase
  adenylate kinase
  artificial kidney

A/K — above knee

A→K — ankle to knee

AKA —
  above-knee amputation
  alcoholic ketoacidosis
  all known allergies
  alpha-allokainic acid
  also known as
  antikeratin antibody

AK amp — above-knee amputation

AKE — acrokeratoelastoidosis

A/kg — amperes per kilogram

AKP — alkaline phosphatase

AKS —
  alcoholic Korsakoff syndrome
  auditory and kinesthetic sensation

AL —
  absolute latency

AL — (continued)
    acinar lumen
    acinar lumina
    acute leukemia
    adaptation level
    albumin
    alcoholism
    alignment
    amyloidosis [amyloid light chain]
    annoyance level
    antihuman lymphocytic [globulin]
    argininosuccinate lysate
    argon laser
    arterial line
    auris laeva (Lat.) left ear
    avian leukosis
    axial length
    axillary loop
    axiolingual
    lethal antigen
Al —
    allantoic
    allergic
    allergy
    aluminum
ALA —
    American Laryngological Association
    American Lung Association
    aminolevulinic acid
    anterior lip of the acetabulum
ALa — axiolabial
Ala — alanine
AL-Ab — antilymphocyte antibody
ALAC — antibiotic-loaded acrylic cement
ALAD —
    abnormal left axis deviation
    aminolevulinic acid dehydrase
ALA-D — aminolevulinic acid dehydrase
ALAG — axiolabiogingival
ALAL — axiolabiolingual
ALARA — as low as reasonably achievable [radiation exposure]

ALARM — adjustable leg and ankle repositioning mechanism
ALAS — 5-aminolevulinate synthetase
ALAT — alanine aminotransferase
ALAX — apical long axis
ALB —
    albumin
    avian lymphoblastosis
alb — albumin
alb. — *albus* (Lat.) white
ALBC — albumin clearance
ALB/GLOB — albumin/globulin [ratio]
ALC —
    absolute lymphocyte count
    acute lethal catatonia
    alcohol
    allogeneic lymphocyte cytotoxicity
    alternate level of care
    Alternative Lifestyle Checklist
    approximate lethal concentration
    avian leukosis complex
    axiolinguocervical
alc —
    alcohol
    alcoholic
    alcoholism
ALCA — anomalous left coronary artery
ALCAA — acetyl-L-carnitine arginyl amide
ALCAPA — anomalous origin of left coronary artery from pulmonary artery
ALCEQ — Adolescent Life Change Event Questionnaire
AlCr — aluminum crown
AlcR — alcohol rub
ALD —
    adrenoleukodystrophy
    alcoholic liver disease
    aldolase
    aldosterone

ALD — *(continued)*
  anterior latissimus dorsi
  Appraisal of Language Disturbance
Ald — aldolase
ALDH — aldehyde dehydrogenase
Aldo — aldosterone
ALE — allowable limits of error
ALEC — artificial lung-expanding compound
ALEP — atypical lymphoepithelioid [cell] proliferation
ALF —
  acute liver failure
  American Liver Foundation
  anterior long fiber
ALFT — abnormal liver function test
ALG —
  Annapolis lymphoblast globulin
  antilymphoblastic globulin
  antilymphocyte globulin
  antithoracic duct lymphocyte globulin
  axiolinguogingival
alg — allergy
ALGOL — algorithmic-oriented language
ALH —
  angiolymphoid hyperplasia
  anterior lobe hormone
  anterior lobe of the hypophysis
ALHE — angiolymphoid hyperplasia with eosinophilia
ALI —
  annual limit of intake
  argon laser iridotomy
A-line —
  arterial catheter
  arterial line
ALIP — abnormal localized immature myeloid precursor
ALK —
  alkaline
  alkylating
ALK-P — alkaline phosphatase

ALL —
  acute lymphatic leukemia
  acute lymphoblastic leukemia
  acute lymphocytic leukemia
  allergy
  anterior longitudinal ligament
all —
  allergy
  allergic
ALLA — acute lymphocytic leukemia antigen
ALLO — atypical *Legionella*-like organism
ALM —
  acral lentiginous melanoma
  alveolar living material
ALME — acetyl-lysine methyl ester
ALMI — anterior lateral myocardial infarction
ALMV — anterior leaflet of the mitral valve
ALN —
  allylnitrile
  anterior lymph node
ALO —
  average lymphocyte output
  axiolinguo-occlusal
Al_2O_3 — aluminum oxide
$Al(OH)_3$ — aluminum hydroxide
ALOS — average length of stay
ALOSH — Appalachian Laboratory for Occupational Safety and Health
ALOX — aluminum oxide
ALP —
  acute leukemia protocol
  acute lupus pericarditis
  alkaline phosphatase
  alveolar proteinosis
  anterior lobe of pituitary
  antilymphocyte plasma
  argon laser photocoagulation
AlPase — alkaline phosphatase
ALPI — alkaline phosphatase isoenzymes
ALPS —
  angiolymphoproliferative syndrome

ALPS — *(continued)*
   Aphasia Language Performance Scale
ALPZ — alprazolam
ALRI — anterolateral rotatory instability
ALROS — American Laryngological, Rhinological, and Otological Society
ALS —
   acute lateral sclerosis
   advanced life support
   afferent loop syndrome
   amyotrophic lateral sclerosis
   angiotensin-like substance
   anterolateral sclerosis
   anticipated life span
   antilymphatic serum
   antilymphocyte serum
   antilymphocytic serum
   antiviral lymphocyte serum
ALSD — Alzheimer's-like senile dementia
ALS-PD — amyotrophic lateral sclerosis–parkinsonism-dementia [complex]
ALT —
   alanine aminotransferase
   alanine transaminase
   argon laser trabeculoplasty
   avian laryngotracheitis
Alt —
   alternate
   altitude
   aluminum tartrate
ALT/AST — ratio of serum alanine aminotransferase to serum aspartate aminotransferase
ALTB — acute laryngotracheobronchitis
alt. dieb. — *alternis diebus* (Lat.) every other day
ALTE — apparent life-threatening event
ALTEE — acetyl-L-tyrosine ethyl ester
alt. hor. — *alternis horis* (Lat.) every other hour

alt. noct. — *alternis nocta* (Lat.) every other night
ALTS —
   acute lumbar traumatic sprain
   acute lumbar traumatic syndrome
ALV —
   Abelson leukemia virus
   adeno-like virus
   alveolar
   alveolus
   ascending lumbar vein
   avian leukosis virus
ALVAD — abdominal left ventricular assist device
alv. adst. — *alvo adstricta* (Lat.) when the bowels are constipated
alv. deject. — *alvi dejectiones* (Lat.) discharge from the bowels
ALVM — alveolar mucosa
ALVT — aortic and left ventricular tunnel
alv vent — alveolar ventilation
ALVX — alveolectomy
ALW — arch-loop-whorl
ALWMI — anterolateral wall myocardial infarct
A-LYM — atypical lymphocyte
AM —
   acrylamide
   actomyosin
   acute myelofibrosis
   adult male
   adult monocyte
   aerospace medicine
   akinetic mutism
   alveolar macrophage
   alveolar mucosa
   amacrine cell
   amalgam
   ambulatory
   amethopterin
   ametropia
   ammeter
   ampere-meter
   ampicillin
   amplitude modulation

AM — (continued)
  amyl
  anovular menstruation
  ante meridiem (Lat.) before noon
  anteromeatal
  arithmetic mean
  arousal mechanism
  arterial mean
  articular manipulation
  artium magister (Lat.) Master of Arts
  atrial myxoma
  Austin-Moore [prosthesis]
  aviation medicine
  axiomesial
  meter angle
  mixed astigmatism
  myopic astigmatism
Am —
  amalgam
  americium
  amnion
  amyl
A/m — amperes per meter
A-m² — ampere-square meter
am —
  ametropia
  amplitude
  amyl
  ante meridiem (Lat.) before noon
  meter angle
  myopic astigmatism
AMA —
  actual mechanical advantage
  Aerospace Medical Association
  against medical advice
  American Medical Association
  antimitochondrial antibody
  antimyosin antibody
  antithyroid microsomal antibody
  apocrine membrane antigen
  Australian Medical Association

AMAD — morning admission
AMA-DE — American Medical Association Drug Evaluation
AMAG — adrenal medullary autograft
AMAL —
  Aeronautical-Medical Acceleration Laboratory
  amalgam
AMAP — as much as possible
AMAT — antimalignant antibody test
A-MAT — amorphous material
AMB —
  ambulate
  ambulatory
  amphotericin B
  anomalous muscle bundle
  avian myeloblastosis
Amb —
  ambulance
  ambulate
  ambulation
  ambulatory
amb —
  ambient
  ambiguous
  ambulance
  ambulate
  ambulatory
ambig — ambiguous
AMBL —
  acute megakaryoblastic leukemia
  acute myeloblastic leukemia
ambul —
  ambulation
  ambulatory
AMC —
  acetylmethyl carbinol
  Animal Medical Center
  antibody-mediated cytotoxicity
  antimalaria campaign
  arm muscle circumference
  Army Medical Corps
  arthrogryposis multiplex congenita

AMC — (continued)
  automated mixture control
  axiomesiocervical
AMCHA — aminomethylcyclo-
  hexane-carboxylic acid
AMCN — anteromedial caudate
  nucleus
AM/CR — amylase to creatinine
  [ratio]
AMD —
  acid maltase deficiency
  acromandibular dysplasia
  actinomycin D
  adrenomyelodystrophy
  age-related macular degenera-
    tion
  Aleutian mink disease
  alpha-methyldopa
  arthroscopic microdiscectomy
  Association for Macular Dis-
    eases
  axiomesiodistal
AMDGF — alveolar macrophage–
  derived growth factor
AMDS — Association of Military
  Dental Surgeons
AME —
  amphotericin methyl ester
  aseptic meningoencephalitis
AMEA — American Medical Electroencephalographic Association
AMEAE — acute monophasic
  experimental autoimmune
  encephalomyelitis
AMEDS — Army Medical Service
AMegL — acute megakaryoblastic
  leukemia
AMet — adenosyl-L-methionine
AMF —
  antimuscle factor
  autocrine motility factor
  automated motility factor
AMFAR — American Foundation
  for AIDS Research
AMG —
  acoustic myography
  aminoglycoside

AMG — (continued)
  amyloglucosidase
  amyloglucoside
  antimacrophage globulin
  axiomesiogingival
A₂MG — alpha₂-macroglobulin
AMH —
  anti-müllerian hormone
  automated medical history
Amh — mixed astigmatism with
  myopia predominating over
  hyperopia
AMHA — Association of Mental
  Health Administrators
AMHT — automated multiphasic
  health testing
AMI —
  acquired monosaccharide in-
    tolerance
  acute myocardial infarction
  amitriptyline
  anterior myocardial infarction
  Association of Medical Illus-
    trators
  Athletic Motivation Inven-
    tory
  axiomesioincisal
AMIA — American Medical Informatics Association
AMKL — acute megakaryoblastic
  leukemia
AML —
  acute monocytic leukemia
  acute mucosal lesion
  acute myeloblastic leukemia
  acute myelocytic leukemia
  acute myelogenous leukemia
  acute myeloid leukemia
  anatomic medullary locking
  anterior mitral leaflet
  automated multitest labora-
    tory
AMLB — alternate monaural loudness balance
AMLC —
  adherent macrophage-like cell
  autologous mixed lymphocyte
    culture

AMLR — autologous mixed lymphocyte reaction

AMLS — antimouse lymphocyte serum

AMLSGA — acute myeloblastic leukemia surface glycoprotein antigen

AMM —
agnogenic myeloid metaplasia
ammonia
antibody to murine cardiac myosin
Association Médicale Mondiale (Fr.) World Medical Association

amm — ammonia

AMML — acute myelomonocytic leukemia

AMMoL — acute myelomonoblastic leukemia

ammon — ammonia

AMN —
adrenomyeloneuropathy
alloxazine mononucleotide
aminonucleoside
anterior median nucleus

amnio — amniocentesis

AMNS — aminonucleoside

AMN SC — amniotic fluid scan

AMO —
assistant medical officer
axiomesio-occlusal

A-mode —
amplitude mode
amplitude modulation [unit]

AMoL —
acute monoblastic leukemia
acute monocytic leukemia

amor — amorphous

AMP —
accelerated mental processes
acid mucopolysaccharide
adenosine monophosphate
aminomonophosphate
amphetamine
ampicillin
ampule
amputation

AMP — *(continued)*
average mean pressure

3',5'-AMP — cyclic adenosine monophosphate

amp —
ampere
amperage
ampicillin
amplification
ampule
amputation
amputee

AMPA — American Medical Publishers Association

AMPAC — American Medical Political Action Committee

AMP-c — cyclic adenosine monophosphate

AMPH — amphetamine

amph — amphoric

amp-hr — ampere-hour

ampl. — *amplus* (Lat.) large

AMPPPE — acute multifocal posterior placoid pigment epitheliopathy

A-M pr — Austin-Moore prosthesis

AMPS —
abnormal mucopolysacchariduria
acid mucopolysaccharide

AMP-S — adenylosuccinic acid

AMPT —
aminopterin
alpha-methylparatyrosine

ampul. — *ampulla* (Lat.) ampule

AMQ — American Medical Qualification (British)

AMR —
acoustic muscle reflex
activity metabolic rate
alternate motion rate
alternating motion reflex

AMRA — American Medical Record Association

AMRI — anteromedial rotational instability

AMRL — Aerospace Medical Research Laboratories

AMRNL — Army Medical Research and Nutrition Laboratory
AMRS — automated medical record system
AMS —
    acute mountain sickness
    aggravated in military service
    altered mental status
    American Meteorological Society
    American Microscopical Society
    amount of substance
    amylase
    antimacrophage serum
    Army Medical Service
    aseptic meningitis syndrome
    Association of Military Surgeons
    atypical measles syndrome
    auditory memory span
    automated multiphasic screening
    automicrobic system
ams — amount of a substance
AMSA —
    acridinylamine methanesulfon-*m*-anisidide
    American Medical Society on Alcoholism
    American Medical Student Association
    amsacrine
AMSC — Army Medical Specialist Corps
AmSECT — American Society of Extra-Corporeal Technology
AMSIT — appearance, mood, sensorium, intelligence, and thought process
AMSRDC — Army Medical Service Research and Development Command
AMT —
    acute military tuberculosis
    alpha-methyltyrosine
    American Medical Technologists

AMT — *(continued)*
    amethopterin
    amitriptyline
    amphetamine
    anxiety management training
    applied medical technology
    Association of Medical Technologists
amt — amount
AMTP — alpha-methyltryptophan
AMU — Army Medical Unit
amu — atomic mass unit
AmuLV —
    Abelson murine leukemia virus
    amphotrophic murine leukemia virus
AMV —
    assisted mechanical ventilation
    avian myeloblastosis virus
AMV_2 — avian myelocytomatosis virus
AMVI — acute mesenteric vascular insufficiency
aMVL — anterior mitral valve leaflet
AMWA —
    American Medical Women's Association
    American Medical Writers' Association
AMX — amoxicillin
AMY — amylase
AMY-SP — amylase urine spot [test]
AN —
    acanthosis nigricans
    acne neonatorum
    acoustic neuroma
    administratively necessary
    adult, normal
    ala nasi
    aminonucleoside
    amyl nitrate
    anesthesia
    aneurysm
    anisometropia

AN — (*continued*)
   anodal
   anode
   anorexia nervosa
   antenatal
   anterior
   antineuraminidase
   aseptic necrosis
   atmosphere normal
   atrionodal
   autonomic neuropathy
   avascular necrosis
A/N —
   artery and/or nerve
   as needed
An —
   actinon
   anatomic
   anatomy response
   aniridia
   anisometropia
   anodal
   anode
   atmosphere normal
A$_n$ — atmosphere normal
ANA —
   acetylneuraminic acid
   American Narcolepsy Association
   American Neurological Association
   American Nurses' Association
   anesthesia (British, anaesthesia)
   anesthetic
   antibody to nuclear antigens
   antinuclear antibody
   aspartyl naphthylamide
ANAD —
   anorexia nervosa with associated disorders
   antinicotinamide adenine dinucleotidase
ANAE — alpha-naphthyl acetate esterase
ANA-FL — antinuclear antibody fluid
ANAG — acute narrow angle glaucoma

anal —
   analgesia
   analgesic
   analysis
   analyst
   analytic
ANAP — agglutination negative, absorption positive
ANAS —
   anastomosis
   auditory nerve–activating substance
anast — anastomosis
anat —
   anatomical
   anatomist
   anatomy
ANB — avascular necrosis of bone
ANC —
   absolute neutrophil count
   acid neutralization capacity
   antigen-neutralizing capacity
   Army Nurse Corps
ANCA — antineutrophil cytoplasmic antibody
AnCC — anodal-closure contraction
anch — anchored
ANCOVA — analysis of covariance
AND —
   administratively necessary days
   algoneurodystrophy
   anterior nasal discharge
And — androgen
ANDA — Abbreviated New Drug Application
Andro — androsterone
AnDTe — anodal-duration tetanus
anes —
   anesthesia
   anesthesiology
   anesthetic
ANESR — apparent norepinephrine secretion rate
anesth —
   anesthesia

anesth — (continued)
   anesthesiology
   anesthetic
an ex — anodal excitation
ANF —
   alpha-naphthoflavone
   American Nurses' Foundation
   antineuritic factor
   antinuclear factor
   atrial natriuretic factor
ANG — angiotensin
ang —
   angiogram
   angiography
   angle
   angular
angio —
   angiocatheter
   angiocatheterization
Ang GR — angiotensin generation rate
ang pect — angina pectoris
anh — anhydrous
ANI — acute nerve irritation
ANIA — automated nephelometric immunoassay
ANIS —
   anisocytosis
   Anorexia Nervosa Inventory for Self-rating
aniso — anisocytosis
ANIT — alpha-naphthyl–isothiocyanate
ank — ankle
ANL — acute nonlymphoblastic leukemia
ANLI — antibody-negative with latent infection
ANLL —
   acute nonlymphoblastic leukemia
   acute nonlymphocytic leukemia
   acute nonlymphoid leukemia
ANM — auxiliary nurse midwife
Ann — annual
ann fib — annulus fibrosus
annot — annotation

ANoA — antinucleolar antibody
AnOC — anodal opening contraction
ANOCL — anodal opening clonus
ANOVA — analysis of variance
ANP —
   acute necrotizing pancreatitis
   Adult Nurse Practitioner
   Advanced Nurse Practitioner
   A-norprogesterone
   atrial natriuretic peptide
A-NPP — absorbed normal pooled plasma
ANRC — American National Red Cross
ANRL — antihypertensive neural renomedullary lipids
ANS —
   acanthion
   American Nutrition Society
   8-anilino-1-naphthalene-sulfonic [acid]
   anterior nasal spine
   antineutrophilic serum
   antirat neutrophil serum
   Army Nursing Service
   arteriolonephrosclerosis
   Associate in Nursing Science
   autonomic nervous system
ans — answer
ANSCII — American National Standard Code for Information Interchange
ANSI — American National Standards Institute
ANT —
   acoustic noise test
   aminoglycoside 2'-O-nucleotidyltransferase
   aminonitrothiazole
   anterior
ant —
   antenna
   anterior
antag — antagonist
ant ax line — anterior axillary line
anti — antidote
ANTI A:AGT — anti-blood group A antiglobulin test

Anti bx — antibiotic
anticoag — anticoagulant
anti-DNA — antibody to deoxyribonucleic acid
anti-DNase B — antideoxyribonuclease B
anti-ENA — antibody to extractable nuclear antigen [test]
anti-GMB — antiglomerular basement membrane
anti-HA — antihepatitis antigen
anti-HAA — antibody to hepatitis-associated antigen
anti-HAV — antibody to hepatitis A virus
anti-HB$_c$ — antibody to hepatitis B core antigen
anti-HB$_e$ — antibody to hepatitis B early antigen
anti-HB$_s$ — antibody to hepatitis B surface antigen
anti-PNM Ab — anti-peripheral nerve myelin antibody
anti-RNP — antiribonucleoprotein
anti-S — anti-sulfanilic acid
anti-SM — anti-Smith [antibody]
anti-SM/RNP — antibody-smooth muscle/ribonucleoprotein
ant. jentac. — *ante jentaculum* (Lat.) before breakfast
ant pit — anterior pituitary
ant. prand. — *ante prandium* (Lat.) before dinner
ANTR — apparent net transfer rate
ant sag D — anterior sagittal diameter
ant sup spine — anterior superior spine
ANTU — alpha-naphthyl-thiourea
ANuA — antinuclear antibody
ANUG — acute necrotizing ulcerative gingivitis
ANV — avian nephritis virus
anx —
    anxiety
    anxious
anx neur — anxiety neurosis

anx reac — anxiety reaction
AO —
    abdominal aorta
    achievement orientation
    acid output
    acridine orange
    ankle orthosis
    anodal opening
    anterior oblique
    aorta
    aortic opening
    ascending aorta
    atomic orbital
    atrioventricular [valve] opening
    auriculoventricular [valve] opening
    average optical [density]
    avoidance of others
    axio-occlusal
    opening of the atrioventricular valves
A-O — acoustic-optic
A/O — analog to digital
A&O — alert and oriented
A&O × 3 — alert and oriented to person, place, and time
A&O × 4 — alert and oriented to person, place, time, and date
Ao — aorta
AOA —
    abnormal oxygen affinity
    Administration on Aging
    American Optometric Association
    American Orthopedic Association
    American Orthopsychiatric Association
    American Osteopathic Association
    average orifice area
AOAA — amino-oxyacetic acid
AOAC — Association of Official Agricultural Chemists
AOAP — as often as possible
AOAS — American Osteopathic Academy of Sclerotherapy

AOB—
  accessory olfactory bulb
  alcohol on breath
AOBS—acute organic brain syndrome
AOC—
  abridged ocular chart
  American Ophthalmological
    Color Chart
  amyloxycarbonyl
  anodal-opening contraction
  antacid of choice
  aortic opening click
  area of concern
AOCA—American Osteopathic
  College of Anesthesiologists
AOCD—
  American Osteopathic College of Dermatology
  anemia of chronic disease
AOCl—anodal-opening clonus
AOCPa—American Osteopathic
  College of Pathologists
AOCPr—American Osteopathic
  College of Proctology
AOCR—
  American Osteopathic College of Radiology
  American Osteopathic College of Rheumatology
AOD—
  Academy of Operative Dentistry
  Academy of Oral Dynamics
  adult-onset diabetes
  alleged onset date
  arterial occlusive disease
  arterial oxygen desaturation
  auriculo-osteodysplasia
AODA—alcohol and other drug
  abuse
AODM—adult-onset diabetes
  mellitus
AODME—Academy of Osteopathic Directors of Medical
  Education
AODP—alcohol and other drug
  problems

AOHA—American Osteopathic
  Hospital Association
ao-il—aorta–iliac artery
AOIVM—angiographically occult
  intracranial vascular malformation
AOL—acro-osteolysis
AOM—
  acute otitis media
  alternatives of management
  azoxymethane
AOMA—American Occupational
  Medical Association
AoMP—aortic mean pressure
AOO—anodal-opening odor
AOP—
  anodal-opening picture
  aortic pressure
AOPA—American Orthotics and
  Prosthetics Association
AoPW—aortic posterior wall
AOR—
  Alvarado Orthopedic Research [instruments]
  auditory oculogyric reflex
AORN—Association of Operating Room Nurses
aor regurg—aortic regurgitation
aor sten—aortic stenosis
AOS—
  acridine orange staining
  American Ophthalmological
    Society
  American Orthodontic Society
  American Otological Society
  anodal-opening sound
  anterior [o]esophageal sensor
AOSD—adult-onset Still's disease
AOSSM—American Orthopedic
  Society for Sports Medicine
AOT—
  accessory optic tract
  anodal-opening tetanus
  antiovotransferrin
  Association of Occupational
    Therapists
AOTA—American Occupational
  Therapy Association

AOTe — anodal-opening tetanus
AOU — apparent oxygen utilization
AoV — aortic valve
AP —
    abdominoperineal
    accessory pathway
    acid phosphatase
    acinar parenchyma
    action potential
    active pepsin
    acute pancreatitis
    acute phase
    acute pneumonia
    acute proliferative
    adenomatous polyposis
    adolescent psychiatry
    after parturition
    alkaline phosphatase
    alum-precipitated
    American Pharmacopeia
    aminopeptidase
    aminopyridine
    amyloid P-component
    angina pectoris
    ante partum (Lat.) before parturition
    antepartum
    ante prandium (Lat.) before dinner
    anterior pituitary
    anteroposterior
    antidromic potential
    antiparkinsonian
    antipyrine
    antral peristalsis
    aortic pressure
    aortopulmonary
    apical pulse
    apothecary
    appendectomy
    appendicitis
    appendix
    area postrema
    arithmetic progression
    arterial pressure
    artificial pneumothorax
    aspiration pneumonia

AP — *(continued)*
    assessment and planning
    association period
    atherosclerotic plaque
    atrial pacing
    atrioventricular pathway
    atrium pace
    attending physician
    axiopulpal
A/P — ascites/plasma [ratio]
A-P —
    analytic-psychologic
    anteroposterior
A&P —
    abdominal and perineal
    active and present
    anatomy and physiology
    anterior and posterior
    assessment and planning
    auscultation and palpation
    auscultation and percussion
A_2P_2 — second aortic sound, second pulmonary sound
$A_2 = P_2$ — aortic second sound equal to pulmonary second sound
$A_2 > P_2$ — aortic second sound greater than pulmonary second sound
$A_2 < P_2$ — aortic second sound less than pulmonary second sound
3-AP — 3-acetylpyridine
4-AP — 4-aminopyridine
Ap — apex
ap —
    apothecary
    attachment point
a p. — *a priori* (Lat.) prior to
aP — apical pulse
APA —
    action potential amplitude
    aldosterone-producing adenoma
    American Pancreatic Association
    American Pharmaceutical Association
    American Physiotherapy Association

APA — (*continued*)

    American Podiatric Association

    American Psychiatric Association

    American Psychoanalytic Association

    American Psychological Association

    American Psychopathological Association

    American Psychotherapy Association

    aminopenicillanic acid

    antiparietal antibody

    antipernicious anemia [factor]

6-APA — 6-aminopenicillanic acid

APAAP — alkaline phosphatase-antialkaline phosphatase [labeling]

APAB — antiphospholipid antibody

APACHE — Acute Physiology and Chronic Health Evaluation

APAD — anterior-posterior abdominal diameter

APAF — antipernicious anemia factor

APAP — acetaminophen [amide of acetic acid and *p*-aminophenol]

APAS — annular phased-array system

APB —

    abductor pollicis brevis

    atrial premature beat

    auricular premature beat

APC —

    acetylsalicylic acid, phenacetin, and caffeine

    activated protein cell

    acute pharyngoconjunctival [fever]

    adenoidal-pharyngeal-conjunctival [virus]

    adenomatous polyposis coli

    all-purpose capsule

    alternative patterns of complement

APC — (*continued*)

    antigen-presenting cell

    antiphlogistic corticoid

    aperture current

    apneustic center

    aspirin-phenacetin-caffeine

    atrial premature complex

    atrial premature contraction

APC$_A$ — antiparietal cell antibody

APC/C — aspirin, phenacetin, and caffeine with codeine

APCD —

    acquired prothrombin complex deficiency [syndrome]

    adult polycystic disease

APCF — acute pharyngo-conjunctival fever

APCG — apex cardiogram

APCKD — adult-type polycystic kidney disease

APD —

    action-potential duration

    acute polycystic disease

    adult polycystic disease

    afferent pupillary defect

    aminohydroxypropylidene diphosphate

    anterior-posterior diameter

    antipsychotic drug

    atrial premature depolarization

    autoimmune progesterone dermatitis

    automated peritoneal dialysis

A-PD — anteroposterior diameter

APDC — anxiety and panic disorder clinic

APDER — anterior-posterior dual energy radiography

APDI — Adult Personal Data Inventory

APE —

    acetone powder extract

    acute polioencephalitis

    acute psychotic episode

    acute pulmonary edema

    airway pressure excursion

APE — (continued)

aminophylline, phenobarbital, and ephedrine

anterior pituitary extract

asthma of physical effort

avian pneumoencephalitis

APECED — autoimmune polyendocrinopathy-candidosis-ectodermal dystrophy

APF —

acidulated phosphofluoride

American Psychological Foundation

anabolism-promoting factor

animal protein factor

antiperinuclear factor

APG —

acid-precipated globulin

animal pituitary gonadotropin

APGAR —

adaptability, partnership, growth, affection, and resolve

American Pediatric Gross Assessment Record

Apgar [score]

APGL — alkaline phosphatase activity of the granular leukocytes

APH —

adult psychiatric hospital

alcohol-positive history

alternative pathway hemolysis

aminoglycoside phosphotransferase

antepartum hemorrhage

anterior pituitary hormone

Association of Private Hospitals

aph — aphasia

APHA —

American Protestant Hospital Association

American Public Health Association

APhA — American Pharmaceutical Association

AP/HC — accreditation program/hospice care

AP/HHC — accreditation program/home health care

APHP — anti-*Pseudomonas* human plasma

API —

alkaline protease inhibitor

Analytical Profile Index

arterial pressure index

atmospheric pressure ionization

Autonomy Preference Index

APIC — Association for Practitioners in Infection Control

APIE — assessment, planning, implementation, and evaluation

APIM — Association Professionnelle Internationale des Médecins

APIP — additional personal injury protection

APIVR — artificial pacemaker–induced ventricular rhythm

APK — antiparkinsonian

APKD — adult-onset polycystic kidney disease

APL —

abductor pollicis longus [muscle]

accelerated painless labor

acute promyelocytic leukemia

animal placenta lactogen

anterior pituitary-like [hormone]

APLA — antiphospholipid antibody

AP&Lat — anteroposterior and lateral

AP/LTC — accreditation program/long-term care

APM —

Academy of Parapsychology and Medicine

Academy of Physical Medicine

Academy of Psychosomatic Medicine

acid-precipitable material

alternating pressure mattress

APM — (continued)
   anterior papillary muscle
   anteroposterior movement
   aspartame
   Association of Professors of
      Medicine
APMR — Association for Physical
   and Mental Retardation
APN —
   acute pyelonephritis
   average peak noise
APO —
   abductor pollicis obliquus
   acquired pendular oscillation
   adverse patient occurrences
   aphoxide
   apolipoprotein
   apomorphine
   apoprotein
apo — apolipoprotein
apoC — apolipoprotein C
apoE — apolipoprotein E
APORF — acute postoperative renal failure
apoth — apothecary
APP —
   acute phase protein
   alum-precipitated protein
   alum-precipitated pyridine
   aminopyrazolopyrimidine
   amyloid peptide precursor
   antiplatelet plasma
   appendix
   aqueous procaine penicillin
   automated physiologic profile
   avian pancreatic polypeptide
app —
   appendix
   applied
   approximate
APPA — American Psychopathological Association
appar —
   apparatus
   apparent
APPG — aqueous procaine penicillin G
appl —
   appliance

appl — (continued)
   applicable
   application
   applied
applan. — applanatus (Lat.) flattened
applicand. — applicandus (Lat.) to
   be applied
appoint — appointment
approx —
   approximate
   approximately
   approximation
appt — appointment
Appx — appendix
appy — appendectomy
APR —
   abdominoperineal resection
   absolute proximal reabsorp-
      tion
   accelerator-produced radio-
      pharmaceuticals
   acute phase reactant
   amebic prevalence rate
   anatomic porous replacement
   anterior pituitary resection
   auropalpebral reflex
aprax — apraxia
APRL — American Prosthetic Research Laboratory
APRO — aprobarbital
AProL —
   acute progranulocytic leuke-
      mia
   acute promyelocytic leukemia
APRP —
   acidic proline-rich protein
   acute phase reactant protein
APRT — adenine phosphoribosyl
   transferase
APS —
   acute physiology score
   adenosine phosphosulfate
   Adult Protective Services
   Adult Psychiatric Service
   American Pediatric Society
   American Physiological Soci-
      ety

APS — (continued)
    American Proctologic Society
    American Prosthodontic Society
    American Psychological Society
    American Psychosomatic Society
    attending physician's statement
    autoimmune polyglandular syndrome
    automated patient system
APSAC — anisoylated plasminogen-streptokinase activator complex
APSD —
    Alzheimer presenile dementia
    aorticopulmonary septal defect
APSGN — acute poststreptococcal glomerulonephritis
APSQ — Abbreviated Parent Symptom Questionnaire
APSS — Association for the Psychophysiological Study of Sleep
APT —
    alum-precipitated toxoid
    aminophenylthioether
APTA —
    American Physical Therapy Association
    aneurysm of persistent trigeminal artery
APTD — Aid to Permanently and Totally Disabled
APTT — activated partial thromboplastin time
aPTT — activated partial thromboplastin time
APTX — acute parathyroidectomy
APUD — amine precursor uptake and decarboxylation
APV — abnormal posterior vector
APVC — anomalous pulmonary venous connection
APVD — anomalous pulmonary venous drainage

APW — alkaline peptone water
AQ —
    accomplishment quotient
    achievement quotient
    any quantity
    aphasia quotient
aq — aqueous
aq. — *aqua* (Lat.) water
aq. ad. — *aquam adde* (Lat.) add water
aq. astr. — *aqua astricta* (Lat.) frozen water [ice]
aq. bull. — *aqua bulliens* (Lat.) boiling water
aq. cal. — *aqua calida* (Lat.) hot water
aq. com. — *aqua communis* (Lat.) common water
aq. dest. — *aqua destillata* (Lat.) distilled water
aq. ferv. — *aqua fervens* (Lat.) hot water
aq. flur. — *aqua fluvialis* (Lat.) river water
aq. font. — *aqua fontana* (Lat.) spring water
aq. frig. — *aqua frigata* (Lat.) cold water
aq. niv. — *aqua nivalis* (Lat.) snow water
aq. mar. — *aqua maris* (Lat.) sea water
aq. pluv. — *aqua pluvialis* (Lat.) rain water
aq. pur. — *aqua pura* (Lat.) pure water
AQS — additional qualifying symptoms
aq. tep. — *aqua tepida* (Lat.) tepid water
aqu — aqueous
AR —
    abnormal record
    achievement ratio
    actinic reticuloid [syndrome]
    active resistance
    acute rejection
    adherence ratio

AR — *(continued)*
  admitting room
  airway resistance
  alarm reaction
  alcohol-related
  alkali reserve
  allergic rhinitis
  alloy restoration
  amplitude ratio
  analytical reagent
  androgen receptor
  anterior root
  aortic regurgitation
  apical-radial [pulse]
  Argyll Robertson [pupil]
  aromatase
  arsphenamine
  articulare
  artificially ruptured
  artificial respiration
  ascorbic reductase
  assisted respiration
  at risk
  atrial rate
  atrial regurgitation
  atrophic rhinitis
  attack rate
  aural rehabilitation
  autoradiography
  autorefractor
  autosomal recessive
A/R —
  accounts receivable
  apical/radial
A-R — apical-radial
A&R —
  adenoidectomy with radium
  advised and released
Ar —
  argon
  articulare
ar — aromatic
ARA —
  Academy of Rehabilitative
    Audiometry
  acetylene reduction activity
  American Rheumatism Asso-
    ciation

ARA — *(continued)*
  antireticulin antibody
  aortic root angiogram
  arabinose
  Associate of the Royal Acad-
    emy
ara — arabinose
ara-A — adenine arabinoside
  [vidarabine]
ara-C — cytosine arabinoside
  [cytarabine]
araC-Hu — cytarabine and hydroxyurea
ARAMIS — American Rheuma-
  tism Association Medical Information System
ARAS — ascending reticular activating system
ara-U — arabinosyluracil
ARB —
  adrenergic receptor binder
  any reliable brand
arb — arbitrary unit
ARBD — alcohol-related birth defects
ARBOR — arthropod-borne [virus]
ARBOW — artificial rupture of
  bag of waters
ARC —
  accelerating rate calorimetry
  acquired immunodeficiency
    syndrome (AIDS)–related
    complex
  active renin concentration
  Addiction Research Center
  AIDS-related complex
  alcohol rehabilitation center
  American Red Cross
  anomalous retinal correspon-
    dence
  antigen-reactive cell
  arcuate
  Arthritis Rehabilitation Cen-
    ter
  Association for Retarded Chil-
    dren
  average response computer
ARCBS — American Red Cross
  Blood Services

arch — archives

ARCA —
    acquired red cell aplasia
    American Rehabilitation Counseling Association

ARCI — Addiction Research Center Inventory

ARCO — antigen-reactive cell opsonization

ARCS — Associate of the Royal College of Science

ARD —
    absolute reaction of degeneration
    acute radiation disease
    acute respiratory disease
    acute respiratory distress
    adult respiratory disease
    adult respiratory distress
    allergic respiratory disease
    anorectal dressing
    antibiotic removal device
    antimicrobial removal device
    aphakic retinal detachment
    arthritis and rheumatic diseases
    atopic respiratory disease

ARDS —
    acute respiratory distress syndrome
    adult respiratory distress syndrome

ARE —
    active-resistive exercises
    AIDS-related encephalitis

AREDYLD — acrorenal field defect, ectodermal dysplasia, lipoatrophic diabetes [syndrome]

ARES — antireticulo-endothelial serum

ARF —
    acute renal failure
    acute respiratory failure
    acute rheumatic fever
    Addiction Research Foundation
    area resource file

ARFC —
    active rosette-forming T-cell
    autologous rosette-forming cell

ARF/CRF — acute renal failure and chronic renal failure

Arg — arginine

arg. — *argentum* (Lat.) silver

ARI —
    acute respiratory infection
    airway reactivity index
    aldose reductase inhibitor
    anxiety reaction, intense

ARIA — automated radioimmunoassay

ARIC — Associate of the Royal Institute of Chemistry

ArKr — argon-krypton [laser]

ARL — average remaining lifetime

ARLD — alcohol-related liver disease

ARM —
    adrenergic receptor material
    aerosol rebreathing method
    allergy relief medicine
    alternating rate of motion
    anorectal manometry
    anxiety reaction, mild
    Armenian [hamster]
    artificial rupture of membranes
    atomic resolution microscopy

ARMH — Academy of Religion and Mental Health

ARMS —
    Adverse Reaction Monitoring System
    amplification refractory mutation system

ARN —
    acute renal necrosis
    acute retinal necrosis
    arcuate nucleus
    Association of Rehabilitation Nurses

ARNMD — Association for Research in Nervous and Mental Diseases

ARNP—Advanced Registered
  Nurse Practitioner
ARO—Association for Research
  in Ophthalmology
AROA—autosomal recessive ocu-
  lar albinism
AROM—
    active range of motion
    artificial rupture of mem-
      branes
arom—aromatic
ARP—
    absolute refractory period
    Advanced Research Projects
    alcohol rehabilitation pro-
      gram
    American Registry of Patholo-
      gists
    assay reference plasma
    assimilation regulatory protein
    at-risk period
    automaticity recovery phase
ARPES—angular resolved photo-
  electron spectroscopy
ARPKD—autosomal recessive
  polycystic kidney disease
ARPT—American Registry of
  Physical Therapists
ARR—aortic root replacement
arr—
    arrest
    arrested
    arrive
ARRC—Associate of the Royal
  Red Cross
ARRS—American Roentgen Ray
  Society
ARRT—
    American Registered Respira-
      tory Therapist
    American Registry of Radio-
      logic Technologists
arry—arrhythmia
ARS—
    acquiescence response scale
    adult recovery services
    adult Reye's syndrome
    AIDS-related syndrome

ARS—*(continued)*
    alizarin red S
    American Radium Society
    American Rhinologic Society
    antirabies serum
    arsphenamine
    arylsulfatase
    autonomously replicating se-
      quence
Ars—
    arsphenamine
    arylsulfatase
ARSA—American Reye's Syn-
  drome Association
Ars-A—arylsulfatase A
ARSACS—autosomal recessive
  spastic ataxia of Charlevoix-
  Saguenay
Ars-B—arylsulfatase B
ARSC—Associate of the Royal
  Society of Chemistry
Ars-C—arylsulfatase C
ARSM—acute respiratory system
  malfunction
ARSPH—Associate of the Royal
  Society for the Promotion of
  Health
ART—
    absolute retention time
    Accredited Record Techni-
      cian
    Achilles [tendon] reflex test
    acoustic reflex test
    acoustic reflex threshold(s)
    algebraic reconstruction tech-
      nique
    arrhythmia research technol-
      ogy
    arterial
    artery
    assisted reproductive tech-
      nique
    autologous reactive T cell
    automated reagin test
    automaticity recovery time
art—
    arterial
    artery

art — (continued)
    articulation
    artificial
arth —
    arthritis
    arthrotomy
arthro — arthroscopy
ARTI — acute respiratory tract illness
artic —
    articulated
    articulation
artif — artificial
art insem — artificial insemination
art line — arterial line
Art T — art therapy
ARV —
    AIDS-related virus
    anterior right ventricle
    avian reovirus
ARVD — arrhythmogenic right ventricular dysplasia
ARVO — Association for Research in Vision and Ophthalmology
ARW — accredited rehabilitation worker
ARWY — airway
AS —
    above scale
    acetylstrophanthidin
    acidified serum
    acoustic stimulation
    activated sleep
    active sarcoidosis
    active sleep
    acute salpingitis
    Adams-Stokes [disease]
    adolescent suicide
    aerosol steroid
    affective style
    alimentary sleep
    Alport syndrome
    alveolar sac
    alveolar space
    amphetamine sulfate
    amyloid substance
    anal sphincter
    androsterone sulfate

AS — (continued)
    Angelman syndrome
    ankylosing spondylitis
    annulospiral
    anovulatory syndrome
    antiserum
    antisocial
    antistreptolysin
    antral spasm
    anxiety state
    aortic sac
    aortic sound
    aortic stenosis
    aqueous solution
    aqueous suspension
    arteriosclerosis
    artificial sweetener
    aseptic meningitis
    astigmatism
    asymmetric
    atherosclerosis
    atrial septum
    atrial stenosis
    atropine sulfate
    audiogenic seizure
    Auto-Suture
    sickle-cell trait
A.S. — auris sinistra (Lat.) left ear
A-S —
    Adams-Stokes [disease]
    ascendance-submission
As —
    acetylstrophanthidin
    arsenic
    astigmatism
    asymptomatic
    atmosphere, standard
A(s) — asplenia syndrome
A·s — ampere-second
A×s — ampere per second
ASA —
    acetylsalicylic acid
    active systemic anaphylaxis
    Adams-Stokes attack
    American Society of Anesthesiologists
    American Standards Association

ASA — (continued)
    American Stomatological Association
    American Surgical Association
    anterior spinal artery
    antibody to surface antigen
    argininosuccinate
    argininosuccinic acid
    arylsulfatase A
    aspirin-sensitive asthma
    atrial septal aneurysm
5-ASA — 5-aminosalicylic acid
Asa — arsenate
ASAA — acquired severe aplastic anemia
ASAAD — American Society for the Advancement of Anesthesia in Dentistry
ASAC — acidified serum–acidified complement
ASACl — American Society of Anesthesiologists' classification
ASA-G — guaiacolic acid ester of acetylsalicylic acid
ASAH — antibiotic-sterilized aortic valve homograft
ASAHP — American Society of Allied Health Professionals
ASAI — aortic stenosis and aortic insufficiency
ASAIO — American Society for Artificial Internal Organs
ASAL — argininosuccinic acid lyase
ASAP —
    American Society for Adolescent Psychology
    as soon as possible
ASAS —
    American Society of Abdominal Surgeons
    argininosuccinate synthetase
ASAT — aspartate aminotransferase
ASB —
    American Society of Bacteriologists

ASB — (continued)
    anencephaly–spina bifida [syndrome]
    anesthesia standby
    Anxiety Scale for the Blind
    asymptomatic bacteriuria
AsB — arylsulfatase B
ASBS — arteriosclerotic brain syndrome
ASBV — avocado sunblotch viroid
ASC —
    acetylsulfanilyl chloride
    adenosine-coupled spleen cell
    altered state of consciousness
    ambulatory surgery center
    American Society of Cytology
    anterior subscapular cataract
    antigen-sensitive cell
    antimony–sulfur colloid
    ascorbate
    ascorbic acid
    asthma symptom checklist
AsC — arylsulfatase C
asc —
    arteriosclerosis
    arteriosclerotic
    ascending
    anterior subcapsular
Asc-A — ascending aorta
ASCAD —
    arteriosclerotic coronary artery disease
    atherosclerotic coronary artery disease
ASCAo — ascending aorta
ASCH — American Society of Clinical Hypnosis
ASCI — American Society for Clinical Investigation
ASCII — American Standard Code for Information Interchange
ascit fl — ascitic fluid
ASCL — arteriosclerosis
ASCLT — American Society of Clinical Laboratory Technicians

ASCMS — American Society of Contemporary Medicine and Surgery

ASCO —
American Society of Clinical Oncology
American Society of Contemporary Ophthalmology

ASCP —
American Society of Clinical Pathologists
American Society of Consulting Pharmacists

ASCPC — American Society of Clinical Pharmacology and Chemotherapy

ASCR — American Society of Chiropodical Roentgenology

ascr. — *ascriptum* (Lat.) ascribed to

ASCT — autologous stem cell transplantation

ASCVD —
arteriosclerotic cardiovascular disease
atherosclerotic cardiovascular disease

ASCURD — arteriosclerotic cardiovascular renal disease

ASD —
aldosterone secretion defect
Alzheimer senile dementia
anterior sagittal dimension
antisiphon device
arthritis syphilitica deformans
arthroscopic subacromial decompression
atrial septal defect

ASDA —
American Society for Dental Aesthetics
American Student Dental Association

ASDC —
American Society of Dentistry for Children
Association of Sleep Disorders Centers

ASDH — acute subdural hematoma

ASDR — American Society of Dental Radiographers

ASE —
acute stress erosion
American Society of Echocardiography
axilla, shoulder, elbow

ASECT — American Society of Extra-Corporeal Technology

ASEP — American Society for Experimental Pathology

ASES — Adult Self-Expression Scale

ASET — American Society of Electroencephalographic Technologists

ASF —
African swine fever
aniline, sulfur, formaldehyde [resin]

ASFR — age-specific fertility rate

ASG —
advanced stage group
American Society for Genetics
Army Surgeon General

ASGBI — Association of Surgeons of Great Britain and Ireland

ASGD — American Society of Geriatric Dentistry

ASGE — American Society for Gastrointestinal Endoscopy

AS/GP — antiserum, guinea pig

ASH —
aldosterone-stimulating hormone
American Society of Hematology
ankylosing spinal hyperostosis
antistreptococcal hyaluronidase
asymmetrical septal hypertrophy
hypermetropic astigmatism
hyperopic astigmatism

AsH — hypermetropic astigmatism

A&Sh — arm and shoulder

ASHA—
>American School Health Association
>
>American Social Health Association
>
>American Speech and Hearing Association

ASHCVD—atherosclerotic hypertensive cardiovascular disease

ASHD—
>arteriosclerotic heart disease
>
>atherosclerotic heart disease
>
>atrial septal heart disease

ASHG—American Society for Human Genetics

ASHI—Association for the Study of Human Infertility

ASHMET—American Society for Health Manpower Education and Training

ASHN—acute sclerosing hyaline necrosis

ASHNS—American Society for Head and Neck Surgery

AS/Ho—antiserum, horse

ASHP—
>American Society of Hospital Pharmacists
>
>American Society for Hospital Planning

ASHPA—American Society for Hospital Personnel Administration

ASHT—American Society of Hand Therapists

ASI—
>addiction severity index
>
>Anxiety Status Inventory
>
>arthroscopic screw installation

ASII—American Science Information Institute

ASIM—American Society of Internal Medicine

ASIS—anterior superior iliac spine

ASK—antistreptokinase

ASKA—antiskeletal antibody

ASL—
>American sign language

ASL—(continued)
>ankylosing spondylitis, lung
>
>antistreptolysin
>
>argininosuccinate lyase

ASLC—acute self-limited colitis

ASLIB—Association of Special Libraries and Information Bureau

ASLM—American Society of Law and Medicine

ASLO—antistreptolysin O

ASL-O—antistreptolysin O

ASLT—antistreptolysin test

ASM—
>airway smooth muscle
>
>American Society for Microbiology
>
>anterior scalenus muscle
>
>myopic astigmatism

ASMA—antismooth muscle antibody

ASMC—arterial smooth muscle cell

ASMD—atonic sclerotic muscle dystrophy

ASME—Association for the Study of Medical Education

ASMI—anteroseptal myocardial infarction

As/Mk—antiserum, monkey

ASMPA—Armed Services Medical Procurement Agency

ASMR—age-standardized mortality ratio

ASMT—American Society for Medical Technology

asmt—assessment

ASN—
>alkali-soluble nitrogen
>
>American Society of Nephrology
>
>American Society of Neurochemistry
>
>arteriosclerotic nephritis
>
>asparagine
>
>Associate in Nursing

Asn—asparagine

ASO—
>allele-specific oligonucleotide

ASO — (continued)
  American Society of Ortho-
    dontics
  antistreptolysin O
  arteriosclerosis obliterans
  automatic stop order
ASOR — asialo-orsomucoid
ASOS — American Society of
    Oral Surgeons
ASOT — antistreptolysin O titer
ASP —
  abnormal spinal posture
  acute suppurative parotitis
  acute symmetric polyarthritis
  African swine pox
  aged substrate plasma
  alkali-stable pepsin
  American Society of Parasitol-
    ogists
  American Society of Patholo-
    gists
  American Society of Perio-
    dontists
  ankylosing spondylitis
  antisocial personality
  aortic systolic pressure
  area systolic pressure
  asparaginase
  aspartic acid
  aspiration
Asp —
  asparaginase
  aspartic acid
asp —
  aspartate
  aspartic acid
  aspirate
  aspiration
ASPA —
  American Society of Physi-
    cian Analysts
  American Society of Podiat-
    ric Assistants
ASPAT — antistreptococcal poly-
    saccharide A test
ASPDM — American Society of
    Psychosomatic Dentistry and
    Medicine

Asper — aspergillosis
ASPET — American Society for
    Pharmacology and Experimen-
    tal Therapeutics
ASPG — antispleen globulin
ASPM — American Society of
    Paramedics
ASPO — American Society for
    Psychoprophylaxis in Obstet-
    rics
ASPP — Association for Sane Psy-
    chiatric Practices
ASPRS — American Society of
    Plastic and Reconstructive
    Surgeons
ASPS — advanced sleep phase syn-
    drome
ASPVD —
  arteriosclerotic peripheral vas-
    cular disease
  atherosclerotic peripheral vas-
    cular disease
ASQ —
  Abbreviated Symptom Ques-
    tionnaire
  Anxiety Scale Questionnaire
ASR —
  aldosterone secretion rate
  aldosterone secretory rate
  antistreptolysin reaction
  atrial septal resection
AS/Rab — antiserum, rabbit
ASRT — American Society of Ra-
    diologic Technologists
ASS —
  acute serum sickness
  acute spinal stenosis
  anterior superior spine
  argininosuccinate synthetase
ASSA — aminopterin-like syn-
    drome sine aminopterin
ASSC — acute splenic sequestra-
    tion crisis
ASSH — American Society for
    Surgery of the Hand
ASSI — Accurate Surgical and Sci-
    entific Instruments
ASSIM — assimilate, assimilation

Assn — association

ASSO — American Society for the Study of Orthodontics

Assoc —
associate
association

assocd — associated [with]

ASSR — adult situation stress reaction

asst — assistant

AST —
allergy serum transfer
angiotensin sensitivity test
anterior spinothalamic tract
antistreptolysin titer
aspartate transaminase
Association of Surgical Technologists
astemizole
astigmatism
audiometry sweep test

Ast. — astigmatism

ASTA — anti-alpha-staphylolysin

ASTC — Association of Science Technology Centers

A sten — aortic stenosis

Asth. — asthenopia

ASTHO — Association of State and Territorial Health Officers

ASTI — antispasticity index

ASTM — American Society for Testing and Materials

ASTMH — American Society of Tropical Medicine and Hygiene

ASTO — antistreptolysin O

as tol — as tolerated

ASTZ — antistreptozyme

ASU —
acute stroke unit
aeromedical staging unit
ambulatory surgical unit

ASUTS — American Society of Ultrasound Technical Specialists

ASV —
anodic stripping voltammetry

ASV — (continued)
antisiphon valve
antisnake venom
arteriosuperficial venous [difference]
avian sarcoma virus

ASVD —
arteriosclerotic vascular disease
arteriosclerotic vessel disease

ASVIP — atrial-synchronous ventricular-inhibited pacemaker

ASVO — American Society of Veterinary Ophthalmology

ASVPP — American Society of Veterinary Physiologists and Pharmacologists

ASW —
artificial seawater
artificial sweetener

Asx —
amino acid that gives aspartic acid after hydrolysis
asymptomatic

asym —
asymmetric
asymmetry

AT —
abdominal tympany
Achard-Thiers [syndrome]
achievement test
Achilles tendon
activity therapy
adaptive thermogenesis
adenine-thymine
adipose tissue
adjunctive therapy
adjuvant therapy
air temperature
air trapping
allergy treatment
alt tuberkulin (Ger.) old tuberculin
aminotransferase
aminotriazole
amitriptyline
anaerobic threshold
anaphylatoxin

AT — *(continued)*
    anionic trypsinogen
    anterior tibia
    antithrombin
    antitrypsin
    antral transplantation
    applanation tonometry
    ataxia-telangiectasia
    atmosphere
    atraumatic
    atresia, tricuspid
    atrial tachycardia
    atropine
    attenuation
    attenuate
    autoimmune thrombocyto-
        penia
    axonal terminal
A-T — ataxia-telangiectasia
AT_7 — hexachlorophene
At_{10} — dihydrotachysterol
AT I — angiotensin I
AT II — angiotensin II
AT III —
    angiotensin III
    antithrombin III
At —
    acidity, total
    astatine
    atrial
    atrium
at —
    atom
    atomic
a.t. —
    airtight
    ampere turn
ATA —
    alimentary toxic aleukia
    American Thyroid Associa-
        tion
    American Tinnitus Associa-
        tion
    aminotriazole
    antithymic activity
    antithyroglobulin antibody
    antithyroid antibody
    anti-*Toxoplasma* antibody

ATA — *(continued)*
    atmosphere absolute
    aurintricarboxylic acid
ATB —
    antibiotic
    atrial tachycardia with block
    atypical tuberculosis
ATC —
    activated thymus cell
    alcoholism therapy classes
    all-terrain cycle
    around the clock
ATCC — American-Type Culture
    Collection
ATCS —
    active trabecular calcification
        surface
    anterior tibial compartment
        syndrome
ATD —
    Alzheimer-type dementia
    anthropomorphic test dummy
    antithyroid drug
    aqueous tear deficiency
    asphyxiating thoracic dystro-
        phy
    autoimmune thyroid disease
ATDC — Association of Thalido-
    mide-Damaged Children
ATE —
    acute toxic encephalopathy
    adipose tissue extract
    autologous tumor extract
ATEE — N-acetyl-L-tyrosine ethyl
    ester
ATEM — analytic transmission
    electron microscopy
Aten — atenolol
A tetra P — adenosine tetraphos-
    phate
ATF — ascites tumor fluid
At fib — atrial fibrillation
ATG —
    adenine-thymidine-guanine
    antihuman thymocyte globu-
        lin
    antithrombocyte globulin
    antithymocyte globulin

ATG — *(continued)*
   antithyroglobulin
ATGAM — antithymocyte gamma
   globulin
AT/GC — adenine-thymine/
   guanine-cytosine [ratio]
ATH — acetyl-tyrosine hydrazide
ATh — Associate in Therapy
ATHC — allotetrahydrocortisol
ATHR — angina threshold heart
   rate
Athsc — atherosclerosis
ATI — abdominal trauma index
ATL —
   Achilles tendon lengthening
   adult T-cell leukemia
   adult T-cell lymphoma
   anterior tricuspid leaflet
   antitension line
   atypical lymphocyte
ATLA — adult T-cell leukemia
   [virus-associated] antigen
ATLL —
   adult T-cell leukemia
   adult T-cell lymphoma
ATLS —
   acute tumor lysis syndrome
   Advanced Trauma Life Sup-
      port [Program]
ATLV — adult T-cell leukemia virus
ATM —
   abnormal tubular myelin
   acute transverse myelitis
   acute transverse myelopathy
   atmosphere
atm —
   atmosphere
   atmospheric
ATMA — antithyroid plasma membrane antibody
At ma — atrial milliampere
atmos — atmospheric
ATN —
   acute tubular necrosis
   augmented transition network
   tyrosinase-negative oculocuta-
      neous albinism

ATNC — atraumatic normocephalic
aTNM — [at] autopsy, tumor,
   nodes, and metastases
at. no. — atomic number
ATNR — asymmetrical tonic neck
   reflex
ATP —
   addiction treatment program
   adenosine triphosphate
   ambient temperature and pres-
      sure
   autoimmune thrombocytope-
      nic purpura
A-TP — absorbed test plasma
AT-P — antitrypsin-Pittsburgh
AtP — attending physician
AT-PAS — aldehyde-thionine-
   periodic acid–Schiff [test]
ATPase — adenosine triphosphatase
ATPD — ambient temperature and
   pressure, dry
ATP-2Na — adenosine triphos-
   phate disodium
ATPS — ambient temperature and
   pressure, saturated
ATPTX — acute thyroparathyroi-
   dectomy
ATR —
   Achilles tendon reflex
   atrial
   attenuated total reflection
atr — atrophy
atr fib — atrial fibrillation
ATRO — atropine
ATS —
   Achard-Thiers syndrome
   acid test solution
   adjustable thigh [antiembo-
      lism] stockings
   alpha-D-tocopherol acid succi-
      nate
   American Therapeutic Soci-
      ety
   American Thoracic Society
   American Trauma Society
   American Trudeau Society

ATS — *(continued)*
    anti-rat thymocyte serum
    antitetanic serum
    antitetanus serum
    antithymocyte serum
    anxiety tension state
    arteriosclerosis
    atherosclerosis
ATSDR — Agency for Toxic Substances and Disease Registry
ATT —
    arginine tolerance test
    aspirin tolerance time
att — attending
ATTR — attached report
ATU —
    alcohol treatment unit
    allylthiourea
ATV —
    atrioventricular
    avian tumor virus
at vol — atomic volume
At wt — atomic weight
ATx — adult thymectomy
atyp — atypical
ATZ — atypical transformation zone
AU —
    ad usum (Lat.) according to custom
    allergenic unit
    Ångstrom unit
    antitoxin unit
    arbitrary unit
    aures unitas (Lat.) both ears together
    auris uterque (Lat.) each ear
    azauridine
Au —
    Australian
    antigen
    gold (Lat., *aurum*)
^{198}Au —
    colloidal gold
    radioactive gold
AUA —
    American Urological Association

AUA — *(continued)*
    Association of University Anesthetists
Au Ag — Australia antigen
AUB — abnormal uterine bleeding
AUC — area under the curve
auct. — *auctorum* (Lat.) of authors
AUD — arthritis of unknown diagnosis
aud — auditory
aud-vis — audiovisual
AUFS — absorbance units, full-scale
AUG —
    acute ulcerative gingivitis
    adenine, uridine, guanosine
    adenosine-uracil-guanine
aug. — *augere* (Lat.) increase
AUGH — acute upper gastrointestinal hemorrhage
AUGIB — acute upper gastrointestinal bleeding
AuHAA — Australia hepatitis–associated antigen
AUI — Alcohol Use Inventory
AUL — acute undifferentiated leukemia
AUM — asymmetrical unit membrane
AUO — amyloid of unknown origin
AuP — Australia antigen protein
AUPHA — Association of University Programs in Health Administration
AUR — acute urinary retention
aur. —
    auris (Lat.) ear
    aurum (Lat.) gold
aur. d. — *auris dextra* (Lat.) right ear
aur fib — auricular fibrillation
auric —
    auricle
    auricular
aurin. — *aurinarium* (Lat.) ear cone
aurist. — *auristillae* (Lat.) ear drops
aur. s. — *auris sinistra* (Lat.) left ear

AUS —
    acute urethral syndrome
    auscultation
ausc — auscultation
AuSH — Australia serum hepatitis
AutoAB — autoantibody
Auto-PEEP — self-controlled posi-
    tive end-expiratory pressure
aux — auxiliary
AV —
    air velocity
    allergic vasculitis
    alveolar duct
    anteroventral
    anteversion
    anteverted
    anticipatory vomiting
    antivirin
    aortic valve
    arteriovenous
    artificial ventilation
    assisted ventilation
    atrioventricular
    audiovisual
    auditory-visual
    augmented vector
    auriculoventricular
    average
    aviation medicine
    avoirdupois
A-V —
    arteriovenous
    atrioventricular
    auriculoventricular
A/V —
    ampere/volt
    arteriovenous
    atrial/ventricular
    auricular/ventricular
Av. —
    average
    avoirdupois
aV — abvolt
av —
    air velocity
    anteverted
    average
    avoirdupois

av — (continued)
    avulsion
AVA —
    activity vector analysis
    American Vocational Associa-
        tion
    antiviral antibody
    aortic valve area
    aortic valve atresia
    arteriovenous anastomosis
    availability
AV/AF — anteverted, anteflexed
AVB — atrioventricular block
AVBR — automated ventricular
    brain ratio
AVC —
    aberrant ventricular conduc-
        tion
    Academy of Veterinary Cardi-
        ology
    allantoin vaginal cream
    Association of Vitamin Chem-
        ists
    associative visual cortex
    atrioventricular canal
    automatic volume control
AVCD — atrioventricular canal de-
    fect
AvCDO$_2$ — arteriovenous oxygen
    content difference
AVCS — atrioventricular conduc-
    tion system
AVD —
    aortic valvular disease
    apparent volume of distribu-
        tion
    arteriovenous difference
    atrioventricular dissociation
    Army Veterinary Department
AVDO$_2$ — arteriovenous oxygen
    saturation difference
AVDP — average diastolic pressure
avdp — avoirdupois
AVE — aortic valve echocardio-
    gram
aver — average
AVF —
    antiviral factor

AVF—(*continued*)
  arteriovenous fistula
aV$_F$—augmented voltage, unipolar left leg lead [electrocardiography]
AVFM—arteriovenous fistulous malformation
AVG—ambulatory visit groups
avg—average
AVH—acute viral hepatitis
AVHB—atrioventricular heart block
AVHD—acquired valvular heart disease
AVI—
  air velocity index
  Association of Veterinary Inspectors
A-V IMA—arteriovenous internal mammary artery [fistula]
AVJ—atrioventricular junction
AVJR—atrioventricular junction rhythm
AVJRe—atrioventricular junctional reentrant
AVJT—atrioventricular junctional tachycardia
AVL—anterior vein of leg
aV$_L$—unipolar augmented voltage, left arm lead [electrocardiography]
AVLINE—Audiovisuals On-Line [data base]
AVM—
  arteriovenous malformation
  arteriovenous malfunction
  atrioventricular malformation
  atrioventricular malfunction
  aviation medicine
AVMA—American Veterinary Medical Association
AVN—
  acute vasomotor nephropathy
  arbitrary valve unit
  arteriovenous nicking
  atrioventricular nodal [conduction]
  atrioventricular node

AVN—(*continued*)
  avascular necrosis
AVND—atrioventricular node dysfunction
AVNFH—avascular necrosis of the femoral head
AVNFRP—atrioventricular node functional refractory period
AVNR—atrioventricular nodal reentry
AVNRT—atrioventricular nodal reentry tachycardia
AVO—atrioventricular opening
A-VO$_2$—arteriovenous oxygen difference
AVP—
  abnormal vasopressin
  ambulatory venous pressure
  antiviral protein
  aqueous vasopressin
  arginine vasopressin
  arteriovenous passage [time]
AVR—
  accelerated ventricular rhythm
  antiviral regulator
  aortic valve replacement
AVr—antiviral regulator
aV$_R$—augmented voltage, unipolar right arm lead [electrocardiography]
AVRB—added viscous resistance to breathing
AVRI—acute viral respiratory infection
AVRP—atrioventricular refractory period
AVRT—
  atrioventricular [nodal] reentrant tachycardia
  atrioventricular reciprocating tachycardia
AVS—
  aneurysm of [membranous] ventricular septum
  aortic valve stenosis
  arteriovenous shunt
  Association for Voluntary Sterilization

AVS — *(continued)*
auditory vocal sequencing
AVSC — aortic valve cusp separation
AVSD — atrioventricular septal defect
AVSS — afebrile, vital signs stable
AVSV — aortic valve stroke volume
AVT —
Abelson virus transformed
Allen vision test
area ventralis of Tsai
arginine vasotocin
atrioventricular tachycardia
atypical ventricular tachycardia
Aviation Medicine Technician
AVTB — absolute volume of trabecular bone
Av3V — anteroventral third ventricle
AVZ — avascular zone
AW —
abdominal wall
able to work
abnormal wave
above waist
abrupt withdrawal
alcohol withdrawal
aluminum wafer
alveolar wall
alveolar wash
anterior wall
atomic warfare
atomic weight
A&W — alive and well
A3W — crystalline amino acid solution
aw —
airway
water activity
AWA —
as well as
away without authorization
AWAKE — Alert, Well, and Keeping Energetic [support group]

AWBM — alveolar wall basement membrane
AWF — adrenal weight factor
AWG — American Wire Gauge
AWI —
anterior wall infarction
authorized walk-in [patient]
AWMI — anterior wall myocardial infarction
AWO — airway obstruction
AWOL — absent without leave
AWP —
airway pressure
average of the wholesale prices
AWRS — anti-whole rabbit serum
AWRU — active wrist rotation unit
AWS — alcohol withdrawal syndrome
AWTA — aniridia–Wilms' tumor association
awu — atomic weight unit
AX — alloxan
ax —
axillary
axial
axis
axon
AXF — advanced x-ray facility
AXG — adult xanthogranuloma
ax grad — axial gradient
AXL — axillary lymphoscintigraphy
AXM — acetoxycyclohexamide
AXR — abdominal x-ray
AXT — alternating exotropia
A^y — yellow [mouse]
AYA — acute yellow atrophy
AYF — antiyeast factor
AYP — autolyzed yeast protein
AYV — aster yellow virus
AZ —
acetazolamide
Aschheim-Zondek [test]
azathioprine
Az — *azote* (Fr.) nitrogen

AZA — azathioprine
5-AZA —
    5-azacitidine
    5-azacytidine
AzC — azacytosine
azg. — azaguanine
azo — indicates presence of the
    group –N:N–
AZQ — diaziquone
AZR — alizarin

AZS — automatic zero set
AZT —
    Aschheim-Zondek test
    azidothymidine
    3'-azido-3'-deoxythymidine
    zidovudine (azidothymidine)
AZT-TP — 3'-azido-3'-deoxythymi-
    dine triphosphate
AZU — 6-azauracil
AZUR — 6-azauridine

B —
    bacillus
    bacitracin
    bacterium
    balneum (Lat.) bath
    bands
    barometric
    base
    baseline
    basophil
    basophilic
    Baumé scale
    behavior
    bel
    Benois scale
    benzoate
    beta (second letter of the
        Greek alphabet), upper-
        case
    bicuspid
    bilateral
    black
    blood
    bloody
    blue
    body
    boils at
    Bolton point
    bone marrow–derived [lym-
        phocyte]
    born
    boron
    both

B — (*continued*)
    bound
    bovine
    break
    bregma
    bronchial
    bronchus
    brother
    bruit
    buccal
    Bucky (film in cassette in Pot-
        ter-Bucky diaphragm)
    bursa cells
    bypass
    gauss (unit of magnetic induc-
        tion)
    magnetic flux density
    magnetic induction
    supramentale (craniometric
        point)
    whole blood
B. —
    Bacillus
    Balantidium
    Bordetella
    Borrelia
    Brucella
B_0 — constant magnetic field in nu-
    clear magnetic resonance
B_1 —
    radiofrequency magnetic field
        in nuclear magnetic reso-
        nance

B_1 — (continued)
    thiamine hydrochloride
B_2 — riboflavin
B4 — before
B_6 — pyridoxine
B_7 — biotin
B_8 — adenosine phosphate
B_{12} — cyanocobalamin
BI — Billroth I [operation]
BII — Billroth II [operation]
b —
    barn
    base
    boils at
    born
    brain
    broth
β —
    an anomer of a carbohydrate
    beta (second letter of the
      Greek alphabet), lowercase
    buffer capacity
    carbon separated from a car-
      boxyl by one other carbon
      in aliphatic compounds
    constituent of a plasma pro-
      tein fraction
    a globin polypeptide chain of
      hemoglobin
    probability of type II error
    substituent group of a steroid
      that projects above the
      plane of the ring
β♀ — black female
β♂ — black male
1-β — power of statistical test
b. —
    balneum (Lat.) bath
    bis (Lat.) twice
BA —
    Bachelor of Arts
    backache
    background activity
    bacterial agglutination
    balneum arenae (Lat.) sand
      bath
    basilar artery
    basion

BA — (continued)
    basket axon
    benzanthracene
    benzyl alcohol
    benzyladenine
    benzylamine
    best amplitude
    betamethasone acetate
    bilateral asymmetrical
    bile acid
    biliary atresia
    biological activity
    blocking antibody
    blood agar
    blood alcohol
    bone age
    boric acid
    bovine albumin
    brachial artery
    breathing apparatus
    bronchial asthma
    bronchoalveolar
    buccoaxial
    buffered acetone
    butyric acid
B.A. — Bachelor of Arts
B&A — brisk and active
B>A — bone greater than air
B<A — bone less than air
Ba —
    barium
    barium enema
    basion
ba — basion
b.a. — balneum arenae (Lat.) sand
    bath
BAA —
    benzoylarginine amide
    branched-chain amino acid
BAB — blood-agar base
Bab —
    Babinski's [reflex]
    baboon
BabK — baboon kidney
BAC —
    bacteria
    bacterial adherent colony
    bacterial antigen complex

BAC — (continued)
  benzalkonium chloride
  blood alcohol concentration
  British Association of Chemists
  bronchoalveolar cells
  buccoaxiocervical
Bac —
  Bacillus
  bacillary
BaCl₂ — barium chloride
Bact. — *Bacterium*
bact —
  bacteria
  bacterial
  bacteriologist
  bacteriology
BAD —
  biological aerosol detection
  bipolar affective disorder
  British Association of Dermatologists
BAE —
  bovine aortic endothelium
  bronchial artery embolization
BaE — barium enema
BAEC — bovine aortic endothelial cells
BAEE —
  benzoyl-argine ethyl ester
  benzylarginine ethyl ester
BaEn — barium enema
BAEP — brainstem auditory evoked potential
BAER — brainstem auditory evoked response
BAG — buccoaxiogingival
BAGG — buffered azide glucose glycerol
BAHS — butoctamide hydrogen succinate
BAI — basilar artery insufficiency
BAIB — beta-aminoisobutyric [acid]
BAIF — bile acid independent flow
BAIT — bacterial automated identification technique

BAL —
  blood alcohol level
  British antilewisite (dimercaprol)
  bronchoalveolar lavage
bal —
  balance
  balsam
bal. aren. — *balneum arenae* (Lat.) sand bath
BALB — binaural alternate loudness balance
bal. cal. — *balneum calidum* (Lat.) hot bath
bal. coen. — *balneum coenosum* (Lat.) mud bath
BALF — bronchoalveolar lavage fluid
bal. frig. — *balneum frigidum* (Lat.) cold bath
B ALL — B-cell acute lymphoblastic leukemia
bal. lact. — *balneum lacteum* (Lat.) milk bath
bal. mar. — *balneum maris* (Lat.) saltwater bath
bal. pneu. — *balneum pneumaticum* (Lat.) air bath
bals. — *balsamum* (Lat.) balsam
BALT — bronchus-associated lymphoid tissue
bal. tep. — *balneum tepidum* (Lat.) warm bath
bal. vap. — *balneum vaporis* (Lat.) steam or vapor bath
BAM —
  basilar artery migraine
  brachial artery mean [pressure]
  bronchoalveolar macrophage
BAm — mean brachial artery [pressure]
BaM — barium meal
Bam — benzamide
BAME — benzoylarginine methyl ester
BAN —
  British Approved Name

BAN — (*continued*)
  British Association of Neurologists
BAND — band neutrophil (stab)
BANS — back, arms, neck, and scalp
BAO —
  basal acid output
  brachial artery output
  British Association of Otolaryngologists
B.A.O. — Bachelor of the Art of Obstetrics
BAO-MAO — basal acid output to maximal acid output [ratio]
BAP —
  bacterial alkaline phosphatase
  basic adaptive process
  Behavior Activity Profile
  beta-amyloid peptide
  blood-agar plate
  bovine albumin in phosphate buffer
  brachial artery pressure
BaP — benzo(a)pyrene
BAPhysMed — British Association of Physical Medicine
BAPI — barley alkaline protease inhibitor
BAPN — beta-amino-propionitrile fumarate
BAPS —
  biomechanical ankle platform system
  bovine albumin phosphate saline
  British Association of Paediatric Surgeons
  British Association of Plastic Surgeons
BAPT — British Association of Physical Training
BAPV — bovine alimentary papilloma virus
BAQ — brain-age quotient
BAR — beta-adrenergic receptor
bar —
  bariatrics

bar — (*continued*)
  barometer
  barometric
μ bar — microbar
BARACCO — balloon angioplasty versus rotational angioplasty in chronic coronary occlusion
Barb —
  barbiturate
  barbituric
BART — bypass angioplasty revascularization investigation
BARN — bilateral acute retinal necrosis
BART — blood-activated recalcification time
BAS —
  balloon atrial septostomy
  benzyl analog of serotonin
  benzyl antiserotonin
  beta-adrenergic stimulation
  Bioanalytical Systems
  boric acid solution
BaS — barium swallow
bas —
  basilar
  basophil
  basophilic
BASA — Boston Assessment of Severe Aphasia
BASE — B27-arthritis-sacroiliitis-extraarticular features [syndrome]
BASH — body acceleration given synchronously with the heartbeat
BASIC — Beginner's All-Purpose Symbolic Introduction Code
Baso — basophil
$BaSO_4$ — barium sulfate
BASO STIP — basophilic stippling
BAT —
  Basic Aid Training
  basic assurance test
  benzilic acid 3α-tropanyl ester
  best available technology
  brain adjacent tumor

BAT — *(continued)*
    brown adipose tissue
batt — battery
BAUS — British Association of
    Urological Surgeons
BAV — bicuspid aortic valve
BAVCP — bilateral abductor vocal
    cord paralysis
BAVFO — bradycardia after arte-
    riovenous fistula occlusion
BAVP — balloon aortic valvu-
    loplasty
BAW — bronchoalveolar washing
BB —
    baby boy
    backboard
    bad breath
    bath blanket
    bed bath
    bed board
    beta blockade
    beta blocker
    BioBreeding [rat]
    blanket bath
    blood bank
    blood buffer (base)
    blow bottle
    blue bloater [emphysema]
    body belt
    both bones
    bowel and bladder
    breakthrough bleeding
    breast biopsy
    brush border
    buffer base
    bundle branch
    isoenzyme of creatinine
        kinase containing two B
        subunits
B/B — backward bending
B&B — bowel and bladder
bb —
    Bolton point
    both bones
BBA — born before arrival
BBB —
    blood-brain barrier
    blood buffer base

BBB — *(continued)*
    bundle branch block
BBBB — bilateral bundle branch
    block
BBC — bromobenzylcyanide
BBD —
    before bronchodilator
    benign breast disease
BBE — *Bacteroides* bile esculin
    [agar]
BBEP — brush border endopepti-
    dase
BBF — bronchial blood flow
BBHB — bundle branch heart
    block
BBI — Bowman-Birk soybean in-
    hibitor
BBM —
    banked breast milk
    brush border membrane
BBMV — brush border membrane
    vesicle
BBN — broad band noise
BBOW — bulging bag of water
BBP — butylbenzyl phthalate
BBPRL — big big prolactin
BBRS — Burks' Behavior Rating
    Scale
BBS —
    Bardet-Biedl syndrome
    bashful bladder syndrome
    benign breast syndrome
    bilateral breath sounds
    bombesin
    brown bowel syndrome
BBT —
    basal body temperature
    Blood Bank Technologist
BB/W — BioBreeding/Worcester
    [rat]
BB to MM — belly button to me-
    dial malleolus
B Bx — breast biopsy
BC —
    Baccalaureus Chirurgiae (Lat.)
        Bachelor of Surgery
    back care
    backcross

BC — *(continued)*
    background counts
    bactericidal concentration
    basal cell
    basket cell
    battle casualty
    bed and chair
    bicarbonate
    biliary colic
    biotin carboxylase
    bipolar cell
    birth control
    blastic crisis
    blood cardioplegia
    blood center
    blood count
    blood culture
    Blue Cross [plan]
    board-certified
    bone conduction
    Bowman's capsule
    brachiocephalic
    bronchial carcinoma
    buccal cartilage
    buccocervical
    buffy coat
    bulbocavernosus
    bulbus chordae
B&C —
    bed and chair
    biopsy and curettage
    board and care
    breathed and cried
b/c — benefit/cost [ratio]
BCA —
    balloon catheter angioplasty
    basal cell atypia
    blood color analyzer
    Blue Cross Association
    brachiocephalic artery
    branchial cleft anomaly
    breast cancer antigen
BCAA — branched-chain amino
    acid
BCAC — Breast Cancer Advisory
    Center
BC>AC — bone conduction
    greater than air conduction

BC<AC — bone conduction less
    than air conduction
BCAT — brachiocephalic arterial
    trunk
BCB —
    blood-cerebrospinal fluid bar-
    rier
    brilliant cresyl blue [stain]
BCBR — bilateral carotid body re-
    section
BC/BS — Blue Cross/Blue Shield
    [plan]
BCC —
    basal cell carcinoma
    biliary cholesterol concentra-
    tion
    Birth Control Clinic
bcc — body-centered-cubic
BCCA — basal cell carcinoma
BCCG — British Cooperative
    Clinical Group
BCCP — biotin carboxyl carrier
    protein
BCD —
    basal cell dysplasia
    binary-coded chemical
BCDDP — Breast Cancer Detec-
    tion Demonstration Project
BCDF — B-cell differentiation fac-
    tor
BCDSP — Boston Collaborative
    Drug Surveillance Program
BCE —
    basal cell epithelioma
    B-cell enriched
    benign childhood epilepsy
    bubble chamber equipment
BCF —
    basophil chemotactic factor
    bioconcentration factor
    breast cyst fluid
BCFP — breast cyst fluid protein
BCG —
    bacille Calmette-Guérin [vac-
    cine]
    ballistocardiogram
    ballistocardiography
    bicolor guaiac [test]

BCG — *(continued)*
  bilateral cystogram
  bromocresol green
BCGF — B-cell growth factor
BCH —
  basal cell hyperplasia
  basal cell hypoplasia
BCh — *Baccalaureus Chirurgiae*
  (Lat.) Bachelor of Surgery
BChD — Bachelor of Dental Surgery
BChir — *Baccalaureus Chirurgiae*
  (Lat.) Bachelor of Surgery
BChL — bacterial chlorophyll
BCHS — Bureau of Community
  Health Services
BCIC — Birth Control Investigation Committee
BCKA — branched-chain keto
  acid
BCKD — branched-chain alpha-keto acid dehydrogenase
BCL — basic cycle length
BCLL — B-cell chronic lymphocytic leukemia
BCLP — bilateral cleft of lip and
  palate
BCLS — basic cardiac life support
BCM —
  birth control medication
  blood-clotting mechanism [effects]
  body cell mass
bcm — billion cubic meters
BCME — bis-chloromethyl ether
BCN —
  basal cell nevus
  bilateral cortical necrosis
BCNP — board-certified nuclear
  pharmacist
BCNS — basal cell nevus syndrome
BCNU — bischloroethylnitrosourea
BCO — biliary cholesterol output
BCOC — bowel care of choice
BCP —
  basic calcium phosphate
  biochemical profile

BCP — *(continued)*
  birth control pill
  blood cell profile
  blood pressure cuff
  Blue Cross Plan
  bromocresol purple
BCP-D — bromocresol purple
  desoxycholate [agar]
BCPS — battery-charging power
  supply
BCPV — bovine cutaneous papilloma virus
BCR —
  B-cell reactivity
  birth control regimen
  bromocriptine
  bulbocavernosus reflex
bcr — breakpoint cluster region
BCRP — Breast Cancer Research
  Program
BCRx — birth control drug
BCS —
  battered child syndrome
  blood cell separator
  British Cardiac Society
  Budd-Chiari syndrome
BCSI — breast cancer screening indicator
BCT —
  brachiocephalic trunk
  branched-chain amino acid
  transferase
BCTF — Breast Cancer Task Force
BCtg — bovine chymotrypsinogen
BCtr — bovine chymotrypsin
BCU — burn care unit
BCV — basal cell vigilance
BCW — biological and chemical
  warfare
BCYE — buffered charcoal yeast
  extract [agar]
BD —
  barbital-dependent
  barbiturate dependence
  base deficit
  base [of prism] down
  basophilic degeneration
  Batten's disease

BD — *(continued)*
    beclomethasone dipropionate
    Becton-Dickinson [spinal nee-
        dle]
    behavioral disorder
    Behçet's disease
    belladonna
    below diaphragm
    benzidine
    benzodiazepine
    bicarbonate dialysis
    bile duct
    binocular deprivation
    birth date
    birth defect
    Black Death
    block design [test]
    blood donor
    blue diaper [syndrome]
    borderline dull
    bound
    brain damage
    brain dead
    brain death
    Briquet disorder
    bronchial drainage
    bronchodilation
    bronchodilator
    buccodistal
    Byler's disease
B&D — bondage and discipline
B-D — Becton-Dickinson
Bd —
    board
    buoyant density
bd —
    band
    bundle
b.d. — *bis in die* (Lat.) twice a day
BDA —
    balloon dilation angioplasty
    British Dental Association
BDAC — Bureau of Drug Abuse
    Control
BDAE — Boston Diagnostic Apha-
    sia Examination
BDB — bis-diazotized-benzidine

BDBS —
    Bonnet-Delchaume-Blanc
        syndrome
    burn-dressing change
BDE —
    bile duct examination
    bile duct exploration
BDentSci — Bachelor of Dental
    Science
BDG —
    bilirubin diglucuronide
    buccal developmental groove
    buffered desoxycholate glu-
        cose
BDI —
    Beck Depression Inventory
    burn depth indicator
BDIBS — Boston Diagnostic In-
    ventory of Basic Skills
BDISF — Beck Depression
    Index—Short Form
BDL —
    below detectable limits
    bile duct ligation
BDLS — Brachmann-de Lange syn-
    drome
BDM —
    Becker's muscular dystrophy
    benzphetamine demethylase
    border detection method
BDP —
    beclomethasone dipropionate
    benzodiazepine
    bilateral diaphragmatic paraly-
        sis
    bronchopulmonary dysplasia
BDR — background diabetic reti-
    nopathy
BDS —
    Bachelor of Dental Surgery
    biological detection system
    Blessed Dementia Scale
b.d.s. — *bis in die summendus* (Lat.)
    to be taken twice a day
BDSc — Bachelor of Dental Sci-
    ence
BDTVMI — Beery Developmental
    Test of Visual-Motor Integra-
    tion

BDU — Biomedical Display Unit
BDUR — bromodeoxyuridine
BDW — buffered distilled water
BE —
    bacillary emulsion [tuberculin]
    bacterial endocarditis
    barium enema
    Barrett's esophagus
    base excess
    below-elbow
    bile-esculin [test]
    board-eligible
    bovine enteritis
    brain edema
    bread equivalent
    breast examination
    bronchoesophagology
B/E — below-elbow
B&E — brisk and equal
Be — beryllium
Bé — Baumé scale
BEA —
    below-elbow amputation
    bioelectrical activity
    bromoethylamine
BEAM — brain electrical activity
    mapping
BEAP — bronchiectasis, eosino-
    philia, asthma, pneumonia
BEAR — Biological Effects of
    Atomic Radiation [commit-
    tee]
BEC —
    bacterial endocarditis
    blood ethanol content
    bromo-ergocryptine
BECF — blood extracellular fluid
BEE — basal energy expenditure
BEEP — both end-expiratory pres-
    sure
BEF — bronchoesophageal fistula
beg. — begin, beginning
beh —
    behavior
    behavioral
BEI —
    back-scattered electron im-
    aging

BEI — (continued)
    Biological Exposure Indexes
    butanol-extractable iodine
BEIR — biological effects of ioniz-
    ing radiation
BEK — bovine embryonic kidney
    [cells]
BEL —
    blood ethanol level
    bovine embryonic lung
BELB — below-elbow
BELIR — beta-endorphin–like im-
    munoreactivity
ben. — *bene* (Lat.) good, well
BENAR — blood eosinophilic non-
    allergic rhinitis
Benz —
    benzene
    benzidine
    benzoate
BEP —
    brain evoked potential
    brainstem evoked potential
    basic element of performance
β-EP — β-endorphin
bepti — bionomics, environment,
    Plasmodium, treatment, and
    immunity
BER — basic electrical rhythm
BERA — brainstem evoked re-
    sponse audiometry
BES — balanced electrolyte solu-
    tion
BESM — bovine embryonic skele-
    tal muscle
BESP — bovine embryonic spleen
    [cells]
BESS — Biomedical Experimental
    Scientific Satellite
BET —
    benign epithelial tumor
    bleeding esophageal varix
    Brunauer-Emmet-Teller
    [method]
betaLP — beta-lipoprotein
bet. — between
BETS — benign epileptiform tran-
    sients of sleep

BEV —
  baboon endogenous virus
  bleeding esophageal varices
BeV — billion electron volts
bev — beverage
Bex — base excess
BF —
  bentonite flocculation [test]
  bile flow
  black female
  blastogenic factor
  blister fluid
  blocking factor
  blood flow
  body fat
  Bolivian hemorrhagic fever
  bone fragment
  bouillon filtré (Fr.) bouillon fil-
    trate [tuberculin]
  breakfast fed
  breast fed
  breast feeding
  buccofacial
  buffered
  burning feet [syndrome]
  butter fat
B/F —
  black female
  bound-free [antigen ratio]
B3F — band 3 cytoplasmic fragment
BFA —
  baby for adoption
  bifemoral arteriogram
BFB —
  biological feedback
  bronchial foreign body
BFC — benign febrile convulsion
BFD — bias flow down
BFDI — bronchodilation following
  deep inspiration
BFDT — Bekesy Functionality Detection Test
BFE — blood flow energy
BFEC — benign focal epilepsy of
  childhood
bFGF — basic fibroblast growth factor

BFH — benign familial hematuria
BFL — bird fancier's lung
BFLS — Börjeson-Forssman-
  Lehmann syndrome
BFM — bendroflumethiazide
BFO —
  balanced forearm orthosis
  ball-bearing forearm orthosis
  blood-forming organ
  buccofacial obturator
BFP — biologic false-positive
BFPR — biologic false-positive reaction
BFPSTS — biologic false-positive
  serological test for syphilis
BFR —
  biologic false-positive reaction
  blood flow rate
  bone formation rate
  buffered Ringer's [solution]
BFS — blood fasting sugar
BFT —
  bentonite flocculation test
  biofeedback training
  bladder flap tube
BFU — burst-forming unit
BFU-E — burst-forming unit–
  erythroid
BFU-ME — burst-forming
  unit–myeloid/erythroid
BFV — bovine feces virus
BG —
  baby girl
  background
  basal ganglion
  basic gastrin
  Bender Gestalt [test]
  beta-galactosidase
  beta-glucuronidase
  bicolor guaiac [test]
  Birbeck's granules
  blood glucose
  blood group (system)
  bone graft
  brilliant green
  buccogingival
B-G — Bordet-Gengou [agar, bacillus, phenomenon]

Bg^J — beige [mouse]
BGA — blue-green algae
BGAg — blood group antigen
BGAV — blue-green algae virus
BGC —
    basal ganglion calcification
    blood group class
BGCA — bronchogenic carcinoma
BGD —
    blood group degrading [enzyme]
    blood group degradation
BGDC — Bartholin gland duct cyst
BGE — butyl glycidyl ether
BGG — bovine gamma globulin
bGH — bovine growth hormone
BGL — blood glucose level
BGLB — brilliant green lactose broth
BGlu — blood glucose
BGMV — bean golden mosaic virus
BGO — bismuth germinate
BGP — beta-glycerophosphatase
BGRS — blood glucose reagent strip
BGS —
    balance, gait, and station
    blood group substance
    British Geriatrics Society
BGSA — blood granulocyte–specific activity
BGT —
    basophil granulation test
    Bender-Gestalt test
    bungarotoxin
BGTT — borderline glucose tolerance test
BH —
    base hospital
    benzalkonium and heparin
    bill of health
    birth history
    Bishop-Harman [instruments]
    Board of Health
    Bolton-Hunter [reagent]
    borderline hypertensive

BH — (continued)
    both hands
    brain hormone
    Braxton-Hicks [contraction]
    breathholding
    bronchial hyperreactivity
    Bryan's high titer
    bundle of His
BH$_4$ — tetrahydrobiopterin
BHA —
    benign/bilateral hilar adenopathy
    bound hepatitis antibody
    butylated hydroxyanisole
BHAT — Beta Blocker Heart Attack Trial
BHB — beta-hydroxybutyrate
bHb — bovine hemoglobin
BHBA — beta-hydroxybutyric acid
BHC — benzene hexachloride
BHCDA — Bureau of Health Care Delivery and Assistance
bhCG — beta-human chorionic gonadotropin
BHF — Bolivian hemorrhagic fever
BHI —
    beef heart infusion
    biosynthetic human insulin
    brain-heart infusion
    British Humanities Index
    Bureau of Health Insurance
BHIA — brain-heart infusion agar
BHI-ac — brain-heart infusion broth with acetone
BHIB — brain-heart infusion broth
BHIBA — brain-heart infusion broth agar
BHIRS — brain-heart infusion and rabbit serum
BHIS — beef heart infusion supplemented [broth]
BHK —
    baby hamster kidney [cells]
    type-B Hong Kong [influenza virus]
BHL —
    bilateral hilar lymphadenopathy

BHL — (*continued*)
  biological half-life
BHM — Bureau of Health Manpower
BHN —
  bephenium hydroxynaphthoate
  bridging hepatic necrosis
  Brinell hardness number
BHP — Basic Health Profile
BHPR — Bureau of Health Professions
BHPRD — Bureau of Health Planning and Resources Development
BHR —
  basal heart rate
  benign hypertrophic prostatitis
BHRD — Bureau of Health Resources Development
BHS —
  Bachelor of Health Science
  beta-hemolytic streptococcus
  breathholding spell
BHT —
  beta-hydroxytheophylline
  breath hydrogen test
  butylated hydroxytoluene
BHU — basic health unit
BHV — bovine herpes virus
BH/VH — body hematocrit–venous hematocrit [ratio]
BHyg — Bachelor of Hygiene
BI —
  background interval
  bacterial or bactericidal index
  bacteriological index
  base-in [prism]
  basilar impression
  bifocal
  biological indicator
  bodily injury
  bone injury
  bowel impaction
  Braille Institute
  brain injury
  burn index

Bi — bismuth
BIA —
  biolectric impedance analysis
  bioimmunoassay
BIAC —
  Beth Israel Ambulatory Center
  Bioinstrumentation Advisory Council
BIB —
  biliointestinal bypass
  brought in by
bib. — *bibe* (Lat.) drink
biblio — bibliography
BIBPD — brought in by police department
BIBRA — British Industrial Biological Research Association
B-IBS — B-immunoblastic sarcoma
BIC — blood isotope clearance
Bic — biceps
BICAO — bilateral internal carotid artery occlusion
bicarb — bicarbonate
BiCNU — carmustine
BICROS — bilateral contralateral routing of signals
BID —
  bibliographic information and documentation
  brought in dead
b.i.d. — *bis in die* (Lat.) twice a day
BIDLB — block in the posteroinferior division of the left branch
BIDS —
  bedtime insulin, daytime sulfonylurea [therapy]
  brittle hair, intellectual impairment, decreased fertility, and short stature [syndrome]
BIG 6 — analysis of 6 serum components
BIGGY — bismuth-glycine-glucose-yeast [agar]

BIH —
> benign intracranial hypertension
> bilateral inguinal hernia

bihor — *bihorium* (Lat.) during 2 hours

BII — butanol-insoluble iodine

BIL —
> basal insulin level
> bilirubin

Bil — bilirubin

bil. — bilateral

BIL/ALB — bilirubin/albumin [ratio]

bilat. — bilateral

BILAT-SLC — bilateral short-leg cane

bilat sxo — bilateral salpingo-oophorectomy

bili — bilirubin

bili-c — conjugated bilirubin

bilirub. — bilirubin

BIMA — bilateral internal mammary artery

BIN — benign intradermal nevus

b.i.n. — *bis in noctus* (Lat.) twice a night

biochem —
> biochemistry
> biochemical

BIOD — bony intraorbital distance

bioeng — bioengineering

BIOETHICSLINE — Bioethical Information On-Line

biof — biofeedback

biol —
> biology
> biological

bioLH — bioassay of luteinizing hormone

biophys —
> biophysics
> biophysical

BIOSIS — BioScience Information Service

BIP —
> Background Interference Procedure

BIP — *(continued)*
> bacterial intravenous protein
> biparietal
> bismuth iodoform paraffin
> Blue Cross interim payment
> brief infertility period

BIPD — biparietal diameter

BIPLED — bilateral, independent, periodic, lateralized epileptiform discharge

BIPM — *Bureau International des Poids et Mesures* (Fr.) International Bureau of Weights and Measures

BIPP —
> bismuth iodoform paraffin paste
> bismuth iodoform petrolatum paste

BIR —
> backward internal rotation
> basic incidence rate
> British Institute of Radiology

BIS —
> bone cement implantation syndrome
> Brain Information Service
> building illness syndrome

BiSP — between ischial spines

bisp — bispinous diameter

BIT — bitrochanteric

BITU — benzylthiourea

BIU — barrier isolation unit

BIV — bovine immunodeficiency-like virus

BIW — biweekly

Biz-PLT — bizarre platelets

BJ —
> Bence Jones [protein, proteinuria]
> biceps jerk
> Bielschowsky-Jansky [disease]
> bones and joints

B&J — bones and joints

BJ, BRJ, TJ — biceps jerk, brachioradialis jerk, and triceps jerk

BJE — bone-joint examination

BJM — bones, joints, and muscles

BJP —
    Bence Jones protein
    Bence Jones proteinuria
BK —
    bekanamycin
    below-knee [amputation]
    bovine kidney [cells]
    bradykinin
    bullous keratopathy
B-K — initials of two patients after
    whom a multiple cutaneous
    nevus [mole] was named
Bk — berkelium
bk — back
BKA — below-knee amputation
BK-A — basophil kallikrein of ana-
    phylaxis
BK amp — below-knee amputation
BKC — blepharokeratoconjunctivitis
bkf — breakfast
Bkg — background
BKO — below-knee orthosis
BKS — beekeeper serum
BKTT — below-knee to toe [cast]
BKV — BK virus
BKWC — below-knee walking cast
BKWP — below-knee walking plas-
    ter
BL —
    bacterial levan
    Baralyme
    Barré-Lieou [syndrome]
    basal lamina
    baseline
    Bessey-Lowry [units]
    black light
    bland
    bleeding
    blind loop
    blood
    blood level
    blood loss
    bone marrow lymphocyte
    borderline lepromatous
    bronchial lavage
    buccolingual
    Burkitt's lymphoma
Bl — black

B-L — bursa-equivalent lympho-
    cyte
bl —
    black
    bland
    bleeding
    blood
    blue
BLa — buccolabial
BLAD — borderline left axis devia-
    tion
blad — bladder
blasto — *Blastomyces*
BLAT — Blind Learning Aptitude
    Test
BLB —
    Baker-Lima-Baker [mask]
    Bessey-Lowry-Brock [method
    or unit]
    black light bulb
    Boothby-Lovelace-Bulbulian
    [oxygen mask]
    bulb [syringe]
BL-BS — bilateral equal breath
    sounds
BLC — beef liver catalase
BlC — blood culture
BLCL — Burkitt's lymphoma cell
    line
bl cult — blood culture
BLD —
    basal liquefactive degenera-
    tion
    benign lymphoepithelial dis-
    ease
    beryllium lung disease
bld — blood
Bld Bk — blood bank
bld chem — blood chemistry
bldg — bleeding
BLDY — grossly bloody
BLE — both lower extremities
BLEED — bleeding time
BLEL — benign lymphoepithelial
    lesion
BLEO — bleomycin
BLEP — Breast Lesion Evaluation
    Project

bleph —
    blepharitis
    blepharoplasty
BLESS — bath, laxative, enema,
    shampoo, and shower
BLFD — buccolinguofacial dyski-
    nesia
BL-FST — blood fasting
BLG — beta-lactoglobulin
BL-GAS — blood gases
blH — biologically active luteiniz-
    ing hormone
BLI — bombesin-like immunoreac-
    tivity
blk — black
BLL —
    below lower limit
    bilateral lower lobe
    brows, lids, and lashes
BLLD — British Library Lending
    Division
BLLS — bilateral leg strength
BLM —
    basolateral membrane
    bilayer lipid membrane
    bimolecular liquid membrane
    black lipid membrane
    bleomycin
    buccolinguomasticatory
BLN — bronchial lymph node
BLOBS — bladder obstruction
BLOT — British Library of Tape
βLP — beta-lipoprotein
BlP — blood pressure
β-LPH — beta-lipoprotein hor-
    mone
βLPO — beta-lactamase producing
    organism
β-LPN — beta-lipotropin
bl. pr. — blood pressure
BLQ — both lower quadrants
BLRA — beta-lactamase-resistant
    antimicrobial
BLROA — British Laryngological,
    Rhinological and Otological
    Association
BLS —
    bare lymphocyte syndrome

BLS — (continued)
    basic life support
    blind loop syndrome
    blood and lymphatic system
    blood sugar
    Bloom's syndrome
    Bureau of Labor Statistics
BlS — blood sugar
BLSD — bovine lumpy skin dis-
    ease
BLST — Bankson Language
    Screening Test
BLT —
    bilateral tubal ligation
    bladder tumor
    bleeding time
    blood-clot lysis time
    blood test
    blood typing
BlT —
    bleeding time
    blood test
    blood type
    blood typing
BLU — Bessey-Lowry unit
BLV —
    blood volume
    bovine leukemia virus
BlV —
    blood viscosity
    blood volume
BLVR — biliverdin reductase
Blx — bleeding time
BM —
    Bachelor of Medicine
    basal medium
    basal metabolism
    basement membrane
    basilar membrane
    Bergersen's medium
    betamethasone
    biomedical
    black male
    blind matching
    blood monocyte
    body mass
    Bohr magneton
    bone marrow

BM — *(continued)*
    bowel movement
    breast milk
    buccal mass
    buccomesial
    Bureau of Medicine
B/M — black male
B2M — beta$_2$-microglobulin
b.m. — *balneum maris* (Lat.) salt-water bath
β_2m — beta$_2$-microglobulin
BMA —
    bone marrow arrest
    bone marrow aspirate
    British Medical Association
BmA — *Brugia malayi* adult antigen
BMAP — bone marrow acid phosphatase
BMB —
    biomedical belt
    bone marrow biopsy
BMBL — benign monoclonal B-cell lymphocytosis
BMC —
    balloon mitral commissurotomy
    blood mononuclear cell
    bone marrow cell
    bone mineral content
BMD —
    Becker's muscular dystrophy
    Boehringer Mannheim Diagnostics
    bone marrow depression
    bone mineral density
    bovine mucosal disease
    Bureau of Medical Devices
BMDC — Biomedical Documentation Center
BME —
    basal medium, Eagle's
    biundulant meningoencephalitis
    brief maximal effort
BMed — Bachelor of Medicine
BMedBiol — Bachelor of Medical Biology

BMedSci — Bachelor of Medical Science
BMET — biomedical equipment technician
BMF — bone marrow failure
BMG — benign monoclonal gammopathy
BMI —
    bicuculline methiodide
    body mass index
BMic — Bachelor of Microbiology
BMJ —
    bones, muscles, and joints
    British Medical Journal
bmk — birthmark
BML — bone marrow lymphocytosis
BMLM — basement membrane–like material
BMLS — billowing mitral leaflet syndrome
BMMP — benign mucous membrane pemphigoid
BMN — bone marrow necrosis
BMNC — blood mononuclear cell
BMNR — bone marrow neutrophil reserve
BMOC — Brinster's medium for ovum culture
Bmod — behavior modification
B-mode — brightness modulation
BMP —
    behavior management plan
    bone marrow pressure
    bone morphogenetic protein
BMPI — bronchial mucus proteinase inhibitor
BMQA — Board of Medical Quality Assurance
BMR —
    basal metabolic rate
    best motor response
BMS —
    Bachelor of Medical Science
    betamethasone
    Biomedical Monitoring System
    bleomycin sulfate

BMS — *(continued)*
    Bureau of Medical Services
    Bureau of Medicine and Surgery
    burning mouth syndrome
BMSA — British Medical Students Association
BMST — Bruce maximum stress test
BMT —
    Bachelor of Medical Technology
    Bailliére's Medical Transparencies
    basement membrane thickening
    benign mesenchymal tumor
    bilateral myringotomy tubes
    bone marrow transplantation
    Buschke's Memory Test
BMTU — bone marrow transplant unit
BMU —
    basic metabolic unit
    basic multicellular unit
BMZ — basement membrane zone
BN —
    bladder neck
    brachial neuritis
    bronchial node
    brown Norway [rat]
BNA — Basle Nomina Anatomica
BNB — blood-nerve barrier
BNC — bladder neck contracture
BNCT — boron neutron capture therapy
BND — barely noticeable difference
BNDD — Bureau of Narcotics and Dangerous Drugs
BNEd — Bachelor of Nursing Education
BNEG — B negative (blood type)
BNF — British National Formulary
BNG — bromonaphthyl-beta-galactoside
BNGase — bromonaphthyl-beta-galactoside

βNGF — beta-nerve growth factor
BNIST — *Bureau National d'Information Scientifique* (Fr.) National Bureau of Scientific Information
BNL — breast needle location
BNMSE — Brief Neuropsychological Mental Status Examination
BNO —
    bladder neck obstruction
    bowels not open
BNPA — binasal pharyngeal airway
BNR —
    bladder neck resection
    bladder neck retraction
BNS — benign nephrosclerosis
BNSc — Bachelor of Nursing Science
BNT —
    Boston Naming Test
    brain neurotransmitter
BNYVV — beet necrotic yellow vein virus
BO —
    Bachelor of Osteopathy
    base [of prism] out
    behavior objective
    body odor
    Bolton's [craniometric point]
    bowel obstruction
    bowels open
    bucco-occlusal
B/O — because of
B&O — belladonna and opium
Bo —
    bohemium
    Bolton's [point]
bo — bowel
BOA —
    behavioral observation audiometry
    born on arrival
    born out of asepsis
    British Orthopaedic Association
BOAT — Balloon Versus Optimal Atherectomy Trial

BOB — ball on back
βOBA — beta-oxybutyric acid
BOC —
    blood oxygen capacity
    Bureau of Census
    butyloxycarbonyl
BOCG — Brudzinski, Oppenheim,
    Chaddock, and Gullaird [re-
    flex and sign]
BOD —
    bilateral orbital decompres-
        sion
    biochemical oxygen demand
    biological oxygen demand
    Bureau of Drugs
Bod — Bodansky [unit]
BOE — bilateral otitis externa
BOEA — ethyl biscoumacetate
βOFA — beta-oncofecal antigen
BOH — Board of Health
bol. — *bolus* (Lat.) pill
BOM — bilateral otitis media
BOMA — bilateral otitis media,
    acute
BONENT — Board of Nephrology
    Examiners for Nursing and
    Technology
BOO — bladder outlet obstruction
BOOP — bronchiolitis obliterans–
    organizing pneumonia
BOP — buffalo orphan prototype
    [virus]
BOR —
    basal optic root
    before time of operation
    bowels open regularly
    branchio-oto-renal [syndrome]
BORD — borderline
BORR — blood oxygen release
    rate
B-O₂S — blood oxygen saturation
BoSM — Bolivian squirrel monkey
BOT —
    base of tongue
    botulinum toxin
Bot —
    botanical
    botany

bot — bottle
BOU — branchio-oto-ureteral [syn-
    drome]
BOW — bag of waters
BOWI — bag of waters intact
BP —
    Bachelor of Pharmacy
    back pressure
    barometric pressure
    basic protein
    bathroom privileges
    bedpan
    before present
    behavior pattern
    Bell's palsy
    benzoyl peroxide
    benzpyrene
    beta-protein
    bioequivalence problem
    biotic potential
    biparietal
    biphenyl
    bipolar
    birthplace
    blood pressure
    body part
    body plethysmography
    boiling point
    Bolton's point
    borderline personality
    British Pharmacopoeia
    bronchopleural
    bronchopulmonary
    buccopulpal
    bullous pemphigoid
    bullous pemphigus
    bypass
B/P — blood pressure
bp —
    base pair
    bedpan
    boiling point
BPA —
    Bauhinia purpura agglutinin
    blood pressure assembly
    boronated phenylalanine
    bovine plasma albumin
    British Paediatric Association

BPA — (continued)
   bronchopulmonary aspergillo-
      sis
   burst-promoting activity
BPAEC — bovine pulmonary artery endothelial cell
BPB —
   bromphenol blue
   biliopancreatic bypass
BPC —
   Behavior Problem Checklist
   bile phospholipid concentra-
      tion
   blood pressure cuff
   British Pharmaceutical Codex
   bronchial provocation chal-
      lenge
B-Pco_2 — blood partial pressure of
   carbon dioxide
BPD —
   biparietal diameter
   blood pressure decreased
   Blood Program Directives
   borderline personality disorder
BPd —
   bronchopulmonary dysplasia
   diastolic blood pressure
BPE — bacterial phosphatidylethanolamine
BPEC —
   benign partial epilepsy of
      childhood
   bipolar electrocoagulation
BPEI — blepharophimosis, ptosis,
   epicanthus inversus
BPES — blepharophimos-ptosis-
   epicanthus inversus syndrome
BPF —
   bradykinin-potentiating factor
   bronchopleural fistula
   burst-promoting factor
BPG —
   benzathine penicillin G
   blood pressure gauge
   bypass graft
BPH —
   Bachelor of Public Health
   benign prostatic hyperplasia

BPH — (continued)
   benign prostatic hypertrophy
BPh —
   British Pharmacopoeia
   buccopharyngeal
Bph — bacteriopheophytin
B-pH — blood pH
BPharm — Bachelor of Pharmacy
BPHEng — Bachelor of Public
   Health Engineering
BPheo — bacteriopheophytin
BPHN — Bachelor of Public
   Health Nursing
BPI —
   Basic Personality Inventory
   beef-pork insulin
   bipolar affective disorder
   blood pressure increased
BPIG — bacterial polysaccharide
   immune globulin
BPL —
   benign proliferative lesion
   benzylpenicilloyl polylysine
   beta-propiolactone
   bone phosphate of lime
BPLA — blood pressure, left arm
BPLN — bilateral pelvic lymph
   nodes
BPLND — bilateral pelvic lymph
   node dissection
BPM —
   beats per minute
   biperidyl mustard
   breaths per minute
   brompheniramine maleate
BPMF — British Postgraduate
   Medical Federation
BPMS — blood plasma measuring
   system
BPN —
   bacitracin, polymyxin B, neo-
      mycin sulfate
   brachial plexus neuropathy
BPO —
   basal pepsin output
   benzylpenicilloyl (polylyxine)
   bilateral partial oophorectomy
   bile phospholipid output

B-PO$_2$ — blood PO$_2$

BPP —
    biophysical profile
    bovine pancreatic polypeptide
    bradykinin-potentiating peptide
    breast parenchymal pattern

BP&P — blood pressure and pulse

BPPN — benign paroxysmal positioning nystagmus

BPPP — bilateral pedal pulses present

BPPRT — blood pressure, pulse, respiration, and temperature

BPPV —
    benign paroxysmal positional vertigo
    bovine paragenital papilloma virus

BPQ — Berne pain questionnaire

BPR —
    blood per rectum
    blood pressure recorder
    blood production rate

BPRA — blood pressure, right arm

BPRS —
    Brief Psychiatric Rating Scale
    Brief Psychiatric Reacting Scale

BPS —
    beats per second
    Behavioral Pharmacological Society
    bilateral partial salpingectomy
    Biophysical Society
    bovine papular stomatitis
    brain protein solvent
    breaths per second

BPs — blood pressure, systolic

BPSA — bronchopulmonary segmental artery

BPSD — bronchopulmonary segmental drainage

BPsTh — Bachelor of Psychotherapy

BPT — benign paroxysmal torticollis

BPTI —
    basic pancreatic trypsin inhibitor
    basic polyvalent trypsin inhibitor

BPV —
    benign paroxysmal vertigo
    benign positional vertigo
    bioprosthetic valve
    bovine papilloma virus

BP(Vet) — British Pharmacopoeia (Veterinary)

Bq — becquerel

BQA — Bureau of Quality Assurance

BQC sol — 2,6-dibromoquinone-4-chlorimide solution

BR —
    barrier-reared [experimental animals]
    baseline recovery
    bathroom
    bed rest
    bedside rounds
    Benzing retrograde
    benzodiazepine receptor
    bilirubin
    biologic response
    blink reflex
    bowel rest
    brachialis
    branchial
    breathing rate
    bridge
    bromine
    bronchial
    bronchitis
    bronchus
    Brucella
    brucellosis

Br —
    breech
    bregma
    bridge
    bromide
    bromine
    bronchitiis
    brown

Br — (*continued*)
   Brucella
   brucellosis
br —
   boiling range
   brachial
   branch
   branchial
   breath
   broiled
   brother
BRA —
   beta-resorcylic acid
   bilateral renal agenesis
   bone-resorbing activity
   brain
   brain-reactive antibody
BRAC — basic rest-activity cycle
Brach — brachial
brady — bradycardia
BRAO — branch retinal artery occlusion
BRAP — burst of rapid atrial pacing
BrAP — brachial artery pressure
BRAT —
   bananas, rice cereal, applesauce, and toast
   Baylor's rapid autologous transfusion [system]
BRATT — bananas, rice, applesauce, tea and toast
BRB —
   blood-retinal barrier
   bright red blood
BRBC — bovine red blood cell
BRBN — blue rubber bleb nevus
BRBNS — blue rubber bleb nevus syndrome
BRBPR — bright red blood per rectum
br bx — breast biopsy
Brc — bromocriptine
BRCM — below right costal margin
BRCS — British Red Cross Society

BRD —
   bladder retraining drill
   bovine respiratory disease
BrdU — bromodeoxyuridine
BrdUrd — bromodeoxyuridine
BRET — bretylium tosylate
BRF — bone-resorbing factor
BRH —
   benign recurrent hematuria
   Bureau of Radiological Health
BRI — Bio-Research Index
BRIC — benign recurrent intrahepatic cholestasis
BRIME — brief repetitive isometric maximal exercise
BRJ — brachial radialis jerk
Brkf — breakfast
BRL —
   Beecham Research Laboratories
   Bethesda Research Laboratories
   Biometrics Research Laboratory
BRM —
   biological response modifier
   biuret-reactive material
BrM — breast milk
BRMP — Biological Response Modification Program
BRN — Board of Registered Nursing
brn — brown
BRO —
   bromocriptine
   bronchoscopy
bro — brother
brom — bromide
bron —
   bronchi
   bronchial
bronch —
   bronchoscope
   bronchoscopy
BRP —
   bathroom privileges

BRP — *(continued)*
  bilirubin production
Brph — bronchophony
BRR —
  baroreceptor reflex response
  breathing reserve ratio
BR RAO — branch retinal artery
  occlusion
BR RVO — branch retinal vein oc-
  clusion
BRS —
  battered root syndrome
  Bibliographic Retrieval Ser-
    vices
  breath sounds
  British Roentgen Society
BrSM — Brazilian squirrel monkey
BRT — Brook reaction test
brth — breath
BRU —
  bone remodeling unit
  bromide urine
BrU — bromouracil
Bruc — *Brucella*
BRVO — branch retinal vein oc-
  clusion
BRW — Brown-Roberts-Wells [ste-
  reotactic system]
BS —
  Bachelor of Science
  Bachelor of Surgery
  Bacillus subtilis
  barium swallow
  Bartter's syndrome
  base strap
  bedside
  before sleep
  Behçet's syndrome
  Bennett's seal
  bilateral symmetrical
  bile salt
  Binet-Simon [test]
  bismuth subsalicylate
  blood sugar
  Bloom's syndrome
  Blue Shield [plan]
  borderline schizophrenia
  bowel sounds

BS — *(continued)*
  breaking strength
  breath sounds
  British Standard
  buffered saline
  Bureau of Standards
B-S —
  Bjork-Shiley [valve prosthesis]
  Binet-Simon [test]
B&S —
  Bartholin's and Skene's glands
  Brown and Sharp [sutures]
bs —
  bedside
  bowel sounds
  breath sounds
b.s. — barium swallow
b × s — brother-sister inbreeding
BSA —
  beef serum albumin
  benzenesulfonic acid
  Biofeedback Society of
    America
  bismuth-sulfite agar
  bis-trimethylsilylacetamide
  Blind Service Association
  body surface area
  bovine serum albumin
  bowel sounds active
bsa — bovine serum albumin
BSAB — Balthazar Scales of Adaptive Behavior
BSAER — brainstem auditory
  evoked response
BSAG — Bristol Social
  Adjustment Guides
BSAM — basic sequential access
  method
BSAP —
  brief short-action potential
  brief, small, abundant poten-
    tials
BSB —
  bedside bag
  body surface burned
BSBC — buffer-soluble binding
  component
BS = BL — breath sounds equal
  bilaterally

BSC —
 bedside care
 bedside commode
 bench scale calorimeter
 bile salt concentration
 Biological Stain Commission
 Biomedical Sciences Corps
 Biomedical Signal Conditioner
 burn scar contracture
Bsc — Bachelor of Science
BSC-1, BS-C-1 — *Cercopithecus* monkey kidney cells
BSCC — British Society of Clinical Cytology
BSCIF — bile salt canalicular independent fraction
BSCP — bovine spinal cord protein
BSD —
 baby soft diet
 bedside drainage
BSDLB — block in the superior division of the left branch
BSE —
 bacillus species enzyme
 behavior summarized evaluation
 bilateral, symmetrical, and equal
 breast self-examination
BSEP — brainstem evoked potential
BSER — brainstem evoked response
BSF —
 back scatter factor
 basal skull fracture
 black single female
 B-lymphocyte–stimulating factor
 busulfan
BSG — brachio-skeleto-genital [syndrome]
βSGA — beta-streptococcus group A
BSH — boron sulfhydryl
BSI —
 Behavior Status Inventory

BSI — *(continued)*
 body substance isolation
 Borderline Syndrome Index
 bound serum iron
 brainstem injury
 British Standards Institution
BSID — Bayley Scale of Infant Development
BSIF — bile salt independent fraction
BSL —
 benign symmetrical lipomatosis
 blood sugar level
BSM — Bachelor of Science in Medicine
BSN —
 Bachelor of Science in Nursing
 bowel sounds normal
BSNA — bowel sounds normal and active
BSNT — breast soft and non-tender
BSO —
 bilateral sagittal osteotomy
 bilateral salpingo-oophorectomy
 bilateral serous otitis
 British School of Osteopathy
BSOM — bilateral serous otitis media
BSOT — Bachelor of Science in Occupational Therapy
BSP —
 body segment parameter
 Bromsulphalein
BSp — bronchospasm
BSPA — bowel sounds present and active
BSPh — Bachelor of Science in Pharmacy
BSPM — body surface potential mapping
BSQ — Behavior Style Questionnaire
BSR —
 basal skin resistance

BSR — *(continued)*
    blood sedimentation rate
    bowel sounds regular
    brain stimulation reinforcement
BSRI — BEM Sex Role Inventory
BSS —
    Bachelor of Sanitary Science
    balanced salt solution
    bedside scale
    Bernard-Soulier syndrome
    bismuth subsalicylate
    black silk suture
    buffered saline solution
    buffered salt solution
    buffered single substrate
B-SS — Bernard-Soulier syndrome
BSSE — bile salt–stimulated esterase
BSSG — sitogluside
BSSI — Basic School Skills Inventory
BSSL — bile salt–stimulated lipase
BSSS — benign sporadic sleep spikes
BST —
    bacteriuria screening test
    bedside testing
    biceps semitendinosus
    blood serologic test
    breast stimulation test
    brief stimulus therapy
BSTFA — bis-trimethylsilyltrifluoroacetamide
BSTP — basophilic stippling
BSU —
    Bartholin, Skene, urethral [glands]
    basic structural unit
    British standard unit
BSV — binocular single vision
BSW — Bachelor of Social Work
BT —
    Bacillus thuringiensis
    base of tongue
    bedtime
    bitemporal
    bitrochanteric

BT — *(continued)*
    bituberous
    Blacky test
    bladder tremor
    bladder tumor
    bleeding time
    blood transfusion
    blood type
    blood typing
    blue tetrazolium
    blue tongue
    body temperature
    borderline tuberculoid
    bovine turbinate [cells]
    brain tumor
    breast tumor
    bulbotruncal
BTA —
    N-benzoyl-L-tyrosine amide
    Blood Transfusion Association
    brief tone audiometry
BTB —
    breakthrough bleeding
    bromothymol blue
BTBC — Boehm Test of Basic Concepts
BTBL — bromothymol blue lactose
BTBV — beat-to-beat variability
BTC —
    basal temperature chart
    bilateral tubal coagulation
    bladder tumor check
    body temperature chart
    by the clock
BTDS — benzoylthiamine disulfide
BTE —
    behind-the-ear
    bovine thymus extract
BTEA — Boston Test for Examining Aphasia
BTF — blenderized tube feeding
BTFS — breast tumor frozen section
βTG — beta-thromboglobulin
BTg — bovine trypsinogen
BThU — British thermal unit
BTL — bilateral tubal ligation

BTLS — basic trauma life support
BTM —
    benign tertian malaria
    bilateral tympanic membranes
BTMD — Batten-Turner muscular
    dystrophy
BTMSA — bis-trimethyl-
    silacetylene
BTP — biliary tract pain
BTPABA — *N*-benzoyl-L-tyrosyl-*p*-
    aminobenzoic acid
BTPD — body temperature, ambi-
    ent pressure, dry
BTPS — body temperature, ambi-
    ent pressure, saturated with
    water vapor
BTR —
    Bezold-type reflex
    biceps tendon reflex
    bladder tumor recheck
BTr — bovine trypsin
BTS —
    bioptic telescopic spectacle
    bithional sulfoxide
    Blood Transfusion Service
    blue toe syndrome
    bradycardia-tachycardia syn-
    drome
BTSG — Brain Tumor Study
    Group
bTSH — beef/bovine thyroid-stim-
    ulating hormone
BTU — British thermal unit
BTV — blue tongue virus
BTX —
    bactrachotoxin
    benzene, toluene, and xylene
    brevetoxin
    bungarotoxin
BTX-B — brevetoxin-B
BTZ —
    benzothiazepine
    Butazolidin
BTZ alka — Butazolidin alka
BU —
    base [of prism] up
    below the umbilicus

BU — *(continued)*
    Bethesda unit
    blood urea
    Bodansky unit
    bromouracil
    burn unit
Bu — butyl
bu — bushel
BUA —
    blood uric acid
    broadband ultrasonic attenua-
    tion
Buc — buccal
BUCAIN — dibucaine number
BUD — budesonide
BUDR — 5-bromodeoxyuridine
BUDS — bilateral upper dorsal
    sympathectomy
BUE —
    both upper extremities
    built-up edge
BUF — buffalo [rat]
BUFA — baby up for adoption
BUG — buccal ganglion
BUI — brain uptake index
BULIT — bulimia test
BULL — buccal or upper lingual
    of lower
Bull — bulletin
bull. — *bulliat* (Lat.) let it boil
BuMed — Bureau of Medicine and
    Surgery
BUMP — Behavioral Regression or
    Upset in Hospitalized Medical
    Patients [scale]
BUN —
    blood urea nitrogen
    bunion
bun br — bundle branch
BUN/CR — blood urea nitrogen/
    creatine ratio
BUO —
    bilateral ureteral occlusion
    bilirubin of unknown origin
    bleeding of unknown origin
    bruising of unknown origin
BUQ — both upper quadrants

BUR — backup rate
bur — bureau
Burd — Burdick [suction]
BURR — burr cells
BUS — Bartholin's, urethral, and Skene's glands
Bus — busulfan
BUSEG — Bartholin's, urethral, and Skene's glands and external genitalia
but —
butyrate
butyric
but. — *butyrum* (Lat.) butter
BV —
bacitracin V
bacterial vaginitis
billion volts
biological value
blood vessel
blood volume
bronchovesicular
buccoversion
bulboventricular
b.v. — *balneum vaporis* (Lat.) bath vapor
BVA —
bioimpedence venous analysis
Blind Veterans Association
British Veterinary Association
BVAD — biventricular assist device
BVAT — Binocular Visual Acuity Test
BVC — British Veterinary Codex
BVD — bovine viral diarrhea
BVDT — Brief Vestibular Disorientation Test
BVDU — bromovinyldeoxyuridine
BVE —
binocular visual efficiency
biventricular enlargement
blood vessel endothelium
blood volume expander
blood volume expansion
BVH — biventricular hypertrophy
BVI —
Better Vision Institute
blood vessel invasion

BVL — bilateral vas ligation
BVM —
bronchovascular markings
Bureau of Veterinary Medicine
BVMGT — Bender Visual-Motor Gestalt Test
BVMOT — Bender Visual-Motor Gestalt Test
BVMS — Bachelor of Veterinary Medicine and Surgery
BVO —
branch vein occlusion
brominated vegetable oil
BVP —
blood vessel prosthesis
blood volume pulse
Bonhoeffer van der Pol
burst of ventricular pacing
BVR — baboon virus replication
BVRT — Benton's Visual Retention Test
BVS — blanked ventricular sense
BVSc — Bachelor of Veterinary Science
BVU — bromoisovalerylurea
BVV — bovine vaginitis virus
BVX — bacitracin V and X
BW —
bacteriological warfare
bed wetting
below waist
biological warfare
biological weapon
birth weight
bite wing
bladder washout
blood Wasserman [reaction]
body water
body weight
B&W — black and white [cascara extract and milk of magnesia]
bw — body weight
BWA — bed wetter admission
BWCS — bagged white-cell study
BWD — bacillary white diarrhea

BWFI — bacteriostatic water for injection

BWRWS — Biological Warfare Rapid Warning System

BWS —
    battered woman (or wife) syndrome
    Beckwith-Wiedemann syndrome

BWST — black widow spider toxin

BWSV — black widow spider venom

BWt — birth weight

BWYV — beet western yellow virus

BX —
    bacitracin X

BX — (continued)
    biopsy

BX BS — Blue Cross and Blue Shield

BXM — B-cell cross match

BXO — balanitis xerotica obliterans

BYDV — barley yellow dwarf virus

BYE — Barile-Yaguchi-Eveland [agar, culture medium]

BZ — benzodiazepine

BZA — benzylamine

BzDz — benzodiazepine

Bzl — benzoyl

BZQ — benzquinamide

Bz-Ty-PABA — benzoyltyrosyl-p-aminobenzoic acid [test]

 ....

C —
    ascorbic acid
    calcitonin-forming [cell]
    calculus
    calorie [large]
    canine tooth
    capacitance
    carbohydrate
    carbon
    cardiac
    cardiovascular disease
    carrier
    cast
    cathodal
    cathode
    Catholic
    Caucasian
    cell
    Celsius
    centigrade
    central
    central electrode placement in electroencephalography

C — (continued)
    centromeric or constitutive heterochromatic chromosome [banding]
    cerebrospinal
    certified
    cervical
    cesarean [section]
    chest [precordial lead in electrocardiography]
    chicken
    chloramphenicol
    cholesterol
    class
    clear
    clearance rate [renal]
    clonus
    closure
    clubbing
    coarse [bacterial colonies]
    cocaine
    coefficient
    color sense
    colored [guinea pig]

C — (continued)
   complement
   complete
   complex
   compliance
   component
   concentration
   conditioned
   conditioning
   condyle
   congius
   constant
   consultation
   contact
   content
   contraction
   contracture
   control
   conventionally reared [experimental animal]
   convergence
   cornea
   cornu
   correct
   cortex
   costa
   coulomb
   Coxsackie [virus]
   creatinine
   crystalline
   cubic
   cubitus
   cup
   curie
   cuspid
   cuticular
   cyanosis
   cylinder
   cylindrical lens
   cysteine
   cytidine
   cytochrome
   cytosine
   heat capacity
   hundred [Roman numeral]
   large calorie
   molar heat capacity
   velocity of light
   velocity of sound of blood

C' — complement
$C1$ —
   first cervical nerve
   first cervical vertebra
   first component of complement
CI — first cranial nerve
C_1 —
   cytochrome 1
   first cervical nerve
   first cervical vertebra
   first rib
$C\bar{1}$ — activated first component of complement
$C1\ INH$ — inhibitor of first component of complement
$C2$ —
   second cervical nerve
   second cervical vertebra
   second component of complement
CII — second cranial nerve
C_2 —
   cytochrome 2
   second rib
$C\bar{2}$ — activated second component of complement
$C3$ —
   third cervical nerve
   third cervical vertebra
   third component of complement
$CIII$ — third cranial nerve
C_3 —
   Collins' solution
   third rib
$C\bar{3}$ — activated third component of complement
$C4$ —
   fourth cervical nerve
   fourth cervical vertebra
   fourth component of complement
$C\bar{4}$ — activated fourth component of complement
CIV — fourth cranial nerve
$C5$ —
   fifth cervical nerve
   fifth cervical vertebra

C5 — (*continued*)
  fifth component of complement
C$\bar{5}$ — activated fifth component of complement
CV — fifth cranial nerve
C6 —
  hexamethonium
  sixth cervical nerve
  sixth cervical vertebra
  sixth component of complement
C$\bar{6}$ — activated sixth component of complement
C-6 — hexamethonium
CVI — sixth cranial nerve
C7 —
  seventh cervical nerve
  seventh cervical vertebra
  seventh component of complement
C$\bar{7}$ — activated seventh component of complement
CVII — seventh cranial nerve
C8 —
  eighth component of complement
  eighth cranial nerve
C$\bar{8}$ — activated eighth component of complement
CVIII — eighth cranial nerve
C9 — ninth component of complement
C$\bar{9}$ — activated ninth component of complement
CIX — ninth cranial nerve
C-10 — decamethonium
CX — tenth cranial nerve
CXI — eleventh cranial nerve
CXII — twelfth cranial nerve
^{14}C — carbon-14 [isotope]
C 14 — carbon-14 [isotope]
^{137}Cs — radioactive cesium
°C — degree Celsius
C. — *congius* (Lat.) gallon
C. —
  Campylobacter
  Candida
  Chlamydia

C. — (*continued*)
  Cimex
  Clostridium
  Corynebacterium
  Cryptococcus
  Culex
c —
  calorie [small]
  candle
  canine tooth
  capacity
  capillary in the blood phase
  carat
  centi-
  centi-complementary [strand]
  concentration
  contact
  cubic
  culture [medium]
  cup
  curie
  cuspid
  cycle
  cyclic
  molar concentration
  specific heat capacity
χ — chi (twenty-second letter of the Greek alphabet), lower-case
χ^2 — chi-squared [distribution]
χ_e — electric susceptibility
χ_m — magnetic susceptibility
$\bar{c}$ — *cum* (Lat.) with
c' —
  coefficient of partage
  pulmonary end-capillary
c. —
  centum (Lat.) hundred
  cibus (Lat.) meal
  circa (Lat.) about
  compositus (Lat.) compound
  congius (Lat.) gallon
  contusus (Lat.) bruised
  cum (Lat.) with
CA —
  anterior commissure
  calcium antagonist
  California [rabbit]
  cancer

CA — (continued)
  cancer antigen
  caproic acid
  carbohydrate antigen
  carbonic anhydrase
  carcinoma
  cardiac arrest
  cardiac arrhythmia
  cardiac-apnea [monitor]
  carotid artery
  cast
  catecholamine
  catecholaminergic
  cathodal
  cathode
  Caucasian adult
  celiac artery
  celiac axis
  cellulose acetate
  cerebral aqueduct
  cerebral atrophy
  Certified Acupuncturist
  cervicoaxial
  Chemical Abstracts
  chemotactic activity
  chloroamphetamine
  cholic acid
  chromosomal aberration
  chronic anovulation
  chronological age
  citric acid
  clotting assay
  coagglutination
  coarctation of the aorta
  Cocaine Anonymous
  coefficient of absorption
  cold agglutinin
  collagen antigen
  collagenolytic activity
  colloid antigen
  commissural-association [zone
    of brain]
  common antigen
  community acquired
  compressed air
  conceptional age
  conditioned abstinance
  coronary angioplasty
  coronary arrest

CA — (continued)
  coronary artery
  corpora allata
  corpora amylacea
  corpus albicans
  cortisone acetate
  Council Accepted
  cricoid arch
  croup-associated [virus]
  cytosine arabinoside
  cytotoxic antibody
C/A — Clinitest and Acetest
C&A — Clinitest and Acetest
CA_2 — second colloid antigen
Ca —
  calcium
  cancer
  carcinoma
  Candida albicans
  carmustine antineoplastic
  cathodal
  cathode
^{45}Ca — radioactive calcium
ca —
  candle
  carcinoma
ca. — circa (Lat.) about
CAA —
  carotid audiofrequency analy-
    sis
  cerebral amyloid angiopathy
  chloracetaldehyde
  circulating anodic antigen
  Clean Air Act
  computer-assisted assessment
  constitutional aplastic anemia
  coronary artery aneurysm
  crystalline amino acids
CAAT — computer-assisted axial
    tomography
CAB —
  captive air bubble
  catheter-associated bacteriuria
  cellulose acetate butyrate
  coronary artery bypass
CABG — coronary artery bypass
    graft
CABGS — coronary artery bypass
    graft surgery

CaBI — calcium bone index
CaBP — calcium-binding protein
CABRI — Coronary Angioplasty Bypass Revascularization Investigation
CABS — coronary artery bypass surgery
CAC —
　　cancer [malignant] cell
　　cardiac arrest code
　　cardiac-accelerator center
　　carotid artery canal
　　chronic active cirrhosis
　　circulating anticoagulant
　　comprehensive ambulatory care
CACB — calcium carbonate
CaCC — cathodal closure contraction
CACI — computer-assisted continuous infusion
CaCl₂ — calcium chloride
$CaCl_2$ — calcium chloride
CaCl(OCl) — chlorinated lime
$CaCO_3$ — calcium carbonate
CaC_2O_4 — calcium oxalate
CACP — cisplatin
CaCTe — cathodal closure tetanus
CaCV — *Calicivirus*
CaCX — cancer of cervix
CAD —
　　cadaver
　　cadaveric
　　cold agglutinin disease
　　compressed air disease
　　computer-assisted design
　　computer-assisted diagnosis
　　congenital abduction deficiency
　　coronary artery disease
　　coronoradiographic documentation
Cad —
　　cadaver
　　cadaveric
CADI — computer-assisted diabetic instruction [system]
CADL — Communicative Abilities in Daily Living

CADTe — cathodal-duration tetanus
CAE —
　　caprine arthritis-encephalitis
　　cellulose acetate electrophoresis
　　contingent after-effects
　　coronary artery embolism
CaE — calcium excretion
CAEC — cardiac arrhythmia evaluation center
CaEDTA —
　　calcium disodium edetate
　　calcium disodium ethylenediaminetetraacetate
　　edathamil calcium disodium
CAEP — cortical auditory evoked potential
caerul. — *caerulens* (Lat.) dark blue, dark green
CAEV — caprine arthritis-encephalitis virus
CAF —
　　cell adhesion factor
　　citric acid fermenters
　　continuous atrial fibrillation
　　continuous atrial flutter
　　contract administration fees
　　Cooley's Anemia Foundation
CaF — correction of area factor
Caf — caffeine
CaF_2 — calcium fluoride
CAFT — Clinitron air fluidized therapy
CAG —
　　cholangiogram
　　cholangiography
　　chronic atrophic gastritis
　　continuous ambulatory gamma-globulin [infusion]
　　coronary angiogram
　　coronary angiography
CaG — calcium gluconate
CAGB — coronary artery graft bypass
CAGE — cut down, annoyed by criticism, guilty about drinking, eye-opener drinks [a test for alcoholism]

CAH —
- central alveolar hypoventilation
- chronic active hepatitis
- chronic aggressive hepatitis
- combined atrial hypertrophy
- congenital adrenal hyperplasia
- congenital adrenogenital hyperplasia
- cyanacetic acid hydrazide

CaHA — calcium hydroxyapatite

CAHC — chronic active hepatitis with cirrhosis

CAHD —
- coronary arteriosclerotic heart disease
- coronary atherosclerotic heart disease

CAHEA — Committee on Allied Health Education and Accreditation

CaH₂O₂ — calcium hydroxide

CAHS — central alveolar hypoventilation syndrome

CAHV — central alveolar hypoventilation

CAI —
- complete androgen insensitivity
- computer-assisted instruction
- confused artificial insemination

CA ION — calcium, ionized

CAIS — complete androgen insensitivity syndrome

CAL —
- café au lait
- calcium [test]
- calculated average life
- callus
- calories
- chronic airflow limitation
- computer-assisted learning
- coracoacromial ligament

Cal. —
- calcium
- large calorie

cal. —
- caliber

cal. — (continued)
- small calorie

C_alb — albumin clearance

Calc — calcium

calc —
- calculate
- calculation

calcif — calcification

cal ct — calorie count

calCd — calculated

CALD — chronic active liver disease

calef. —
- calefac (Lat.) make warm
- calefactus (Lat.) warmed

CALGB — cancer and leukemia group B

calgi swab — calcium alginate swab

CALH — chronic active lupoid hepatitis

calib — calibrated

cALL — common null cell acute lymphocytic leukemia

CALLA — common acute lymphoblastic leukemia antigen

CALM — café-au-lait macules

CAM —
- calf aortic microsome
- carminomycin
- Caucasian adult male
- cell adhesion molecule
- cell-associating molecule
- chorioallantoic membrane
- computer-assisted myelography
- contralateral axillary metastasis

CaM — calmodulin

C_am — amylase clearance

CAMAC — computer-automated measurement and control

CAMP —
- Christie-Atkins-Munch-Petersen [test]
- computer-assisted menu planning
- concentration of adenosine monophosphate

cAMP — cyclic adenosine monophosphate
c. amplum — *cochleare amplum*
(Lat.) heaping spoonful
CAMS —
cellular-adhesion molecules
computer-assisted monitoring
system
CAMU —
cardiac ambulatory monitoring unit
coronary arrhythmia monitoring unit
CaMV — cauliflower mosaic virus
CAN — cord (umbilical) around
neck
CA/N — child abuse and neglect
Can —
cancer
Candida
Cannabis
CANA — circulating antineuronal
antibody
canc — cancelled
CANCERLIT — Cancer Literature
CANCERPROJ — Cancer Re-
search Projects
CANDID — *Candida* yeast
CANP — calcium-activated neu-
tral protease
CANS — central auditory nervous
system
CAO —
chronic airflow obstruction
chronic airway obstruction
coronary artery obstruction
CaO — calcium oxide
CaO$_2$ — arterial oxygen concentra-
tion
CaOC — cathodal opening con-
traction
CaOCL — cathodal opening clo-
nus
CAOD — coronary artery occlu-
sive disease
Ca(OH)$_2$ — calcium hydroxide
CAOM — chronic adhesive otitis
media

CaOTe — cathodal opening tetanus
Ca ox — calcium oxalate
CAP —
camptodactyly-arthropathy-
pericarditis [syndrome]
cancer of prostate
capillary blood
capsule
captopril
catabolite [gene] activator protein
cell-attachment protein
cellular acetate propionate
cellulose acetate phthalate
central apical part
chloramphenicol
chloroacetophenone
cholesteric analysis profile
chronic alcoholic pancreatitis
College of American Pathologists
community-acquired pneumonia
complement-activated plasma
compound action potentials
computerized automated psychophysiologic [device]
coupled atrial pacing
cyclic AMP–binding protein
cystine aminopeptidase
Ca/P — calcium to phosphorus
[ratio]
cap. — *capiat* (Lat.) let [the
patient] take
cap —
capacity
capillary
capsule
CAPA —
caffeine, alcohol, pepper, and
aspirin
cancer-associated polypeptide
antigen
CAPB — central auditory processing battery
CAPC — calcium phosphate
CAPD —
chronic ambulatory peritoneal
dialysis

CAPD — *(continued)*
  continuous abdomino-peritoneal dialysis
  continuous ambulatory peritoneal dialysis
CAPERS — Computer-assisted Psychiatric Evaluation and Review System
capiend. — *capiendus* (Lat.) to be taken
cap. moll. — *capsula mollis* (Lat.) soft capsule
$Ca_3(PO_4)_2$ — tribasic calcium phosphate
CAPPS — Current and Past Psychopathology Scale
cap. quant. vult — *capiat quantum vult* (Lat.) let [the patient] take as much as he wants
CAPR — calcium pyrophosphate
CAPRCA — chronic, acquired, pure red cell aplasia
CAPRI — Cardiopulmonary Research Institute
CAPS — caffeine, alcohol, pepper, and spicy foods
caps —
  capsule
  capsules
CAP test — cholesteric analysis profile test
CAPYA — child and adolescent psychoanalysis
CAR —
  Canadian Association of Radiologists
  cancer-associated retinopathy
  cardiac ambulation routine
  chronic articular rheumatism
  computer-assisted research
  conditioned avoidance response
car — carotid
CARA — chronic aspecific respiratory ailment
CARB —
  carbohydrate
  coronary artery bypass [graft]

carb —
  carbohydrate
  carbonate
CARBAM — carbamazepine
carbo — carbohydrate
CARD — cardiac automatic resuscitative device
card —
  cardiac
  cardiology
card insuff — cardiac insufficiency
cardiol — cardiology
CARE — computerized adult and records evaluation [system]
CARF — Commission on Accreditation of Rehabilitation Facilities
CAROT — carotene
CARS —
  Childhood Autism Rating Scale
  Children's Affective Rating Scale
CART — computer-assisted real time transcription
cart — cartilage
CARTOS — computer-assisted reconstruction by tracing of serial sections
CAS —
  calcarine sulcus
  calcific aortic stenosis
  Cancer Attitude Survey
  carbohydrate-active steroid
  cardiac adjustment scale
  cardiac surgery
  carotid artery stenosis
  carotid artery system
  casein
  Celite-activated normal serum
  Center for Alcohol Studies
  cerebral arteriosclerosis
  cerebral atherosclerosis
  Chemical Abstracts Service
  chronic anovulation syndrome
  Civil Air Surgeon
  cold agglutinin syndrome

CAS — *(continued)*
 congenital alcoholic syndrome
 congenital asplenia syndrome
 control adjustment strap
 coronary artery spasm
Cas — casualty
cas —
 castrated
 castration
CASA — Computer-Assisted Self-Assessment
CASANOVA — Carotid Artery Stenosis with Asymptomatic Narrowing Operation Versus Aspirin
casc — cascara
CASE — computer-assisted sensory examination
CASH —
 Commission for Administrative Services in Hospitals
 corticoadrenal stimulating hormone
 cruciform anterior spinal hyperextension
CASHD —
 coronary arteriosclerotic heart disease
 coronary atherosclerotic heart disease
CASMD — congenital atonic sclerotic muscular dystrophy
CaSO₄ — calcium sulfate
CA-SP — calcium urine spot [test]
CAS-REGN — Chemical Abstracts Service Registry Number
CASRT — corrected adjusted sinus node recovery time
CASS —
 computer-aided sleep system
 Coronary Artery Surgery Study
CASSIS — Classification and Search Support Information System [Patent Office]

CAST —
 cardiac arrhythmia suppression trial
 Children of Alcoholism Screening Test
 Clearinghouse Announcements in Science and Technology
C-AST — cytoplasmic aspartate aminotransferase
CASTNO — cast number [urinalysis]
CAT —
 California Achievement Test
 capillary agglutination test
 catalase
 cataract
 catecholamine
 cellular atypia
 Children's Apperception Test
 chloramphenicol acetyltransferase
 chlormerodrin accumulation test
 choline acetyltransferase
 chronic abdominal tympany
 classified anaphylatoxin
 Cognitive Abilities Test
 computed abdominal tomography
 computed axial tomography
 computer-aided transcription
 computer-assisted tomography
 computerized axial tomography
cat —
 catalysis
 catalyst
 cataract
CAT-A-KIT — Catecholamine Radioenzymatic Assay Kit
CAT'ase — catalase
CATCH —
 Child and Adolescent Trial of Cardiovascular Health
 Community Actions to Control High Blood Pressure
cat c̄ IL — cataract with intraocular lens

cath. — *catharticus* (Lat.) cathartic
cath —
    catheter
    catheterization
    catheterize
    cathode
    catholic
CATLINE — Catalog On-line
CAT-S — Children's Apperception
    Test, Supplemental
CAT scan — computed axial to-
    mography scan
CATT — calcium tolerance test
Cauc — Caucasian
caud — caudal
caut — cauterization
CAV —
    computer-assisted ventilation
    congenital absence of vagina
    congenital adrenal virilism
    constant angular velocity
    croup-associated virus
cav — cavity
CAVB — complete atrioventricular
    block
CAVC — common arterioventricu-
    lar canal
CAVD —
    complete atrioventricular dis-
      sociation
    completion, arithmetic prob-
      lems, vocabulary, and fol-
      lowing directions [test]
$C(a\text{-}VDO_2)$ — arteriovenous oxy-
    gen difference
CAVEAT — coronary angioplasty
    versus excisional atherectomy
    trial
CAVH — continuous arteriove-
    nous hemofiltration
CAVHD —
    continuous arteriovenous he-
      modialysis
    continuous arteriovenous he-
      mofiltration (with) dialysis
CA virus — croup-associated virus
CAVLT — Children's Auditory
    Verbal Learning Test

CAVO — common atrioventricular
    orifice
$C(a\text{-}v)O_2$ — arteriovenous oxygen
    content difference
CAVS — Conformance Assess-
    ment to Voluntary Standards
CAVU — continuous arteriove-
    nous ultrafiltration
CAW — central airways
C_{AW} — airway conductance
CAWO — closing abductory
    wedge osteotomy
CAZ — ceftazidime
CB —
    calcium blocker
    carbenicillin
    carbonated beverage
    carotid body
    catheterized bladder
    ceased breathing
    cesarean birth
    chair and bed
    chest-back
    Chirurgiae Baccalaureus (Lat.)
      Bachelor of Surgery
    chocolate blood [agar]
    chromatin body
    chronic bronchitis
    circumflex branch
    code blue
    color blind
    compensated base
    conjugated bilirubin
    contrast baths
    coracobrachial
    cytochalasin B
C&B —
    chair and bed
    crown and bridge
C-B — chest-back
CB_{11} — phenadoxone hydrochlo-
    ride
Cb — (columbium) niobium
CBA —
    carcinoma-bearing animal
    chronic bronchitis and
      asthma
    competitive-binding assay

CBA — (continued)
cost-benefit analysis
CBAB — complement-binding antibody
CBADAA — Certifying Board of the American Dental Assistants Association
CB agar — chocolate blood agar
CBAT — Coulter battery
CBB — Coomassi brilliant blue (stain)
CBBB — complete bundle branch block
CBC —
 carbenicillin
 cerebrobuccal connective
 child behavior characteristics
 complete blood (cell) count
cbc — complete blood count
CBCL — Child Behavior Checklist
CBCL/2–3 — Child Behavior Checklist for ages 2–3
CBCME — computer-based continuing medical education
CBCN — carbenicillin
CBD —
 cannabidiol
 carotid body denervation
 closed bladder drainage
 common bile duct
 community-based distribution
CBDC — chronic bullous disease of childhood
CBDE — common bile duct exploration
CBDL — chronic bile duct ligation
CBDS — Carcinogenesis Bioassay Data System
CBE — Council of Biology Editors
CBET — certified biomedical equipment technician
CBF —
 capillary blood flow
 cerebral blood flow
 ciliary beat frequency
 coronary blood flow

CBF — (continued)
 cortical blood flow
CBFS — cerebral blood flow studies
CBFV — cerebral blood flow velocity
CBG —
 capillary blood gases
 capillary blood glucose
 coronary bypass graft
 corticosteroid-binding globulin
 cortisol-binding globulin
CBG_v — corticosteroid-binding globulin variant
CBH —
 chronic benign hepatitis
 cutaneous basophilic hypersensitivity
CBI —
 close-binding-intimate
 continuous bladder irrigation
CBIL — conjugated bilirubin
CBIP — Canter Background Interference Procedure
CBIPBG — Canter Background Interference Procedure for Bender Gestalt [test]
C3b ina — C3b inactivator
CBL —
 circulating blood lymphocytes
 cord blood leukocytes
Cbl — cobalamin
cbl — chronic blood loss
CBM — capillary basement membrane
CBMMP — chronic benign mucous membrane pemphigus
CBMT — capillary basement membrane thickness
CBMW — capillary basement membrane width
CBN —
 cannabinol
 central benign neoplasm
 chronic benign neutropenia
 Commission on Biological Nomenclature

CBO — Congressional Budget Office

CBOC — completion bed occupancy care

CBP —
calcium-binding protein
carbohydrate-binding protein
chlorobiphenyl
cobalamin-binding protein

CBPA — competitive protein-binding assay

CBPS — coronary bypass surgery

CBR —
carotid bodies resected
chemical, biological, and radiological [warfare]
chemically bound residue
chronic bed rest
crude birth rate

C_{BR} — bilirubin clearance

CBRAM — controlled partial rebreathing — anesthesia method

CBS —
cervicobrachial syndrome
chronic brain syndrome
conjugated bile salts
Cruveilhier-Baumgarten syndrome
culture-bound syndrome
cystathionine beta-synthase

CBT —
carotid body tumor
cognitive behavior therapy
computed body tomography

CBV —
capillary blood [flow] velocity
catheter balloon valvuloplasty
central blood volume
cerebral blood velocity
cerebral blood volume
circulating blood volume
corrected blood volume
cortical blood volume
Coxsackie B virus

CBVD — cerebrovascular disease

CBW —
chemical and biological warfare

CBW — (continued)
critical bandwidth [range of frequencies]

CBX — computer-based examination

CBZ — carbamazepine

Cbz — carbobenzoxy chloride

CC —
calcaneal-cuboid
calcium cyclamate
cardiac catheterization
cardiac contusion
cardiac cycle
cardiovascular clinic
carotid-cavernous
case coordinator
canal catheterization
cell culture
cellular compartment
central compartment
cerebral commissure
cerebral concussion
cerebral cortex
cervical collar
chest circumference
chief complaint
cholecalciferol
chondrocalcinosis
choriocarcinoma
chronic complainer
ciliated cell
circulatory collapse
classical conditioning
clean catch [of urine]
Clinical Center [NIH]
clinical course
clomiphene citrate
closed up
closing capacity
coefficient of correlation
colony count
colorectal cancer
columnar cells
commission-certified [stain]
common cold
complications and comorbidities
compound cathartic

CC — (continued)
  computer calculated
  concave
  congenital cardiopathy
  consumptive coagulopathy
  continuing care
  contractile component
  contrast cystogram
  conversion complete
  coracoclavicular
  cord compression
  coronary collateral
  corpora cardiaca
  corpus callosum
  costochondral
  Coulter counter
  craniocaudad
  craniocervical
  creatinine clearance
  critical care
  critical condition
  Cronkhite-Canada [syndrome]
  crus cerebri
  crus communis
  cubic centimeter
  cup cell
  current complaint
  current contents
  cytochrome C
  with correction (with glasses)
C-C — convexo-concave
C/C —
  chief complaint
  cholecystectomy and (opera-
    tive) cholangiogram
  complete upper and lower
    dentures
C&C —
  cold and clammy
  confirmed and compatible
Cc — concave
cc —
  carbon copy
  chest circumference
  concave
  condylocephalic
  corrected
  cubic centimeter

cc — (continued)
  with correction
  with spectacles
c̄c̄ — with meals
CCA —
  cephalin cholesterol antigen
  chick cell agglutination
  chimpanzee coryza agent
  choriocarcinoma
  circulating cathodic antigen
  circumflex coronary artery
  colitis colon antigen
  common carotid artery
  concentrated care area
  congenital contractural arach-
    nodactyly
C-C-A —
  cytidyl-cytidyl-adenyl
  constitutional chromosome
    abnormality
CCAP — capsule cartilage articular preservation
CCAT —
  Canadian Coronary Atherec-
    tomy Trial
  chick cell agglutination test
  conglutinating complement
    absorption test
CCB — calcium channel blocker
CCBV — central circulating blood
  volume
CCC —
  calcium cyanamide (carbi-
    mide) citrated
  Cancer Care Center
  care-cure coordination
  cathodal closure contraction
  central counteradaptive
    changes
  child care clinic
  chronic calculous cholecystitis
  chronic catarrhal colitis
  citrated calcium carbimide
  Commission on Clinical
    Chemistry
  comprehensive cancer center
  comprehensive care clinic
  consecutive case conference

CCC — *(continued)*
  continuing community care
  critical care complex
  cylindrical confronting cister-
    nae
CC&C — colony count and culture
CCCC — centrifugal countercurrent chromatography
cccDNA — covalently closed circular deoxyribonucleic acid
CCCl — cathodal closure clonus
CCCP — carbonyl cyanide *m*-chlo-
  rophenyl-hydrazone
CCCR —
  closed-chest cardiac resuscita-
    tion
  closed-chest cardiopulmonary
    resuscitation
CCCS — condom catheter collecting system
CCCT — closed craniocerebral
  trauma
CCCU —
  comprehensive cardiac care
    unit
  comprehensive cardiovascular
    care unit
CCD —
  calibration curve data
  charge-coupled device
  childhood celiac disease
  cortical collecting duct
  countercurrent distribution
  cumulative cardiotoxic dose
CCDC — Canadian Communicable Disease Center
CCDN — Central Council for District Nursing
ccDNA — closed circle deoxyribonucleic acid
CCE —
  carboline-carboxylic acid ester
  chamois contagious ecthyma
  clear-cell endothelioma
  clubbing, cyanosis, and edema
  countercurrent electrophoresis
CCEI — Crown-Crisp Experimental Index

CCF —
  cancer coagulation factor
  cardiolipin complement fixa-
    tion
  carotid-cavernous fistula
  centrifuged culture fluid
  cephalin-cholesterol floccula-
    tion
  compound comminuted frac-
    ture
  congestive cardiac failure
  crystal-induced chemotactic
    factor
CCFA — cycloserine-cefoxitin-
  fructose agar
CCFAS — compact colony-forming active substance
CCFE — cyclophosphamide, cisplatin, fluorouracil, and estra-
  mustine
CCFMG — Cooperating Committee on Foreign Medical Graduates
CCG —
  cholecystogram
  cholecystography
CCGC — capillary column gas
  chromotography
CCGG — cytosine-cytosine gua-
  nine-guanine
CCH —
  C-cell hyperplasia
  chronic cholestatic hepatitis
CCh — carbamylcholine
CCHD — cyanotic congenital
  heart disease
CCHE — Central Council for
  Health Education
CCHMS — Central Committee
  for Hospital Medical Services
CCHP — Consumer Choice
  Health Plan
CCHS — congenital central hypo-
  ventilation syndrome
CCI —
  chronic coronary insufficiency
  corrected count increment
CCJ —
  costochondral junction

CCJ — *(continued)*
craniocervical junction
CCK — cholecystokinin
CCK-8 — cholecystokinin octapeptide
CCK-GB — cholecystokinin-gallbladder [cholecystogram]
CCKLI — cholecystokinin-like immunoreactivity
CCK-OP — cholecystokinin octapeptide
CCK-PZ — cholecystokinin-pancreozymin
CCL —
carcinoma cell line
cardiac catheterization laboratory
certified cell line
Charcot-Leyden crystal
critical carbohydrate level
critical condition list
CCl_4 — carbon tetrachloride
$CCl_3CH(OH)_2$ — chloral hydrate
CCLI — composite clinical and laboratory index
CCM —
calcium-citrate-malate
cerebrocostomandibular [syndrome]
congestive cardiomyopathy
contralateral competing message
craniocervical malformation
critical care medicine
c cm — cubic centimeter
CCMC — Committee on the Costs of Medical Care
CCME — Coordinating Council on Medical Education
CCMS —
cerebrocostomandibular syndrome
clean-catch midstream [urine]
clinical care management system
CCMSU — clean-catch midstream urine
CCMSUA — clean-catch midstream urinalysis

CCMT — catechol-O-methyltransferase
CCMU — critical care medical unit
CCN —
caudal central nucleus
coronary care nursing
critical care nursing
CCNS — cell cycle nonspecific [agent]
CCNSC — Cancer Chemotherapy National Service Center
CCNU —
chloroethylcyclohexlnitrosourea [lomustine]
N-(2-chloroethyl)-N'-cyclohexyl-N-nitrosourea
CCO — cytochrome C oxidase
CcO_2 — pulmonary end-capillary blood oxygen concentration
CCOF — chromosally competent ovarian failure
C-collar — cervical collar
CCOT — cervical compression overloading test
CCP —
chronic calcifying pancreatitis
ciliocytophthoria
Crippled Children's Program
cytidine cyclic phosphate
CCPD —
continuous cycling peritoneal dialysis
crystalline calcium pyrophosphate dihydrate
CCPDS — Centralized Cancer Patient Data System
CCPR — crypt cell production rate
CCR — complete continuous remission
C_{cr} — creatinine clearance
CCRC — continuing care residential community
CCRIS — Chemical Carcinogenesis Research Information System
CCRN — Critical Care Registered Nurse

CCRS — carotid chemoreceptor stimulation

CCRU — critical care recovery unit

CCS —
Canadian Cardiovascular Society
casualty clearing station
cell cycle–specific
cholecystosonography
chronic cerebellar stimulation
chronic compartment syndrome
Clinical Sleep Society
cloudy cornea syndrome
concentration camp syndrome
costoclavicular syndrome
Crippled Children's Society
Critical Care Services

CC&S — cornea, conjunctiva, and sclera

CCSA — central chemosensitive area

CCSCS — central cervical spinal cord syndrome

CCSE — Cognitive Capacity Screening Examination

CCSG — Children's Cancer Study Group

CCT —
calcitriol
carotid compression tomography
central conduction time
cerebrocranial trauma
chocolate-coated tablet
clear, creamy layer on top
closed cerebral trauma
coated compressed tablet
combined cortical thickness
composite cyclic therapy
computerized cranial tomography
congenitally corrected transposition [of great vessels]
controlled cord traction
coronary care team
cranial computed tomography

CCT — (continued)
crude coal tar
cyclocarbothiamine

cct — circuit

CCTe — cathodal closure tetanus

CCTGA — congenitally corrected transposition of the great arteries

CCT in PET — crude coal tar in petroleum

CCTP — coronary care training program

CCTV — closed-circuit television

CCU —
cardiac care unit
cardiovascular care unit
Cherry-Crandall unit
color-changing unit
community care unit
coronary care unit
critical care unit

CCUA — clean-catch urinalysis

CCUP — colpocystourethropexy

CCV —
channel catfish virus
conductivity cell volume

CCVD — chronic cerebrovascular disease

CCVM — congenital cardiovascular malformation

CCW —
chest wall compliance
childcare worker
counterclockwise

CCX — complications

CD —
cadaveric donor
canine distemper
canine dose
carbohydrate dehydratase
carbonate dehydratase
carbon dioxide
cardiac disease
cardiac dullness
cardiac dysrhythmia
cardiovascular deconditioning
cardiovascular disease
Carrel-Dakin [fluid]

CD — (continued)
  Castleman's disease
  caudad
  caudal
  celiac disease
  cell dissociation
  central deposition
  cervicodorsal
  cesarean delivery
  channel down
  character disorder
  chemical dependency
  chemotactic difference
  childhood disease
  circular dichroism
  cluster designation
  cluster of differentiation
  colloid droplet
  combination drug
  common duct
  communicable disease
  communication deviance
  communication disorders
  completely denaturated
  complicated delivery
  conduct disorder
  conduction disorder
  conjugata diagonalis (Lat.) diag-
    onal conjugate diameter (of
    pelvis)
  consanguineous donor
  contact dermatitis
  contagious disease
  continuous drainage
  control diet
  conventional dialysis
  convulsive disorder
  convulsive dose
  coroneal dystrophy
  Cotrel-Dubousset [rod]
  covert dyskinesia
  Crohn's disease
  crossed diagonal
  curative dose
  current diagnosis
  cutdown
  cystic duct
  Czapek-Dox [agar]

CD_{50} — median curative dose
C/D —
    cigarettes per day
    cup to disc [ratio]
C&D —
    curettage and desiccation
    cystoscopy and dilatation
Cd —
    cadmium
    caudal
    coccygeal
    condylion
    drug coefficient
^{115}Cd — radioactive cadmium
cd —
    candela
    caudal
    coccygeal
    cord
c/d — cigarettes per day
c.d. — conjugata diagonalis (Lat.) di-
    agonal conjugate diameter (of
    pelvis)
CDA —
    Canadian Dental Assocation
    Certified Dental Assistant
    chenodeoxycholic acid
    ciliary dyskinesia activity
    complement-dependent anti-
      body
    completely denatured alcohol
    congenital dyserythropoietic
      anemia
CDAA — chlorodiallylacetamide
    [herbicide]
CDAI — Crohn's Disease Activity
    Index
CDAK — Cordis Dow Artificial
    Kidney
C&DB — cough and deep breath
CDC —
    calculated date of confine-
      ment
    cancer detection center
    cancer diagnosis center
    capillary diffusion capacity
    cardiac diagnostic center
    cell division cycle

CDC — (continued)
  Centers for Disease Control
  chenodeoxycholate
  chenodeoxycholic [acid]
  child development clinic
  Communicable Disease Center
  complement-dependent cytotoxicity
  Crohn's disease of the colon
CD-C — controlled
  drinker — control
CDCA — chenodeoxycholic acid
CDCF — Clostridium difficile culture filtrate
CDCP — Centers for Disease Control and Prevention
CDD —
  certificate of disability for discharge
  choledochoduodenostomy
  chronic degenerative disease
  chronic degenerative disease
  chronic disabling dermatosis
  critical degree of deformation
CDDP — cis-diaminedichloroplatinum
CDE —
  canine distemper encephalitis
  Certified Diabetes Educator
  chlordiazepoxide
  common duct exploration
CD-E — controlled
  drinker — experimental
CDEC — Comprehensive Developmental Evaluation Chart
CDF — chondrodystrophia foetalis
cdF — cumulative distribution function
CDG — central developmental groove
CDGD — constitutional delay in growth and development
cDGS — complete form of DiGeorge's syndrome
CDH —
  ceramide dihexoside
  chronic daily headache

CDH — (continued)
  chronic disease hospital
  congenital diaphragmatic hernia
  congenital dislocation of hip
  congenital dysplasia of hip
CDI —
  cell-directed inhibitor
  central diabetes insipidus
  Children's Depression Inventory
  chronic diabetes insipidus
CDILD — chronic diffuse interstitial lung disease
CDK — climatic droplet keratopathy
CDL — chlordeoxylincomycin
CDLE — chronic discoid lupus erythematosus
CDLS — Cornelia de Lange syndrome
CDM —
  chemically defined medium
  clinical decision making
cDNA —
  circular deoxyribonucleic acid
  complementary deoxyribonucleic acid
  copy deoxyribonucleic acid
CDNB — 1-chloro-2,4-dinitrobenzene
CDP —
  chlordiazepoxide
  chronic destructive periodontitis
  collagenase-digestible protein
  constant distending pressure
  continuing distending pressure
  Coronary Drug Project
  cytidine diphosphate
  cytosine diphosphate
CDPC — cytidine diphosphate choline
CDPS — common duct pigment stones
CDPX — X-linked chondrodysplasia punctata

CDQ — corrected development quotient
CDR —
calcium-dependent regulator
chronologic drinking record
complementarity-determining region
computed digital radiography
computerized digital radiography
continuing disability review
cup/disk ratio
CDR(H) — cup to disk ratio, horizontal
CDRS — Children's Depression Rating Scale
CDRS-R — Children's Depression Rating Scale — Revised
CDR(V) — cup to disk ratio, vertical
CDS —
catechol-3,5-disulfonate
caudal dysplasia syndrome
Chemical Data Systems
Christian Dental Society
cul-de-sac
cumulative duration of survival
CDSC — Communicable Diseases Surveillance Centre [London]
CDSM — Committee on Dental and Surgical Materials
cd-sr — candela-steradian
CDSS — clinical decision support system
CDT —
carbon dioxide therapy
Certified Dental Technician
Clostridium difficile toxin
combined diphtheria tetanus
CDTe — cathode duration tetanus
CDU —
chemical dependency unit
cumulative dose unit
CDV — canine distemper virus
CDX — chlordiazepoxide
Cdyn — dynamic compliance
C_{dyn} — dynamic compliance

CDZ —
chlordiazepoxide
conduction delay zone
CE —
California encephalitis
cardiac emergency
cardiac enlargement
cardioesophageal
catamenial epilepsy
cataract extraction
cell extract
central episiotomy
chemical energy
chick embryo
chloroform-ether
cholera exotoxin
cholesterol esters
cholinesterase
chorioepithelioma
chromatoelectrophoresis
ciliated epithelium
clinical emphysema
columnar epithelium
community education
conjugated estrogens
constant error
constant estrus
continuing education
contractile element
contrast echocardiology
converting enzyme
crude extract
cytopathic effect
C-E — chloroform-ether
C&E —
consultation and examination
cough and exercise
curettage and electrodesiccation
Ce — cerium
^{58}Ce — radioactive cerium
CEA —
carcinoembryonic antigen
carotid endarterectomy
cholesterol-esterifying activity
cholinesterase
cost-effectiveness analysis
crystalline egg albumin

CEARP — Continuing Education Approval and Recognition Program

CEAT — chronic ectopic atrial tachycardia

CEB — cotton elastic bandage

CEBD — controlled extrahepatic biliary drainage

cEBV — chronic Epstein-Barr virus [infection]

CEC —
ciliated epithelial cell
contractile electrical complex

CECT — contrast-enhanced computed tomography

CED —
chondroectodermal dysplasia
cultural/ethnic diversity

CEDIA — cloned enzyme donor immunoassay

CEE —
Central European encephalitis
chick embryo extract

CEEA — curved end-to-end anastomosis [stapler]

CEEC — calf esophagus epithelial cell

CEEG — computer-analyzed electroencephalography

CeeNU — lomustine

CEEV — Central European encephalitis virus

CEF —
centrifugal extractable fluid
chick embryo fibroblast
constant electric field

CEFMG — Council on Education for Foreign Medical Graduates

CEG — chronic erosive gastritis

CEH — cholesterol ester hydrolase

CEHC — calf embryonic heart cell

CEI —
character education inquiry
continuous extravascular infusion
converting enzyme inhibitor
corneal epithelial involvement

CEID — crossed electroimmunodiffusion

CEJ —
cardioesophageal junction
cement-enamel junction

CEK — chick embryo kidney

CEL —
cardiac exercise laboratory
Celsius

Cel — Celsius

Cell — celluloid

CELO — chick embryo lethal orphan [virus]

CELOV — chick embryo lethal orphan virus

CEM —
computerized electroencephalographic map
conventional transmission electron microscope

cemf — counterelectromotive force

CEN —
Certificate for Emergency Nursing
Comité European de Normalisation [standards]
continuous enteral nutrition

cen —
central
centromere

CENP — centromere protein

cent —
centigrade
centimeter
central

CEO —
chick embryo origin
Chief Executive Officer
chloroethylene oxide

CEOT — calcifying epithelial odontogenic tumor

CEP —
chronic eosinophilic pneumonia
chronic erythropoietic porphyria
cognitive evoked potential
congenital erythropoietic porphyria

CEP — (continued)
  continuing education program
  cortical evoked potential
  countercurrent electrophoresis
  counter-electrophoresis
CEPA — chloroethane phosphoric
  acid
CEPB — Carpentier-Edwards porcine bioprosthesis
CEPH —
  cephalic
  cephalin
  cephalosporin
ceph —
  cephalin
  cephalosporin
CEPH FLOC — cephalin flocculation
CEQ — Council on Environmental Quality
CER —
  capital expenditure review
  ceramide
  conditioned emotional re-
    sponse
  control electrical rhythm
  cortical evoked response
CE&R — central episiotomy and
  repair
CERA — cortical evoked response
  audiometry
CERCLA — The Comprehensive
  Environmental Response,
  Compensation, and Liability
  Act
CERD — chronic end-stage renal
  disease
Cert —
  certificate
  certified
cert —
  certificate
  certified
CERULO — ceruloplasmin
cerv —
  cervical
  cervix
CES —
  cat's eye syndrome

CES — (continued)
  cauda equina syndrome
  chronic electrophysiological
    study
  cognitive environmental stim-
    ulation
  conditioned escape response
ces — central excitatory state
CESD — cholesterol ester storage
  disease
CES-D — Center for Epidemiologic Studies — Depression
CET —
  capital expenditure threshold
  congenital eyelid tetrad
  controlled environment treat-
    ment
CETE — Central European tick-
  borne encephalitis
CETI — Communication with Ex-
  traterrestrial Intelligence
CEU —
  congenital ectropion uveae
  continuing education unit
CEV —
  California encephalitis virus
  Citrus exocortis viroid
CEX — clinical evaluation exercise
CEZ — cefazolin
CF —
  calcium folinate (calcium leu-
    covorin)
  calf blood flow
  calibration factor
  cancer-free
  carbolfuchsin
  carbon-filtered
  cardiac failure
  carotid foramen
  carrier-free
  cascade filtration
  case file
  Caucasian female
  centrifugal force
  cephalothin
  certainty factor
  characteristic frequency

CF — (continued)
chemotactic factor
chest and left leg [lead in electrocardiography]
Chiari-Frommel [syndrome]
chick fibroblast
choroid fissure
Christmas factor
citrovorum factor
climbing fiber
clotting factor
colicin factor
collected fluid
colonization factor
colony-forming
color and form
complement fixation
completely follicular
computed fluoroscopy
constant frequency
contractile force
coronary flow
cough frequency
count fingers
counting finger
coupling factor
cycling fibroblast
cystic fibrosis
C&F —
cell and flare
curettage and fulguration
C'F — complement fixing
CFII — Cohn fraction II
Cf —
californium
carrier of ferrum (iron)
cf —
centrifugal force
cf. — confer (Lat.) bring together, compare
CFA —
clofibric acid
colonization factor antigen
colony-forming assay
common femoral artery
complement-fixing antibody
complete Freund's adjuvant
configuration frequency analysis

CFA — (continued)
cryptogenic fibrosing alveolitis
CFAC — complement-fixing antibody consumption
C-factor — cleverness factor
CFB — central fibrous body
CFC —
capillary filtration coefficient
cardiofaciocutaneous [syndrome]
chlorofluorocarbon
colony-forming capacity
colony-forming cell
continuous flow centrifugation
CFCCT — Committee for Freedom of Choice in Cancer Therapy
CFCL — continuous flow centrifugation leukapheresis
CFC-S — colony-forming cells — spleen
CFD —
cephalofacial deformity
Concern for the Dying
craniofacial dysostosis
CFDS — craniofacial dysostosis
CFF —
critical flicker frequency
critical flicker [test]
critical flicker fusion frequency [test]
cystic fibrosis factor
Cystic Fibrosis Foundation
cff —
critical flicker fusion
critical fusion frequency
CFFA — cystic fibrosis factor activity
Cf-Fe — carrier-bound iron
CFH — Council on Family Health
CFI —
cardiac function index
chemotactic factor inactivator
complement fixation inhibition
confrontation fields intact
CFIDS — chronic fatigue and immune dysfunction syndrome

CFM —
    chlorofluoromethane
    close-fitting mask
    craniofacial microsomia
cfm — cubic feet per minute
CFMA — Council for Medical Affairs
CFMG — Commission on Foreign Medical Graduates
CFND — craniofrontonasal dysostosis
CFNS —
    chills, fever, night sweats
    craniofrontonasal syndrome
CFO — chief financial officer
CFP —
    cerebrospinal fluid protein
    chronic false positive
    Clinical Fellowship Program
    cystic fibrosis of pancreas
    cystic fibrosis patients
    cystic fibrosis protein
CFPP — craniofacial pattern profile
CFPR — Canadian Familial Polyposis Registry
CFR —
    case-fatality ratio
    citrovorum-factor rescue
    Code of Federal Regulations
    complement-fixation reaction
    coronary flow reserve
    correct fast reaction
    cyclic flow reduction
CFS —
    call for service
    cancer family syndrome
    Chiari-Frommel syndrome
    chronic fatigue syndrome
    contoured femoral stem
    craniofacial stenosis
    crush fracture syndrome
    culture fluid supernatant
    Cystic Fibrosis Society
cfs — cubic feet per second
CFSE — crystal field stabilization energy

CFSTI — Clearinghouse for Federal Scientific and Technical Information
CFT —
    cardiolipin flocculation test
    clinical full-time
    complement-fixation test
    complement-fixing titer
CFTCR — cystic fibrosis transmembrane conductance regulator
CFU —
    colony-forming unit
    color-forming unit
CFU-C — colony-forming unit — culture
CFU-E —
    colony-forming unit — erythrocyte
    colony-forming unit — erythroid
CFU_{EOS} — colony-forming unit — eosinophil
CFU-F — colony-forming unit — fibroblastoid
CFU_F — colony-forming unit — fibroblastoid
CFU_{GM} — colony-forming unit — granulocyte-macrophage
CFU_L — colony-forming unit — lymphoid
CFU_M — colony-forming unit — megakaryocyte
CFU_{MEG} — colony-forming unit — megakaryocyte
CFU/mL — colony-forming units per milliliter
CFU_{NM} — colony-forming unit — neutrophil-monocyte
CFU-S — colony-forming unit — spleen
CFV — continuous flow ventilation
CFW —
    cancer-free white [mouse]
    Carworth farm [mouse], Webster strain

CFWM —
    cancer-free white mouse
    Carworth farm mouse [Webster strain]
CFX —
    cefoxitin
    circumflex [coronary artery]
CFZ — capillary-free zone
CFZC — continuous-flow zonal centrifugation
CG —
    calcium gluconate
    cardiography
    Cardio-Green
    center of gravity
    central gray
    choking gas (phosgene)
    cholecystogram
    cholecystography
    choriogenic gynecomastia
    chorionic gonadotropin
    chromogranin
    chronic glomerulonephritis
    cingulate gyrus
    colloidal gold
    contact guarding
    control group
    cryoglobulin
    cystine guanine
cg —
    center of gravity
    centrigram
    chemoglobulin
CGA — catabolite gene activator
CGAS — Children's Global Assessment Scale
CGB —
    chronic gastrointestinal bleeding
    chronic gonadotropin beta-unit
CGC — Certified Gastrointestinal Clinician
CGD —
    chromosomal gonadal dysgenesis
    chronic granulomatous disease
    commissural gastric driver

CGDE — contact glow discharge electrolysis
CGFH — congenital fibrous histiocytoma
CGFNS — Commission on Graduates of Foreign Nursing Schools
CGH — chorionic gonadotropic hormone
CGI —
    chronic granulomatous inflammation
    Clinical Global Impression [scale]
    computer-generated imagery
CGKD — complex glycerol kinase deficiency
CGL —
    chronic granulocytic leukemia
    correction with glasses
c gl — correction with glasses
CGM — central gray matter
cgm — centigram
CGMMV — cucumber green mottle mosaic virus
cGMP — cyclic guanosine monophosphate
CGN — chronic glomerulonephritis
CGNB — composite ganglioneuroblastoma
CG/OQ — cerebral glucose-oxygen quotient
CGP —
    choline glycerophosphatide
    chorionic growth hormone-prolactin
    circulating granulocyte pool
    N-carbobenzoxy-glycyl-L-phenylalanine
CGRN — coarsely granular
CGRP — calcitonin gene-related peptide
CGS —
    cardiogenic shock
    catgut suture
    centimeter-gram-second [system]

cgs — centimeter-gram-second
  [system]
CGT —
  chorionic gonadotropin
  cyclodextrin glucanotransfer-
    ase
  N-carbobenzoyl-α-glutamyl-L-
    tyrosine
CGTT —
  cortisol glucose tolerance test
  cortisone glucose tolerance
    test
cGy — centigray
CH —
  case history
  casein hydrolysate
  Chédiak-Higashi [syndrome]
  chest
  chiasma
  chief
  child
  children
  Chinese hamster
  chirurgia (Lat.) surgery
  chloral hydrate
  cholesterol
  Christchurch chromosome
  chronic
  chronic hepatitis
  chronic hypertension
  Clarke-Hatfield [syndrome]
  cluster headache
  common hepatic [duct]
  communicating hydrocele
  community health
  completely healed
  congenital hypothyroidism
  Conradi-Hünermann [syn-
    drome]
  continuous heparin [infusion]
  convalescent hospital
  crown-heel [length of fetus]
  cycloheximide
  cystic hygroma
  wheelchair
C&H —
  cocaine and heroin
  coarse and harsh [breathing]

CH_4 — methane
C_2H_2 — acetylene
C_2H_4 — ethylene
C_6H_6 — benzene
$C'H_{50}$ — 50% hemolyzing dose of
  complement
C_H —
  constant domain of H chain
  constant region
Ch —
  chest
  Chido [antibody]
  chief
  child
  cholesterol
  choline
  Christchurch [syndrome]
  chromosome
Ch^1 — Christchurch chromosome
cH^+ — hydrogen ion concentration
ch —
  chest
  chief
  child
  choline
  chronic
CHA —
  Catholic Hospital Association
  Chinese hamster
  chronic hemolytic anemia
  common hepatic artery
  congenital hypoplasia of adre-
    nal glands
  congenital hypoplastic anemia
  continuously heated aerosol
  cyclohexyladenosine
  cyclohexylamine
ChA — choline acetylase
ChAC — choline acetyltransferase
ChAct — choline acetyltransferase
CHAD — cyclophosphamide, hexamethylmelamine, Adriamycin (doxorubicin), and cisplatin
CHAI — continuous hepatic artery infusion
CHAID — chi-square automatic
  interaction detection

CHAL — chronic haloperidol
CHAMP — Children's Hospital Automated Medical Program
CHAMPUS — Civilian Health and Medical Program of Uniformed Services
CHAMPVA — Civilian Health and Medical Program of Veterans Administration
CHANDS — curly hair–ankyloblepharon–nail dysplasia syndrome
Chang C — Chang conjunctiva cells
Chang L — Chang liver cells
CHAP —
    Certified Hospital Admission Program
    Child Health Assessment Program
CHARGE — coloboma, heart disease, atresia choanae, retarded growth and retarded development and/or CNS anomalies, genital hypoplasia, and ear anomalies and/or deafness [syndrome]
chart. — *charta* [Lat.] paper
CHAS — Center for Health Administration Studies
ChAT — choline acetyltransferase
CHB —
    chronic hepatitis B
    complete heart block
    congenital heart block
Ch.B. — *Chirurgiae Baccalaureus* (Lat.) Bachelor of Surgery
CHBHA — congenital Heinz body hemolytic anemia
C_2H_5Br — ethyl bromide
CHC —
    community health center
    community health computing
    community health council
CH_3CCNU — semustine
$CHCl_3$ — chloroform
$C_2H_4Cl_2$ — ethylene chloride
C_2H_5Cl — ethyl chloride

CHCM — cellular hemoglobin concentration mean
$C_2H_5CO_2NH_2$ — ethyl carbamate
$(CH_3 \cdot CO)_2O$ — acetic anhydride
$CH_3 \cdot COOH$ — acetic acid
$C_4H_9 \cdot COOH$ — valeric acid
CHcm — cellular hemoglobin concentration, mean
CHCP — correctional health care program
CHD —
    center hemodialysis
    Chédiak-Higashi disease
    childhood disease(s)
    chronic hemodialysis
    common hepatic duct
    congenital heart disease
    congenital hip dislocation
    congenital hip dysplasia
    congestive heart disease
    constitutional hepatic dysfunction
    coordinate home care
    coronary heart disease
    cyanotic heart disease
Ch.D. — *Chirurgiae Doctor* (Lat.) Doctor of Surgery
CHDM — comprehensive hospital drug monitoring
ChE —
    cholesterol ester
    cholinesterase
che — a gene involved in chemotaxis
CHEC — community hypertension evaluation clinic
CHEF — Chinese hamster embryo fibroblast
chem —
    chemical
    chemistry
    chemotherapy
ChemID — Chemical Identification
CHEMLINE — Chemical Dictionary On-line
chemo — chemotherapy
CHEMTREC — Chemical Transportation Emergency Center

CHERSS — continuous high-amplitude EEG rhythmical synchronous slowing

CHEST — Chick Embryotoxicity Screening Test

CHF —
chick heart fibroblast
chronic heart failure
congenital hepatic fibrosis
congestive heart failure
Crimean hemorrhagic fever

CHFD — controlled high flux dialysis

CHFV — combined high-frequency ventilation

chg —
change
changed
charge

Ch Gn — chronic glomerulonephritis

CHH — cartilage-hair hypoplasia

CHI —
closed head injury
creatinine height index

CHI_3 — iodoform

C_2H_5I — ethyl iodide

chi — chimera

Chi-A — chimpanzee leukocyte antigen

CHILD — congenital hemidysplasia with ichthyosiform erythroderma and limb defects [syndrome]

CHIME — coloboma, heart anomaly, ichthyosis, mental retardation, ear abnormality

CHINA —
chronic infectious neuropathic agent
chronic infectious neurotropic agent

CHINS —
child in need of service
children in need of service

CHIP —
comprehensive health insurance plan

CHIP — (continued)
comprehensive hospital infections project

CHIPASAT — Children's Paced Auditory Serial Addition Task

CHIPS — catastrophic health insurance plans

Chir. Doct. — Chirurgiae Doctor (Lat.) Doctor of Surgery

chirurg. — chirurgicalis (Lat.) surgical

chix — chickenpox

CHL —
Chinese hamster lung
chlorambucil
chloramphenicol
crown-heel length

Chl —
chloroform
chlorophyll

CHLA — cyclohexyl linoleic acid

Chlb — chlorobutanol

CHLD — chronic hypoxic lung disease

chlor —
chloride
chloroform

chloro — chloramphenicol

Ch.M. — Chirurgiae Magister (Lat.) Master of Surgery

CHMD — clinical hyaline membrane disease

CHN —
carbon, hydrogen, and nitrogen
central hemorrhagic necrosis
Certified Hemodialysis Nurse
child neurology
Chinese [hamster]
community health network
community health nurse

$C_6H_5NH_2$ — aniline

$C_3H_5(NO_3)_3$ — glyceryl trinitrate (nitroglycerin)

$C_5H_4N_4O_3$ — uric acid

$C_5H_{11}NO_2$ — amyl nitrite

C_8H_9NO — acetanilid

$C_9H_9NO_3$ — hippuric acid

$C_6H_2(NO_2)_3OH$ — trinitrophenol (picric acid)

CHO —
> carbohydrate
> Chinese hamster ovary
> cholesterol
> chorea

CH_2O — formaldehyde

CH_2O_2 — formic acid

CH_4O — methyl alcohol

$C_2H_2O_4$ — oxalic acid

$C_2H_4O_2$ — acetic acid

C_2H_6O — ethyl alcohol

C_3H_6O — acetone

$C_3H_6O_3$ — lactic acid

$C_3H_8O_3$ — glycerin

$C_4H_6O_2$ — crotonic acid

$C_4H_6O_5$ — malic acid

$C_4H_6O_6$ — tartaric acid

$C_4H_8O_2$ — butyric acid; isobutyric acid

$C_4H_{10}O$ — ether (ethyl ether)

$C_5H_{10}O_2$ — valeric acid

$C_5H_{12}O$ — amyl alcohol

C_6H_6O — phenol

$C_6H_8O_7$ — citric acid

$C_6H_{12}O_6$ — dextrose (D-glucose)

$C_7H_4O_7$ — meconic acid

$C_7H_6O_2$ — benzoic acid

$C_7H_6O_3$ — salicylic acid

$C_7H_6O_5$ — gallic acid

$C_{12}H_{22}O_{11}$ — cane sugar

$C_{15}H_{10}O_4$ — chrysophanic acid

$C_{18}H_{34}O_2$ — oleic acid

$C_{18}H_{36}O_2$ — stearic acid

Cho — choline

C_{H_2O} — water clearance

choc — chocolate

CHOI — considered characteristic of osteogenesis imperfecta

C_6H_5OH — phenol

CHOL — cholesterol

chol — cholesterol

c̄hold — withhold

chole — cholecystectomy

chol est — cholesterol esters

$(C_6H_{10}O_5)$ — starch, glycogen, or other hexose polymers

CHP —
> capillary hydrostatic pressure
> charcoal hemoperfusion
> Chemical Hygiene Plan
> child psychiatry
> comprehensive health planning
> coordinating hospital physician
> cutaneous hepatic porphyria

ChP — chest physician

chpx — chickenpox

CHQ — chloroquinol

CHR —
> Cercarien-Hüllen Reaktion [test]
> cerebrohepatorenal [syndrome]

Chr. — *Chromobacterium*

chr —
> chromosome
> chronic

c hr — candle hour

c-hr — curie-hour

ChRBC — chicken red blood cell

ChrBrSyn — chronic brain syndrome

Chr.ETOH — chronic ethanolism

CHRIS — Cancer Hazards Ranking and Information System

chron —
> chronic
> chronological

CHRPE — congenital hypertrophy of the retinal pigment epithelium

CHRS —
> cerebrohepatorenal syndrome
> congenital hereditary retinoschisis

CHS —
> central hypoventilation syndrome
> Chédiak-Higashi syndrome
> cholinesterase
> chondroitin sulfate
> compression hip screw
> congenital hypoventilation syndrome

CHS — (continued)
  contact hypersensitivity
CHSD — Children's Health Services Division
CHSS — cooperative health statistics system
CHT —
  closed head trauma
  combined hormone therapy
  contralateral head turning
ChTg — chymotrypsinogen
ChTK — chicken thymidine kinase
CHU —
  centigrade heat unit
  closed head unit
CHV — canine herpesvirus
CI —
  cardiac index
  cardiac insufficiency
  cell immunity
  cell inhibition
  cephalic index
  cerebral infarction
  cesium implant
  chain-initiating
  chemical ionization
  chemotactic index
  chemotherapeutic index
  chromatid interchange
  chronic infection
  chronically infected
  clinical impression
  clinical investigation
  clinical investigator
  clomipramine
  clonus index
  cochlear implant
  coefficient of intelligence
  colloidal iron
  colony inhibition
  color index
  Colour Index
  complete iridectomy
  confidence interval
  contamination index
  continued insomnia
  continuous infusion

CI — (continued)
  convergence insufficiency
  coronary insufficiency
  corrected count increment
  crystalline insulin
  cumulative incidence
  cytotoxic index
  first cranial nerve
Ci — curie
CIA —
  canine inherited ataxia
  chemiluminescent immunoassay
  chronic idiopathic anhidrosis
  chymotrypsin inhibitor activity
  colony-inhibiting activity
  congenital intestinal aganglionosis
CIAA — competitive insulin autoantibodies
CIAED — collagen-induced autoimmune ear disease
CIB —
  crying-induced bronchospasm
  cytomegalic inclusion bodies
cib. — cibus (Lat.) food
CIBD — chronic inflammatory bowel disease
CIBHA — congenital inclusion-body hemolytic anemia
CIBP — chronic intractable benign pain
CIBPS — chronic intractable benign pain syndrome
CIC —
  cardiac inhibitory center
  cardioinhibitor center
  Certified Infection Control
  chronic inactive cirrhosis
  circulating immune complex
  constant initial concentration
  coronary intensive care
  crisis intervention center
CICA — cervical internal carotid artery
CICE — combined intracapsular cataract extraction

CICU —
    cardiac intensive care unit
    cardiovascular inpatient care
       unit
    coronary intensive care unit
CID —
    cellular immunodeficiency
    Central Institute for the Deaf
    central integrative deficit
    cervical immobilization de-
       vice
    chick infective dose
    combined immunodeficiency
       disease
    cytomegalic inclusion disease
CIDEP — chemically induced dy-
    namic electron polarization
CIDNP — chemically induced dy-
    namic nuclear polarization
CIDP —
    chronic idiopathic polyradicu-
      lopathy
    chronic inflammatory demye-
      linating polyradiculoneu-
      ropathy
CIDS —
    cellular immunodeficiency
      syndrome
    circular intensity differential
      scattering
    continuous insulin delivery
      system
CIE —
    cellulose ion exchange
    countercurrent immunoelec-
      trophoresis
    counterimmunoelectrophore-
      sis
    crossed immunoelectrophore-
      sis
CIEA — continuous infusion, epi-
    dural anesthesia
CIEBM — Committee on the In-
    terplay of Engineering with Bi-
    ology and Medicine
CIE-C — counterimmunoelectro-
    phoresis — colorimetric
CIE-D — counterimmunoelectro-
    phoresis — densitometric

CIEP —
    counterimmunoelectrophore-
      sis
    crossed immunoelectrophore-
      sis
CIF —
    cartilage induction factor
    claims inquiry form
    cloning inhibiting factor
    cloning inhibitory factor
CIFC — Council for the Investiga-
    tion of Fertility Control
CIG —
    cigarette
    cold-insoluble globulin
CIg — intracytoplasmic immuno-
    globulin
cIgM — cytoplasmic immunoglobu-
    lin M
CIH —
    carbohydrate-induced hyper-
      glyceridemia
    Certificate in Industrial
      Health
    children in hospital
CIHD — chronic ischemic heart
    disease
Ci-hr — curie-hour
CIHS — central infantile hypo-
    tonic syndrome
CII —
    Carnegie Interest Inventory
    controlled substance, class
      two
    second cranial nerve
CIIA — common internal iliac ar-
    tery
CIII — third cranial nerve
CIIP — chronic idiopathic intesti-
    nal pseudo-obstruction
CIIS — Cattell Infant Intelligence
    Scale
CIL — Center for Independent
    Living
CIM —
    cimetidine
    cortical induction of move-
      ment

CIM — *(continued)*
cortically induced movement
Cumulated Index Medicus
Ci/ml — curies per milliliter
CIMS —
chemical ionization mass spectrometry
Conflict in Marriage Scale
CIN —
central inhibition
cerebriform intradermal nevus
cervical intraepithelial neoplasia
chronic interstitial nephritis
cinoxacin
C_{in} — inulin clearance
CIN 1 or I — cervical intraepithelial neoplasia, grade 1 [mild dysplasia]
CIN 2 or II — cervical intraepithelial neoplasia, grade 2 [moderate–severe]
CIN 3 or III — cervical intraepithelial neoplasia, grade 3 [severe dysplasia and carcinoma in situ]
CINCA — chronic infantile neurological cutaneous and auricular [syndrome]
CINE —
chemotherapy-induced nausea and emesis
cineangiogram
CIOMS — Council for International Organizations of Medical Sciences
CIOP — chromosally incompetent ovarian failure
CIP —
Carcinogen Information Program
Cardiac Injury Panel
cellular immunocompetence profile
chronic idiopathic polyradiculoneuropathy
chronic inflammatory polyneuropathy

CIP — *(continued)*
chronic intestinal pseudo-obstruction
Collection de l'Institut Pasteur
CIPD —
chronic inflammatory polyneuropathy, demyelinating
chronic intermittent peritoneal dialysis
CIPF — clinical illness-promoting factor
CIPN — chronic inflammatory polyneuropathy
CIPSO — chronic intestinal pseudo-obstruction
cir —
circuit
circular
circumference
circ —
circuit
circular
circulatory
circulation
circumcised
circumcision
circumference
circ & sens — circulation and sensation
circum — circumcision
CIRR — cirrhosis
CIS —
Cancer Information Service
carcinoma in situ
catheter-induced spasm
central inhibitory state
Chemical Information System
clinical information system
CI-S — calculus index, simplified
CiS — cingulate sulcus
cis-DPP — cisplatin
CISP — chronic intractable shoulder pain
CIT —
citrate
combined intermittent therapy

CIT — *(continued)*
conjugated-immunoglobulin
technique
conventional immunosuppressive therapy
conventional insulin therapy
cit — citrate
cit. disp. — *cito dispensetur* (Lat.)
dispense quickly
CIU — chronic idiopathic urticaria
CIV —
Chloriridovirus
common iliac vein
continuous intravenous [infusion]
fourth cranial nerve
CIVII — continuous intravenous
insulin infusion
CIX — ninth cranial nerve
CIXU — constant infusion excretory urogram
CJ — conjunctivitis
CJD — Creutzfeldt-Jakob disease
CJR — centric jaw relationship
CJS — Creutzfeldt-Jakob syndrome
CK —
calf kidney
check
chicken kidney
cholecystokinin
choline kinase
contralateral knee
creatine kinase
cytokinin
CK_1, CK_2, CK_3 — isoenzymes of
creatine kinase
ck —
check(ed)
contralateral knee
CK-BB —
creatine kinase—BB band
isoenzyme of creatine kinase
with brain subunits
CKC — cold-knife conization
CKG —
cardiokymograph
cardiokymography

CK-ISO — creatine kinase isoenzyme
CK-MB — isoenzyme of creatine
kinase with muscle and brain
subunits
CK-MM — isoenzyme of creatine
kinase with muscle subunits
CK-PZ — cholecystokinin-pancreozymin
CKS — classic form of Kaposi's sarcoma
CKW — clockwise
CL —
capacity of the lung
capillary lumen
cardinal ligament
cardiolipin
cell line
center line
centralis lateralis
chemiluminescence
chest and left arm [lead in
electrocardiography]
cholelithiasis
cholesterol-lecithin [test]
chronic leukemia
cirrhosis of liver
clamp lamp
clavicle
clear liquid
clearance
cleft lip
clinical laboratory
clomipramine
cloudy
complex loading
compliance of the lungs
composite lymphoma
confidence level
confidence limit
contact lens
continence line
corpus luteum
cricoid lamina
criterion level
critical list
cutis laxa
cycle length

CL — *(continued)*
cytotoxic lymphocyte
lung compliance
C-L — consultation-liaison
CL1–CL5 — Papanicolaou classes
1 through 5
C_L —
compliance of the lungs
constant domain of L chain
constant region
Cl —
chloride
chlorine
clavicle
clear
clinic
clonus
Clostridium
closure
colistin
cl —
centiliter
clarified
clavicle
clean
clear
cleft
clinic
clinical
clonus
closure
clotting
cloudy
corpus luteum
CLA —
Certified Laboratory Assistant
cervicolinguoaxial
community living arrange-
ments
contralateral local anesthesia
cyclic lysine anhydride
CLA(ASCP) — Clinical Laboratory Assistant (American Society of Clinical Pathologists)
ClAc — chloroacetyl
CLAH — congenital lipoid adrenal hyperplasia
C Lam — cervical laminectomy

CLAS — congenital localized absence of skin
class — classification
classif — classification
clav — clavicle
CLB —
chlorambucil
curvilinear body
CLBBB — complete left bundle
branch block
CLBP — chronic low back pain
CLC —
Charcot-Leyden crystal
Clerc-Levy-Critesco [syn-
drome]
cork, leather, and celastic [or-
thotic]
ClC·CHO — chloral
ClCN — cyanogen chloride
CL/CP — cleft lip/cleft palate
CLD —
central language disorder
chronic liver disease
chronic lung disease
congenital limb deficiency
crystal ligand field
cld —
cleared
colored
CLDH — choline dehydrogenase
CLDM — clindamycin
cldy — cloudy
CLE —
centrilobular emphysema
continuous lumbar epidural
[anesthesia]
CLED — cystine-lactose electro-
lyte-deficient [agar]
CLF —
cardiolipin fluorescent [anti-
body]
cholesterol-lecithin flocculation
CLH —
chronic lobular hepatitis
corpus luteum hormone
cutaneous lymphoid hyperplasia

CLI — corpus luteum insufficiency

CLIA — Clinical Laboratories Improvement Act

CLIF —
cloning inhibitory factor
Crithidia luciliae immunofluorescence

clin —
clinic
clinical

Clin Path — clinical pathology

Clin Proc — clinical procedure(s)

CLINPROT — Clinical Cancer Protocols

CLIP —
cerebral lipidosis
corticotropin-like intermediate lobe peptide

CLL —
cholesterol-lowering lipid
chronic lymphatic leukemia
chronic lymphocytic leukemia
cow lung lavage

CLLE — columnar-lined lower esophagus

cl liq — clear liquid

CL LYS — clot lysis

CLMA — Clinical Laboratory Management Association

CLML — Current List of Medical Literature

CLMN — complete lower motor neuron [lesion]

clmp — clumped

CLMV — cauliflower mosaic virus

CLN — computer liaison nurse

CLO — cod liver oil

clo — "clothing" (a unit of thermal insulation)

CLOF — clofibrate

CLON — clonidine

Clon — *Clonorchis*

Clostr — *Clostridium*

CLOT R — clot retraction

CLP —
chymotrypsin-like protein
cleft lip with cleft palate
cycle length, paced

CL(P) — cleft lip without cleft palate

CL&P — cleft lip and palate

ClP — clinical pathology

Clpal — cleft palate

CLR — chloride test

CLRO — community leave for reorientation

CLS —
Clinical Laboratory Scientist
Coffin-Lowry syndrome
Cornelia de Lange syndrome

CLSE — calf lung surfactant extract

CLSH — corpus luteum–stimulating hormone

CLSL — chronic lymphosarcomatous leukemia

CLSP — clinical laboratory specialist

CLT —
Certified Laboratory Technician
chronic lymphocytic thyroiditis
clinical laboratory technician
clinical laboratory technologist
clot-lysis time
clotted
clotting time
total lung compliance

CL_{TB} — total body clearance

CLT(NCA) — Laboratory Technician Certified by the National Certification Agency for Medical Laboratory Personnel

CLV —
cassava latent virus
constant linear velocity

CL VOID — clean voided specimen [urine]

CLX — cloxacillin

CLZ — clozapine

CM —
California mastitis [test]
calmodulin
capreomycin

CM — (*continued*)
carboxymethyl
cardiac monitor
cardiac muscle
cardiomyopathy
carpometacarpal
Caucasian male
causa mortis (Lat.) cause of
death
cavernous malformation
cell membrane
center of mass
centrum medianum
cerebral malaria
cerebral mantle
cervical mucosa
cervical mucus
chemotactic migration
Chick-Martin [coefficient]
Chirurgiae Magister (Lat.) Master in Surgery
chloroquine-mepacrine
chondromalacia
chopped meat [medium]
chylomicron
circular muscle
circulating monocyte
circumferential measurement
clindamycin
clinical medicine
clinical modification
coccidioidal meningitis
cochlear microphonic(s)
common migraine
competing message
complete medium
complications
conditioned medium
congenital malformation
congestive myocardiopathy
continuous murmur
contrast medium
copulatory mechanism
costal margin
cow's milk
crête manche (Fr.) narrow-diameter endosseous screw implant

CM — (*continued*)
culture medium
cystic mesothelioma
cytometry
cytoplasmic membrane
C/M — counts per minute
C&M — cocaine and morphine
Cm —
capreomycin
curium
maximum clearance
C_m — maximum clearance
cM — centimorgan
cm —
centimeter
costal margin
c.m. — *cras mane* (Lat.) tomorrow morning
cm^2 — square centimeter
cm^3 — cubic centimeter
CMA —
Canadian Medical Association
Candida metabolic antigen
Certified Medical Assistant
chronic metabolic acidosis
compound myopic astigmatism
cow's milk allergy
cultured macrophages
CMAF — centrifuged microaggregate filter
CMAmg — corticomedial amygdaloid [nucleus]
CMAP —
compound motor action potential
compound muscle action potential
Cmax — maximum concentration
C_{max} — maximum concentration
CMB —
carbolic methylene blue
Central Midwives' Board
chloromercuribenzoate
CMBBT — cervical mucus basal body temperature

CMC —
  carboxymethylcellulose
  care management continuity
  carpometacarpal
  cell-mediated cytolysis
  cell-mediated cytotoxicity
  chloramphenicol
  Chloromycetin
  chronic mucocutaneous candidiasis
  critical micelle concentration
CMCC — chronic mucocutaneous candidiasis
CMCt — care management continuity [across settings]
CMD —
  cartilage matrix deficiency
  cerebromacular degeneration
  childhood muscular dystrophy
  comparative mean dose
  congenital muscular dystrophy
  count median diameter
  cytomegalic disease
CME —
  cervical mediastinal exploration
  cervical mucous extract
  continuing medical education
  Council on Medical Education
  crude marijuana extract
  cystic macular edema
  cystoid macular edema
CMER — current medical evidence of record
CMF —
  calcium-magnesium free
  catabolite modular factor
  chondromyxoid fibroma
  Christian Medical Fellowship
  cold mitten fraction
  cortical magnification factor
  craniomandibulofacial
CMFE — calcium and magnesium–free plus ethylenediaminetetraacetic acid
CMFT — cardiolipin microflocculation test

CMG —
  canine myasthenia gravis
  chopped meat–glucose [medium]
  congenital myasthenia gravis
  cyanmethemoglobin
  cystometrogram
  cystometrography
CMGN — chronic membranous glomerulonephritis
CMGS — chopped meat-glucose-starch [medium]
CMGT — chromosome-mediated gene transfer
CMH — congenital malformation of the heart
CMHC — community mental health center
CMHN — Community Mental Health Nurse
cm H_2O — centimeters of water [cuff pressure]
CMI —
  carbohydrate metabolism index
  care management integration
  cell-mediated immunity
  cell multiplication inhibition
  chronically mentally ill
  chronic mesenteric ischemia
  circulating microemboli index
  colonic motility index
  Commonwealth Mycological Institute
  computer-managed instruction
  Cornell Medical Index
CMID — cytomegalic inclusion disease
c/min — cycles per minute
CMIR — cell-mediated immune response
CMIT — Current Medical Information and Terminology
CMJ —
  carpometacarpal joint
  Committee on Medical Journalism

CMK —
    chloromethyl ketone
    congenital multicystic kidney
CML —
    cell-mediated lymphocyto-
        toxicity
    cell-mediated lympholysis
    cell-mediated lysis
    chronic myelocytic leukemia
    chronic myelogenous leuke-
        mia
    chronic myeloid leukemia
    cross midline
    count median length
CMM —
    cell-mediated mutagenesis
    cutaneous malignant mela-
        noma
cmm — cubic millimeter
cm/m^2 — centimeters per square
    meter
CMME — chloromethyl methyl
    ether
CMML — chronic myelomono-
    cytic leukemia
CMMoL — chronic myelomono-
    cytic leukemia
CMMS — Columbia Mental Matu-
    rity Scale
CMMT — Columbia Mental Ma-
    turity Test
CMN —
    caudal mediastinal node
    cystic medial necrosis
CMNA — complement-mediated
    neutrophil activation
CMN-AA — cystic medial necro-
    sis of ascending aorta
CMO —
    calculated mean organism
    cardiac minute output
    card made out
    Chief Medical Officer
    comfort measures only
    corticosterone methyloxidase
cMO — centimorgan
CMoL —
    chronic monoblastic leukemia

CMoL — (continued)
    chronic monocytic leukemia
CMOMC — cell meeting our mor-
    phologic criteria
CMOR — craniomandibular
    orthopedic repositioning
    [device]
CMOS — complementary metal-
    oxide semiconductor [logic]
CMP —
    cardiomyopathy
    cervical mucus penetration
    chondromalacia patellae
    competitive medical plan
    comprehensive medical plan
    cytidine monophosphate
    cytidine-5'-phosphate
CMPD — chronic myeloprolifera-
    tive disorder
cmp'd — compound
CMP-FX — complement fixation
CMPGN — chronic membrano-
    proliferative glomerulonephri-
    tis
cmps — centimeters per second
CMPT — cervical mucus penetra-
    tion test
CMR —
    carpometacarpal ratio
    cerebral metabolic rate
    Certified Medical Representa-
        tive
    chief medical resident
    common mode rejection
    crude mortality ratio
CMRG — cerebral metabolic rate
    of glucose
CMRglu — cerebral metabolic rate
    of glucose
CMRL — cerebral metabolic rate
    of lactate
CMRNG — chromosomally medi-
    ated resistant *Neisseria gonor-
    rhoeal*
CMRO — cerebral metabolic rate
    of oxygen
CMRO$_2$ — cerebral metabolic rate
    of oxygen

CMRR — common mode rejection ratio

CMS —
cardiomediastinal silhouette
central material section
central material supply
cervical mucous solution
Christian Medical Society
chromosome modification site
chronic myelodysplastic syndrome
circulation, motion, and sensation
circulation, muscle sensation
clean, midstream [urine]
click murmur syndrome
clofibrate-induced muscular syndrome
Clyde Mood Scale
complement-mediated solubility
Council of Medical Staffs

c.m.s. — *cras mane sumendus* (Lat.) to be taken tomorrow morning

cm/s — centimeters per second

cm/sec — centimeters per second

CMSS —
circulation, motor ability, sensation, and swelling
Council of Medical Specialty Societies

CMSUA — clean, midstream urinalysis

CMT —
California mastitis test
cancer multistep therapy
catechol-O-methyltransferase
Certified Medical Transcriptionist
cervical motion tenderness
Charcot-Marie-Tooth [syndrome]
chronic motor tic
circus movement tachycardia
complex motor test
continuous memory test
Council on Medical Television

CMT — (*continued*)
current medical terminology

CMTC — cutis marmorata telangiectatica congenita

CMTD — Charcot-Marie-Tooth disease

CMTS — Charcot-Marie-Tooth syndrome

CMU —
cardiac monitoring urea
chlorophenyldimethylurea
complex motor unit

CMUA — continuous motor unit activity

CMV —
continuous mechanical ventilation
controlled mechanical ventilation
conventional mechanical ventilation
cool mist vaporizer
cucumber mosaic virus
cytomegalic (inclusion) virus
cytomegalovirus

CMVIG — cytomegalovirus immune globulin

CMV-MN — cytomegaloviral mononucleosis

CMVS — culture midvoid specimen

CMX — cefmenoxime

CMZ — carbamazepine

CN —
caudate nucleus
cellulose nitrate
charge nurse
child nutrition
chloroacetophenone
clinical nursing
cochlear nucleus
congenital nephrosis
congenital nystagmus
cranial nerve
Crigler-Najjar [syndrome]
cyanide anion
cyanogen
cyanosis neonatorum

C/N —
  carbon/nitrogen [ratio]
  carrier/noise [ratio]
  contrast/noise [ratio]
CNII-XII — cranial nerves II
  through XII
Cn —
  color naming
  cyanide
c.n. — *cras nocte* (Lat.) tomorrow
  night
CNA —
  calcium nutrient agar
  Canadian Nurses' Association
  chart not available
CNAF — chronic nonvalvular
  atrial fibrillation
CNAG — chronic narrow angle
  glaucoma
CNAP —
  cochlear nucleus action poten-
    tial
  compound nerve action po-
    tential
CNB — cutting needle biopsy
CNBr — cyanogen bromide
CNC —
  clear, no creamy [layer]
  Critical Nursing Conference
CNCbl — cyanocobalamin
CND —
  canned
  cannot determine
CNDC —
  chronic nonspecific diarrhea
    of childhood
  chronic nonsuppurative de-
    structive cholangitis
CNE —
  chronic nervous exhaustion
  concentric needle electrode
  could not establish
CNEMG — concentric needle
  electromyography
CNES — chronic nervous exhaustion syndrome
CNF —
  chronic nodular fibrositis

CNF — (*continued*)
  congenital nephrotic (syn-
    drome) of the Finnish
    [type]
CNH —
  central neurogenic hyperpnea
  central neurogenic hyperven-
    tilation
  community nursing home
  contract nursing home
CNHD — congenital nonsphero-
  cytic hemolytic disease
CNHI — Committee for National
  Health Insurance
CNI —
  center of nuclear imaging
  chronic nerve irritation
CNK — cortical necrosis of kidneys
CNL —
  cardiolipin natural lecithin
  chronic neutrophilic leukemia
CNM —
  Certified Nurse-Midwife
  computerized nuclear morpho-
    metry
CNMT — Certified Nuclear Medicine Technologist
CNN — congenital nevocytic nevus
CNOH — cyanic acid
CNOR — Certified Nurse, Op-
  erating Room
CNP —
  community nurse practitioner
  continuous negative pressure
  cranial nerve palsy
  2′,3′-cyclic nucleotide 3′-
    phosphodiesterase
CNPase — 2′,3′-cyclic nucleotide
  3′-phosphohydrolase
CNPV — continuous negative
  pressure ventilation
CNR —
  Civil Nursing Reserve
  Council of National Represen-
    tatives [of International
    Council of Nurses]

CNRN — Certified Neuroscience Registered Nurse

CNRS — citrated normal rabbit serum

CNRT — corrected sinus node recovery time

CNS —
central nervous system
Chief, Nursing Services
clinical nurse specialist
coagulase-negative staphylo-cocci
computerized notation system
congenital nephrotic syn-drome
cyanide sulfonate (sulfocya-nate)

c.n.s. — *cras nocte sumendus* (Lat.) to be taken tomorrow night

CNSD — chronic nonspecific diar-rhea

CNSHA — congenital nonsphero-cytic hemolytic anemia

CNS-L — central nervous system leukemia

CNSLD — chronic nonspecific lung disease

CNSN — Certified Nutrition Sup-port Nurse

CNT —
could not test
current night terrors

CNTF — ciliary neurotrophic fac-tor

CNV —
choroidal neovascularization
colistimethate, nystatin, van-comycin
conative negative variation
contingent negative variation
cutaneous necrotizing vasculi-tis

CO —
candidal onychomycosis
carbon monoxide
cardiac output
castor oil
casualty officer

CO — *(continued)*
centric occlusion
cervical orthosis
cervicoaxial
choline oxidase
coccygeal
coenzyme
community organization
compound
control
corneal opacity
corpus (referring to uterus)
crossover

C/O —
check out
complains of
under care of

CO_2 — carbon dioxide

$C_{\bar{v}}O_2$ — mixed venous oxygen con-tent

Co —
cobalt
coccygeal
coenzyme

Co I — coenzyme I

Co II — coenzyme II

^{57}Co — cobalt isotope

Co 57 — cobalt isotope

^{60}Co — cobalt isotope

Co 60 — cobalt isotope

co — cutoff

co. — *compositus* (Lat.) com-pounded, a compound

COA —
calculated opening area
Canadian Ophthalmological Association
Canadian Orthopaedic Asso-ciation
cervico-oculo-acusticus [syn-drome]
condition on admission

CoA —
coarctation of the aorta
coenzyme A

COAD —
chronic obstructive airway dis-ease

COAD — *(continued)*
 chronic obstructive arterial disease
COAG — chronic open-angle glaucoma
coag —
 coagulate
 coagulation
COAG PD — coagulation profile — diagnosis
COAG PP — coagulation profile — presurgery
COAG SC — coagulation screen
coarc — coarctation (of aorta)
CoA SH — uncombined coenzyme A
CoA-SPC — coenzyme A-synthesizing protein complex
COAT — Children's Orientation and Amnesia Test
COB —
 chronic obstructive bronchitis
 coordination of benefits
coban — cohesive bandage
COBOL — common business-oriented language
COBRA — Consolidated Omnibus Budget Reconciliation Act
COBS —
 cesarean-obtained barrier-sustained [animals]
 chronic organic brain syndrome
COBT — chronic obstruction of the biliary tract
COC —
 calcifying odontogenic cyst
 cathodal opening clonus
 cathodal opening contraction
 coccygeal
 combination oral contraceptive
coc — coccygeal
Cocci — coccidioidomycosis
cochl. — *cochleare* (Lat.) a spoonful
cochl. amp. — *cochleare amplum* (Lat.) a heaping spoonful

cochl. mag. — *cochleare magnum* (Lat.) a tablespoonful
cochl. med. — *cochleare medium* (Lat.) a dessert spoonful
cochl. mod. — *cochleare modicum* (Lat.) a dessert spoonful
cochl. parv. — *cochleare parvus* (Lat.) a teaspoonful
COCI — Consortium on Chemical Information
COCl — cathodal opening clonus
COCM — congestive cardiomyopathy
coct. — *coctio* (Lat.) boiling
COD —
 cause of death
 chemical oxygen demand
 codeine
 condition on discharge
cod — codeine
CODATA — Committee on Data for Science and Technology
COD-MD — cerebro-ocular dysplasia — muscular dystrophy [syndrome]
COE — court-ordered examination
coeff — coefficient
COEPS —
 cortically originating extrapyramidal symptoms
 cortically originating extrapyramidal system
COF — cutoff frequency
CoF —
 cobra (venom) factor
 cofactor
C of A — coarctation of aorta
COFS — cerebro-oculofacial-skeletal [syndrome]
COG —
 Central Oncology Group
 clinical obstetrics and gynecology
 cognitive [function tests]
CoGME — Council on Graduate Medical Education
COGN — cognition
COGTT — cortisone-primed oral glucose tolerance test

COH — carbohydrate
COHB — carboxyhemoglobin
C$_4$O$_6$H$_4$NaK — potassium sodium tartrate
COHSE — Confederation of Health Service Employees
COI — Central Obesity Index
CoI — coenzyme I
COIF — congenital onychodysplasia of the index finger
CoII — coenzyme II
COL —
    collection
    collagen
    colony
    color
    colored
    column
    cost of living
Col — colicin
col. — *cola* (Lat.) strain
colat. — *colatus* (Lat.) strained
COLD — chronic obstructive lung disease
COLD A — cold agglutinin titer
cold agg — cold agglutinin titer
colet. — *coletur* (Lat.) let it be strained
COLL —
    collateral
    collect
    collection
    collective
    college
    colloidal
collat — collateral
collun. — *collunarium* (Lat.) nosewash
collut. — *collutorium* (Lat.) mouthwash
coll vol — collective volume
collyr. — *collyrium* (Lat.) eyewash
col/ml — colonies per milliliter
color. — *coloretur* (Lat.) let it be colored
color — colorimetry
colp —
    colporrhaphy

colp — *(continued)*
    colposcopy
colpo —
    colporrhaphy
    colposcopy
COM —
    chronic otitis media
    College of Osteopathic Medicine
    computer-output on microfilm
com —
    comminuted
    commitment
COMA — Certified Ophthalmic Medical Assistant
comb —
    combination
    combine
COMC — carboxymethylcellulose
comf — comfortable
com fix — complement fixation
comm —
    commission
    commissioner
    committee
    communicable
commun — communicable
commun dis — communicable disease
COMP —
    complication
    compound
comp —
    comparable
    comparative
    compare
    compensated
    compensation
    complaint
    complete
    composition
    compound
    compounded
    comprehension
    compress
    compression
    computer
comp. — *compositus* (Lat.) compound

compl —
>   complaint
>   complement
>   complete
>   completed
>   completion
>   complicated
>   complication

complic —
>   complicated
>   complication

compn — composition

compr — compression

COMS —
>   cerebro-oculomuscular syndrome
>   chronic organic mental syndrome

COMT — catechol-O-methyltransferase

COMTRAC — computer-based (case) tracing

COMUL — complement fixation murine leukosis [test]

CON — certificate of need

Con — concanavalin

con. — *contra* (Lat.) against

ConA — concanavalin A

Con A-HRP — concanavalin A–horseradish peroxidase

C-onc — cellular oncogene

conc. —
>   concentrate
>   concentrated
>   concentration

concis. — *concisus* (Lat.) cut

cond —
>   condensed
>   condensation
>   condition
>   conditional
>   conditioned
>   conductivity
>   conductor

cond ref — conditioned reflex

cond resp — conditioned response

conf —
>   conference

conf — (*continued*)
>   confined
>   confinement
>   confirmed
>   confusion

cong —
>   congenital
>   congested, congestion
>   congress

cong. — *congius* (Lat.) gallon

congr — congruent

$CO(NH_2)_2$ — urea

coniz — conization

conj —
>   conjunctiva
>   conjunctival

conjug —
>   conjugated
>   conjugation

cons. — *conserva* (Lat.) keep

cons —
>   conservation
>   conservative
>   conserve

consperg. — *consperge* (Lat.) dust, sprinkle

const — constant

constit —
>   constituent
>   constitution

consult —
>   consultant
>   consultation

cont. —
>   containing
>   contains
>   contents
>   continuation
>   continue
>   continuous
>   *contra* (Lat.) against
>   contusion
>   *contusus* (Lat.) bruised

contag —
>   contagion
>   contagious

conter. — *contere* (Lat.) rub together

contin. — *continuetur* (Lat.) let it be continued

contr —
contracted
contraction

contra — contraindicated

contralat — contralateral

cont. rem. — *continuetur remedium* (Lat.) let the medicine be continued

contrib — contributory

contrit. — *contritus* (Lat.) broken down

contrx — contraction

contus. — *contusus* (Lat.) bruised

conv —
convalescence
convalescent
convalescing
conventional [rat]
convergence
convergent
convulsions
convulsive

converg —
convergence
convergent

CONV HOSP — convalescent hospital

conv strab — convergent strabismus

COOD — chronic obstructive outflow disease

COOP — cooperative

coord —
coordinated
coordination

COP —
capillary osmotic pressure
change of plaster
cicatricial ocular pemphigoid
coefficient of performance
colloid oncotic pressure
colloid osmotic pressure

COPA — Council on Postsecondary Accreditation

COPC — community-oriented primary care

COPD — chronic obstructive pulmonary disease

COPE — chronic obstructive pulmonary emphysema

COPI — California Occupational Preference Inventory

COP_i — colloid osmotic pressure in interstitial fluid

COP_p — colloid osmotic pressure in plasma

COPRO —
coproporphyria
coproporphyrin

CoQ — coenzyme Q

coq. — *coque* (Lat.) boil

coq. in s. a. — *coque in sufficiente aqua* [Lat.] boil in sufficient water

coq. s. a. — *coque secundum artem* (Lat.) boil properly

coq. simul — *coque simul* (Lat.) boil together

COR —
cardiac output recorder
comprehensive outpatient rehabilitation [facility]
conditioned orientation reflex
consensual ophthalmotonic reaction
coroner
corpus
corrosion·
corrosive
cortisone
cortex
custodian of records

CoR — Congo red

cor —
coronary
corrected
correction

cor. — *corpus* (Lat.) body

CORA — conditioned orientation reflex audiometry

CORD —
chronic obstructive respiratory disease
Commissioned Officer Residency Deferment

corr —
   corrected
   correspondence
   corresponding
CORT —
   Certified Operating Room
      Technician
   corticosterone
Cort —
   cortex
   cortical
cort. — *cortex* (Lat.) bark
CORTIS — cortisol
COS —
   Canadian Ophthalmological
      Society
   cheiro-oral syndrome
   chief of staff
   Clinical Orthopaedic Society
   clinically observed seizures
cos — change of shift
COSATI — Committee on Scientific and Technical Information
COSMIS — Computer System for Medical Information Systems
COSTAR — Computer-stored Ambulatory Record
COSTEP — Commissioned Officer Student Training and Extern Program
COT —
   cathodal opening tetanus
   colony overlay test
   content of thought
   continuous oxygen therapy
   contralateral optic tectum
   critical off-time
CO_2T — total carbon dioxide content
COTA — Certified Occupational Therapy Assistant
COTD — cardiac output by thermodilution
COTe — cathodal opening tetanus
COTH — Council of Teaching Hospitals
COTRANS — Coordinated Transfer Application System

COTX — cast off, take x-ray
COU — cardiac observation unit
coul — coulomb
COV — cross-over value
COVESDEM — costovertebral segmentation defect with mesomelia [syndrome]
CoVF — cobra venom factor
COWAT — Controlled Oral Word Association Test
COWS — cold to opposite and warm to same side
COX —
   cast-off x-ray
   coxsackievirus
   cytochrome C oxidase
CP —
   C peptide
   candle power
   capillary pressure
   carbamoyl phosphate
   cardiac pacing
   cardiac performance
   cardiac pool
   cardiopulmonary
   cardiopulmonary performance
   caudate putamen
   cell passage
   central pit
   centric position
   cerebellopontine
   cerebral palsy
   certified prosthetist
   ceruloplasmin
   cervical probe
   chemically pure
   chest pain
   child psychiatry
   child psychology
   chloramphenicol
   chloropurine
   chloroquine-primaquine
   chondrodysplasia punctata
   chondromalacia patellae
   chronic pain
   chronic pancreatitis
   chronic polyarthritis
   chronic pyelonephritis

CP — (continued)
  cicatricial pemphigoid
  circular polarization
  cleft palate
  clinical pathology
  clock pulse
  closing pressure
  clottable protein
  cochlear potential
  code of practice
  cold pressor
  color perception
  combination product
  combining power
  compensated base
  complete physical
  compound
  compressed
  congenital porphyria
  constant pressure
  coproporphyria
  coproporphyrin
  cor pulmonale
  coracoid process
  cortical plate
  costal plaque
  creatine phosphate
  creatine phosphokinase
  cross-linked protein
  crude protein
  current practice
  cyclophosphamide
  cystosarcoma phyllodes
  cytosol protein
C/P —
  cardiopulmonary
  cholesterol-phospholipid [ratio]
C&P —
  compensation and pension
  complete and pain-free [range of motion]
  cytoscopy and pyelography
Cp —
  ceruloplasmin
  chickenpox
  Corynebacterium parvum
  peak concentration

Cp — (continued)
  phosphate clearance
C_p —
  constant pressure
  phosphate clearance
cp —
  candle-power
  centipoise
  chemically pure
  compare
c_p — constant pressure
CPA —
  Canadian Psychiatric Association
  carboxypeptidase A
  cardiophrenic angle
  cardiopulmonary arrest
  carotid phonoangiography
  carotid photoangiography
  cerebellar-pontine angle
  chlorophenylalanine
  chronic pyrophosphate arthropathy
  circulating platelet aggregate
  complement proactivator
  costophrenic angle
  cyclophosphamide
  cyproterone acetate
C3PA — complement-3 proactivator
C3PAse — complement-3 proactivator convertase
CPAF — chlorpropamide-alcohol flushing
Cpah — *para*-aminohippuric acid clearance
C_{pah} — *para*-aminohippurate clearance
CPAI — central principal axis of inertia
CPAN — Certified Post-anesthesia Nurse
CPA/OPG — carotid phonoangiography/oculoplethysmography
CPAP — continuous positive airway pressure
c. parvum — *cochleare parvum* (Lat.) teaspoonful

CPB —
    cardiopulmonary bypass
    cetylpyridinium bromide
    competitive protein binding
    [assay]
CPBA — competitive protein-
    binding analysis
CPBS — cardiopulmonary bypass
    surgery
CPBV — cardiopulmonary blood
    volume
CPC —
    central posterior curve
    cerebellar Purkinje cell
    cerebral palsy clinic
    cetylpyridinium chloride
    chronic passive congestion
    circumferential pneumatic
      compression
    clinicopathological confer-
      ence
    committed progenitor cell
CPCL — congenital pulmonary
    cystic lymphangiectasia
CPCN — capitated primary care
    network
CPCP — chronic progressive coc-
    cidioidal pneumonitis
CPCR — cardiopulmonary-
    cerebral resuscitation
CPCS —
    circumferential pneumatic
      compression suit
    clinical pharmacokinetics con-
      sulting service
CPD —
    calcium pyrophosphate deposi-
      tion
    calcium pyrophosphate dihy-
      drate
    cephalopelvic disproportion
    childhood polycystic disease
    chorioretinopathy and pitu-
      itary dysfunction
    chronic peritoneal dialysis
    chronic protein deprivation
    citrate phosphate dextrose
    compound

CPD — (continued)
    congenital polycystic disease
    contact potential difference
    contagious pustular dermatitis
    critical point drying
    cyclopentadiene
cpd —
    compound
    cycles per degree
CPDA-1 — citrate phosphate dex-
    trose adenine
CPDD —
    calcium pyrophosphate deposi-
      tion disease
    cis-platinum-diammine-
      dichloride
cpd E — compound E
cpd F — compound F
CPDL — cumulative population
    doubling level
CPDX — cefpodoxime
CPDX-PR — cefpodoxime proxetil
CPE —
    cardiac pulmonary edema
    cardiogenic pulmonary edema
    chronic pulmonary emphy-
      sema
    compensation, pension, and
      education
    complete physical examina-
      tion
    complex partial epilepsy
    corona-penetrating enzyme
    cytopathic effect
    cytopathogenic effect
CPed — Certified Pedorthist
CPEHS — Consumer Protection
    and Environmental Health
    Service
CPEO — chronic progressive exter-
    nal ophthalmoplegia
CPF —
    clot-promoting factor
    contraction peak force
CP&FD — cephalopelvic distor-
    tion and fetal distress
CPG —
    capillary blood gases

CPG — *(continued)*
   cardiopneumographic [recording]
   carotid phonoangiogram
   coproporphyrinogen
CPGN —
   chronic progressive glomerulonephritis
   chronic proliferative glomerulonephritis
CPH —
   Certificate in Public Health
   chronic paroxysmal hemicrania
   chronic persistent hepatitis
   chronic primary headache
CPH 5 — Cutter protein hydrolysate 5% in water
CPHA — Committee on Professional and Hospital Activities
CPHA-PAS — Commission on Professional and Hospital Activities — Professional Activity Study
CPI —
   California Personality Inventory
   Cancer Potential Index
   congenital palatopharyngeal incompetence
   constitutional psychopathic inferiority
   coronary prognostic index
   cysteine proteinase inhibitor
CPIB — chlorophenoxyisobutyrate
CPID — chronic pelvic inflammatory disease
CPIP —
   chronic pulmonary insufficiency of prematurity
   common peak-developed isovolumetric pressure
CPIR — cephalic-phase insulin release
CPK — creatine phosphokinase
CPKD — childhood polycystic kidney disease
CPKI — creatinine phosphokinase isoenzyme(s)

CPKISO — creatinine phosphokinase isoenzyme(s)
CPL —
   caprine placental lactogen
   conditioned pitch level
   congenital pulmonary lymphangiectasia
C/PL — cholesterol/phospholipid [ratio]
cpl —
   complete
   completed
CPLM — cysteine-peptone-liver (infusion) medium
CPM —
   central pontine myelinosis
   chlorpheniramine maleate
   clinical practice model
   cognitive-perceptual-motor
   colored progressive matrices
   continue present management
   continuous passive motion
   counts per minute
   cyclophosphamide
cpm —
   counts per minute
   cycles per minute
CPmax — peak (maximum) serum concentration
CPMDI — computerized pharmacokinetic model — driven (drug) infusion
CPMG — Carr-Purcell-Meiboom-Gill (spin-echo [technique])
CPMI — central principal moments of inertia
CP min — trough (minimum) serum concentration
CPMM — constant passive motion machine
CPMP — computer-patient management problems
CPMS —
   chronic progressive multiple sclerosis
   Clozaril patient management system
CPMV — cowpox mosaic virus

CPN —
  carboxypeptidase N
  chronic polyneuropathy
  chronic pyelonephritis
CPNM — corrected perinatal mortality
CPNP/A — Certified Pediatric Nurse Practitioner/Associate
CPP —
  cancer proneness phenotype
  canine pancreatic polypeptide
  carboxy terminus of propressophysin
  cerebral perfusion pressure
  chronic pigmented purpura
  Collaborative Perinatal Project
  cryoprecipitate
  cyclopentenophenanthrene
  DL-2[3-(2'-chlorophenoxy)-phenyl] propionic [acid]
CPPB —
  constant positive-pressure breathing
  continuous positive-pressure breathing
CPPD —
  calcium pyrophosphate deposition
  calcium pyrophosphate dihydrate
  chest percussion and postural drainage
  cisplatin
CP&PD — chest percussion and postural drainage
CPPT — coronary primary prevention trial
CPPV — continuous positive-pressure ventilation
CPR —
  cardiac and pulmonary rehabilitation
  cardiac pulmonary reserve
  cardiopulmonary reserve
  cardiopulmonary resuscitation
  centripetal rub
  cerebral cortex perfusion rate

CPR — (continued)
  chlorophenyl red
  cochleopalpebral reflex
  cortisol production rate
  cumulative patency rate
  customary, prevailing, and reasonable [rate]
c-PR — cyclopropyl
CPRAM — controlled partial rebreathing anesthesia method
CPRCA — constitutional pure red cell aplasia
CPRD — Committee on Prosthetics Research and Development
CPRS —
  Children's Psychiatric Rating Scale
  Comprehensive Psychiatric Rating Scale
  Comprehensive Psychopathological Rating Scale
CPS —
  carbamyl phosphate synthetase
  cardioplegic perfusion solution
  cardiopulmonary support
  centipoise
  cervical pain syndrome
  characters per second
  chest pain syndrome
  Child Personality Scale
  Child Protective Services
  chloroquine, pyrimethamine, and sulfisoxazole
  chronic prostatitis syndrome
  clinical performance score
  Clinical Pharmacy Services
  clinical pharmacokinetics service
  coagulase-positive *Staphylococcus*
  complex partial seizures
  constitutional psychopathic state
  contagious pustular stomatitis
  C-polysaccharide

CPS — (*continued*)
    cumulative probability of success
    current population survey
cps —
    counts per second
    cycles per second
CPSC —
    congenital paucity of secondary synaptic clefts [syndrome]
    Consumer Products Safety Commission
CPSP — central poststroke pain
CPT —
    carnitine palmityl transferase
    carotid pulse tracing
    chest physiotherapy
    child protection team
    choline phosphotransferase
    ciliary particle transport
    clinical pharmacokinetics team
    cold pressor test
    cold pressure test
    combining power test
    concentration performance test
    continuous performance task
    continuous performance test
    continuous primary tests
    Current Procedural Terminology
CPTH —
    chronic post-traumatic headache
    C-terminal parathyroid hormone
CPTN — culture-positive toxin-negative
CPTP — culture-positive toxin-positive
CPTX — chronic parathyroidectomy
CPU —
    caudate putamen
    central processing unit
CPUE — chest pain of unknown etiology

CPV —
    canine parvovirus
    cytoplasmic polyhidrosis virus
CPVD — congenital polyvalvular disease
CPX — complete physical examination
CPZ —
    cefoperazone
    chlorpromazine
    Compazine
CQ —
    chloroquine
    chloroquine-quinine
    circadian quotient
    conceptual quotient
CQA — concurrent quality assurance
CQI — continuous quality improvement
CQM — chloroquine mustard
CQUCC — Commission on Quantities and Units in Clinical Chemistry
CR —
    calcification rate
    calculus removal
    calculus removed
    calorie-restricted
    cardiac rehabilitation
    cardiac resuscitation
    cardiac rhythm
    cardiorespiratory
    cardiorrhexis
    caries-resistant
    cartilage residue
    case report
    cathode ray
    central ray
    centric relation
    chest and right arm [lead in electrocardiography]
    chest roentgenogram
    chest roentgenography
    chief resident
    child-resistant [bottle top]
    chloride
    choice reaction

CR — (continued)
  chromium
  chronic rejection
  clinical record
  clinical research
  closed reduction
  clot retraction
  coefficient (of fat) retention
  colon resection
  colonization resistance
  colony-reared [animal]
  colorectal
  complement receptor
  complete recanalization
  complete remission
  complete responders
  complete response
  conditioned reflex
  conditioned response
  congenital rubella
  Congo red
  contact record
  continuous reinforcement
  controlled reflex
  controlled release
  controlled respiration
  controlled response
  conversion ratio
  cooling rate
  correct response
  corticoresistant
  cranial
  creamed
  creatinine
  cremaster reflex
  cresyl red
  critical ratio
  crown-rump [measurement]
C&R —
  cardiac and respiratory
  convalescence and rehabilitation
  cystoscopy and retrograde
CR$_1$ — first cranial nerve
CR$_2$ — second cranial nerve
CR3 — complement receptor
  type 3
Cr —
  chromium

Cr — (continued)
  cranial
  cranium
  cream
  creatinine
  crown
^{51}Cr — chromium isotope
Cr 51 — chromium isotope
cr. — cras (Lat.) tomorrow
CRA —
  central retinal artery
  Chinese restaurant asthma
  chronic rheumatoid arthritis
  colorectal adenocarcinoma
  colorectal anastomosis
  constant relative alkalinity
CRABP — cellular retinoic acid-
  binding protein
CRAG — cerebral radionuclide angiography
CRAMS — circulation, respiration, abdomen, motor, and
  speech
cran —
  cranial
  cranium
CRAO — central retinal artery occlusion
crast. — crastinus (Lat.) for tomorrow
CRB — chemical, radiological, and
  biological
CRBBB — complete right bundle
  branch block
CRBC — chicken red blood cell
CRBP — cellular retinol-binding
  protein
Cr&Br — crown and bridge
CRC —
  calomel, rhubarb, and colo-
  cynth [cathartic]
  cardiac reconditioning center
  cardiovascular reflex conditioning
  child-resistant container
  clinical research center
  colorectal carcinoma
  concentrated red (blood) cell

CRC — (continued)
    Crisis Resolution Center
    cross-reacting cannabinoids
CR&C — closed reduction and cast
CrCl — creatinine clearance
CRCS — cardiovascular reflex conditioning system
CRD —
    childhood rheumatic disease
    child-restraint device
    chorioretinal degeneration
    chronic renal disease
    chronic respiratory disease
    colorectal distension
    completely randomized design
    complete reaction of degeneration
    cone-rod dystrophy
    congenital rubella deafness
    crown-rump distance
CR-DIP — chronic relapsing demyelinating inflammatory polyneuropathy
CRE — cumulative radiation effect
Cre — creatinine
CREA-S — creatinine urine spot [test]
creat — creatinine
CREG — cross-reactive group
crem — cremaster
CRENA — crenated
crep — crepitation
crep. — *crepitus* (Lat.) crepitation
CREST — calcinosis cutis, Raynaud's phenomenon, esophageal dysfunction, sclerodactyly, and telangiectasia [syndrome]
CRF —
    case report form
    chronic renal failure
    chronic respiratory failure
    citrovorum rescue factor
    coagulase-reacting factor
    continuous reinforcement
    corticotropin-releasing factor
CRFK — Crandell feline kidney [cells]

CRG — cardiorespirogram
CRH — corticotropin-releasing hormone
CRHL — Collaborative Radiological Health Laboratory
CRHV — cottontail rabbit herpesvirus
CRI —
    Cardiac Risk Index
    catheter-related infection
    chemical rust-inhibiting
    chronic renal insufficiency
    chronic respiratory insufficiency
    cold running intelligibility [test]
    Composite Risk Index
    concentrated rust inhibitor
    congenital rubella infection
    cross-reactive idiotype
CRIE — crossed radioimmunoelectrophoresis
CRIS — controlled release infusion syndrome
CRISP — Computer Retrieval of Information on Scientific Projects
Crit — critical
crit — hematocrit
CRL —
    cell repository line
    Certified Record Librarian
    complement receptor location
    complement receptor lymphocyte
    crown-rump length
CRM —
    certified raw milk
    Certified Reference Materials
    contralateral remote masking
    counting rate meter
    cross-reacting material
    crown-rump measurement
CRMO — chronic recurrent multifocal osteomyelitis
CRN —
    complement-requiring neutralization

CRN — (continued)
cranial nerves
CRNA — Certified Registered Nurse Anesthetist
cRNA —
chromosomal ribonucleic acid
complementary ribonucleic acid
CRNF — chronic rheumatoid nodular fibrositis
CRNI — Certified Registered Nurse Intravenous
cr nn — cranial nerves
CRNP — Certified Registered Nurse Practitioner
cr ns — cranial nerves
crns — cranial nerves
CRO —
cathode ray oscillograph
cathode ray oscilloscope
centric relation occlusion
CROM — cervical range of motion
CROS —
contralateral routing of signal
contralateral routing of signs
CRP —
chronic relapsing pancreatitis
confluent reticulate papillomatosis
corneal-retinal potential
coronary rehabilitation program
C-reactive protein
cross-reacting protein
cyclic (adenosine monophosphate, AMP) receptor protein
CrP — creatine phosphate
CRPA — C-reactive protein antiserum
CRPD — chronic restrictive pulmonary disease
CRPF —
chloroquine-resistant *Plasmodium falciparum*
contralateral renal plasma flow

CRRT — Certified Respiratory Therapy Technician
CRS —
catheter-related sepsis
caudal regression syndrome
Chinese restaurant syndrome
colon and rectum surgery
compliance of the respiratory system
congenital rubella syndrome
CRSM — cherry red spot myoclonus
CRSP — comprehensive renal scintillation procedure
CrSp — craniospinal
CRST —
calcinosis, cutis, Raynaud's phenomenon, sclerodactyly, telangiectasia [syndrome]
corrected sinus recovery time
CRT —
cadaver renal transplant
cardiac resuscitation team
cathode-ray tube
central reaction time
certified
Certified Record Technique
choice reaction time
chromium release test
complex reaction time
computed renal tomography
copper reduction test
corrected
corrected retention time
cortisone resistant thymocyte
cranial radiation therapy
crt — hematocrit
CRTP — Consciousness Research and Training Project
CrTr — crutch training
CRTT — Certified Respiratory Therapy Technician
CRTX — cast removed, take to x-ray
CRU —
cardiac rehabilitation unit
clinical research unit

CRV — central retinal vein
CRVF — congestive right ventricular failure
CRVO — central retinal vein occlusion
CRY-AB — cryptococcal antibody
CRY-AG — cryptococcal antigen
CRY N — crystal number [on urinalysis]
cryo —
    cryogenic
    cryoglobulin
    cryoprecipitate
    cryosurgery
    cryotherapy
CRYPTO — *Cryptococcus*
Crys —
    crystal
    crystalline
    crystallinized
CS —
    calf serum
    camptomelic syndrome
    carcinoid syndrome
    cardiogenic shock
    caries-susceptible
    carotid sheath
    carotid sinus
    cat scratch [disease]
    celiac sprue
    central service
    central supply
    cerebrospinal
    cervical spine
    cervical stimulation
    cesarean section
    chemical sympathectomy
    chest strap
    chief of staff
    cholesterol stone
    chondroitin sulfate
    chorionic somatomammotropin
    Christian Scientist
    chronic schizophrenia
    cigarette smoke [solution]
    cigarette smoker
    citrate synthase

CS — *(continued)*
    climacteric syndrome
    clinical (laboratory) scientist
    clinical stage
    clinical state
    close supervision
    Cockayne syndrome
    colistin
    colla sinistra (Lat.) with the left hand
    Collet-Sicard [syndrome]
    completed stroke
    completed suicide
    compression syndrome
    concentrated strength [of solution]
    conditioned stimulus
    congenital syphilis
    conjunctival secretion
    conjunctiva-sclera
    conscious
    consciousness
    constant spring
    consultation service
    contact sensitivity
    continue same [treatment]
    continuing smoker
    continuous stripping
    contrast sensitivity
    control serum
    convalescence
    convalescent
    convalescent status
    coronary sclerosis
    coronary sinus
    corpus striatum
    cortical spoking
    corticoid-sensitive
    corticosteroid
    cover screen
    crush syndrome
    current smoker
    current strength
    Cursdmann-Steinert [syndrome]
    Cushing's syndrome
    cycloserine
    cyclosporine

C-S — cervical spine
C/S —
> cesarean section
> Cost-Stirling [antibody]
> culture and sensitivity
> cycles per second
> standard clearance

C&S —
> calvarium and scalp
> conjunctiva and sclera
> cough and sneeze
> culture and sensitivity
> culture and susceptibility

CS_2 — carbon disulfide
CS IV — clinical stage 4
C4S — chondroitin-4-sulfate
Cs —
> case
> cell surface
> cesium
> consciousness
> cyclosporine
> standard clearance

^{137}Cs — cesium-137 [isotope]
C_s —
> standard clearance
> static (respiratory) compliance

cS — centistoke
cs —
> case
> chromosome
> conscious
> consciousness

c/s — cycles per second
CSA —
> canavaninosuccinic acid
> carbonyl salicylamide
> cell surface antigen
> chondroitin sulfate A
> colon-specific antigen
> colony-stimulating activity
> compressed spectral assay
> computerized spectral analysis
> controlled substance analog
> cross-section area

CsA — cyclosporin A
CSAA — Child Study Association of America

CSAD — cysteine sulfinic acid decarboxylase
CSAP — colon-specific antigen protein
CSAS — central sleep apnea syndrome
CSAVP — cerebral subarachnoid venous pressure
CSB —
> caffeine–sodium benzoate
> chemical screening battery I and II
> Cheyne-Stokes breathing
> contaminated small bowel

CSB I&II — Chemistry Screening Batteries I and II
csb — chromosome break
CSBF — coronary sinus blood flow
CSBO — complete small bowel obstruction
CSBS — contaminated small bowel syndrome
CSC —
> central serous choroidopathy
> cigarette smoke condensate
> collagen sponge contraceptive
> cornea, sclera, and conjunctiva
> corticostriatocerebellar
> *coup sur coup* (Fr.) blow on blow (administration of drug in small doses in short intervals)
> cryogenic storage container

C/S & CC — culture and sensitivity and colony count
CSCD — Center for Sickle Cell Disease
CSCI — continuous subcutaneous infusion
CSCR — Central Society for Clinical Research
CSCT — comprehensive support care team
CSD —
> carotid sinus denervation
> cat scratch disease
> combined system disease

CSD — (continued)
   conditionally streptomycin-
      dependent
   conduction system disease
   cortically spreading depression
   craniospinal defect
   critical stimulus duration
CS&D — cleaned, sutured, and
      dressed
CSDB — cat scratch disease bacil-
      lus
CSE —
   clinical symptom/self-evalua-
      tion [questionnaire]
   cone-shaped epiphysis
   cross-sectional echocardiogra-
      phy
C sect — cesarean section
C section — cesarean section
CSEP — cortical somatosensory
      evoked potential
CSER — cortical somatosensory
      evoked response
CSF —
   cancer family syndrome
   cerebrospinal fluid
   circumferential shortening
      fraction
   cold stability factor
   colony-stimulating factor
   coronary sinus flow
CSFH — cerebrospinal fluid hypo-
      tension
CSFP — cerebrospinal fluid pres-
      sure
CSFV — cerebrospinal fluid vol-
      ume
CSF-WR — cerebrospinal fluid–
      Wassermann reaction
csg — chromosome gap
CSGBI — Cardiac Society of
      Great Britain and Ireland
CSGBM — collagenase-soluble
      glomerular basement mem-
      brane
CSH —
   carotid sinus hypersensitivity
   chronic subdural hematoma

CSH — (continued)
   cortical stromal hyperplasia
C-Sh — chair shower
CSHH — congenital self-healing
      histiocytosis
CSI —
   calculus surface index
   cancer serum index
   cavernous sinus infiltration
   cholesterol saturation index
   computerized severity of ill-
      ness [index]
   coronary sinus intervention
CSICU — cardiac surgery inten-
      sive care unit
CSII — continuous subcutaneous
      insulin infusion
CSIIP — continuous subcutaneous
      insulin infusion pump
CSIN — Chemical Substances In-
      formation Network
CSIS — clinical supplies and in-
      ventory system
CSL —
   cardiolipin synthetic lecithin
   corticosteroid liposome
CSLM — confocal scanning mi-
      croscopy
CSLU — chronic stasis leg ulcer
CSM — carotid sinus massage
   cerebrospinal meningitis
   circulation, sensation, motion
   Committee on Safety of Medi-
      cines
   Consolidated Standards Man-
      ual
   corn-soy milk
CSMA — chronic spinal muscular
      atrophy
CSMB — Center for the Study of
      Multiple Births
CSME — cotton-spot macular
      edema
CSMMG — Chartered Society of
      Massage and Medical Gym-
      nastics
CSMP — chloramphenicol-
      sensitive microsomal protein

CSMT — chorionic somatomammotropin
CSN —
cardiac sympathetic nerve
carotid sinus nerve
CSNA — congenital sensory neuropathy with anhidrosis [syn-
drome]
CSNB — congenital stationary
night blindness
CS(NCA) — Clinical (Laboratory) Scientist certified by the
National Certification
Agency
CSNRT — corrected sinus node recovery time
CSNS — carotid sinus nerve stimulation
CSO —
claims services only
common source outbreak
copied standing orders
CSOM —
chronic serous otitis media
chronic suppurative otitis media
CSOP — coronary sinus occlusion
pressure
CSP —
carotid sinus pressure
cavum septi pellucidi
cavum septum pellucidum
cell surface protein
cellulose sodium phosphate
cerebrospinal protein
Chartered Society of Physiotherapy
chemistry screening profile
chondroitin sulfate protein
Cooperative Statistical Program
criminal sexual psychopath
cyclosporine
CSPI — Center for Science in the
Public Interest
C-spine — cervical spine
CSPS — continual skin peeling
syndrome

CSR —
central supply room
Cheyne-Stokes respiration
continued stay review
corrected sedimentation rate
corrected survival rate
corrective septorhinoplasty
cortical secretion rate
cortisol secretion rate
cumulative survival rate
CSRT — corrected sinus (node) recovery time
CSS —
Cancer Surveillance System
carotid sinus stimulation
carotid sinus syndrome
cavernous sinus syndrome
central sterile supply
chewing, sucking, swallowing
chronic subclinical scurvy
Churg-Strauss syndrome
coronary sinus stimulation
cranial sector scan
CSSD — central sterile supply department
CST —
cardiac stress test
cavernous sinus thrombosis
certified surgical technician
Christ-Siemens-Touraine [syn-
drome]
compliance, static
Compton scatter tomography
contraction stress test
convulsive shock therapy
corticospinal tract
cosyntropin stimulation test
Cst — static compliance
C_{st} — static compliance
cST — centistoke
C_{stat} — static compliance
CSTI — Clearinghouse for Scientific and Technical Information
CSTT — cold-stimulation time
test
CSU —
cardiac surgery unit

CSU — (continued)
    cardiac surveillance unit
    cardiovascular surgery unit
    casualty staging unit
    catheter specimen of urine
    Central Statistical Unit
    clinical specialty unit
CSUF — continuous slow ultrafil-
    tration
CSV — chick syncytial virus
CSW —
    Certified Social Worker
    current sleepwalker
CT —
    calcitonin
    calf testis
    cardiac tamponade
    cardiothoracic [ratio]
    Cardiovascular Technologist
    carotid tracing
    carpal tunnel
    cationic trypsinogen
    cellular therapy
    center thickness
    cerebral thrombosis
    cerebral tumor
    cervical traction
    cervicothoracic
    chemotaxis
    chemotherapy
    chest tube
    chicken tumor
    Chlamydia trachomatis
    chloramine T
    chlorothiazide
    cholera toxin
    cholesterol, total
    chordae tendineae
    chronic thyroiditis
    chymotrypsin
    circulating time
    circulation time
    classic technique
    closed thoracotomy
    clotting time
    coagulation time
    coated tablet
    cobra toxin

CT — (continued)
    cognitive therapy
    coil test
    collecting tubule
    colon, transverse
    combined tumor
    compressed tablet
    computed tomography
    computerized tomography
    connective tissue
    continue treatment
    continuous-flow tub
    contraceptive technique
    contraction time
    controlled temperature
    Coombs' test
    corneal thickness
    corneal transplant
    coronary thrombosis
    corrected transposition
    corrective therapist
    corrective therapy
    cortical thickness
    cough threshold
    crest time
    crutch training
    cystine-tellurite [medium]
    cytotechnologist
    cytotoxic therapy
C/T —
    compression/traction [ratio]
    cross-match/transfusion [ratio]
C&T — color and temperature
Ct — carboxyl terminal
    Ctenocephalides [genus of fleas]
$C_{T\text{-}1824}$ — T-1824 (Evans blue)
    clearance
ct —
    carat
    chromatid
    count
CTA —
    Canadian Tuberculosis Associ-
      ation
    chemotactic activity
    chromotropic acid
    clear to auscultation
    Committee on Thrombolytic
      Agents

CTA — (continued)
  computed tomographic angiography
  congenital trigeminal anesthesia
  cyanotrimethyl-androsterone
  cyproterone acetate
  cystine trypticase agar
  cytoplasmic tubular aggregate
  cytotoxic assay
Cta — catamenia (Gr., katamenia) menses
CTAB — cetyltrimethyl-ammonium bromide
C-TAB — cyanide tablet
CTAC —
  Cancer Treatment Advisory Committee
  Carrow Test for Auditory Comprehension
  cetyltrimethylammonium chloride
cTAL — cortical thick ascending limb
c. tant. — cum tanto (Lat.) with the same amount
CTAP —
  computed tomography during arterial portography
  connective tissue–activating peptide
CT(ASCP) — Cytotechnologist (American Society of Clinical Pathologists)
CTAT — computerized transaxial tomography
CTB — ceased to breathe
CTBA — cetrimonium bromide
ctb — chromated break
CTBM — cetyltrimethylammonium bromide (cetrimonium bromide)
CTC —
  chlortetracycline
  Clinical Trial Certificate
  computer-aided tomographic cisternography
  cultured T cells

CTCL —
  cutaneous T-cell leukemia
  cutaneous T-cell lymphoma
$ctCO_2$ — total carbon dioxide concentration
CTD —
  carpal tunnel decompression
  chest tube drainage
  congenital thymic dysplasia
  connective tissue disease
  Corrective Therapy Department
CT&DB — cough, turn, and deep breathe
ctDNA — chloroplast deoxyribonucleic acid
CTDW — continues to do well
CTE —
  calf thymus extract
  cultured thymic epithelium
CTEM — conventional transmission electron microscopy
C-terminal — carboxyl terminal
CTF —
  cancer therapy facility certificate
  Colorado tick fever
  cytotoxic factor
ctf — certificate
CTFE — chlorotrifluoroethylene
CTFS — complete testicular feminization syndrome
CTG —
  cardiotocography
  cervicothoracic ganglion
  chymotrypsinogen
C/TG — cholesterol-triglyceride [ratio]
ctg — chromated gap
CTGA — complete transposition of great arteries
CTH —
  ceramide trihexoside
  chronic tension headache
  clot to hold
CTh — carrier-specific T-helper [cell]
CTHD — chlorthalidone

CTI — certification of terminal illness

CTIU — cardiac-thoracic intensive care unit

CTL —
cervico-thoraco-lumbar
cytotoxic thymus-dependent lymphocyte
cytotoxic T-lymphocyte

ctl — contact lens

CTLD — chlorthalidone

CTLL — cytotoxic T-lymphocyte line

CTLSO — cervicothoracolumbosacral orthosis

CTM —
cardiotachometer
Chlamydia transport media
Chlor-Trimeton
continuous tone masking
cricothyroid muscle

CTMM — computed tomographic metrizamide myelography

CTMM-SF — California Test of Mental Maturity — Short Form

CT/MPR — computed tomography with multiplanar reconstructions

CTN —
calcitonin
computer tomography number
continuous noise

C&TN BLE — color and temperature normal, both lower extremities

cTNM — tumor-node-metastasis (staging of neoplasms by clinical examination)

CTP —
California Test of Personality
comprehensive treatment plan
cytidine triphosphate
cytosine triphosphate

CTP-³H — cytidine triphosphate, tritium-labeled

C-TPN — cyclic total parenteral nutrition

CTPP — cerebral tissue perfusion pressure

CTPV — coal tar pitch volatiles

CTPVO — chronic thrombotic pulmonary vascular obstruction

CTR —
cardiothoracic ratio
carpal tunnel release
central tumor registry

ctr —
center
central
centric

CTRB — chymotrypsinogen B

CTRX — ceftriaxone

CTS —
carpal tunnel syndrome
composite treatment score
computed tomographic scan
computed tomographic scanner
computed topographic scan
computed topographic scanner
contralateral threshold shift
corticosteroid

CTSNFR — corrected time of sinoatrial node function recovery

CTSP — called to see patient

CTT —
cefotetan
central tegmental tract
central transmission time
compressed tablet triturate
computed transaxial tomography
critical tracking time

CTU —
cardiac-thoracic unit
centigrade thermal unit
constitutive transcription unit

CTUWSD — chest tube underwater-seal drainage

CTV —
clinical target volume
cervical and thoracic vertebrae

CTW —
  central terminal of Wilson
  combined testicular weight
CTX —
  cefotaxime
  cerebrotendinous xanthoma-
    tosis
  chemotaxis
  chemotoxins
  contraction
  Cytoxan
CTx —
  cardiac transplantation
  conotoxin
CTXN — contraction
CTZ —
  chemoreceptor trigger zone
  chlorothiazide
CU —
  Campylobacter urease [test]
  cardiac unit
  casein unit
  cause undetermined
  cause unknown
  chymotrypsin unit
  clinical unit
  color unit
  contact urticaria
  control unit
  convalescent unit
  curie
Cu — copper (Lat., *cuprum*)
Cu-7 — Copper-7 [intrauterine
  contraceptive device]
^{61}Cu — radioactive copper
^{64}Cu — radioactive copper
C_u — urea clearance
cu —
  cubic
  curie
CuB — copper band
CUC — chronic ulcerative colitis
cu cm — cubic centimeter
CUD —
  cause undetermined
  congenital urinary deformity
CuD — copper deficiency
CUE — cumulative urinary excretion

cu ft — cubic foot
CUG —
  cystourethrogram
  cystourethrography
  cytidine-uridine-guanosine
CuHVL — copper half-value
  layer
CUI — Cox-Uphoff International
  [tissue expander]
cu in — cubic inch
cuj. — *cujus* (Lat.) of which
cuj. lib. — *cujus libet* (Lat.) of whatever you please
cult — culture
cu m —
  cubic meter
  cubic micrometer
cum — cumulative
CUMITECH — Cumulative Techniques and Procedures in Clinical Microbiology
cu mm — cubic millimeter
CuO — cupric oxide
Cu_2O — cuprous oxide
CUP — carcinoma, unknown primary
CUPS — carcinoma of unknown
  primary site
CUR —
  curettage
  cystourethrorectal
cur —
  curative
  cure
  current
curat. — *curatio* (Lat.) dressing
CURN — Conduct and Utilization
  of Research in Nursing
CUS —
  carotid ultrasound examina-
    tion
  catheterized urine specimen
  chronic undifferentiated
    schizophrenia
  contact urticaria syndrome
CuS — copper supplement
CUSA — Cavitron ultrasonic aspirator

cusp. — cuspid
CUT — chronic undifferentiated type [schizophrenia]
CuTS — cubital tunnel syndrome
CUX — checkup x-ray
cu yd — cubic yard
CV —
  cardiac volume
  cardiovascular
  carotenoid vesicle
  cell volume
  central venous
  cerebrovascular
  cervical vertebra
  chikungunya virus
  closed vitrectomy
  closing volume
  coefficient of variation
  color vision
  concentrated volume
  conducting vein
  conduction velocity
  consonant-vowel [syllable]
  contrast ventriculography
  conventional ventilation
  conversational voice
  corpuscular volume
  costovertebral
  Coxsackie virus
  cresyl violet
  critical value
  crystal violet
  curriculum vitae
  cutaneous vasculitis
  fifth cranial nerve
C.V. —
  conjugata vera (Lat.) true conjugate [diameter of pelvic inlet]
  cras vespere (Lat.) tomorrow evening
C/V — coulomb per volt
Cv — specific heat at constant volume
C$_v$ — constant volume
cv — cultivar
CVA —
  cardiovascular accident

CVA — (continued)
  cerebrovascular accident
  cervicovaginal antibody
  chronic villous arthritis
  costovertebral angle
  cresyl violet acetate
CVAH — congenital virilizing adrenal hyperplasia
CVAP — cerebrovascular amyloid peptide
C-Vasc — cerebral vascular [profile study]
CVAT — costovertebral angle tenderness
CVB — chorionic villi biopsy
CVC —
  central venous catheter
  consonant-vowel-consonant [syllable]
CV cath — central venous catheter
CVCT — cardiovascular computed tomography
CVD —
  cardiovascular disease
  cerebrovascular disease
  cerebrovascular disorder
  collagen vascular disease
  color vision deviant
  craniovertebral decompression
cvd — curved
CVE — cerebrovascular evaluation
CVF —
  cardiovascular failure
  central visual field
  cervicovaginal fluid
  cobra venom factor
CVG —
  contrast ventriculography
  coronary venous graft
CVH —
  cerebroventricular hemorrhage
  cervicovaginal hood
  combined ventricular hypertrophy
  common variable hypogammaglobulinemia

CVHD — chronic valvular heart disease

CVI —
- cardiovascular incident
- cardiovascular insufficiency
- cerebrovascular incident
- cerebrovascular insufficiency
- chronic venous insufficiency
- common variable immunodeficiency
- continuous venous infusion
- sixth cranial nerve

CVID — common variable immunodeficiency

CVII — seventh cranial nerve

CVIII — eighth cranial nerve

CVL — clinical vascular laboratory

CVLT — California Verbal Learning Test

CVM —
- cardiovascular monitor
- cerebral venous malformation

CVMP — Committee on Veterans Medical Problems

CVN — central venous nutrient

CVO —
- central vein occlusion
- central venous oxygen
- Chief Veterinary Officer
- circumventricular organs
- *conjugata vera obstetrica* (Lat.) obstetric conjugate [diameter of pelvic inlet]

C_VO_2 — mixed venous oxygen content

CVOD — cerebrovascular obstructive disease

CVOR — cardiovascular operating room

CVP —
- cardiac valve procedure
- cardioventricular pacing
- cell volume profile
- central venous pressure
- cerebrovascular profile

CVP lab — cardiovascular-pulmonary laboratory

$cvPO_2$ — cerebral venous partial pressure of oxygen

CVR —
- cardiovascular resistance
- cardiovascular review
- cardiovascular-renal
- cardiovascular-respiratory
- cephalic vasomotor response
- cerebrovascular resistance

CVRD — cardiovascular renal disease

CVRI — cardiovascular resistance index

CVRR — cardiovascular recovery room

CVS —
- cardiovascular surgery
- cardiovascular system
- cerebral vasospasm
- challenge virus strain
- chorionic villus sampling
- clean-voided specimen
- current vital signs

CVSF — conduction velocity of slower fibers

CVSU — cardiovascular specialty unit

CVT —
- central venous temperature
- congenital vertical talus

CVT-ICU — cardiovascular-thoracic intensive care unit

CVTR — charcoal viral transport medium

CVTS — cardiovascular-thoracic surgery

CVUG — cystoscopy and voiding urethrogram

CW —
- cardiac work
- careful watch
- case worker
- casework
- cell wall
- chemical warfare
- chemical weapon
- chest wall
- children's ward
- clockwise
- compare with

CW — (*continued*)
    continuous wave
    cotton wool (spots)
    crutch walking
C/W —
    compare with
    compatible with
    consistent with
    crutch walking
cw — clockwise
c/w —
    compatible with
    consistent with
    crutch walking
CWBTS — capillary whole blood
    true sugar
CWD —
    cell wall defect
    continuous-wave Doppler
CWDF — cell wall–deficient form
    [bacteria]
CWE — cotton wool exudates
CWF — Cornell Word Form
CWH — cardiomyopathy and
    wooly hair-coat [syndrome]
CWHB — citrated whole human
    blood
CWI — cardiac work index
CWL — cutaneous water loss
CWMS — color, warmth, move-
    ment, sensation
CWOP — childbirth without pain
CWP —
    centimeters of water pressure
    childbirth without pain
    coal workers' pneumoconiosis
CWPEA — Childbirth Without
    Pain Education Association
CWS —
    cell wall skeleton
    chest wall stimulation
    Child Welfare Service
    cold water–soluble
    comfortable walking speed
    cotton wool spots
CWT — cold water treatment
cwt — hundredweight
CWXSP — Coal Workers' X-ray
    Surveillance Program

CX —
    cancel
    cerebral cortex
    cervix
    chest x-ray [film]
    circumflex artery
    cloxacillin
    critical experiment
    culture
    cylinder axis
    tenth cranial nerve
Cx —
    cancel
    cervix
    circumflex
    chest x-ray [film]
    clearance
    complaint
    complex
    complication
    contraction
    convex
    cylinder axis
CXI — eleventh cranial nerve
CXII — twelfth cranial nerve
CXM —
    cefuroxime
    cycloheximide
CxMT — cervical motion tender-
    ness
CXR — chest x-ray [film]
CXTX — cervical traction
CY —
    calendar year
    casein-yeast autolysate [me-
    dium]
    cyanogen
    cyclophosphamide
Cy —
    cyanogen
    cyclonium
    cyclophosphamide
    cyst
    cytarabine
CyA — cyclosporin A
cyan — cyanosis
cyath. — *cyathus* (Lat.) a glassful
cyath. vin. — *cyathus vinarius*
    (Lat.) wineglass

cyborg — cybernetic organism
CYC — cyclophosphamide
cyc —
    cyclazocine
    cycle
    cyclotron
cyclic AMP — cyclic adenosine
    monophosphate
cyclic GMP — cyclic guanosine
    monophosphate
Cyclo —
    cyclophosphamide
    cyclopropane
Cyclo C — cyclocytidine hydro-
    chloride
Cyd — cytidine
CYE — charcoal yeast extract
    [agar]
CYFL — cyst fluid
CYL — casein yeast lactate
cyl —
    cylinder
    cylindrical lens
CYN — cyanide
CYNAP — cytotoxicity negative,
    absorption positive
CYP — cyproheptadine
CYS — cystoscopy
Cys —
    cyclosporine
    cysteine

Cys-Cys — cystine
cysto —
    cystogram
    cystoscopic
    cystoscopy
CYT — cytochrome
Cyt —
    cytoplasm
    cytosine
cyt —
    cytological
    cytology
    cytoplasm
    cytoplasmic
cytol —
    cytological
    cytology
CYTOMG — cytomegalovirus
Cyt Ox — cytochrome oxidase
cyt sys — cytochrome system
CZ —
    carzinophilin
    cefazolin
Cz — central midline placement of
    electrodes in electroencepha-
    lography
CZD — cefazedone
CZI — crystalline zinc insulin
CZN — chlorzotocin
C_{Zn} — zinc clearance
CZP — clonazepam

D —
    absorbed dose aspartic acid
    cholecalciferol
    coefficient of diffusion
    dacron
    dalton
    date
    daughter
    day
    dead
    dead air space

D — (continued)
    debye
    deciduous
    decimal reduction time
    decreased
    degree
    density
    dental
    dermatologic
    dermatologist
    dermatology

D — (continued)

    detur (Lat.) let it be given
    deuterium
    deuteron
    development
    deviation
    dexter (Lat.) right
    dextra (Lat.) right
    dextrorotary
    dextrose
    diagnosis
    diagonal
    diameter
    diarrhea
    diastole
    diathermy
    didymium
    died
    difference
    diffusing capacity
    diffusion
    dihydrouridine
    dilution [rate]
    diopter
    diplomate
    disease
    dispense
    displacement [loop]
    distal
    diuresis
    diurnal
    divergence
    diverticulum
    divorced
    doctor
    dog
    dominant
    donor
    dorsal vertebrae (D1 through
      D12)
    doubtful
    drive
    drug
    dual
    duct
    duodenum, duodenal
    duration
    dwarf [colony]

D — (continued)

    dyne
    electric displacement
    mean dose
    vitamin D unit
Δ — delta (fourth letter of the Greek alphabet), uppercase
$\overline{D}$ — mean dose
$\frac{1}{D}$ — diffusion resistance
D_1 — diagonal one
$\overline{D}$ — mean dose
D_{CO} — diffusing capacity for carbon monoxide
D_L — diffusing capacity of lung
D1–D12 — first through twelfth dorsal vertebra
1-D — one-dimensional
D_2 — diagonal two
2-D — two-dimensional
2,4-D — 2,4-dichlorophenoxyacetic acid
D/3 — distal third
3-D —
    delayed double diffusion [test]
    three-dimensional
D4 — fourth digit
D_{10} — decimal reduction time
D — dead space gas
d —
    atomic orbital with angular momentum quantum number 2
    day
    dead
    deceased
    decigram
    decrease
    decreased
    degree
    density
    deoxy
    deoxyribose
    deuteron
    dextrorotatory
    diameter
    diarrhea
    died
    diopter

d — (continued)
  distal
  diurnal
  divorced
  dorsal
  dose
  doubtful
  duration
  dyne
δ —
  delta (fourth letter of the
    Greek alphabet), lowercase
  immunoglobulin D
d. —
  da (Lat.) give
  dentur (Lat.) let them be
    given
  detur (Lat.) let it be given
  dexter (Lat.) right
  dies (Lat.) day
  dosis (Lat.) dose
1/d — once a day
2/d — twice a day
D 860 — tolbutamide
DA —
  dark adaptation
  dark agouti [rat]
  daunomycin
  decubitus angina
  degenerative arthritis
  delayed action
  delivery awareness
  dental assistant
  deoxyadenosine
  developmental age
  diabetic acidosis
  diagnostic arthroscopy
  differential analyzer
  differentiation antigen
  diphenylchlorarsine
  Diploma in Anesthetics
  direct admission
  direct agglutination
  disability assistance
  disaggregated
  dispense as directed
  District Administrator
  dopamine

DA — (continued)
  dopaminergic
  drug addict
  drug addiction
  ductus arteriosus
D/A —
  date of accident
  date of admission
  digital-to-analog [converter]
  discharge and advise
D-A — donor-acceptor
D&A — dilatation and aspiration
Da — dalton
dA —
  day of admission
  deoxyadenosine
da —
  daughter
  day
d.a. — detur ad (Lat.) let it be
  given to
DAA —
  decompensated autonomous
    adenoma
  dehydroacetic acid
  dementia associated with alco-
    holism
  dialysis-associated amyloidosis
  diaminoanisole
DA/A — drug/alcohol addiction
DAAO — diaminoacid oxidase
DAB —
  days after birth
  3,3'-diaminobenzidine
  dimethylaminoazobenzene
  dysrhythmic aggressive behav-
    ior
DABA — 2,4-diaminobutyric acid
DAC —
  diazacholesterol
  digital-to-analog converter
  Disablement Advisory Com-
    mittee
  Disaster Assistance Center
  Division of Ambulatory Care
dac — dacryon
DACA —
  dissecting aneurysm of coro-
    nary artery

DACA — (continued)
Drug Abuse Control Amendments

DACL — Depression Adjective Check List

DACM — N-(7-diethylamino-4-methyl-3-coumarinyl) maleimide

DACS — data acquisition and control system

DACT — dactinomycin

DAD —
delayed afterdepolarization
diffuse alveolar damage
dispense as directed
drug administration device

DADA — dichloroacetic acid diisopropylammonium salt

DADAVS — Deputy Assistant Director Army Veterinary Services

DADDS — diacetyldiaminodiphenylsulfone

DADMS — Deputy Assistant Director of Medical Services

dADP — deoxyadenosine diphosphate

DADS — Director of Army Dental Service

DAE —
diphenylanthracene endoperoxide
diving air embolism

DAF —
decay antibody-accelerating factor
delayed auditory feedback
Draw-A-Family [test]
drug-adulterated food

DAG —
diacylglycerol
dianhydrogalactitol

DAGT — direct antiglobulin test

DAH — disordered action of the heart

DAHEA — Department of Allied Health Education and Accreditation

DAHM — Division of Allied Health Manpower

DAI — diffuse axonal injury

DAL — drug analysis laboratory

daL — decaliter

DALA — delta-aminolevulinic acid

DALE — Drug Abuse Law Enforcement

DAM —
data-associated message
degraded amyloid
diacetyl monoxime
diacetylmorphine
discriminant analytic model

dam — decameter

DAMA — discharged against medical advice

dAMP —
deoxyadenosine monophosphate
deoxyadenylate adenosine monophosphate

DANA — drug-induced antinuclear antibodies

D and C —
dilatation and curettage
dilation and curettage

dand. — dandus (Lat.) to be given

DANS — 1-dimethylaminonaphthalene-5-sulfonyl chloride

DAO —
diamine oxidase
duly authorized officer

DAo — descending aorta

DAP —
data acquisition processor
delayed after polarization
depolarizing afterpotential
diabetes-associated peptide
diaminopimelic acid
diastolic aortic pressure
dihydroxyacetone phosphate
dipeptidylaminopeptidase
direct agglutination pregnancy [test]
Director of Army Psychiatry

DAP — (continued)
  Draw-a-Person [test]
  dynamic aortic patch
DAP&E — Diploma of Applied
  Parasitology and Entomology
DAPRE — daily adjustable progressive resistive exercise
DAPRU — Drug Abuse Prevention Resource Unit
DAPST — Denver Auditory Pho-
  neme Sequencing Test
DAPT —
  diaminophenylthiazole
  direct agglutination preg-
    nancy test
Dapt — Daptazole
dAPT — deoxyadenosine triphosphate
DAQ — Diagnostic Assessment
  Questionnare
DAR —
  daily affective rhythm
  death after resuscitation
  diacereine
  differential absorption ratio
  dual asthmatic reaction
DARF — direct antiglobulin rosette-forming
DARP — drug abuse rehabilitation
  program
DARTS — Drug and Alcohol Rehabilitation Testing System
DAS —
  data acquisition system
  dead air space
  death anxiety scale
  delayed anovulatory syndrome
  developmental aproxia of
    speech
  dextroamphetamine sulfate
DASA — distal articular set angle
DASD — direct access storage device
DASH — Distress Alarm for the
  Severely Handicapped
DASI — Developmental Activities
  Screening Inventory
DASP — double antibody solid
  phase

DAT —
  delayed-action tablet
  dementia of the Alzheimer's
    type
  dental aptitude test
  diacetylthiamine
  diet as tolerated
  differential agglutination titer
  differential antibody titer
  differential aptitude test
  dipeptidyl amino peptidase
  diphtheria antitoxin
  direct agglutination test
  direct antiglobulin test
  Disaster Action Team
DATATOP — Deprenyl and tocopherol antioxidative therapy of Parkinsonism
DATE — dental auxiliary teacher
  education
dATP — deoxyadenosine triphosphate
DATTA — diagnostic and therapeutic technology assessment
DAU —
  3-deazauridine
  Dental Auxiliary Utilization
dau — daughter
DAV —
  data valid
  Disabled American Veterans
  duck adenovirus
DAVIT — Danish Verapamil In-
  farction Trial
DAVM — dural arteriovenous mal-
  formation
DAvMED — Diploma in Aviation
  Medicine
DAVP — deamino-arginine vaso-
  pressin
DAV and RS — Director of Army
  Veterinary and Remount Ser-
  vices
DAvMed — Diploma in Aviation
  Medicine
DAW — dispense as written
DB —
  Baudelocque's diameter

DB — *(continued)*
 database
 date of birth
 deep breath
 dense body
 dextran blue
 diabetes
 diabetic
 diagonal band
 diet beverage
 direct bilirubin
 disability
 distobuccal
 double-blind [study]
 dry bulb
 duodenal bulb
 Dutch belted [rabbit]
D/B — date of birth
Db —
 diabetes
 diabetic
dB — decibel
DBA —
 Diamond-Blackfan anemia
 dibenzanthracene
 Dolichos biflorus agglutinin
DBAE — dihydroxyboryl-
 aminoethyl
DBC —
 dibencozide
 dye-binding capacity
DB&C — deep breathing and
 coughing
DBCL — dilute blood clot lysis
 [method]
DBCP — dibromochloropropane
DBD —
 definitive brain damage
 dibromodulcitol
DBDG — distobuccal developmental groove
DBE —
 deep breathing exercise
 dibromoethane
DBED — dibenzylethylenediamine
 dipenicillin (penicillin G benzathine)
DBF — disturbed bowel function

DBH — dopamine beta-hydroxy-
 lase
DBI — development-at-birth
 index
DBIL — direct bilirubin
DBIOC — data base input/output
 control
DBIR — Director of Biotechnology
 Information Resources
dBk — decibels above 1 kilowatt
dbl — double
DBM —
 database management
 decarboxylase base Moeller
 diabetic management
 dibromomannitol
 dobutamine
dBm — decibels above 2 milliwatt
DBMS — data base management
 systems
DBO — distobucco-occlusal
db/ob — diabetic obese [mouse]
DBP —
 demineralized bone powder
 diastolic blood pressure
 dibutylphthalate
 distobuccopulpal
 Döhle body panmyelopathy
 vitamin D–binding protein
DBQ — debrisoquin
DBR —
 direct bilirubin
 distorted breathing rate
DBS —
 deep brain stimulation
 Denis Browne splint
 despeciated bovine serum
 Diamond-Blackfan syndrome
 dibromosalicil
 diminished breath sounds
 direct bonding system
 Division of Biological Standards
DBT —
 disordered breathing time
 dry blood temperature
 dry bulb temperature
DBW — desirable body weight

dBW — decibels above 1 watt
DB2 — dibenzamine
DC —
    daily census
    data communication
    date conversion
    decarboxylase
    decrease
    deep compartment
    degenerating cell
    Dental Corps
    deoxycholate
    descending colon
    dextran charcoal
    diagnostic center
    diagnostic code
    diagonal conjugate
    differentiated cell
    diffuse cortical
    digit copying
    digital computer
    dilatation and curettage
    dilation and curettage
    dilation catheter
    diphenylamine chlorarsine
    diphenylarsine cyanide
    direct and consensual
    direct Coombs' [test]
    direct current
    discharge
    discharged
    discontinue
    discontinued
    distal colon
    distocervical
    Doctor of Chiropractic
    donor cells
    dorsal column
    dressing change
    duodenal cap
    Dupuytren contracture
    dyskeratosis congenita
    electric defibrillator using DC
        discharge
D/C —
    decrease
    diarrhea/constipation
    discharge

D/C — (continued)
    discontinue
    disseminated intravascular co-
        agulation
D&C —
    dilatation and curettage
    dilation and curettage
    direct and consensual
    drugs and cosmetics
DC65 — Darvon compound 65
Dc — critical dilution rate
dC — deoxycytidine
dc —
    decrease
    direct current
    discharged
    discontinue
    discontinued
DCA —
    deoxycholate-citrate agar
    deoxycholic acid
    desoxycorticosterone acetate
    dicarboxylic acid
    dichloroacetate
    dichloroacetic acid
DCABG — double coronary artery
    bypass graft
DCAG — double coronary artery
    graft
DCAMP — dibutyryl cyclic adeno-
    sine monophosphate
DC and B — dilation, curettage,
    and biopsy
DCB —
    dichlorobenzidine
    dilutional cardiopulmonary
        bypass
DCBE — double contrast barium
    enema
DCBF — dynamic cardiac blood
    flow
DCC —
    day care center
    detected in colon cancer
    dextran-coated charcoal
    N,N'-dicyclohexylcarbodi-
        imide
    Disaster Control Center

DCC — *(continued)*
 dorsal cell column
DCc — double concave
DCCF — dural carotid cavernous fistula
DC_{CO2} — diffusing capacity for carbon dioxide
DCCT — Diabetes Control and Complications Trial
DCD — Diploma in Chest Diseases
D/c'd — discontinued
DCDA — deuterium with cesium dihydrogen arsenate
dCDP — deoxycytidine diphosphate
DCE —
 delayed contrast enhancement
 dichloroethylene
DCET — dicarboxyethoxythiamine
DCF —
 deoxycoformycin
 direct centrifugal flotation
 dopachrome conversion factor
DCFM — Doppler color flow mapping
DCG —
 deoxycorticosterone glucoside
 disodium cromoglycate
 dynamic electrocardiography
DCH —
 delayed cutaneous hypersensitivity
 Diploma in Child Health
DCh — *Doctor Chirurgiae* (Lat.) Doctor of Surgery
DCHFB — dichlorohexafluorobutane
DCHN — dicyclohexylamine nitrite
DChO — Doctor of Ophthalmic Surgery
DCI —
 dichloroisoprenaline
 dichloroisoproterenol
DCIP — dichlorophenolindophenol
DCIS — ductal carcinoma in situ
DCL —
 dicloxacillin

DCL — *(continued)*
 diffuse or disseminated cutaneous leishmaniasis
 digital counter/locator
DCLS — deoxycholate citrate lactose saccharose
DCM —
 dichloromethane
 dichloromethotrexate
 dilated cardiomyopathy
 Doctor of Comparative Medicine
 dyssynergia cerebellaris myoclonica
DCML — dorsal column medial lemniscus
dCMP —
 deoxycytidine monophosphate
 deoxycitidine-5'-phosphate
DCMT — Doctor of Clinical Medicine of the Tropics
DCMX — 2,4-dichloro-m-xylenol
DCMXT — dichloromethotrexate
DCN —
 Data Collection Network
 deep cerebral nucleus
 delayed conditional necrosis
 depressed, cognitively normal
 dorsal column nucleus
 dorsal cutaneous nerve
DCNU — chlorozotocin
DCO — Diploma of the College of Optics
D_{CO} — diffusing capacity for carbon monoxide
DCOG — Diploma of the College of Obstetricians and Gynaecologists (British)
DCOME — Dworkin/Culatta Oral Mechanism Examination
DCP —
 decentralized pharmacy
 dicalcium phosphate
 dichlorophene
 Diploma in Clinical Pathology
 Diploma in Clinical Psychology

DCP — (continued)
  discharge planner
  District Community Physician
  dynamic compression plate
DCPN — direction-changing positional nystagmus
DCPU — dorsal caudate putamen
DCR —
  dacryocystorhinostomy
  data conversion receiver
  delayed cutaneous reaction
  direct cortical response
DCS —
  decompression sickness
  dense canalicular system
  diffuse cortical sclerosis
  disease control serum
  dorsal column stimulation
  dorsal column stimulator
  dynamic condylar screw
  dyskinetic cilia syndrome
DCSA — double contrast shoulder arthrography
DCT —
  deep chest therapy
  diastolic control team
  direct Coombs' test
  distal convoluted tubule
  diurnal cortisol test
  dynamic computed tomography
dct. — decoctum (Lat.) boiled down
3D-CTA — three dimensional computed tomographic angiography
DCTM — delay computer tomographic myelography
DCTMA — desoxycorticosterone trimethylacetate
dCTP — deoxycytidine triphosphate
DCTPA — desoxycorticosterone triphenylacetate
DCU — dichloral urea
DCVO — Deputy Chief Veterinary Officer
DCX — double charge exchange

DCx — double convex
DD —
  dangerous drug
  data definition
  day of delivery
  de die (Lat.) daily
  degenerated disc
  degenerative disease
  delusional disorder
  dependent drainage
  detrusor dyssynergia
  developmental disability
  dialysis dementia
  diaper dermatitis
  died of the disease
  differential diagnosis
  digestive disorder
  Di Guglielmo's disease
  discharge diagnosis
  discharged dead
  disk diameter
  distortion of Dots
  dog danger
  double diffusion
  double dose
  drug dependence
  dry dressing
  Duchenne's dystrophy
  Dupuytren's disease
D/D — differential diagnosis
D&D — diarrhea and dehydration
D6D — delta-6-desaturase
d/D — day of discharge
dd — disc diameter
d.d. —
  de die (Lat.) daily
DDA —
  Dangerous Drugs Act
  dideoxyadenosine
ddA — 2′,3′-dideoxyadenosine
DDAVP — 1-deamino(8-D-arginine) vasopressin
DDC —
  dangerous drug cabinet
  Developmental Disability Council
  dideoxycytidine
  diethyl dithiocarbamic acid

DDC — *(continued)*
dihydrocollidine
direct display console
diverticular disease of the colon
DDc — double concave
DDCT — dideoxycytidine
DDD —
AV universal [pacemaker]
defined daily dose
degenerative disk disease
dehydroxydinaphthyl disulfide
dense deposit disease
Denver dialysis disease
dichlorodiphenyl-dichloro-
ethane
dihydroxydinaphthyl disulfide
Dowling Degos disease
DDD CT — double-dose–delay
computed tomography
DDE — dichlorodiphenyldichloro-
ethylene
DDG — deoxy-D-glucose
DDH —
Diploma in Dental Health
dissociated double hypertropia
Division of Dental Health
DDHT — double dissociated hypertropia
DDI —
dressing dry and intact
dideoxyinosine
DDIB — Disease Detection Information Bureau
d.d. in d. — *de die in diem* (Lat.)
from day to day
DDM —
Diploma in Dermatological
Medicine
Doctor of Dental Medicine
Dyke Davidoff-Masson [syn-
drome]
DDMS — Deputy Director of Med-
ical Services
dDNA — denatured deoxyribonu-
cleic acid
DDNTP — dideoxynucleoside tri-
phosphate

DDO — Diploma in Dental Ortho-
paedics
DDP —
cis-diaminodichloroplatinum
cisplatin
density-dependent phospho-
protein
difficult denture patient
digital data processing
distributed data processing
DDPA — Delta Dental Plans Association
DDR —
diastolic descent rate
Diploma in Diagnostic Radiology
DDRB — Doctors and Dentists'
Review Body
DDS —
damaged disc syndrome
Demos Dropout Scale
dendrodendritic synaptosome
dental distress syndrome
depressed DNA synthesis
dialysis disequilibrium syndrome
diaminodiphenylsulfone
directional Doppler sonography
Director of Dental Services
disability determination service
Disease-disability Scale
Doctor of Dental Surgery
dodecyl sulfate
double decidual sac
dystrophy-dystocia syndrome
DDSc — Doctor of Dental Science
DDS4,4′ — diaminodiphenylsulfone
DDSI — digital damage severity index
DDSO — diaminodiphenylsulfoxide
DDST — Denver Developmental
Screening Test
DDT —
dichlorodiphenyltrichloro-
ethane
ductus deferens tumor

DDTN — dideoxy-didehydro-
thymide
DDTP — drug dependence treatment program
ddTTP — dideoxythymidine triphosphate
DDU — dermo-distortive urticaria
DDV — dichlorvos
DDVP — dimethyldichlorovinyl
phosphate
D/DW — dextrose in distilled water
D 5% DW — 5% dextrose in distilled water
DDx — differential diagnosis
DE —
dendritic expansion
deprived eye
diagnostic error
dialysis encephalopathy
digestive energy
dose equivalent
dream elements
duodenol exclusion
duration of ejection
D&E —
diet and elimination
diet and excretion
dilation and evacuation
D₅E₄₈ — 5% dextrose and electrolyte 48% [solution]
2DE — two-dimensional echocardiography
DEA —
dehydroepiandrosterone
diethanolamine
Drug Enforcement Agency
DEAE —
diethylaminoethanol
diethylaminoethyl [cellulose]
DEAE-D — diethylaminoethyl
dextran
dearg. pil. — *deargentur pilulae*
(Lat.) let the pills be silver-
ized
deaur. pil. — *deaurentur pilulae*
(Lat.) let the pills be gilded
DEB —
diepoxybutane

DEB — *(continued)*
diethylbutanediol
Division of Environmental Biology
dystrophic epidermolysis bullosa
deb — débridement
DEBA — diethylbarbituric acid
debil — debilitation
DEBRA — Dystrophic Epidermolysis Bullosa Research Association
DEBS — dominant epidermolysis
bullosa simplex
deb. spis. — *debita spissitudine*
(Lat.) of the proper consistency
DEC —
deceased
deciduous
decimal
decimeter
decompose
decomposition
decrease
dendritic epidermal cell
deoxycholate citrate
diethylcarbamazine
dynamic environmental conditioning
dec. — *decanta* (Lat.) pour off
DECEL — deceleration
decd — decreased
DECO — decreasing consumption
of oxygen
decoct. — *decoctum* (Lat.) a decoction
decomp —
decompose
decomposition
decon — decontamination
decr —
decrease
decreased
decub. — *decubitus* (Lat.) lying
down
DED —
date of expected delivery

DED — *(continued)*
  defined exposure dose
  delayed erythema dose
de d. in d. — *de die in diem* (Lat.)
  from day to day
DEEG —
  depth electroencephalogram
  depth electroencephalography
  depth electrography
DEET — diethyltoluamide
DEF — decayed, extracted, or
  filled
def —
  defecation
  deferred
  deficiency
  deficient
  define
  definition
defib
  defibrillate
  duck embryo fibroblast
  defibrillation
defic —
  deficiency
  deficit
deform —
  deformed
  deformity
DEFT — direct epifluorescent filter
  technique
DEG — diethylene glycol
Deg —
  degeneration
  degenerative
  degree
degen —
  degeneration
  degenerative
deglut. — *deglutiatur* (Lat.) let it be
  swallowed
DEH — dysplasia epiphysealis hem-
  imelica
DEHFT — developmental hand
  function test
DEHP — di(2-ethylhexyl)phtha-
  late
DEHS — Division of Emergency
  Health Services

dehyd —
  dehydrated
  dehydration
DEJ — dentoenamel junction
del —
  deletion
  delivery
  delusion
deliq —
  deliquescence
  deliquescent
delt — deltoid
deltaTG — delta triglyceride incre-
  ments
DEM —
  Department of Emergency
    Medicine
  diethylmaleate
Dem. — Demerol
DEN —
  denervation
  dengue
  dermatitis exfoliativa neonato-
    rum
  diethylnitrosamine
denat — denatured
denom — denominator
DENT — Dental Exposure Nor-
  malization Technique
Dent —
  dental
  dentist
  dentistry
  dentition
dent. — *dentur* (Lat.) let them be
  given
dent. tal. dos. — *dentur tales
  doses* (Lat.) let such doses be
  given
DEP —
  diethyl pyrocarbonate
  diethylpropanediol
  dilution end point
dep. — *depuratus* (Lat.) purified
dep —
  dependents
  deposit
DEPA — diethylene phosphoram-
  ide

DEPC — diethyl pyrocarbonate
depr —
    depressed
    depression
depr. neur. — depressive neurosis
DEPS — distal effective potassium
    secretion
DEP ST SEG — depressed ST seg-
    ment
Dept. — department
DEQ — Depression Experiences
    Questionnaire
DER —
    disulfiram-ethanol reaction
    dual energy radiography
DeR — degeneration reaction
der — derivative chromosome
deriv —
    derivative of
    derived from
Derm. —
    dermatitis
    dermatological
    dermatologist
    dermatology
    dermatome
DES —
    dermal-epidermal separation
    dialysis encephalopathy syn-
        drome
    diethylstilbestrol
    diffuse esophageal spasm
    disequilibrium syndrome
    Doctor's Emergency Service
desat — desaturated
desc —
    descendant
    descending
Desc Ao — descending aorta
DESI — drug efficacy study imple-
    mentation
desq — desquamation
DEST —
    Denver Eye Screening Test
    dichotic environmental
        sounds test
dest. —
    destilla (Lat.) distill

dest. — (continued)
    destillatus (Lat.) distilled
    destil. (Lat.) distill
DET —
    diethyltryptamine
    dipyridamole echocardiogra-
        phy test
det. — detur (Lat.) let it be given
Det-6 — detroid-6 [human sternal
    marrow cells]
determ —
    determination
    determined
det. in dup. — detur in duplo (Lat.)
    let twice as much be given
detn — detention
detox — detoxification
d. et s. — detur et signetur (Lat.) let
    it be given and labeled
DEUC — direct electronic urethro-
    cystometry
DEV —
    deviant
    deviation
    duck embryo [rabies] vaccine
dev —
    develop
    development
    deviate
    deviation
    develop
devel — development
DevPd — developmental pediatrics
DEVR — dominant exudative
    vitreoretinopathy
DEX — dexamethasone
dex —
    dexterity
    dextrorotatory
    dextrose
    Dextrostix
dex. — dexter (Lat.) right
DEXA — dual-energy x-ray absorp-
    tiometry
DF —
    decapacitation factor
    decayed and filled
    decontamination factor

DF — (*continued*)
 deferoxamine
 deficiency factor
 defined flora [animal]
 degree of freedom
 dengue fever
 Dermatology Foundation
 desferrioxamine
 diabetic father
 diaphragmatic function
 diastolic filling
 dietary fiber
 digital fluoroscopy
 discriminant function
 disseminated foci
 distribution factor
 dorsiflexion
 drug-free
 dye-free
Df — *Dermatophagoides farinae*
df —
 decayed and filled
 degree of freedom
DFA —
 diet for age
 direct fluorescent antibody
  [test]
 dorsiflexion assistance
DFB —
 dinitrofluorobenzene
 dysfunctional bleeding [uterine]
DFC —
 developmental field complex
 dry-filled capsule
DFD —
 defined formula diets
 degenerative facet disease
 diisopropyl phosphorofluoridate
DFDD — difluoro-diphenyl-dichloroethane
DFDT — difluorodiphenyltrichloroethane
DFE —
 diffuse fasciitis with eosinophilia
 distal femoral epiphysis

DFECT — dense fibroelastic connective tissue
DFG — direct forward gaze
DFHom — Diploma of the Faculty of Homeopathy
DFI — disease-free interval
DFM — decreased fetal movement
DFMC — daily fetal movement count
DFMO — difluoromethylornithine
DFMR — daily fetal movement record
DFOM — deferoxamine
DFP —
 diastolic filling period
 diisopropyl fluorophosphate
 diisopropyl fluorophosphonate
DF^{32}P — radiolabeled diisopropyl fluorophosphonate
DFPP — double filtration plasmapheresis
DFR —
 diabetic floor routine
 dialysate filtration rate
DFRC — deglycerolized frozen red cells
DFS —
 disease-free survival
 dynamic flow study
DFSP — dermatofibrosarcoma protuberans
DFT —
 diagnostic function test
 defibrillation threshold
 discrete Fourier transforms
DFT$_3$ — dialyzable fraction of triiodothyronine
DFT$_4$ — dialyzable fraction of thyroxine
DFU —
 dead fetus in utero
 dideoxyfluorouridine
DFV — diarrhea with fever and vomiting
DFX — desferrioxamine
DG —
 dark ground
 dentate gyrus

DG — (continued)
   deoxyglucose
   diagnosis
   diastolic gallop
   diglyceride
   distogingival
   Duchenne-Griesinger [disease]
2DG — 2-deoxy-D-glucose
Dg — diagnosis
dg. — decigram
dG — deoxyguanosine
DGAVP — desglycinamide-9-[Arg-8]-vasopressin
DGBG — dimethylglyoxal bisguanyl hydrazone
DGCI — delayed gamma camera image
dGDP — deoxyguanosine diphosphate
DGE —
   delayed gastric emptying
   density gradient electrophoresis
dge — drainage
DGF — duct growth factor
DGI — disseminated gonococcal infection
DGL — deglycyrrhized licorice
DGLA — dihomogamma-linolenic acid
DGM — ductal glandular mastectomy
dgm — decigram
dGMP —
   deoxyguanosine monophosphate
   deoxyguanosine-5'-phosphate
DGMS — Division of General Medical Sciences
DGN — diffuse glomerulonephritis
DGO — Diploma in Gynaecology and Obstetrics
DGP —
   deoxyglucose phosphate
   2,3-diglycerophosphate
DGPG — diffuse proliferative glomerulonephritis
DGS —
   developmental Gerstmann's syndrome

DGS — (continued)
   diabetic glomerulosclerosis
   Di George's syndrome
dGTP — deoxyguanosine triphosphate
DGV — dextrose-gelatin-veronal [buffer]
DGVB — dextrose, gelatin, veronal buffer
DH —
   daily habits
   day hospital
   dehydrocholate
   dehydrocholic acid
   dehydrogenase
   delayed hypersensitivity
   dental habits
   dental hygienist
   dermatitis herpetiformis
   developmental history
   diaphragmatic hernia
   diffuse histiocytic [lymphoma]
   disseminated histoplasmosis
   dominant head
   dorsal horn
   drug hypersensitivity
   ductal hyperplasia
   Dunkin-Hartley [guinea pig]
D/H — deuterium/hydrogen [ratio]
DHA —
   dehydroacetic acid
   dehydroascorbic acid
   dehydroepiandrosterone
   dihydroacetic acid
   dihydroxyacetone
   district health authority
   docosahexaenoic acid
DHAC — dihydro-5-azacytidine
DHAD — dihydroxybisamino-anthraquinone dihydrochloride (mitoxantrone hydrochloride)
DHAP — dihydroxyacetone phosphate
DHAP-AT — dihydroxyacetone phosphate acyltransferase
DHAS — dehydroepiandrosterone sulfate

DHB — duct hepatitis B
DHBE — dihydroxybutyl ether
DHBG — dihydroxybutyl guanine
DHBS — dihydrobiopterin synthetase
DHBV — duck hepatitis B virus
DHC —
> dehydrocholate
> dehydrocholesterol
> dehydrocholic acid

DHCA — deep hypothermia and circulatory arrest
DHCC — dihydroxycholecalciferol
DHD — district health department
DHE — dihematoporphyrin ether
DHE 45 — dihydroergotamine
DHEA — dehydroepiandrosterone
DHEAS — dehydroepiandrosterone sulfate
DHEC — dihydroergocryptine
DHES — Division of Health Examination Statistics
DHESN — dihydroergosine
DHEW — Department of Health, Education, and Welfare
DHF —
> dengue hemorrhagic fever
> dihydrofolate
> dihydrofolic acid
> dorsihyperflexion

DHF/DSS — dengue hemorrhagic fever/dengue shock syndrome
DHFR — dihydrofolate reductase
DHFS — dengue hemorrhagic fever shock [syndrome]
DHg — Doctor of Hygiene
DHGG — deaggregated human gammaglobulin
DHHS — Department of Health and Human Services
DHI —
> Dental Health International
> dihydroisocodeine
> dihydroxyindole

DHIA — dehydroisoandrosterone
DHIC — dihydroisocodeine
DHK — dihydroergocryptine
DHL — diffuse histiocytic lymphoma

DHM — dihydromorphinone
DHMA — 3,4-dihydroxymandelic acid
DHMSA — Diploma of History of Medicine, Society of Apothecaries
DHN — Department of Hospital Nursing
DHO —
> deuterium hydrogen oxide
> dihydroergocornine

DHO 180 — dihydroergocornine
DHP —
> dehydrogenated polymer
> dihydroprogesterone
> dihydropyridines
> dihydroxyacetone phosphate

DHPA — dihydroxypropyl adenine
DHPc — dorsal hippocampus
DHPG —
> 3,4-dihydroxyphenylglycol
> 9-(1,3-dihydroxy-2-propoxy methyl) guanine
> dihydroxyproproxymethylguanine

DHPR — dihydropteridine reductase
dhPRL — decidual prolactin
DHR — delayed hypersensitivity reaction
DHS —
> delayed hypersensitivity
> Department of Human Services
> diabetic hyperosmolar state
> dihydrostreptomycin
> duration of hospital stay
> dynamic hip screw

D-5-HS — 5% dextrose in Harman's solution
DHSM — dihydrostreptomycin
DHSS —
> Department of Health and Social Security
> dihydrostreptomycin sulfate

DHST — delayed hypersensitivity test

DHT —
 dihydroergotoxine
 dihydrotachysterol
 dihydrotestosterone
 dihydrothymine
 dihydroxytryptamine
 dissociated hypertropia
DHTB — dihydroteleocidin B
DHTP — dihydrotestosterone propionate
DHTR — dihydrotestosterone receptor
DHyg — Doctor of Hygiene
DHZ — dihydralazine
DI —
 date of injury
 Debrix Index
 defective interfering [particle]
 degradation index
 dentinogenesis imperfecta
 deoxyribonucleic acid index
 depression inventory
 desorption ionization
 deterioration index
 detrusor instability
 diabetes insipidus
 diagnostic imaging
 dialyzed iron
 disability insurance
 distal intestine
 distoincisal
 dorsal interosseous
 dorsoiliac
 double indemnity
 drug information
 drug interactions
 dyskaryosis index
 dyspnea index
D&I —
 débridement and irrigation
 dry and intact
D_1 — inulin dialysance
Di — didymium
DIA —
 depolarization-induced auto-
  maticity
 diabetes
 diazepam

DIA — (continued)
 Drug Information Association
DiA — Diego antigen
dia —
 diakinesis
 diathermy
diab. —
 diabetes
 diabetic
DIAC — diiodothyroacetic acid
diag. —
 diagonal
 diagnosis
 diagnostic
 diagram
diam. — diameter
diaph. —
 diaphragm
 diaphragmatic
DIAR — dextran-induced anaphy-
 lactoid reaction
dias. —
 diastole
 diastolic
diath. — diathermy
Diath SW — diathermy short
 wave
DIAZ — diazepam
DIB —
 Diagnostic Interview for Bor-
  derlines
 disability insurance benefits
 dot immunobinding
 duodenoileal bypass
diBR-HQ — 5,7-dibromo-8-
 hydroxyquinidine
DIC —
 dicarbazine
 differential interference contrast [microscopy]
 diffuse intravascular coagulation
 diffuse intravascular coagulopathy
 disseminated intravascular coagulation
 disseminated intravascular
  coagulopathy

DIC — (*continued*)
Drug Information Center
dic. — dicentric
DICD — dispersion-induced circular dichroism
diclox — dicloxacillin
DID —
dead of intercurrent disease
delayed ischemia deficit
double immunodiffusion
DIDD — dense intramembranous deposit disease
DIDMOA — diabetes inspidius, diabetes mellitus and optic atrophy [syndrome]
DIDMOAD — diabetes insipidus, diabetes mellitus, optic atrophy and deafness [syndrome]
DIE —
died in Emergency Room
direct injection enthalpimetry
dieb. alt. — *diebus alternis* (Lat.) on alternate days
dieb. secund. — *diebus secundis* (Lat.) every second day
dieb. tert. — *diebus tertiis* (Lat.) every third day
DIEDA — diethyliminodiacetic acid
Diet. Tech. — Dietetic Technician
DIF —
diffuse interstitial fibrosis
diflunisal
direct immunofluorescence
dose increase factor
DIFF — differential [blood count]
diff —
difference
different
difficult
diff. diag. — differential diagnosis
DIFP —
diffuse interstitial fibrosing pneumonitis
diisopropyl fluorophosphonate
dig —
digitalis
digitoxin

dig — (*continued*)
digoxin
drug-induced galactorrhea
dig. — *digeratur* (Lat.) let it be digested
dig tox — digitalis toxicity
DIH —
died in hospital
Diploma in Industrial Health
DIHE — drug-induced hepatic encephalopathy
DIHPPA — diiodohydroxyphenylpyruvic acid
DIJOA — dominantly inherited juvenile optic A
DIL —
Dilantin
drug-induced lupus
dil. — *dilue* (Lat.) dilute or dissolve
dilat —
dilatation
dilated
DILD —
diffuse infiltrative lung disease
diffuse interstitial lung disease
dild — diluted
DILE — drug-induced lupus erythematosus
diln — dilution
diluc. — *diluculo* (Lat.) at daybreak
dilut. — *dilutus* (Lat.) diluted
DIM — divalent ion metabolism
dim —
dimension
diminish
diminutive
dim. —
dimidius (Lat.) one half
diminutus (Lat.) diminished
dosis infectionis media (Lat.) medium infective dose
DIME — Division of International Medical Education
DIMIT — 3,5-dimethyl-3'-isopropyl-L-thyronine
DIMOAD — diabetes insipidus, diabetes mellitus, optic atrophy, and deafness [syndrome]

DIMS — disorders of initiating and maintaining sleep

DIMSA — disseminated intravascular multiple systems activation

din — damage inducible [gene]

DIND — delayed ischemic neurological deficit

d. in dup. — *detur in duplo* (Lat.) give twice as much

d. in p. aeq. — *dividetur in partes aequales* (Lat.) divide into equal parts

diopt — diopter

DIP —
    desquamative interstitial pneumonia
    desquamative interstitial pneumonitis
    diisopropyl phosphate
    diisopropylamine
    diphtheria
    distal interphalangeal
    drip-infusion pyelogram
    drug-induced parkinsonism
    dual-in-line package

Dip —
    diploma
    diplomate

dip —
    diploid
    diplotene

DIPA — diisopropylamine

DipBact — Diploma in Bacteriology

DIPC — diffuse interstitial pulmonary calcification

DipChem — Diploma in Chemistry

DipClinPath — Diploma in Clinical Pathology

DIPF — diisopropylphosphofluoridate

diph. — diphtheria

diph-tet — diphtheria-tetanus [toxoid]

diph-tox AP — alum-precipitated diphtheria toxoid

DIPJ — distal interphalangeal joint

DipMicrobiol — Diploma in Microbiology

DipSocMed — Diploma in Social Medicine

DIR — double isomorphous replacement

dir —
    direct
    direction
    director

dir. — *directio* (Lat.) direction

DIRD — drug-induced renal disease

DIRLINE — Directory of Information Resources On-line

dir. prop. — *directione propria* (Lat.) with proper direction

DIS — Diagnostic Interview Schedule

DI-S — Debris Index, Simplified

dis —
    disability
    disabled
    disease
    dislocation
    distal
    distance
    distribution

DISC — Diagnostic Interview Schedule for Children

disc. — discontinue

disch. —
    discharge
    discharged

DISH —
    diffuse idiopathic skeletal hyperostosis
    disseminated idiopathic skeletal hyperostosis

DISI — dorsal intercalated segmental instability

disinfect — disinfection

disloc —
    dislocated
    dislocation

D$_5$Is.M — dextrose 5% in Isolyte M

disod — disodium

disp —
    dispense

disp — *(continued)*
    dispensary
disp. — *dispensia* (Lat.) to dispense
diss —
    dissolve
    dissolved
dissem —
    disseminated
    dissemination
dist —
    distal
    distance
    distill
    distillation
    distilled
    distribution
    disturbance
    disturbed
dist. — *distilla* (Lat.) distill
dist. H_2O — distilled water
DIT —
    deferoxamine infusion test
    diet-induced thermogenesis
    diiodotyrosine
    drug-induced thrombocyto-
      penia
dITP — deoxyinosine triphosphate
DIV — double-inlet ventricle
div —
    divergence
    divergent
    divide
    divided
    division
    divorced
    double-inlet ventricle
div. — *divide* (Lat.) divide
div. in par. aeq. — *dividetur in partes aequales* (Lat.) divide into
equal parts
DIVA — digital intravenous angiography
DIVBC — disseminated intravascular blood coagulation
DIVC — disseminated intravascular coagulation
DJD — degenerative joint disease
DJOA — dominant juvenile optic
atrophy

DJS — Dubin-Johnson syndrome
DK —
    decay
    degeneration of keratinocytes
    Dejerine-Klumpke [syndrome]
    diabetic ketoacidosis
    diet kitchen
    diseased kidney
    dog kidney [cells]
Dk — diffusion coefficient
dk —
    dark
    deka-
DKA — diabetic ketoacidosis
DKB — deep knee bends
DKDP — deuterium with potas-
sium dihydrogen phosphate
dkg — dekagram
dkl — dekaliter
dkm — dekameter
DKP —
    dibasic potassium phosphate
    dikalium phosphate
    diketopiperazine
DKTC — dog kidney tissue culture
DKV — deer kidney virus
DL —
    danger list
    dansyl lysine
    De Lee [catheter]
    deep lobe
    developmental level
    diagnostic laparoscopy
    diagnostic laparotomy
    difference limen
    diffuse lymphoma
    diffusion lung [capacity]
    direct laryngoscopy
    directed listening
    disabled list
    distolingual
    Donath-Landsteiner [test]
    drug level
    equimolecular mixture of the
      dextrorotatory and levorota-
      tory enantiomorphs
d.l. — *dosis lethalis* (Lat.) lethal
dose

D$_L$ — diffusing capacity of the lungs

dl — deciliter

DLa — distolabial

D-L Ab — Donath-Landsteiner antibody

DLaI — distolabioincisal

DLaP — distolabiopulpal

DL&B — direct laryngoscopy and bronchoscopy

DLBD — diffuse Lewy body disease

DLC —
    Dental Laboratory Conference
    differential leukocyte count
    dual-lumen catheter

DL$_{CO_2}$ — carbon dioxide diffusion in the lungs

DL$_{CO}$^{SB} — single-breath carbon monoxide diffusing capacity of the lungs

DL$_{CO}$^{SS} — steady-state carbon monoxide diffusing capacity of the lungs

DLE —
    delayed light emission
    dialyzable leukocyte extract
    discoid lupus erythematosus
    disseminated lupus erythematosus

D$_1$LE — diagonal 1 lower extremity

D$_2$LE — diagonal 2 lower extremity

DLF —
    digitalis-like factor
    digoxin-like factor
    Disabled Living Foundation
    dorsolateral funiculus

DLG — distolingual groove

DLI —
    distolinguoincisal
    double label index

DLIF — digoxin-like immunoreactive factor

DLIS — digoxin-like immunoreactive substance

DLL — dihomo-gammalinoleic acid

DLLI — dulcitol lysine lactose iron

DLMP — date of last menstrual period

DLNMP — date of last normal menstrual period

DLO —
    Diploma in Laryngology and Otology
    distinguo-occlusal

DLO_2 — diffusing capacity of the lungs for oxygen

DLP —
    delipidized serum protein
    developmental learning problems
    direct linear plotting
    dislocation of patella
    distolinguopulpal
    dysharmonic luteal phase

D$_5$LR — dextrose 5% in lactated Ringer's solution

DLS — daily living skills

DLT — dihydroepiandrosterone loading test

DLTS — digoxin-like immunoreactive substance

DLV — defective leukemia virus

DLVO — Derjaguin-Landau-Verwey-Overbeek [theory]

DLW — dry lung weight

DLWD — diffuse lymphocytic, well differentiated

DM —
    dermatomyositis
    Descemet's membrane
    dextromaltose
    dextromethorphan
    diabetes mellitus
    diabetic mother
    diastolic murmur
    diffuse mixed [lymphoma]
    diphenylaminearsine chloride
    diphenylamine chlorarsine
    distant metastases
    dopamine
    dorsomedial
    dose modification
    double minute [chromosome]

DM — (continued)
   dry matter
   duodenal mucosa
D.M. — Doctor Medicinae (Lat.)
   Doctor of Medicine
dM — decimorgan
D_M — membrane component of diffusion
dm. — decimeter
dm^2 — square decimeter
dm^3 — cubic decimeter
DMA —
   dimethyladenosine
   dimethylamine
   dimethylaniline
   dimethylarginine
   direct memory access
DMAB — dimethylaminobenzaldehyde
DMAC — dimethylacetamide
DMAE — dimethylaminoethanol
DMAPN — dimethylaminopropionitrile
DMARD — disease-modifying anti-rheumatic drug
DMAS — dimethylamine sulfate
DMB — deep medial branch
DMBA — 7,12-dimethylbenz[a]anthracene
DMC —
   demeclocycline
   di(p-chlorophenyl)methylcarbinol
   direct microscopic count
   duration of muscle contraction
DMCC — direct microscopic clump count
DMCL — dimethylclomipramine
DMCM — dimethoxyethylcarboline carboxylate
DMCT — dimethylchlortetracycline
DMD —
   disease-modifying drug
   Doctor of Dental Medicine
   Duchenne's muscular dystrophy
   dystonia musculorum deformans

DMDC — dimethyldithiocarbamate
DMDS — dimethyl disulfide
DMDT — dimethoxydiphenyl trichloroethane
DMDZ — desmethyldiazepam
DME —
   degenerative myoclonus epilepsy
   dextromethorphan
   dimethyl diester
   dimethyl ether
   diphasic meningoencephalitis
   Director of Medical Education
   dropping mercury electrode
   drug-metabolizing enzyme
   Dulbecco's modified Eagle's [medium]
   durable medical equipment
DMEM — Dulbecco's modified Eagle's medium
DMF —
   decayed, missing, or filled [teeth]
   dimethylformamide
   diphasic milk fever
DMFO — eflornithine
DMG — dimethylglycine
DMGBL — dimethyl-gamma-butyrolactone
DMH —
   Department of Mental Health
   Department of Mental Hygiene
   diffuse mesangial hypercellularity
   dimethylhydralazine
DMHS — Director of Medical and Health Services
DMI —
   defense mechanism inventory
   desipramine
   Diagnostic Mathematies Inventory
   Diagnostic Medical Instruments
   diaphragmatic myocardial infarction

DMI — (*continued*)
   direct migration inhibition
dmin — double minute
DMJ — Diploma in Medical Jurisprudence
DMKA — diabetes mellitus ketoacidosis
DML —
   diffuse mixed lymphoma
   distal motor latency
DMM —
   dimethylmyleran
   disproportionate micromelia
DMN —
   dimethylnitrosamine
   dorsal motor nucleus
   dysplastic melanocytic nevus
DMNA — dimethylnitrosamine
DMNL — dorsomedial hypothalamic nucleus lesion
DMO — 5,5-dimethyl-2,4-oxazolidinedione (dimethadione)
DMO_2 — membrane diffusing capacity for oxygen
DMOA — diabetes mellitus–optic atrophy [syndrome]
DMOOC — diabetes mellitus out of control
DMP —
   diffuse mesangial proliferation
   dimercaprol
   dimethylphosphate
   dimethylphthalate
   dura mater prosthesis
DMPA — depomedroxyprogesterone acetate
DMPE — 3,4-dimethoxyphenylethylamine
DMPP — dimethylphenylpiperazinium
DMPS — dysmyelopoietic syndrome
DMR —
   Diploma in Medical Radiology
   Directorate of Medical Research

DMRD — Diploma in Medical Radiodiagnosis (British)
DMRE — Diploma in Medical Radiology and Electrology
DMRF — dorsal medullary reticular formation
DMRT — Diploma in Medical Radio-therapy (British)
DMS —
   delayed match-to-sample
   delayed microembolism syndrome
   demarcation membrane system
   dense microsphere
   Department of Medicine and Surgery
   dermatomyositis
   Diagnostic Medical Sonography
   diffuse mesangial sclerosis
   dimethyl sulfate
   dimethyl sulfoxide
   Director of Medical Services
   District Management Team (British)
   Doctor of Medical Science
   dysmyelopoietic syndrome
dms — double minute sphere
DMSA —
   2,3-dimercaptosuccinic acid
   disodium monomethanarsonate
DMSLT — daytime multiple sleep latency test
DMSO — dimethyl sulfoxide
DMSS — Director of Medical and Sanitary Services
DMT —
   dermatophytosis
   dimethyltryptamine
   Doctor of Medical Technology
DMTU — dimethylthiourea
DMU —
   dimethanolurea
   dimethyluracil
DMV — Doctor of Veterinary Medicine

DMWP — distal mean wave pressure

DMX — diathermy, massage, and exercise

DN —
dextrose-nitrogen [ratio]
diabetic neuropathy
dibucaine number
dicrotic notch
Dieter's nucleus
dinitrocresol
Diploma in Nursing
Diploma in Nutrition
District Nurse
Doctor of Nursing
dysplastic nevus

D/N — dextrose/nitrogen [ratio]

D&N — distance and near [vision]

Dn. — dekanem

dn. — decinem

DNA —
deoxyribonucleic acid
did not answer
does not apply

DNAP — deoxyribonucleic acid phosphorus

DNAR — do not attempt resuscitation

DNase — deoxyribonuclease

DNB —
dinitrobenzene
Diplomate of the National Board of Medical Examiners
dorsal nonadrenergic bundle

DNBP — dinitrobutylphenol

DNC —
did not come
dinitrocarbanilide
dinitrocresol
Disaster Nursing Chairman

DNCB — dinitrochlorobenzene

DND — died a natural death

DNE —
Director of Nursing Education
Doctor of Nursing Education

DNFB — dinitrofluorobenzene

DNI — do not intubate

DNKA — did not keep appointment

DNL —
diffuse nodular lymphoma
disseminated necrotizing leukoencephalopathy

DNLL — dorsal nucleus of lateral lemniscus

DNMS — Director of Naval Medical Services

DNO — District Nursing Officer

DNOC — dinitro-o-cresol

DNP —
deoxyribonucleoprotein
dinitrophenol

DNPH — dinitrophenylhydrazine

DNPM — dinitrophenol morphine

DNR —
daunorubicin
did not respond
do not resuscitate
dorsal nerve root

DNS —
de nova synthesis
deviated nasal septum
diaphragmatic nerve stimulation
did not show
Doctor of Nursing Services
do not substitute
dysplastic nevus syndrome

D$_5$NSS — 5% dextrose in normal saline solution

DNT — did not test

DNTM — disseminated nontuberculous mycobacterial [infection]

DNTP — diethylnitrophenyl thiophosphate

dNTP — deoxyribonucleoside triphosphate

DNV — dorsal nucleus of vagus [nerve]

DO —
diamine oxidase
digoxin
Diploma in Ophthalmology
Diploma in Osteopathy

DO — (continued)
   dissolved oxygen
   disto-occlusal
   Doctor of Ophthalmology
   Doctor of Optometry
   Doctor of Osteopathy
   doctor's orders
   drugs only
D/O — disorder
D_O — oxygen diffusion
D_{O_2} — oxygen delivery
do — ditto (from Lat. *dictus*, said)
d/o — died of
DOA —
   date of admission
   date of arrival
   dead on arrival
   Department of Agriculture
   differential optical absorption
   dominant optic atrophy
   duration of action
DOAC — Dubois oleic albumin
   complex
DOB —
   date of birth
   dobutamine
   doctor's order book
DObstRCOG — Diploma of the
   Royal College of Obstetricians and Gynaecologists
   (British)
DOC —
   date of conception
   deoxycholate
   11-deoxycorticosterone
   diabetes out of control
   died of other causes
   diet of choice
   disorders of cornification
   dissolved organic carbon
doc —
   doctor
   document
   documentation
DOCA — deoxycorticosterone acetate
DOCG — deoxycorticosterone glucoside

DOCLINE — Documents On-line
DOCS — deoxycorticosteroids
DOcSc — Doctor of Ocular Science
DOC-SR — deoxycorticosterone
   secretion rate
DOD —
   date of death
   date of discharge
   dementia syndrome of depression
   died of disease
   dissolved oxygen deficit
DOE —
   date of examination
   desoxyephedrine
   direct observation evaluation
   dyspnea on exercise
   dyspnea on exertion
DOES — disorders of excessive
   sleepiness
DOET — dimethoxyethylamphetamir
DOFOS — disturbance of function
   occlusion syndrome
DOH — Department of Health
DOH b — Döhle bodies
DOHyg — Diploma in Occupational Hygiene
DOI —
   date of injury
   died of injuries
DOL — day of life
dol — dolorimetric unit
dol. — *dolor* (Lat.) pain
DOLLS — [Lee's] double-loop locking suture
DOLV — double outlet–left ventricle
DOM —
   deaminated *o*-methyl metabolite
   Department of Medicine
   2,5-dimethoxy-4-methyl-
   amphetamine
   dissolved organic matter
   dominance
   dominant
dom — domestic

DOMA — dihydroxymandelic acid

DOMF — 2,7'-dibromo-4'(hydroxymercuri)fluorescein

DOMS —
  Doctor of Orthopedic Medicine and Surgery
  Diploma in Ophthalmic Medicine and Surgery

DON —
  diazo-oxonorleucine
  Director of Nursing

don. — *donec* (Lat.) until

donec alv. sol. fuerit — *donec alvus soluta fuerit* (Lat.) until the bowels are opened (until a bowel movement occurs)

Dooc — diabetes out of control

DOOR — deafness, onycho-osteodystrophy, mental retardation [syndrome]

DOP — dopamine

DOPA — dihydroxyphenylalanine (methyldopa)

DOPAC — dihydroxyphenyl acetic acid

dopase — dihydroxyphenylalanine oxidase

DOPC — determined osteogenic precursor cell

DOph — Doctor of Ophthalmology

DOPP — dihydroxyphenylpyruvate

DOPS —
  diffuse obstructive pulmonary syndrome
  dihydroxyphenylserine

DORNA — desoxyribonucleic acid

Dors — dorsal

DOrth —
  Diploma in Orthodontics
  Diploma in Orthoptics

DORV — double-outlet right ventricle

DoRx — date of treatment

DOS —
  day of surgery
  deoxystreptamine
  disk operating system

DOS — (*continued*)
  Division of Occupational Safety
  Doctor of Ocular Science
  Doctor of Optical Science

dos — dosage

dos. — *dosis* (Lat.) dose

DOSC — Dubois oleic serum complex

DOSS —
  Department of Social Services
  dioctyl sodium sulfosuccinate
  distal overshoulder strap
  docusate sodium

DOT —
  died on (operating) table
  date of transfer
  Dictionary of Occupational Titles
  Doppler ophthalmic test

DOTC — Dameshek's oval target cell

DOU — direct observation unit

DOV — discharged on visit

Dox — doxorubicin

DP —
  data processing
  deep pulse
  definitive procedure
  degradation product
  degree of polymerization
  deltopectoral
  dementia praecox
  dementia pugillistica
  dense plate
  dental prosthesis
  dental prosthodontics
  dexamethasone pretreatment
  diaphragmatic plaque
  diastolic pressure
  diffuse precipitation
  diffusion pressure
  digestible protein
  diphosgene
  diphosphate
  dipropionate
  direct puncture
  directional preponderance

DP — *(continued)*
  directione propria (Lat.) with proper direction
  disability pension
  discrimination power
  disopyramide phosphate
  displaced person
  distal pancreatectomy
  distal phalanx
  distal pit
  distopulpal
  Doctor of Pharmacy
  Doctor of Podiatry
  donor's plasma
  dorsalis pedis
D-P — Depo-Provera
D_p — pattern difference
Dp — dyspnea
DPA —
  Department of Public Assistance
  dextroposition of aorta
  diphenylalanine
  dipicolinic acid
  dipropylacetic acid
  D-penicillamine
  dual photoabsorptiometry
  dynamic physical activity
DPB —
  days post-burn
  diffuse panbronchiolitis
DPBP — diphenylbutylpiperidine
DPC —
  delayed primary closure
  desaturated phosphatidylcholine
  diethylpyrocarbonate
  direct patient care
  discharge planning coordinator
  distal palmar crease
DPCRT — double-blind placebo-controlled randomized clinical trial
DPD —
  Department of Public Dispensary
  desoxypyridoxine

DPD — *(continued)*
  diffuse pulmonary disease
  diphenamid
  Diploma in Public Dentistry
DPDA — phosphorodiamidic anhydride
DPDL — diffuse, poorly differentiated lymphoma
dpdt — double-pole double-throw [switch]
DPE —
  Death Personification Exercise
  dipiperidinoethane
DPF —
  Dental Practitioners' Formulary
  diisopropyl fluorophosphate
DPFC — distal flexion palmar crease
DPFR — diastolic pressure-flow relationship
DPG —
  2,3-diphosphoglycerate
  displacement placentogram
2,3-DPG — 2,3-diphosphoglycerate
DPGM — diphosphoglycerate mutase
DPGN — diffuse proliferative glomerulonephritis
DPGP — diphosphoglycerate phosphatase
DPH —
  Department of Public Health
  diphenhydramine
  diphenylhexatriene
  diphenylhydantoin
  Diploma in Public Health
  Doctor of Public Health
  Doctor of Public Hygiene
  dopamine betahydrolase
DPhC — Doctor of Pharmaceutical Chemistry
DPhc — Doctor of Pharmacology
DPHN — Doctor of Public Health Nursing
DPhys — Diploma in Physiotherapy

DPhysMed — Diploma in Physical Medicine

DPI —
    daily permissible intake
    days post-inoculation
    dietary protein intake
    diphtheria-pertussis immunization
    drug prescription index
    Dynamic Personality Inventory

Dpi — *Dermatophagoides pteronyssinus*

DPIF — Drug Product Information File

DPJ — dementia paralytica juvenilis

DPL —
    diagnostic peritoneal lavage
    dipalmitoyl lecithin

DPLa — distopulpolabial

DPLN — diffuse proliferative lupus nephritis

DPM —
    Diploma in Psychological Medicine
    dipyridamole
    disabling pansclerotic morphea
    discontinue previous medication
    Doctor of Physical Medicine
    Doctor of Podiatric Medicine
    Doctor of Preventive Medicine
    Doctor of Psychiatric Medicine
    dopamine
    drops per minute

dpm — disintegrations per minute

DPN —
    dermatosis papulosa nigra
    diabetic polyneuropathy
    diphosphopyridine nucleotide
    disabling pansclerotic morphea

DPNase — diphosphopyridine nucleotide

DPNB — dorsal penile nerve block

DPNH — diphosphopyridine nucleotide [reduced form]

DPO — dimethoxyphenyl penicillin

DPP —
    differential pulse polarography
    dimethoxyphenyl penicillin
    dimethylphenylpenicillin

DPPC —
    dipalmitoylphosphatidylcholine
    double-blind placebo-controlled trial

DPS —
    descending perineum syndrome
    dimethylpolysiloxane
    dysesthetic pain syndrome

dps — disintegration per second

DPSS — Department of Public Social Service

dpst — double-pole single-throw [switch]

DPT —
    Demerol, Phenergan, and Thorazine
    dichotic pitch discrimination test
    diphosphothiamine
    diphtheria, pertussis, and tetanus [vaccine]
    diphtheritic pseudotabes
    dipropyltryptamine
    dumping provocation test

Dpt — house dust mite [*Dermatophagoides pteronyssinus*]

DPTA — diethylenetriaminepentaacetic acid

DPTI — diastolic pressure time index

DPTPM — diphtheria, pertussis, tetanus, poliomyelitis and measles [vaccine]

Dptr — diopter

DPU — delayed pressure urticaria

DPUD — duodenal peptic ulcer disease

DPV — disabling positional vertigo

DPVNS — diffuse pigmented villonodular synovitis

DPVS — Denver peritoneovenous shunt

DPW — distal phalangeal width

DPX — dextropropoxyphene

DQ —
deterioration quotient
developmental quotient

DQE — detective quantum efficiency

DR —
daunorubicin
degeneration reaction
Dejerine-Roussey syndrome
delivery room
deoxyribose
diabetic retinopathy
diagnostic radiology
direct repeat
distribution ratio
diurnal rhythm
division of rootlets
doctor
donor-related
dorsal raphe
dorsal root
dose ratio
drug receptor
reaction of degeneration

Dr. — doctor

dr —
dorsal root
drachm
drain
dram
dressing

DRA —
despite resuscitation attempts
dextran-reactive antibody
disease-resistant antigen
drug-related admission

DRACOG — Diploma of Royal Australian College of Obstetricians and Gynaecologists

DRACR — Diploma of Royal Australasian College of Radiologists

DRAM — dynamic random access memory

dr ap — dram, apothecary

DRAT — differential rheumatoid agglutination test

DRB — daunorubicin

DRBC —
denatured red blood cell
dog red blood cell
donkey red blood cell

DRC —
damage risk criteria
dendritic reticulum cell
digitorenocerebral [syndrome]
dog red cell
dorsal root, cervical

dRCA — distal right coronary artery

DRCOG — Diploma of Royal College of Obstetricians and Gynaecologists

DRCPath — Diploma of Royal College of Pathologists

DRD — dorsal root dilator

DRE — digital rectal examination

DREF — dose rate effectiveness factor

DREZ — dorsal root entry zone

DRF —
Daily Rating Form
daily replacement factor
Deafness Research Foundation
dose-reduction factor

DRFB — doubly refractile fat bodies

DRG —
Diagnosis-Related Group
Division of Research Grants [NIH]
dorsal respiratory group
dorsal root ganglion
duodenal-gastric reflux gastropathy

drg — drainage

DrHyg — Doctor of Hygiene
DRI — Discharge Readiness Inventory
dRib — deoxyribose
DRIC — Dental Research Information Center
DRID —
    double radial immunodiffusion
    double radioisotope derivative
DRL —
    dorsal root, lumbar
    drug-related lupus
D5RL — 5% dextrose in Ringer's lactate [solution]
DRME — Division of Research in Medical Education
Dr Med — Doctor of Medicine
DRMS — drug reaction monitoring system
DrMT — Doctor of Mechanotherapy
DRN — dorsal raphe nucleus
DRNDP — diribonucleoside-3'3'-diphosphate
DRnt — diagnostic roentgenology
DRO —
    differential reinforcement of other behavior
    Disablement Resettlement Officer
DRP —
    digoxin reduction product
    dorsal root potential
dRp — deoxyribose-phosphate
DrPH — Doctor of Public Health
    Doctor of Public Hygiene
DRQ — discomfort relief quotient
DRR —
    Division of Research Resources [NIH]
    dorsal root reflex
DRS —
    descending rectal septum
    Division of Research Services [NIH]
    drowsiness
    Duane retraction syndrome

DRS — (continued)
    dynamic renal scintigraphy
    Dyskinesia Rating Scale
DRs — dorsal root, sacral
drsg — dressing
DRT — dorsal root, thoracic
DRUJ — distal radioulnar joint
DS —
    dead air space
    dead space
    Debré-Sémélaigne [syndrome]
    deep sedative
    deep sleep
    defined substrate
    dehydroepiandrosterone sulfate
    Dejerine-Sottas [syndrome]
    delayed sensitivity
    dendritic spine
    density standard
    dental surgery
    deprivation syndrome
    dermatan sulfate
    dermatology and syphilology
    desynchronized sleep
    Devic's syndrome
    dextran sulfate
    dextrose-saline
    dextrose stick
    diaphragm stimulation
    diastolic murmur
    difference spectroscopy
    differential stimulus
    diffuse scleroderma
    digit span
    dihydrostreptomycin
    dilute strength
    dioptric strength
    Disaster Services
    discharge summary
    discrimination score
    discriminative stimulus
    disoriented
    disseminated sclerosis
    dissolved solids
    Doctor of Science
    donor's serum
    Doppler sonography

DS — *(continued)*
  double-stranded
  double strength
  Down's syndrome
  drug store
  dry swallow
  dumping syndrome
  duration of systole
D-S — Doerfler-Stewart [test]
D/S —
  day of surgery
  dextrose/saline
  dextrose/sodium chloride
D&S —
  dominance and submission
  dermatology and syphilology
  dilation and suction
D-5-S — 5% dextrose in saline solution
ds — double-stranded
DSA —
  digital subtraction angiography
  digital subtraction arteriography
  disease-susceptible antigen
DSACT — direct sinoatrial conduction time
DSAP — disseminated superficial actinic porokeratosis
DSAS — discrete subaortic stenosis
Dsb — single-breath diffusion capacity
DSBB — double-sheath bronchial brushing
DSBL — disabled
DSBT — donor-specific blood transfusion
DSC —
  De Sanctis-Cacchione [syndrome]
  differential scanning colorimeter
  disodium chromoglycate
  Doctor of Surgical Chiropody
  Down's syndrome child
DSc — Doctor of Science

DSCF — Doppler-shifted constant frequency
DSCG — disodium chromoglycate
DSCT — dorsal spinocerebellar tract
DSD —
  depression spectrum disease
  depression sine depression
  discharge summary dictated
  dry sterile dressing
DSDB — direct self-destructive behavior
DSDDT — double-sampling dye dilution technique
dsDNA — double-stranded deoxyribonucleic acid
DSE —
  digital subtraction echocardiogram
  Doctor of Sanitary Engineering
d. seq. — *die sequente* (Lat.) on the following day
DSF —
  disulfiram
  dry sterile fluff
DSG — dry sterile gauze
dsg. — dressing
DSH —
  deliberate self-harm
  dexamethasone suppressible hyperaldosteronism
DSHR — delayed skin hypersensitivity reaction
DSI —
  deep shock insulin
  Depression Status Inventory
  digital subtraction imaging
  Down Syndrome International
DSIM — Doctor of Science in Industrial Medicine
DSIP — delta sleep-inducing peptide
DSL — distal sensory latency
DSL M-U — distal sensory latency — median-ulnar
dslv — dissolved

DSM —
> dextrose solution mixture
> Diagnostic and Statistical Manual [of Mental Disorders]
> dihydrostreptomycin
> Diploma in Social Medicine

DSO — distal subungual onychomycosis

DSP —
> decreased sensory perception
> delayed sleep phase
> dibasic sodium phosphate
> digital subtraction phlebography
> digital signal processor

D5p — digit span

DSPC — disaturated phosphatidylcholine

D/spine — dorsal spine

DSPN —
> distal sensory polyneuropathy
> distal symmetrical polyneuropathy

DSR —
> daily symptom report
> distal splenorenal
> double simultaneous recording
> dynamic spatial reconstructor

DSRF — drainage (of) subretinal fluid

dsRNA — double-stranded ribonucleic acid

DSRS — distal splenorenal shunt

DSS —
> dengue shock syndrome
> Developmental Sentence Scoring
> dioctyl sodium sulfosuccinate
> Disability Status Scale
> docusate sodium
> double simultaneous stimulation

DSSc — Diploma in Sanitary Science

DSSEP — dermatomal somatosensory evoked potential

DSST — digit symbol substitutional test

DST —
> desensitization test
> desensitization time
> dexamethasone suppression test
> dihydrostreptomycin
> disproportionate septal thickening
> donor-specific transfusion

D-S test — Doerfler-Stewart test

D-stix — Dextrostix

DSU —
> day surgery unit
> double setup

DSUH — directed suggestion under hypnosis

DSur — Doctor of Surgery

DSV — digital subtraction ventriculography

DSVP — downstream venous pressure

DSWI — deep surgical wound infection

DSX — Dextrostix

DT —
> defibrillation threshold
> Dejerine-Thomas [syndrome]
> delirium tremens
> dental technician
> depression of transmission
> dietetic technician
> digitoxin
> diphtheria and tetanus [toxoid]
> discharge tomorrow
> dispensing tablet
> distance test
> diversional therapy
> dorsalis tibialis
> double tachycardia
> doubling time
> duration of tetany
> dye test

D/T — date of treatment

D&T — diagnosis and treatment

Dt —
> duration tetany
> total ratio of death

dT —
    deoxythymidine
    due to
dt — dystonic
DTA — differential thermal analysis
DTaP — diphtheria and tetanus toxoids and acellular pertussis [vaccine]
DTB — dedicated time block
DTBC — D-tubocurarine
DTBN — di-*tert*-butyl nitroxide
DTBP — di-*tert*-butyl peroxide
DTC —
    day treatment center
    differential thyroid carcinoma
dTc — D-tubocurarine
DTCD — Diploma in Tuberculosis and Chest Diseases
DTCH — Diploma in Tropical Child Health
d.t.d. —
    datur talis dosis (Lat.) give such a dose
    dosis therapeutica die (Lat.) daily therapeutic dose
dTDP — deoxythymidine diphosphate
DTE — desiccated thyroid extract
2-D TEE — two-dimensional transesophageal echocardiography
DTF — detector transfer function
DTGA — dextrotransposition of great arteries
DTH —
    delayed-type hypersensitivity
    Diploma in Tropical Hygiene
DTI — dipyridamole-thallium imaging
DTIC — dimethyltriazeno-imidazole carboxamide (dacarbazine)
DTICH — delayed traumatic intracerebral hemorrhage
D time — dream time
DTLA — Detroit Test of Learning Aptitude
DTM —
    dermatophyte test medium

DTM — *(continued)*
    Diploma in Tropical Medicine
DTMA — deoxycorticosterone trimethylacetate
DTM&H — Diplomate of Tropical Medicine and Hygiene
DTMP — deoxythymidine monophosphate
dTMP — thymidine-5'-phosphate
DTMV — diastolic transmembrane voltage
DTN — diphtheria toxin, normal
DTNB — 5,5'-dithiobis-(2-nitrobenzoic) acid
DTO — deodorized tincture of opium
d. tox. — *dosis toxica* (Lat.) toxic dose
DTP —
    diphtheria, tetanus toxoids, and pertussis [vaccine]
    distal tingling on percussion
DTPA — diethylenetriamine-penta-acetic acid
DTPH — Diploma in Tropical Public Health
DTR — deep tendon reflex
DTRTT — digital temperature recovery time test
DTS —
    dense tubular system
    diphtheria toxin sensitivity
    discrete time sample
    donor transfusion, specific
DTs — delirium tremens
DTT —
    diagnostic and therapeutic team
    diphtheria-tetanus toxoid
    direct transverse traction
dTTP — deoxythymidine triphosphate
DTUS — diathermy, traction, and ultrasound
DT-VAC — diphtheria-tetanus vaccine
DTVM — Diploma in Tropical Veterinary Medicine

DTVMI — Developmental Test of Visual Motor Integration
DTVP — Developmental Test of Visual Perception
DTX — detoxification
DTZ — diatrizoate
DU —
  decubitus ulcer
  density unknown
  deoxyuridine
  dermal ulcer
  diabetic urine
  diagnosis undetermined
  diazouracil
  diffuse and undifferentiated
  dog unit
  dose unit
  duodenal ulcer
  duroxide uptake
  Dutch [rabbit]
Du — urea dialysance
dU — deoxyuridine
d.u. — dial unit
DUA — dorsal uterine artery
DUB —
  Dubowitz [score]
  dysfunctional uterine bleeding
dUDP — deoxyuridine diphosphate
D₁UE — diagonal 1 upper extremity
D₂UE — diagonal 2 upper extremity
DUF —
  Doppler ultrasonic flowmeter
  drug use forecast
DUI — driving under the influence
DUID — driving under the influence of drugs
DUL — diffuse undifferentiated lymphoma
dulc. — *dulcis* (Lat.) sweet
DUM — dorsal unpaired median [axon]
DUMC — Duke University Medical Center
dUMP — deoxyuridine monophosphate

DUNHL — diffuse undifferentiated non-Hodgkin's lymphoma
duod. —
  duodenal
  duodenum
DUP — deoxyuridine-5′-phosphate
dup —
  duplicate
  duplication
DUR — Drug Use Review
dur —
  duration
  during
dur. — *duris* (Lat.) hard
dur. dolor. — *durante dolore* (Lat.) while the pain lasts
DUS — Doppler ultrasound stethoscope
DUSN — diffuse unilateral subacute neuroretinitis
dUTP — deoxyuridine triphosphate
DUV — damaging ultraviolet [radiation]
DV —
  dependent variable
  difference in volume
  digital vibration
  dilute volume
  distant vision
  distemper virus
  domiciliary visit
  dorsoventral
  double vibrations
  double vision
D&V —
  diarrhea and vomiting
  disks and vessels
d.v. —
  double vibrations
  double vision
DVA —
  Department of Veterans Affairs
  developmental venous anomaly
  distance visual acuity
  duration of voluntary apnea

DVA — (continued)
vindesine
D/V$_A$ — diffusion per unit of alveolar volume
DVB — divinylbenzene
DVC —
  direct visualization of vocal cords
  divanillylcyclohexane
DVCC — Disease Vector Control Center
DVD —
  dissociated vertical deviation
  dissociated vertical divergence
  double vessel disease
DV&D — Diploma in Venereology and Dermatology
DVDALV — double vessel disease with abnormal left ventricle
dVDAVP — 1-deamine-4-valine-D-arginine vasopressin
DVE — duck virus enteritis
DVH —
  Diploma in Veterinary Hygiene
  Division for the Visually Handicapped
DVI —
  digital vascular imaging
  Doppler velocity index
  AV sequential [pacemaker]
DVIS — digital vascular imaging system
DVIU — direct-vision internal urethrotomy
DVL — deep vastus lateralis
DVM —
  digital voltmeter
  Doctor of Veterinary Medicine
DVMS — Doctor of Veterinary Medicine and Surgery
DVN — dorsal vagal nucleus
DVR —
  Department of Vocational Rehabilitation
  derotational varus osteotomy
  digital vascular reactivity

DVR — (continued)
  Doctor of Veterinary Radiology
  double valve replacement
  double ventricular response
DVS —
  Division of Vital Statistics
  Doctor of Veterinary Science
  Doctor of Veterinary Surgery
DVSA — digital venous subtraction angiography
DVT —
  deep vein thrombosis
  deep venous thrombosis
DVTS — deep venous thrombo-scintigram
DVXI — direct vision times one
DW —
  daily weight
  deionized water
  dextrose in water
  distilled water
  doing well
  dry weight
D/W —
  dextrose in water
  doing well
  dry to wet
D$_5$W — 5% dextrose in water
D10W — 10% aqueous dextrose solution
dw — dwarf [mouse]
DWA — died from wounds by the action of the enemy
DWD — died with disease
DWDL — diffuse well-differentiated lymphocytic lymphoma
DWI —
  driving while impaired
  driving while intoxicated
DWMI — deep white matter infarct
DWRT — delayed work recall test
DWS —
  Dandy-Walker syndrome
  disaster warning system
DWT — dichotic word test
dwt. — pennyweight

DX —
    dextran
    dicloxacillin
Dx — diagnosis
Dxd — discontinued
DXM — dexamethasone
DXR —
    deep x-ray
    doxorubicin
DXT —
    deep x-ray therapy
    dextrose
dXTP — deoxyxanthine triphosphate
D-XYL — D-xylose
DY —
    dense parenchyma
    Dyke-Young [syndrome]
Dy — dysprosium

dy — dystrophia muscularis [mouse]
dyn —
    dynamic
    dynamometer
    dyne
dysp — dyspnea
DZ —
    diazepam
    dizygotic
    dizygous
    dizziness
dz —
    disease
    dozen
DZM — dorsal zone of membranelle
DZP — diazepam
DZT — dizygotic twins

E —
    air dose
    average beta energy
    cortisone (compound E)
    each
    edema
    einstein [unit of energy]
    elastance
    electric affinity
    electric charge
    electric field vector
    electric intensity
    electrode potential
    electromagnetic force
    electromotive force
    electron
    embryo
    emmetropia
    encephalitis
    endangered [animal]
    endogenous
    endoplasm
    enema

E — (continued)
    energy
    engorged
    Entamoeba
    Enterococcus
    enterococcus
    entgegen (Ger.) stereodescriptor to indicate the configuration at a double bond
    enzyme
    eosinophil
    epicondyle
    epinephrine
    epsilon (fifth letter of the Greek alphabet), uppercase
    error
    erythrocyte
    erythroid
    erythromycin
    Escherichia
    esophagus
    esophoria
    ester

E — (continued)
   estradiol
   ethanol
   ethmoid [sinus]
   ethyl
   etiocholanolone
   etiology
   examination
   examiner
   exercise
   expectancy
   expected frequency in a cell
      of a contingency table
   experiment
   experimental
   experimenter
   expiration
   expired
   expired air
   extension
   extinction [coefficient]
   extract
   extracted
   extraction
   extraction fraction
   extraction ratio
   extralymphatic
   eye
   glutamic acid
   internal energy
   kinetic energy
   kinetic energy of a particle
   mathematical expectation
   redox potential
   standard electrode potential
   vectorcardiography electrode
      [midsternal]
   vitamin E
E^* — lesion on the erythrocyte
   cell membrane at the site of
   complement fixation
E' — esophoria [for near]
$E°$ —
   standard electrode potential
   standard potential
   standard reduction potential
E_0 —
   electric affinity

E_0 — (continued)
   skin dose [of radiation]
$E_0{}^+$ — oxidation-reduction potential
E^+ — positron [positive electron]
E^- — negative electron
E_1 — estrone
E_2 —
   17 beta-estradiol
   estradiol
E_3 — estriol
E_4 — estetrol
E_h — redox potential
$4E$ — four-plus edema
E. —
   Entamoeba
   Enterococcus
   Escherichia
$_E$ — expired gas
e —
   base of natural logarithms
   early
   egg transfer
   electric charge
   electron
   elementary charge
   emergency area
   erg
   exchange
$e-$ — electron
$e+$ — positron
ϵ —
   chain of hemoglobin
   dielectric constant
   epsilon (the fifth letter of the
      Greek alphabet), lowercase
   fifth in a series or group
   heavy chain of immunoglobu-
      lin E
   molar absorption coefficient
   molar absorptivity
   molar extinction coefficient
   permittivity
   specific absorptivity
η —
   absolute viscosity
   eta (the seventh letter of the
      Greek alphabet), lowercase

EA —
early antigen
educational age
egg albumin
elbow aspiration
electric affinity
electroacupuncture
electroanesthesia
electrophysiologic abnormality
electrophysiological abnormality
embryonic antibody
embryonic antigen
emergency area
endocardiographic amplifier
Endometriosis Association
enteral alimentation
enteroanastomosis
enzymatic active
enzymatically active
epiandrosterone
erythrocyte antibody
erythrocyte antisera
esophageal atresia
esterase activity
estivoautumnal [malaria]
ethacrynic acid

E→A — "E to A" [in pulmonary consolidation, all vowels including "e" heard as "a"]

E&A — evaluate and advise

E$_\alpha$ — kinetic energy of alpha particles

ea. — each

EAA —
electroacupuncture analgesia
electrothermal atomic absorption
Epilepsy Association of America
essential amino acid
extrinsic allergic alveolitis

EAB —
elective abortion
Ethics Advisory Board
extra-anatomic bypass

EABV — effective arterial blood volume

EAC —
Ehrlich ascites carcinoma
electroacupuncture
epithelioma adenoides cysticum
erythema action [spectrum]
erythema annulare centrifugum
erythrocyte, antibody, and complement
external auditory canal

EACA — epsilon-aminocaproic acid

EACD — eczematous allergic contact dermatitis

EAD —
early afterdepolarization
extracranial arterial disease

ead. — eadem (Lat.) the same

EA-D — early antigen diffuse [component]

E-ADD — epileptic attentional deficit disorder

EADS — early amnion deficit spectrum or syndrome

EAE —
experimental allergic encephalitis
experimental allergic encephalomyelitis
experimental autoimmune encephalitis
experimental autoimmune encephalomyelitis

EAEC — enteroadherent Escherichia coli

EAF — emergency assistance to families

EAG —
electroantennogram
electroarteriography
electroatriogram

EAHF — eczema, asthma, and hay fever [complex]

EAHLG — equine antihuman lymphoblast globulin

EAHLS — equine antihuman lymphoblast serum

EAI —
  Emphysema Anonymous, Inc.
  Employment and Adaptation
    Index
  erythrocyte antibody inhibi-
    tion
EAK — ethyl amyl ketone
EAL — electronic artificial larynx
EAM —
  external acoustic meatus
  external auditory meatus
EAMG — experimental autoimmune myasthenia gravis
EAN — experimental allergic neuritis
EANG — epidemic acute nonbacterial gastroenteritis
EAO — experimental allergic orchitis
EAP —
  electric acupuncture
  electroacupuncture
  epiallopregnanolone
  erythrocyte acid phosphatase
  evoked action potential
EAQ — eudismic affinity quotient
e⁻ (aq) — aqueous electron
EAR —
  electroencephalographic audi-
    ometry
  expired air resuscitation
Ea. R. — *Entartungs-Reaktion*
  (Ger.) reaction of degeneration
ear ox — ear oximetry
EARR — extended aortic root replacement
EAST —
  elevated-arm stress test
  Emory angioplasty versus sur-
    gery trial
  external rotation, abduction
    stress test
EAT —
  Eating Attitudes Test
  ectopic atrial tachycardia
  Edinburgh Articulation Test
  Education Apperception Test

EAT — (*continued*)
  Ehrlich ascites tumor
  electro-aerosol therapy
  epidermolysis acuta toxica
  experimental autoimmune
    thymitis
  experimental autoimmune
    thyroiditis
EATC — Ehrlich ascites tumor
  cell
EAU — experimental autoimmune
  uveitis
EAV —
  equine abortion virus
  extra-alveolar vessel
EAVC — enhanced arterioventricular conduction
EAVM — extramedullary arteriovenous malformation
EAVN — enhanced arterioventricular nodal [conduction]
EB —
  elbow bearing
  elective abortion
  elementary body
  endometrial biopsy
  epidermolysis bullosa
  Epstein-Barr [virus]
  esophageal body
  estradiol benzoate
  ethidium bromide
  Evans blue [dye]
E-B — Epstein-Barr [virus]
E_2B — estradiol benzoate
EBA —
  epidermolysis bullosa acquisita
  epidermolysis bullosa atrophi-
    cans
  orthoethoxybenzoic acid
  extrahepatic biliary atresia
EBAA — Eye Bank Association of
  America
EBAB — equal breath sounds bilaterally
EBC — esophageal balloon catheter
EBCDIC — Extended Binary
  Coded Decimal Interchange
  Code

EBCT — electron beam computed tomography

EBD — epidermolysis bullosa dystrophica

EBDD — epidermolysis bullosa dystrophica, dominant

EBDR — epidermolysis bullosa dystrophica, recessive

EBEA — Epstein-Barr [virus] early antigen

EBF — erythroblastosis fetalis

EBG —
electroblepharogram
electroblepharography

EBI —
elective brain irradiation
emetine bismuth iodide
erythroblastic island
estradiol binding index

EBK — embryonic bovine kidney

EBL —
enzootic bovine leukosis
erythroblastic leukemia
estimated blood loss

eBL — endemic Burkitt's lymphoma

EBL/S — estimated blood loss during surgery

EBM —
electrophysiologic behavior modification
expressed breast milk

EBNA — Epstein-Barr [virus-associated] nuclear antigen

EBNe — Epstein-Barr nasopharyngeal carcinoma

E/BOD — electrolyte biochemical oxygen demand

EBP —
epidural blood patch
estradiol-binding protein

EBRT —
electron beam radiotherapy
electron beam radiation therapy

EBS —
elastic back strap
electric brain stimulation

EBS — (continued)
electric brain stimulator
Emergency Bed Service
epidermolysis bullosa simplex

EBSS — Earle's balanced salt solution

EBT —
early bedtime
ethylsulfonylbenzaldehyde thiosemicarbazone (subathizone)
external beam (photon) therapy

EBV —
effective blood volume
Epstein-Barr virus

EB-VCA — Epstein-Barr viral capsid antigen

EBVDNA — Epstein-Barr virus–determinated nuclear antigen

EBVEA — Epstein-Barr virus, early antigen

EBVNA — Epstein-Barr virus, nuclear antigen

EBZ — epidermal basement zone

EC —
econazole
effect of closing [of eyes in electroencephalography]
effective concentration
ejection click
electrochemical
electron capture
Ellis-van Creveld [syndrome]
embryonal carcinoma
emetic center
endemic cretinism
endocrine cells
endothelial cell
energy charge
enteric-coated
entering complaint
enterochromaffin
entorhinal cortex
entrance complaint
environmental complexity
Enzyme Commission [of International Union of Biochemistry]

EC — *(continued)*
    enzyme-treated cell
    epidermal cell
    epidermal cyst
    epithelial cell
    equalization-cancellation
    Erb-Charcot [syndrome]
    error correction
    Escherichia coli
    esophageal carcinoma
    ether-chloroform [mixture]
    excitation-contraction
    excitatory center
    experimental control
    expiratory center
    external carotid [artery]
    external conjugate
    extracellular
    extracellular compartment
    extracellular concentration
    extracranial
    extruded cell
    eye care
    eyes closed

E/C —
    endoscopy/cystoscopy
    estriol/creatinine [ratio]
    estrogen/creatinine [ratio]

E-C —
    ether-chloroform [mixture]
    excitation-contraction

Ec — ectoconchion

EC_{50} — median effective concentration

ECA —
    electric control activity
    electrocardioanalyzer
    endothelial cytotoxic activity
    enterobacterial common antigen
    epidemiologic catchment area
    ethacrynic acid
    ethylcarboxylate adenosine
    external carotid artery

E-CABG — endarterectomy and coronary artery bypass graft

ECAD — extracranial carotid arterial disease

ECAO — enteric cytopathogenic avian orphan [virus]

ECAT — emission computed axial tomography

ECB — electric cabinet bath

ECBD — exploration of common bile duct

ECBO — enteric cytopathogenic bovine orphan [virus]

ECBV — effective circulating blood volume

ECC —
    edema, clubbing, and cyanosis
    electrocorticogram
    electrocorticography
    embryonal cell carcinoma
    emergency cardiac care
    endocervical cone
    endocervical curettage
    estimated creatinine clearance
    external cardiac compression
    extracorporeal circulation
    extrusion of cell cytoplasm

ECCE — extracapsular cataract extraction

ECCLS — European Committee for Clinical Laboratory Standards

ECCO — enteric cytopathogenic cat orphan [virus]

$ECCO_2R$ — extracorporeal carbon dioxide removal

ECD —
    electrochemical detector
    electron capture detector
    endocardial cushion defect
    enzymatic cell dispersion

ECDB — encourage to cough and deep breathe

ECDEU — early clinical drug evaluation unit

ECDO — enteric cytopathogenic dog orphan [virus]

ECE —
    early childhood education
    endocervical ecchymosis
    equine conjugated estrogen

ECEMG — evoked compound electromyography

ECEO — enteric cytopathogenic
  equine orphan [virus]
ECF —
  East Coast fever
  effective capillary flow
  eosinophil chemotactic factor
  erythroid colony formation
  Escherichia coli filtrate
  extended care facility
  extracellular fluid
ECF-A — eosinophil chemotactic
  factor of anaphylaxis
ECF-C — eosinophil chemotactic
  factor–complement
ECFMG —
  Educational Commission on
    Foreign Medical Graduates
  Educational Council for For-
    eign Medical Graduates
ECFMS — Educational Council
  for Foreign Medical Students
ECFV — extracellular fluid volume
ECG —
  electrocardiogram
  electrocardiography
ECGF — endothelial cell growth
  factor
ECGS — endothelial cell growth
  supplement
ECH —
  epichlorohydrin
  extended care hospital
ECHINO — echinocyte
ECHO —
  echocardiogram
  echocardiography
  echoencephalogram
  echoencephalography
  echogram
  enteric cytopathogenic hu-
    man orphan [virus]
Echo-VM — echoventriculometry
ECHSCP — Exeter Community
  Health Services Computer
  Project
ECI —
  electrocerebral inactivity
  eosinophilic cytoplasmic in-
    clusion

ECI — (*continued*)
  extracorporeal irradiation
ECIB — extracorporeal irradiation
  of blood
EC-IC — extracranial-intracranial
ECIL — extracorporeal irradiation
  of lymph
ECIS — equipment control information system
ECK — extracellular kalium (potassium)
ECL —
  electrogenerated chemilu-
    minescence
  emitter-coupled logic
  enterochromaffin-like [type]
  euglobulin clot lysis
  extent of cerebral lesion
  extracapillary lesions
eclec. — eclectic
ECLT — euglobulin clot lysis time
ECM —
  embryonic chick muscle
  erythema chronicum migrans
  experimental cerebral malaria
  external cardiac massage
  external chemical messenger
  extracellular material
  extracellular matrix
E-C mixture — ether-chloroform
  mixture
ECMO —
  enteric cytopathogenic mon-
    key orphan [virus]
  extracorporeal membrane oxy-
    genation
ECMP — enterocoated micro-
  spheres of pancrelipase
ECN — extended care nursery
EC No. — Enzyme Commission
  Number
ECochG — electrocochleography
ECOG — Eastern Cooperative Oncology Group
ECoG —
  electrocorticogram
  electrocorticography
E. coli — *Escherichia coli*

ECP —
  ectrodactyly-cleft palate [syndrome]
  effector cell precursor
  electronic claims processing
  endocardial potential
  eosinophil cationic protein
  erythrocyte coproporphyrin
  erythroid committed precursor
  Escherichia coli polypeptide
  estradiol cyclopentanepropionate
  external cardiac pressure
  external counterpulsation
  free cytoporphyrin in erythrocytes
ECPD — external counterpressure device
ECPO — enteric cytopathogenic porcine orphan [virus]
ECPOG — electrochemical potential gradient
ECPR — external cardiopulmonary resuscitation
ECR —
  effectiveness-cost ratio
  electrocardiographic response
  emergency chemical restraint
ECRB — extensor carpi radialis brevis
ECRL — extensor carpi radialis longus
ECRO — enteric cytopathogenic rodent orphan [virus]
ECS —
  elective cosmetic surgery
  electrocerebral silence
  electroconvulsive shock
  electronic claims submission
  electroshock
  extracellular space
ECSO — enteric cytopathogenic swine orphan [virus]
ECSP — epidermal cell surface protein
ECT —
  electroconvulsive therapy
  emission computed tomography

ECT — (*continued*)
  enhanced computed tomography
  enteric-coated tablet
  euglobulin clot test
  European compression technique [bone screw and internal fixation]
  extracellular tissue
ect —
  ectopic
  ectopy
ECTA — Everyman's Contingency Table Analysis
ECTEOLA — epichlorohydrin and triethanolamine
ECU —
  environmental control unit
  extended care unit
  extensor carpi ulnaris
ECV —
  epithelial cell vacuolization
  extracellular volume
  extracorporeal volume
ECVD — extracellular volume of distribution
ECVE — extracellular volume expansion
ECW — extracellular water
ED —
  early differentiation
  ectodermal dysplasia
  ectopic depolarization
  effective dose
  Ehlers-Danlos [syndrome]
  elbow disarticulation
  electrodiagnosis
  electrodialysis
  electron diffraction
  elemental diet
  embryonic death
  emergency department
  emotional disorder
  emotional disturbance
  emotionally disturbed
  end diastole
  entering diagnosis
  Entner-Doudoroff [metabolic pathway]

ED — *(continued)*
    enzyme deficiency
    epidural
    epileptiform discharge
    equilibrium dialysis
    equine dermis [cells]
    erythema dose
    ethyl dichlorarsine
    ethylenediamine
    ethynodiol
    evidence of disease
    exertional dyspnea
    extensive disease
    extensor digitorum
    external diameter
    external dyspnea
    extra-low dispersion
E-D — ego-defense
ED_{50} — median effective dose
E_d — depth dose
ed — edema
EDA —
    electrodermal activity
    electrodermal audiometry
    electrolyte-deficient agar
    electron donor acceptor
    end-diastolic area
EDAM — electron-dense amorphous material
EDAP — Emergency Department Approval for Pediatrics
EDAS — encephaloduroarterio synangiosis
EDAX — energy dispersive x-ray analysis
EDB —
    early dry breakfast
    electron-dense body
    ethylene dibromide
    extensor digitorum brevis
EDBP — erect diastolic blood pressure
EDC —
    effective dynamic compliance
    electrodesiccation and curettage
    emergency decontamination center

EDC — *(continued)*
    end-diastolic count
    estimated date of conception
    estimated date of confinement
    expected date of confinement
    expected delivery, cesarean
    extensor digitorum communis
ED&C — electrodessication and curettage
EDCF — endothelium-derived contracting factor
EDCI — energetic dynamic cardiac insufficiency
EDCS —
    end-diastolic chamber stiffness
    end-diastolic circumferential stress
EDCT — early distal proximal tubule
EDD —
    effective drug duration
    electron-dense deposit
    end-diastolic dimension
    enzyme-digested delta
    estimated discharge date
    estimated due date
    expected date of delivery
EDDA — expanded duty dental auxiliary
edent —
    edentia
    edentulous
EDF —
    end-diastolic flow
    extradural fluid
EDG — electrodermography
EDH —
    epidural hematoma
    extradural hematoma
EDICP — electron-dense iron-containing particle
EDIM —
    epidemic disease of infant mice
    epizootic diarrhea of infant mice
E-diol — estradiol

EDL —
    end-diastolic length
    end-diastolic load
    estimated date of labor
    extensor digitorum longus
ED/LD — emotionally disturbed
    and learning disabled
EDM —
    early diastolic murmur
    extramucosal duodenal myot-
        omy
EDMA — ethylene glycol dimetha-
    crylate
EDMD — Emery-Dreifuss muscular
    dystrophy
EDN —
    electrodesiccation
    eosinophil-derived neurotoxin
EDNA — Emergency Department
    Nurses Association
EDNF — endogenous digitalis–like
    natriuretic factor
EDOC — estimated date of con-
    finement
EDP —
    electron-dense particle
    electronic data processing
    emergency department physi-
        cian
    end-diastolic pressure
EDPA — ethyldiphenylpropenylamine
EDQ — extensor digiti quinti
EDR —
    early diastolic relaxation
    edrophonium
    effective direct radiation
    electrodermal response
    electrodialysis (with) reversed
        (polarity)
EDRF — endothelium-derived re-
    laxing factor
EDS —
    edema disease of swine
    egg drop syndrome
    Ego Development Scale
    Ehlers-Danlos syndrome
    Emery-Dreifuss syndrome
    energy-dispersive spectrometry

EDS — (continued)
    epigatric distress syndrome
    excessive daytime sleepiness
    extended data stream
    extradimensional shift
EDSS — expanded disability status
    scale
EDT —
    end-diastolic thickness
    erythrocyte density test
EDTA —
    edathamil
    edetic acid
    ethylenediaminetetraacetic
        acid
    European Dialysis and Trans-
        plant Association
EdU — eating disorder unit
Educ — education
EDV — end-diastolic volume
EDVI — end-diastolic volume in-
    dex
EDW — estimated dry weight
EDWGT — emergency drinking
    water germicidal tablet
EDWTH — end-diastolic wall
    thickness
EDX — electrodiagnosis
EDXA — energy-dispersive x-ray
    analysis
EE —
    embryo extract
    end expiration
    end-to-end [anastomosis]
    end-to-end [bite, occlusion]
    energy expenditure
    Enterobacteriaceae enrich-
        ment [broth]
    equine encephalitis
    ethynyl estradiol
    expressed emotion
    external ear
    eye and ear
E-E —
    erythema-edema [reaction]
    erythematous-edematous [re-
        action]
E&E — eye and ear

EEA —
>   electroencephalic audiometry
>   elemental enteral alimentation
>   end-to-end anastomosis

EEC —
>   ectrodactyly-ectodermal dysplasia-clefting [syndrome]
>   enteropathogenic *Escherichia coli*

EECD — endothelial-epithelial corneal dystrophy

EECG —
>   electroencephalogram
>   electroencephalography

EEDQ — ethoxycarbonylethoxy-dihydroquinoline

EEE —
>   eastern equine encephalomyelitis [virus]
>   edema, erythema, and exudate
>   experimental enterococcal endocarditis
>   external eye examination

EEEP — end-expiratory esophageal pressure

EEEV — eastern equine encephalomyelitis virus

EEG —
>   electroencephalogram
>   electroencephalography

EEGA — electroencephalographic audiometry

EEG-CSA — electroencephalography with computerized spectral analysis

EEG T — Electroencephalographic Technologist

EELS — electron energy loss spectroscopy

EEM —
>   ectodermal dysplasia, ectrodactyly, macular dystrophy [syndrome]
>   erythema exudativum multiforme
>   external elastic membrane

EEME — ethynylestradiol methyl ether

EEMG — evoked electromyogram

EENT — eyes-ears-nose-throat

EEP —
>   end-expiratory pressure
>   equivalent effective photon

EEPI — extraretinal eye position information

EER —
>   electroencephalic response
>   electroencephalographic response

EERP — extended endocardial resection procedure

EES —
>   erythromycin ethylsuccinate
>   ethyl ethanesulfate

EESG — evoked electrospinogram

EEV — encircling endocardial ventriculotomy

EF —
>   ectopic focus
>   edema factor
>   ejection factor
>   ejection fraction
>   elastic fiber
>   elastic fibril
>   electric field
>   elongation factor
>   embryo-fetal
>   embryo fibroblast
>   emergency facility
>   emotional factor
>   encephalitogenic factor
>   endothoracic fascia
>   endurance factor
>   eosinophilic fasciitis
>   epithelial focus
>   equivalent focus
>   erythroblastosis fetalis
>   erythrocyte fragmentation
>   essential findings
>   etiologic fraction
>   exophthalmic factor
>   exposure factor
>   extended field (radiotherapy)
>   extrafine

EF — (continued)
    extra food
    extrinsic factor
EFA —
    Epilepsy Foundation of
        America
    essential fatty acids
    extrafamily adoptee
EFAD — essential fatty acid defi-
    ciency
EFAS — embryofetal alcohol syn-
    drome
EFBW — estimated fetal body
    weight
EFC —
    elastin fragment concentra-
        tion
    endogenous fecal calcium
    ephemeral fever of cattle
EFDA — expanded function den-
    tal assistant
EFE — endocardial fibroelastosis
eff —
    effect
    efferent
    efficiency
    efficient
    effusion
effect — effective
effer — efferent
EFFU — epithelial focus-forming
    unit
EF-G — elongation factor G
EFH — explosive follicular hyper-
    plasia
EFHBM — eosinophilic fibrohisti-
    ocytic (lesion of) bone mar-
    row
EFL —
    effective focal length
    external fluid loss
EFM —
    elderly fibromyalgia
    electronic fetal monitoring
    external fetal monitor
EFP —
    early follicular phase
    effective filtration pressure

EFP — (continued)
    endoneural fluid pressure
EFPS — epicardial fat pad sign
EFR — effective filtration rate
E FRAG — erythrocyte fragility
    [test]
EFS —
    electric field stimulation
    event-free survival
EFT — Embedded Figures Test
EFV — extracellular fluid volume
EFVC — expiratory flow-volume
    curve
EFW — estimated fetal weight
EF/WM — ejection fraction/wall
    motion
EG —
    enteroglucagon
    Erb-Goldflam [syndrome]
    esophagogastrectomy
    esophagogastric
    external genitalia
e.g. — exempli gratia (Lat.) for ex-
    ample
EGA — estimated gestational age
EGAT — Educational Goal Attain-
    ment Tests
EGBPS — equilibrium-gated blood
    pool study
EGBUS — external genitalia, Bar-
    tholin, urethral, Skene's
    glands
EGC —
    early gastric cancer
    epithelioid globoid cell
EGCT — extragonadal germ cell
    tumor
EGD — esophagogastroduodenoscopy
EGDF — embryonic growth and
    development factor
EGF — epidermal growth factor
EGF-R — epidermal growth factor
    receptor
EGF-URO — epidermal growth
    factor—urogastrone
EGG —
    electrogastrogram
    electrogastrography

EGH — equine growth hormone

EGJ — esophagogastric junction

EGL — eosinophilic granuloma of the lung

EGLT —
  euglobin lysis time
  euglobulin lysis time

EGM —
  electrogram
  extracellular granular material

EGME — ethylene glycol mono-methyl ether

EGN — experimental glomerulonephritis

EGOT — erythrocyte glutamic oxaloacetic transaminase

EGR — erythema gyratum repens

E-GR — erythrocyte glutathione reductase

EGRA — equilibrium-gated radionuclide angiography

EGRAC — erythrocyte glutathione reductase activity coefficient

EGRET — Epidemiological Graphics, Estimation, and Testing

EGS —
  electric galvanic stimulation
  ethylene glycol succinate
  external guide sequence

EGT — ethanol gelation test

EGTA —
  egtazic acid
  esophageal gastric tube airway
  ethylene glycol tetraacetic acid

EH —
  early healed
  educationally handicapped
  emotionally handicapped
  enlarged heart
  enteral hyperalimentation
  environment and heredity
  epidermolytic hyperkeratosis
  epoxide hydratase
  essential hypertension
  extramedullary hematopoiesis

E/H — environment and heredity

E&H — environment and heredity

eH — oxidation-reduction potential

eh — enlarged heart

EHA —
  Emotional Health Anonymous
  Environmental Health Agency

EHAA — epidemic hepatitis–associated antigen

EHB — elevate head of bed

EHBA — extrahepatic biliary atresia

EHBD — extrahepatic bile duct

EHBF —
  estimated hepatic blood flow
  exercise hyperemia blood flow
  extrahepatic blood flow

EHC —
  enterohepatic circulation
  enterohepatic clearance
  essential hypercholesterolemia
  ethylhydrocupreine hydrochloride
  extended health care
  extrahepatic cholestasis

EH-CF — *Entamoeba histolytica*–complement fixation

EHD —
  electrohemodynamics
  epizootic hemorrhagic disease

EHDA — ethanehydroxydiphosphonic acid (etidronate sodium)

EHDP —
  ethane hydroxydiphosphate
  ethane-1-hydroxy-1,1-diphosphonate

EHDV — epizootic hemorrhagic disease virus

EHE — epithelioid hemangioendothelioma

EHEC — enterohemorrhagic *Escherichia coli*

EHF —
  electrohydraulic fragmentation
  epidemic hemorrhagic fever

EHF — (*continued*)
  exophthalmos-hyperthyroid factor
  extreme high frequency
  extremely high factor
EHH — esophageal hiatal hernia
EHL —
  effective half-life
  electrohydraulic lithotripsy
  endogenous hyperlipidemia
  Environmental Health Laboratory
  essential hyperlipemia
  essential hyperlipidemia
  extensor hallucis longus
EHME — Employee Health Maintenance Examination
EHMS — electrohemodynamic ionization mass spectrometry
EHO — extrahepatic obstruction
EHP —
  di-(2-ethylhexyl) hydrogen phosphate
  Environmental Health Perspectives
  excessive heat production
  extra-high potency
EHPAC — Emergency Health Preparedness Advisory Committee
EHPH — extrahepatic portal hypertension
EHPT — Eddy hot plate test
EHSDS — Experimental Health Services Delivery System
EHT —
  electrohydrothermoelectrode
  essential hypertension
EHV —
  electric heart vector
  equine herpesvirus
EI —
  electrolyte imbalance
  electron impact
  electron ionization
  emotionally impaired
  enzyme inhibitor
  eosinophilic index

EI — (*continued*)
  excretory index
  external intervention
E/I — expiration/inspiration [ratio]
E&I — endocrine and infertility
EIA —
  electroimmunoassay
  Electronics Industries Association
  enzyme immunoassay
  enzyme-linked immunosorbent assay
  equine infectious anemia
  erythroimmunoassay
  exercise-induced asthma
EIAB — extracranial-intracranial arterial bypass
EIAV — equine infectious anemia virus
EIB —
  electrophoretic immunoblotting
  exercise-induced bronchoconstriction
  exercise-induced bronchospasm
EIC —
  elastase inhibition capacity
  enzyme inhibition complex
EICDT — Ego-Ideal and Conscience Development Test
EICT — external isovolumic contraction time
EID —
  egg infective dose
  electroimmunodiffusion
  electronic induction desorption
  electronic infusion device
  emergency infusion device
EIEC — enteroinvasive *Escherichia coli*
EIEE — early infantile epileptic encephalopathy
EIF —
  erythrocyte initiation factor
  eukaryotic initiation factor
EIM — excitability-inducing material

EIMS — electron ionization mass spectrometry

EIN — esophageal intraepithelial neoplasia

EIP —
  elective interruption of pregnancy
  end-inspiratory pause
  end-inspiratory pressure
  extensor indicis proprius

EIPS — endogenous inhibitor of prostaglandin synthase

eIPV — enhanced-potency inactivated polio vaccine

EIRnv — extra incidence rate in nonvaccinated groups

EIRP — effective isotropic radiated power

EIRv — extra-incidence rate in vaccinated [groups]

EIS —
  endoscopic injection scleropathy
  Environmental Impact Statement
  Epidemic Intelligence Service

EISA — electroencephalogram interval spectrum analysis

EIT —
  erythrocyte iron turnover
  erythroid iron turnover

EIV — external iliac vein

EIVA — equine infectious viral anemia

EJ —
  ejection [fraction]
  elbow jerk
  external jugular

EJB — ectopic junctional beat

EJP —
  excitation junction potential
  excitatory junction potential

ejusd. — *ejusdem* (Lat.) of the same

EK —
  enterokinase
  erythrokinase

EKC — epidemic keratoconjunctivitis

EKG —
  electrocardiogram
  electrocardiography

EKS — epidemic Kaposi sarcoma

EKV — erythrokeratodermia variabilis

EKY —
  electrokymogram
  electrokymography

EL —
  early latent
  Eaton-Lambert [syndrome]
  egg lecithin
  elbow
  electroluminescence
  elixir
  erythroleukemia
  exercise limit
  external lamina

E-L —
  Eaton-Lambert [syndrome]
  external lids

El — elastase

el. —
  elbow
  elixir

ELA —
  elastomer-lubricating agent
  endotoxin-like activity

ELAM — expression of a leukocyte-adhesion molecule 1

ELAS — extended lymphadenopathy syndrome

ELAT — enzyme-linked antiglobulin test

ELB — early light breakfast

elb. — elbow

ELBW — extremely low birth weight

ELD — egg lethal dose

El Dx — electrodiagnosis

elec —
  electric
  electricity
  electuary

elect — elective

ELEM — equine leukoencephalomalacia

elem — elementary
elev —
    elevated
    elevation
    elevator
ELF —
    elective low forceps [delivery]
    extremely low frequency
ELG — eligible
ELH —
    egg-laying hormone
    endolymphatic hydrops
ELI —
    endomyocardial lymphocytic
        infiltrates
    Environmental Language In-
        ventory
    exercise lability index
ELIA —
    enzyme-labeled immunoassay
    enzyme-linked immunoassay
ELICT — enzyme-linked immuno-
    cytochemical technique
ELIEDA — enzyme-linked immu-
    noelectrodiffusion assay
ELISA — enzyme-linked immuno-
    sorbent assay
elix. — *elixir* (Lat.) elixir
ELLIP — elliptocyte
ELM —
    Early Language Milestone
        [scale]
    external limiting membrane
    extravascular lung mass
ELN — electronic noise
ELOP — estimated length of pro-
    gram
ELOS —
    estimated length of stay
    extralymphatic organ site
ELP —
    early labeled peak
    elastase-like protein
    electrophoresis
    endogenous limbic potential
    Estimated Learning Potential
ELPS — excessive lateral pressure
    syndrome

ELR — Equal Listener Response
    [scale]
ELS —
    Eaton-Lambert syndrome
    electron loss spectroscopy
    extracorporeal life support
    extralobar sequestration
ELSO — Extracorporeal Life Sup-
    port Organization
ELSS — emergency life support sys-
    tem
ELT —
    endless loop tachycardia
    euglobulin lysis test
    euglobulin lysis time
ELU — extended length of utter-
    ance
ELV — erythroid leukemia virus
elx — elixir
elytes — electrolytes
EM —
    early memory
    echo measurement
    effective masking
    ejection murmur
    electromagnetic
    electromechanical
    electron micrograph
    electron microscope
    electron microscopy
    electrophoretic mobility
    Embden-Meyerhof [pathway]
    emergency medicine
    emmetropia
    emotional disorder
    emotionally disturbed
    emphysema
    ergonovine maleate
    erythema migrans
    erythema multiforme
    erythrocyte mass
    erythromycin
    esophageal manometry
    esophageal motility
    excreted mass
    extensive metabolizers
    external monitor
    extracellular matrix

E/M —
   electron microscope
   electron microscopy
E-M — Embden-Meyerhof [pathway]
E&M — endocrine and metabolic
Em — emmetropia
E_m — midpoint redox potential
em — electromagnetic
e/m — ratio of charge to mass
EMA —
   antiepithelial membrane antigen
   electronic microanalyzer
   emergency assistance
   emergency assistant
   emergency medical attendant
   endomysial antibody
   epithelial membrane antigen
EMAD — equivalent mean age at death
EMAP — evoked muscle action potential
EMB —
   embryology
   endometrial biopsy
   endomyocardial biopsy
   engineering in medicine and biology
   eosin-methylene blue
   ethambutol (Myambutol)
   explosive mental behavior
   explosive motor behavior
Emb —
   embolus
   embryo
   embryology
EMBASE — Excerpta Medica Database
EMBL — European Molecular Biology Laboratory
embryol — embryology
EMC —
   electron microscopy
   emergency medical care
   emergency medical coordinator
   encephalomyocarditis [virus]

EMC — (continued)
   endometrial curettage
   essential mixed cryoglobulinemia
EMC&R — emergency medical care and rescue
EMCRO — Experimental Medical Care Review Organization
EMCV — encephalomyocarditis virus
EMD —
   electromechanical dissociation
   Emery-Dreifuss muscular dystrophy
   esophageal motility disorder
EMEM — Eagle's minimal essential medium
EMER — electromagnetic molecular electronic resonance
emer. — emergency
EMF —
   electromagnetic flowmeter
   electromotive force
   Emergency Medicine Foundation
   endomyocardial fibrosis
   erythrocyte maturation factor
   evaporated milk formula
emf — electromotive force
EMG —
   electromyelogram
   electromyelography
   electromyogram
   electromyography
   essential monoclonal gammopathy
   exomphalos, macroglossia, gigantism [syndrome]
   eye movement gauge
EMGN — extramembranous glomerulonephritis
EMGORS — electromyogram sensors
EMI —
   Electric and Musical Industries [scan]
   electromagnetic interference

EMI — (continued)
emergency medical information

EMIC — emergency maternal and infant care

EMIC BACK — Environmental Mutagen Information Center Backfile

E-MICR — electron microscopy

EMIP — European Myocardial Infarction Project

EMIT — Enzyme-Multiplied Immunoassay Technique

EMJH — Ellinghausen-McCullough-Johnson-Harris [medium]

EML —
effective mandibular length
erythema nodosum leprosum

EMLB — erythromycin lactobionate

EMLD — external muscle layer damaged

EMM — erythema multiforme major

EMMA — eye movement measuring apparatus

EMMIA — enzyme modulator–mediated immunoassay

EMMV — extended mandatory minute ventilation

EMO —
Epstein-Macintosh-Oxford [inhaler]
exophthalmos, myxedema circumscriptum praetibiale, and osteoarthropathia hypertrophicans [syndrome]

emot —
emotion
emotional

EMP —
electric membrane property
electromagnetic pulse
Embden-Meyerhof pathway
epimacular proliferation
external membrane potential or protein

EMP — (continued)
extramedullary plasmacytoma

Emp. —
emplastrum (Lat.) a plaster
ex modo prescripto (Lat.) as directed, after the manner prescribed

EMPEP —
erythrocyte membrane protein electrophoretic pattern

emph — emphysema

EMPP — ethylmethylpiperidinopropiophenone

EMPS — exertional muscle pain syndrome

emp. vesic. — emplastrum vesicatorium (Lat.) a blistering plaster

EMR —
educable mentally retarded
electromagnetic radiation
emergency mechanical restraint
empty, measure, and record
essential metabolism ratio
ethanol metabolic rate
eye movement record

EMRA — Emergency Medicine Residents Association

EMRC — European Medical Research Council

EMS —
early morning specimen
early morning stiffness
electrical muscle stimulation
Electronic Medical Service
Emergency Medical Service
endometriosis
eosinophilia myalgia syndrome
ethyl methane-sulfonate
extramedullary site

EMT —
Emergency Medical Tag
Emergency Medical Team
Emergency Medical Technician
emergency medical treatment

EMTA — endomethylene tetrahydrophthalic acid

EMT-A — Emergency Medical Technician—Ambulance

EMT-I — Emergency Medical Technician—Intermediate

EMT-M — Emergency Medical Technician—Military

EMT-P — Emergency Medical Technician—Paramedic

EMU — early morning urine

emu — electromagnetic unit

emul. — *emulsum* (Lat.) emulsion

EMV — eye, motor, voice (Glasgow coma scale)

EMVC — early mitral valve closure

EMW — electromagnetic waves

EN —
  electronarcosis
  endocardial
  endoscopy
  enrolled nurse
  enteral nutrition
  epidemic nephritis
  erythema nodosum

en. — enema

E 50% N — extension 50% of normal

ENA —
  extractable nuclear antibodies
  extractable nuclear antigen

ENC — environmental control

END —
  early neonatal death
  elective node dissection
  endocrinology
  endorphin
  enhancement Newcastle disease

end. — endoreduplication

ENDO — endoscopy

Endo —
  endocardial
  endocardium
  endocrine
  endocrinology
  endodontics
  endotracheal

ENDOR — electron nuclear double resonance

endos — endosteal

ENE — ethylnorepinephrine

ENeG — electroneurography

enem. — enema

ENF — Enfamil

ENG —
  electroneurography
  electronystagmogram
  electronystagmography
  engorged

Eng — English

ENI — elective neck irradiation

ENK — enkephalin

ENL —
  erythema nodosum leprosum
  erythema nodosum leproticum

enl. — enlargement

ENNS — Early Neonatal Neurobehavior Scale

Eno — enolase

ENOG — electroneurography

ENP —
  ethyl-*p*-nitrophenylthiobenzene phosphate
  extractable nucleoprotein

ENR —
  eosinophilic nonallergic rhinitis
  extrathyroidal neck radioactivity

ENS —
  enteral nutritional support
  enteric nervous system
  ethylnorsuprarenin

ENT —
  ear, nose, and throat
  enzootic nasal tumor
  extranodular tissue

ent A — enterotoxin A

Entom — entomology

ENU — *N*-ethyl-nitrosourea

env — envelope [of cell]

environ —
  environment
  environmental

enz. —
  enzymatic
  enzyme

EO —
    effect of opening [eyes]
    elbow orthosis
    eosinophil
    eosinophilia
    eosinophils
    ethylene oxide
    eyes open

EOA —
    effective orifice area
    erosive osteoarthritis
    esophageal obturator airway
    examination, opinion, and advice

EOB — emergency observation bed

EOCA — early onset cerebellar ataxia

EOC — enema of choice

EO CT — eosinophil count

EOD —
    electrical organ discharge
    entry on duty

e.o.d. — every other day

EOE — ethiodized oil emulsion

EOF —
    end of field
    end of file

E of M — error of measurement

EOG —
    electro-oculogram
    electro-oculography
    electro-olfactogram
    electro-olfactography

EOGBS — early onset group B streptococcal [infection]

EOJ — extrahepatic obstructive jaundice

EOL — end of life

EOM —
    end of message
    equal ocular movement
    error of measurement
    external otitis media
    extraocular movement
    extraocular muscle

EOMA — emergency oxygen mask assembly

EOM F & Conj — extraocular movements full and conjugate

EOMI — extraocular muscles intact

EOM NL — extraocular eye movements normal

EOP —
    efficiency of plating
    emergency outpatient
    endogenous opioid peptides

EOR — emergency operating room

EORA — elderly onset rheumatoid arthritis

EORTC — European Organization for Research and Treatment of Cancer

EOS —
    eligibility on-site
    end of study
    eosinophil
    European Orthodontic Society

eos. — eosinophil

Eosm — effective osmolarity

EOT — effective oxygen transport

EOU — epidemic observation unit

EOWPVT — Expressive One-Word Picture Vocabulary Test

EP —
    ectopic pregnancy
    edible portion
    electrophoresis
    electrophysiologic
    electrophysiology
    electroprecipitin
    elopement precaution
    emergency physician
    emergency procedure
    end point
    endogenous pyrogen
    endoperoxide
    endorphin
    enteropeptidase
    environmental protection
    enzyme product
    eosinophilic pneumonia
    ependymal [cell]
    epicardial

EP — *(continued)*
    epithelial
    epithelium
    epoxide
    erythrocyte protoporphyrin
    erythrophagocytosis
    erythropoietic porphyria
    erythropoietin
    esophageal pressure
    esophoria
    evoked potential
    extreme pressure
E&P — estrogen and progesterone
Ep — erythropoietin
EPA —
    eicosapentaenoic acid
    empiric phrase association
    Environmental Protection
      Agency
    erect posterior-anterior
      [projection]
    erythroid potentiating activity
    ethylphenacemide
    exophthalmos-producing ac-
      tivity
    extrinsic plasminogen activa-
      tor
EPAP — expiratory positive airway
    pressure
EPAQ — Extended Personal Attri-
    butes Questionnaire
EPA/RCRA — Environmental Pro-
    tection Agency Resource Con-
    servation and Recovery Act
EPB —
    Environmental Pre-Language
      Battery
    extensor pollicis brevis
EPC —
    electronic pain control
    end-plate current
    epilepsia partialis continua
    external pneumatic compres-
      sion
EPCA — external pressure circula-
    tory assistance
EPCG — endoscopic pancreato-
    cholangiography

EPD — effective pressor dose
EPDML —
    epidemiological
    epidemiologist
    epidemiology
EPE — erythropoietin-producing
    enzyme
EPEA — expense per equivalent
    admission
EPEC — enteropathogenic *Esche-
    richia coli*
EPEG — etoposide
EPF —
    early pregnancy factor
    endocarditis parietalis fibro-
      plastica
    endothelia proliferating factor
    Enfamil premature formula
    estrogenic positive feedback
    exophthalmos-producing fac-
      tor
EPG —
    eggs per gram [count]
    electropneumogram
    electropneumography
    ethanolamine phosphoglycer-
      ide
EPH —
    edema-proteinuria-
      hypertension
    extensor proprius hallucis
EPI —
    Emotional Profile Index
    epilepsy
    epileptic
    epinephrine
    epithelial
    epithelioid [cells]
    epithelium
    epitympanic
    evoked potential index
    exocrine pancreatic insuffi-
      ciency
    Expanded Programme of Im-
      munization [WHO]
    extrapyramidal involvement
    Eysenck Personality Inventory
Epi —
    epicardium

Epi — (continued)
    epiglottis
Epi. — epinephrine
epid — epidemic
epig — epigastric
epil —
    epilepsy
    epileptic
EPIS —
    episiotomy
    episode
    epistaxis
epistom — *epistomium* (Lat.) stopper [on mouth of bottle]
epith. —
    epithelial
    epithelium
EPK — early prenatal karyotype
EPL —
    effective patient's life
    essential phospholipid
    extensor pollicis longus
    external plexiform layer
    extracorporeal piezoelectric lithotriptor
EPM —
    electron probe microanalysis
    electronic pacemaker
    electrophoretic mobility
    energy-protein malnutrition
EPN — *O*-ethyl *O*-*p*-nitrophenylphosphyonothionate
EPO —
    erythropoiesis
    erythropoietin
    evening primrose oil
    exclusive provider organization
    expiratory port occlusion
EPP —
    end-plate potential
    equal pressure point
    erythropoietic protoporphyria
EPPB — end positive-pressure breathing
EPPS — Edwards Personal Preference Schedule
EPQ — Eysenck Personality Questionnaire

EPR —
    early progressive resistance
    electron paramagnetic resonance
    electrophrenic respiration
    emergency physical restraint
    estradiol production rate
    extraparenchymal resistance
EPROM — erasable programmable read-only memory
EPS —
    elastosis perforans serpiginosa
    electrophysiologic study
    enzyme pancreatic secretion
    exophthalmos-producing substance
    expressed prostatic secretion
    extracellular polysaccharide
    extrapyramidal side effect
    extrapyramidal symptom
    extrapyramidal syndrome
EPSD — E-point to septal distance
EPSDT — early periodic screening, diagnosis, and treatment
EPSE — extrapyramidal side effects
EPSEM — equal probability of selection method
EPSP — excitatory postsynaptic potential
EPSS — E-point septal separation
EPT —
    early pregnancy test
    Eidetic Parents Test
    endoscopic papillotomy
EPTE — existed prior to enlistment
EPTFE — expanded polytetrafluoroethylene
EPTS — existed prior to service
EPV — entomopoxvirus
EPXMA — electron probe x-ray microanalyzer
EQ —
    educational quotient
    encephalization quotient
    energy quotient
    equal to
Eq. —
    equation

Eq. — *(continued)*
    equivalent
eq —
    equal
    equilibrium
EQA — external quality assessment
equip — equipment
equiv —
    equivalency
    equivalent
    equivocal
ER —
    early reticulocyte
    efficacy ratio
    efficiency ratio
    ejection rate
    electroresection
    emergency room
    endoplasmic reticulum
    enhanced reactivation
    enhancement ratio
    environmental resistance
    epigastric region
    equine rhinopneumonia
    equivalent roentgen [unit]
    erbium
    erythrocyte
    erythrocyte receptor
    esophageal rupture
    estradiol receptor
    estrogen receptor
    etretinate
    evoked response
    expiratory reserve
    extended release [tablet]
    extended resistance
    external reduction
    external resistance
    external rotation
    extraction ratio
    eye research
ER^- — decreased estrogen receptor
ER^+ — increased estrogen receptor
ER + — estrogen receptor-positive
E&R —
    equal and reactive
    examination and report

Er —
    erbium
    erythrocyte
er — endoplasmic reticulum
ERA —
    electrical response activity
    electrical response audiometry
    electroencephalic response audiometry
    Electroshock Research Association
    estradiol receptor assay
    estrogen receptor assay
    evoked response audiometry
ERB — ethnic relational behavior
ERBF — effective renal blood flow
ERC —
    endoscopic retrograde cholangiography
    enteric cytopathic human orphan-rhino-coryza [virus]
    equal, reactive, and contracting [pupils]
    erythropoietin-responsive cell
Erc — erythrocyte
ERCP —
    endoscopic retrograde cannulation of pancreatic [duct]
    endoscopic retrograde cholangiopancreatography
    endoscopic retrograde choledochopancreatography
ERD —
    early retirement with disability
    evoked response detector
ERDA — Energy Research and Development Administration
ERE — external rotation in extension
ERF —
    Education and Research Foundation
    external rotation in flexion
    Eye Research Foundation
erf — error function
ERFC — erythrocyte rosette–forming cell

E-RFC — E-rosette–forming cell

ERFS — electrophysiological ring-finger splinting

ERG —
 electrolyte replacement with glucose
 electron radiography
 electroretinogram
 electroretinography

erg — energy unit

ERGO — Euthanasia Research and Guidance Organization

ERH — egg-laying release hormone

ERHD — exposure-related hypothermia death

ERI —
 Environmental Response Inventory
 E-rosette inhibitor
 erythrocyte rosette inhibitor

ERIA — electroradioimmunoassay

ERIC — Educational Resource Information Clearinghouse

ERISA — Employee Retirement Income Security Act

ERL — effective refractory length

ERM —
 electrochemical relaxation method
 extended radical mastectomy

ERP —
 early receptor potential
 effective refractory period
 emergency room physician
 endocardial resection procedure
 endoscopic retrograde pancreatography
 enzyme-releasing peptide
 equine rhinopneumonitis
 estrogen receptor protein
 event-related potential

ERPF — effective renal plasma flow

ERPLV — effective refractory period of the left ventricle

ERR — error

ERS — endoscopic retrograde sphincterectomy

ERSP — event-related slow-brain potential

ERT —
 esophageal radionuclide transit
 estrogen replacement therapy
 external radiation therapy

ERU — endorectal ultrasound

ERV —
 equine rhinopneumonitis virus
 expiratory reserve volume

ERY — erysipelas

Ery — *Erysipelothrix*

eryth —
 erythema
 erythrocyte

ES —
 Ego Strength [test]
 ejection sound
 elastic suspensor
 electrical stimulation
 electrical stimulus
 electroshock
 elopement status [psychology]
 emergency service
 emission spectrometry
 end stage
 end systole
 endometritis-salpingitis
 endoscopic sclerosis
 endoscopic sphincterotomy
 end-to-side
 environmental stimulation
 enzyme substrate
 epileptic syndrome
 esophageal scintigraphy
 esophagus
 esophoria
 esterase
 exfoliation syndrome
 Expectation Score
 experimental study
 exsmoker
 exterior surface
 extrasystole

E-S — end-to-side (anastomosis)

Es —
einsteinium
electrical stimulation
estriol

e.s. — *enema saponis* (Lat.) soap enema

ESA —
Electrolysis Society of America
end-to-side anastomosis
esterase

ESAP — evoked sensory (nerve) action potential

ESB — electrical stimulation to brain

ESC —
electromechanical slope computer
endosystolic count
end-systolic count
erythropoietin-sensitive stem cell

ESCA — electron spectroscopy for chemical analysis

ESCC —
electrolyte steroid cardiopathy by calcification
epidural spinal cord compression

ESCH — electrolyte steroid-produced cardiopathy characterized by hyalinization

Esch. — *Escherichia*

ESCN —
electrolyte and steroid cardiopathy with necrosis
electrolyte- and steroid-produced cardiopathy characterized by necrosis

ESCS — Early Social Communication Scale

ESD —
electronic summation device
electron-stimulated desorption
electrostatic discharge
emission spectrometric detector

ESD — *(continued)*
end-systolic dimension
environmental sex determination
esophagus, stomach, and duodenum
esterase-D
exoskeletal device

ESE — *electrostatische Einheit* (Ger.) electrostatic unit

ESEP — elbow sensory potential

ESF —
electrosurgical filter
erythropoietic-stimulating factor
external skeletal fixation

ESFL — end-systolic force-length relationship

ESG —
electrospinogram
estrogen
exfoliation syndrome glaucoma

ESI —
Ego State Inventory
enzyme substrate inhibitor
epidural steroid injection
extent of skin involvement

ES-IMV — expiration-synchronized intermittent mandatory ventilation

ESL —
end-systolic length
English as a second language
extracorporeal shockwave lithotripsy

ESLD — end-stage liver disease

ESLF — end-stage liver failure

ESM —
ejection systolic murmur
endothelial specular microscope
ethosuximide

ESMIS — Emergency (Medical) Services Management Information System

ESMO — European Society for Medical Oncology

ESN —
    educationally subnormal
    estrogen-stimulated neurophy-
        sin
ESN(M) — educationally
    subnormal—moderate
ESN(S) — educationally
    subnormal—severe
ESO — electrospinal orthosis
eso. —
    esophagoscopy
    esophagus
ESP —
    early systolic paradox
    effective sensory projection
    effective systolic pressure
    electrosensitive point
    endometritis-salpingitis-
        peritonitis
    end-systolic pressure
    eosinophil stimulation pro-
        moter
    epidermal soluble protein
    evoked synaptic potential
    extrasensory perception
esp — especially
ESPA — electrical stimulation–
    produced analgesia
ESPQ — Early School Personality
    Questionnaire
ESR —
    Einstein stroke radius
    electric skin resistance
    electron spin resonance
    erythrocyte sedimentation
        rate
esr — electron spin resonance
ESRD — end-stage renal disease
ESRF — end-stage renal failure
ESRS — extrapyramidal symptom
    rating scale
ESS —
    empty sella syndrome
    endostreptosin
    erythrocyte-sensitizing sub-
        stance
    euthyroid sick syndrome
    excited skin syndrome

ess. —
    essence
    essential
ess. neg. — essentially negative
EST —
    electric shock therapy
    electroshock therapy
    electroshock threshold
    endodermal sinus tumor
    endoscopic sphincterectomy
    esterase
    exercise stress test
est. —
    ester
    estimated
    estimation
esth — esthetic
e.s.u. —
    electrostatic unit
    electrosurgical unit
E-sub — excitor substance
ESV —
    end-systolic [ventricular] vol-
        ume
    esophageal valve
ESVEM — Electrophysiologic
    Study versus Electrocardio-
    graph Monitoring
ESVI — end-systolic volume index
ESVS — epiurethral suprapubic vag-
    inal suspension
ESWL — extracorporeal shock-
    wave lithotripsy
ESWS — end-systolic wall stress
ET —
    Ebbinghaus test
    edge thickness
    educational therapy
    effective temperature
    ejection time
    electroneurodiagnostic tech-
        nologist
    embryo transfer
    endothelin
    endotoxin
    endotracheal
    endotracheal tube
    end-tidal

ET — *(continued)*
    endurance time
    enterostomal therapist
    enterostomal therapy
    enterotoxin
    epidermolytic toxin
    epithelial tumor
    esotropia
    esotropic
    essential thrombocythemia
    essential tremor
    ethanol
    ethyl
    etiocholanolone test
    etiology
    eustachian tube
    exchange transfusion
    exercise test
    exercise treadmill
    exfoliative toxin
    expiration time
    extracellular tachyzoite
ET′ — esotropia for near
E(T) — intermittent esotropia
E/T — effector-to-target ratio
ET_1 — esotropia at near
ET_3 — erythrocyte triiodothyronine
ET_4 — effective thyroxine [test]
Et —
    ethyl
    etiology
et — *et* (Lat.) and
ETA —
    eicosatetraenoic acid
    electron transfer agent
    endotracheal airway
    endotracheal aspirates
    estimated time of arrival
    ethionamide
ETAB — extrathoracic-assisted breathing
ETAF — epithelial thymic-activating factor
et al. —
    et alibi (Lat.) and elsewhere
    et alii (Lat.) and others
E_2TBG — estradiol-testosterone-binding globulin

ETC —
    electron transport chain
    estimated time of conception
ET_c — corrected ejection time
etc. — *et cetera* (Lat.) and so forth
E_TCO_2 — end-tidal carbon dioxide concentration
ETD — eustachian tube dysfunction
ETE — end-to-end (anastomosis)
ETEC — enterotoxic *Escherichia coli*
ETF —
    electron transferring flavoprotein
    eustachian tube function
ETH —
    elixir of terpin hydrate
    ethanol
    ethionamide
    ethmoid
    ethnoid
    Ethrane (enflurane)
eth. — ether
ETH/C — elixir of terpin hydrate with codeine
ETI — ejective time index
ETIBACK — Environmental Teratology Information Center Backfile
ETIO — etiocholanolone
etiol. — etiology
ETK — erythrocyte transketolase
ETKTM — every test known to mankind
ETL — expiratory threshold load
ETM — erythromycin
Et_3N — triethylamine
ET-NANB — enterically transmitted non-A, non-B hepatitis
ETNU — ethyl nitrosourea
ETO —
    estimated time of ovulation
    eustachian tube obstruction
Eto — ethylene oxide
Et_2O — ether
ETOH —
    ethanol

ETOH — (continued)
  ethyl alcohol
ETOX — ethylene oxide
ETP —
  elective termination of pregnancy
  electron transfer particle
  electron transport particle
  entire treatment period
  ephedrine, theophylline, and phenobarbital
  eustachian tube pressure
ETR —
  effective thyroxine ratio
  epitympanic recess
  estimated thyroid ratio
ETS —
  Educational Testing Service
  electrical transcranial stimulation
  end-to-side (anastomosis)
ETT —
  endotracheal tube
  epinephrine tolerance test
  esophageal transit time
  exercise tolerance test
  exercise treadmill test
  extrapyramidal thyroxine
  extrathyroidal thyroxine
ETTN — ethyltrimethyloltrimethane trinitrate
ETU —
  Emergency and Trauma Unit
  Emergency Treatment Unit
ETV —
  educational television
  extravascular thermal volume
ETX — ethosuximide
ETYA — eicosatetroenoic acid
EU —
  Ehrlich unit
  emergency unit
  endotoxin unit
  entropy unit
  enzyme unit
  esophageal ulcer
  esterase unit
  etiology unknown

EU — (continued)
  excretory urography
  expected utility
Eu —
  europium
  euryon
EUA — examination under anesthesia
EUCD — emotionally unstable character disorder
EUG — extrauterine gestation
EUL — expected upper limit
EUM — external urethral meatus
EUP — extrauterine pregnancy
EUROHEP — European Concerted Action on Viral Hepatitis
EURONET — European On-Line Network
EUROTOX — European Committee on Chronic Toxicity Hazards
EUS —
  endoscopic ultrasound
  external urethral sphincter
Eust — eustachian
EUV — extreme ultraviolet laser
EV —
  emergency vehicle
  enterovirus
  epidermodysplasia verruciformis
  esophageal varices
  estradiol valerate
  eversion
  evoked potential [response]
  excessive ventilation
  expected value
  extravascular
eV — electron volt
ev —
  eversion
  ever
EVA —
  ethylene vinyl acetate
  ethyl violet azide
evac. —
  evacuate

evac. — *(continued)*
    evacuated
    evacuation
eval. —
    evaluate
    evaluated
    evaluation
evap. —
    evaporated
    evaporation
EVB — esophageal variceal bleeding
EVC — Ellis–van Creveld [syndrome]
EVCI — expected value of clinical information
EVD —
    external ventricular drainage
    extravascular (lung) density
eve — evening
ever. —
    eversion
    everted
EVF — ethanol volume fraction
EVFMG — exchange visitor foreign medical graduate
EVG —
    electroventriculogram
    electroventriculography
EVI — endocardial, vascular, interstitial
evisc. — evisceration
EVLW — extravascular lung water
EVM —
    electronic voltmeter
    extravascular mass
evol — evolution
EVP —
    episcleral venous pressure
    evoked visual potential
EVR —
    endocardial viability ratio
    evoked visual response
EVRS — early ventricular repolarization syndrome
EVS — endoscopic variceal sclerosis
EVSD — Eisenmenger's ventricular septal defect

EVTV — extravascular thermal volume
EW — Emergency Ward
E-W — Edinger-Westphal [nucleus]
ew. — elsewhere
EWB — estrogen withdrawal bleeding
EWHO — elbow-wrist-hand orthosis
EWI — Experiential World Inventory
EWL —
    egg-white lysozyme
    evaporation water loss
EWSCLs — extended-wear soft contact lenses
EWT — erupted wisdom teeth
EX —
    exfoliation
    exsmoker
E(X) — expected value of the random variable X
ex —
    exacerbation
    exaggerated
    examination
    examine
    example
    excision
    exercise
    exophthalmos
    exposure
    extraction
ex aff. — *ex affinis* (Lat.) out of affinity
EXAFS — extended x-ray absorption fine structure [spectroscopy]
exag. — exaggerated
exam. —
    examination
    examine
    examined
ex aq. — *ex aqua* (Lat.) out of water
EXBF — exercise hyperemia blood flow
exc. —
    except

exc. — *(continued)*
  excision
exch. — exchange
excr. — excretion
EXD — ethylxanthic disulfide
exec. — executive
ExEF — ejection fraction during exercise
EXELFS — extended electron–loss line fine structure
exer. — exercise
EXGBUS — external genitalia, Bartholin [gland], urethral [gland], and Skene [gland]
ex gr. — *ex grupa* (Lat.) of the group of
exhib. — *exhibeatur* (Lat.) let it be given
exist. — existing
EXO —
  exonuclease
  exophoria
exog — exogenous
exoph — exophthalmia
exos. — exostosis
EXP —
  experienced
  expose
Exp —
  expect
  expiration
  expiratory
  expire
  exploration
  exploratory
  exponent
exp. —
  expansion
  expectorant
  experiment
  experimental
  exponential function
  exposure
ExPGN — extracapillary proliferative glomerulonephritis
exp. lap. — exploratory laparotomy

EXREM — external radiation-emission man [dose]
EXS —
  externally supported
  extrinsically supported
exsicc. — *exsiccatus* (Lat.) dried out
EXT —
  exercise testing
  extraction
ext —
  extension
  extensive
  extensor
  exterior
  external
  extract
  extreme
  extremity
ext. —
  extende (Lat.) spread
  extractum (Lat.) extract
ext aud — external auditory
extd —
  extended
  extracted
ext fd — fluid extract
Ext FHR — external fetal heart rate [monitoring]
extr — extremity
extrap —
  extrapolate
  extrapolation
extrav — extravasation
ext. rot. — external rotation
extub — extubation
EXU — excretory urogram
exud —
  exudate
  exudation
EY —
  egg yolk
  epidemiological year
EYA — egg yolk agar
Ez. — eczema

F —

bioavailability

a cell that donates F factor in bacterial conjugation

a conjugative plasmid in F+ bacterial cells

degree of fineness of abrasive particles

facial

facies

factor

Fahrenheit

failure

fair

false

family

farad

Faraday

fascia

fasting

fat

father

fecal

feces

Fellow

female

feminine

fermentation

fertility

fetal

fibroblast

fibrous

Ficol

field of vision

filament

fine

finger

firm

flexed

flexion

flow

fluid

fluoride

fluorine

F — (continued)

flutter wave

flux

focal length

focus

foil

fontanel

foramen

force

form

forma

formula

formulary

fornix

fossa

fraction

fractional

fracture

fragment [of an antibody]

free

French [catheter size]

frequency

frontal

frontal electrode placement in electroencephalography

function

fundus

fusion beat

gilbert [unit of magnetomotive force]

Helmholtz free energy

hydrocortisone (compound F)

inbreeding coefficient

left foot electrode in vectorcardiography

phenylalanine

variance ratio

visual field

F. —

Filaria

Fusarium

Fusiformis

Fusobacterium

F₁ — first filial generation

F$_2$ — second filial generation
F$_3$-TFT — trifluorothymidine
FI–FXIII — factors I through XIII
F344 — Fischer 344 [rat]
μF — microfarad
°F — degree on the Fahrenheit
　　scale
F$_0$ — emitted frequency
F′ — a hybrid F plasmid
F$^-$ —
　　a bacterial cell lacking an F
　　　plasmid
　　poor form response
F$^+$ —
　　a bacterial cell having an F
　　　plasmid
　　good form response
f —
　　atomic orbital with angular
　　　momentum quantum num-
　　　ber 3
　　breathing frequency
　　farad
　　father
　　female
　　femto-
　　fiber
　　fibrous
　　fingerbreadth
　　fission
　　flexion
　　fluid
　　focal length [of a lens]
　　foot
　　form
　　formula
　　fostered [experimental animal]
　　fraction
　　fracture
　　fragment
　　frequency
　　frequently
　　frontal
　　function
　　fundus
f — numerical expression of the
　　relative aperture of a
　　camera lens

f. —
　　fiant (Lat.) let them be made
　　fiat (Lat.) let there be made
　　forma (Lat.) form
f-12 — Freon
FA —
　　false aneurysm
　　Families Anonymous
　　Fanconi's anemia
　　far advanced
　　fatty acid
　　febrile antigen
　　femoral artery
　　fertilization antigen
　　fetal age
　　fibrinolytic activity
　　fibroadenoma
　　fibrosing alveolitis
　　field ambulance
　　filterable agent
　　filtered air
　　first aid
　　fluorescein angiography
　　fluorescence assay
　　fluorescent antibody
　　fluoroalanine
　　folic acid
　　follicular area
　　food allergy
　　foramen
　　forearm
　　fortified aqueous [solution]
　　free acid
　　Freund's adjuvant
　　Friedreich's ataxia
　　functional activity
　　fusaric acid
　　fusidic acid
F/A — fetus active
fa — fatty [rat]
FAA —
　　folic acid antagonist
　　formaldehyde, acetic acid, al-
　　　cohol
FAAD — fetal activity accelera-
　　tion determination
FAAP — Family Assessment
　　Adjustment Pass

FAB —
>   fast atom bombardment
>   formalin ammonium bromide
>   fragment antigen-binding [of
>   immunoglobulin G]
>   French-American-British
>   [Leukemia Classification]
>   functional arm brace

Fab — fragment, antigen-binding
>   [of immunoglobulin G]

$F(ab')_2$ — fragment, antigen-binding [of immunoglobulin G] [after digestion with enzyme pepsin]

Fabc — fragment, antigen, and complement binding [of immunoglobulins]

FABER — flexion, abduction, and external rotation

FABERE — flexion, abduction, external rotation, and extension

FABF — femoral artery blood flow

FAB/MS — fast atom bombardment mass spectrometry

FABP —
>   fatty acid-binding protein
>   folic acid-binding protein
>   folate-binding protein

FAC —
>   familial adenomatosis coli
>   femoral arterial cannulation
>   ferric ammonium citrate
>   fetal abdominal circumference
>   foamy alveolar cast
>   fractional area changes
>   fractional area concentration
>   free available chlorine

Fac — factor

fac — facility

fac. — *facere* (Lat.) to make

FACA —
>   Fellow of the American College of Anesthesiologists
>   Fellow of the American College of Angiology
>   Fellow of the American College of Apothecaries

FACAI — Fellow of the American College of Allergy and Immunology

FACAL — Fellow of the American College of Allergy

FACAS — Fellow of the American College of Abdominal Surgeons

Facb — fragment, antigen-and-complement binding

FACC — Fellow of the American College of Cardiologists

FACCP — Fellow of the American College of Chest Physicians

FACCPC — Fellow of the American College of Pharmacology and Chemotherapy

FACD — Fellow of the American College of Dentists

FACEB — Federation of American Societies for Experimental Biology

FACES — unique facies, anorexia, cachexia, and eye and skin lesions [syndrome]

FACFP — Fellow of the American College of Family Physicians

FACFS — Fellow of the American College of Foot Surgeons

FACG — Fellow of the American College of Gastroenterology

FACH — forceps to after-coming head

FACHA — Fellow of the American College of Hospital Administrators

FACLM — Fellow of the American College of Legal Medicine

FACMTA — Federal Advisory Council on Medical Training Aids

FACN — Fellow of the American College of Nutrition

FACNHA — Foundation of American College of Nursing Home Administrators

FACNP — Fellow of the American College of Neuropsychopharmacology

FACO — Fellow of the American College of Otolaryngology

FACOG — Fellow of the American College of Obstetricians and Gynecologists

FACOS — Fellow of the American College of Orthopedic Surgeons

FACOSH — Federal Advisory Committee on Occupational Safety and Health

FACP — Fellow of the American College of Physicians

FACPM — Fellow of the American College of Preventive Medicine

FACR — Fellow of the American College of Radiology

FACS —
　　Fellow of the American College of Surgeons
　　fluorescence-activated cell sorter

FACSM — Fellow of the American College of Sports Medicine

FACT — Flannagan Aptitude Classification Test

Factor VII — proconvertin

FACWA — familial amyotrophic chorea with acanthocytosis

FAD —
　　familial Alzheimer's dementia
　　familial autonomic dysfunction
　　Family Assessment Device
　　fetal abdominal diameter
　　fetal activity-acceleration determination
　　flavin adenine dinucleotide

FADF — fluorescent antibody darkfield

$FADH_2$ — flavin adenine dinucleotide [reduced form]

FADIR — flexion, adduction, and internal rotation

FADIRE — flexion, adduction, internal rotation, and extension

FADN — flavin adenine dinucleotide

FADS — fetal akinesia deformation sequence

FADU — fluorometric analysis of DNA unwinding

FAE — fetal alcohol effect

FAF —
　　fatty acid–free
　　fibroblast-activating factor

FAGA — full-term appropriate for gestational age

FAH — Federation of American Hospitals

Fahr. — Fahrenheit

FAI —
　　first aid instruction
　　free androgen index
　　functional aerobic impairment
　　functional assessment inventory

FAIDS — feline AIDS

FAIT — First Aid Instructor Trainer

FAJ — fused apophyseal joint

FALG — fowl anti-mouse lymphocyte globulin

FALP — fluorography-assisted lumbar puncture

Fam —
　　familial
　　family

FAMA —
　　Fellow of the American Medical Association
　　fluorescent antibody to membrane antigen [test]

FAME — fatty acid methyl ester

fam. doc. — family doctor

fam. hist. — family history

FAMMM — familial atypical multiple mole-melanoma [syndrome]

fam. per. par. — familial periodic paralysis

Fam. Phys. — Family Physician

FAN — fuchsin, amido black, and naphthol yellow

FANA — fluorescent antinuclear antibody

FANCAP — fluids, aeration, nutrition, communication, activity, and pain

FANCAS — fluids, aeration, nutrition, communication, activity, and stimulation

F and C — foam and condom

F and R — force and rhythm [of pulse]

FANPT — Freeman Anxiety Neurosis and Psychosomatic Test

FANS — Fellow of the American Neurological Society

FANY — First Aid Nursing Yeomanry

FAP —
  familial adenomatous polyposis
  familial amyloid polyneuropathy
  fatty acid–poor
  fatty acids polyunsaturated
  femoral artery pressure
  fibrillating action potential
  fixed action potential
  frozen animal procedure

FAPA —
  Fellow of the American Psychiatric Association
  Fellow of the American Psychoanalytical Association

FAPHA — Fellow of the American Public Health Association

FAQ — Family Attitudes Questionnaire

FAR — fractional albumin rate

Far — immediate good function followed by accelerated rejection

far. —
  farad
  faradic

FARE — Federation of Alcoholic Rehabilitation Establishments

FARS — Fatal Accident Reporting system

FAS —
  fatty acid synthetase
  Federation of American Scientists
  fetal alcohol syndrome

FASC — Free-Standing Ambulatory Surgical Center

fasc —
  fasciculation
  fascicle

fasc. — *fasciculus* (Lat.) bundle

FASEB — Federation of American Societies for Experimental Biology

FASF — Factor Analyzed Short Form

FASHP — Federation of Associations of Schools of the Health Professions

FAST —
  Filtered Audiometer Speech Test
  flow-assisted, short-term [balloon catheter]
  fluorescent allergosorbent test
  fluorescent antibody staining technique
  fluoro-allergosorbent test
  Frenchay Aphasia Screening Test

FAT —
  family attitudes test
  fast axoplasmic transport
  fluorescent antibody technique
  fluorescent antibody test
  Food Awareness Training

FATG — fat globules

F_1ATPase — F_1 adenosine triphosphatase

FATSA — Flowers Auditory Test of Selective Attention

FAV —
  feline ataxia virus
  floppy aortic valve
  fowl adenovirus

FAX — facsimile
FAZ —
    Fanconi-Albertini-Zellweger [syndrome]
    foveal avascular zone
    fragmented atrial activity zone
FB —
    Factor B
    fasting blood [sugar]
    feedback
    fiberoptic bronchoscopy
    fingerbreadth
    foreign body
    Fusobacterium
F/B — forward bending
f-b — face-bow
FBA —
    fecal bile acid
    Fellow of the British Academy
FBC —
    full blood count
    functional bacterial concentration
FBCOD — foreign body of the cornea, oculus dexter [right eye]
FBCOS — foreign body of the cornea, oculus sinister [left eye]
FBCP — familial benign chronic pemphigus
FBD —
    fibrocystic breast disease
    functional bowel disorder
FbDP — fibrin degradation products
FBE —
    full blood examination
    full body examination
FBEC — fetal bovine endothelial cell
FBF — forearm blood flow
FBG —
    fasting blood glucose
    fibrinogen
    foreign body [type] granuloma
fbg — fibrinogen
FBH — familial benign hypercalcemia

FBHH — familial benign hypocalciuric hypercalcemia
FBI — flossing, brushing, and irrigation
FBL —
    fecal blood loss
    follicular basal lamina
FBM — fetal breathing movement
FBN — Federal Bureau of Narcotics
FBP —
    femoral blood pressure
    fibrinogen breakdown products
FBPsS — Fellow of the British Psychological Society
FBR — *Frischblut* (Ger.) fresh-blood reaction
FBRCM — fingerbreadth below right costal margin
FBS —
    fasting blood sugar
    feedback signal
    feedback system
    fetal bovine serum
FBSS — failed back surgery syndrome
FBU — fingers below umbilicus
FBW — fasting blood work
FC —
    family conference
    fasciculus cuneatus
    fast component [of a neuron]
    febrile convulsions
    fecal coli [broth]
    feline conjunctivitis
    ferric citrate
    fever and chills
    fibrocystic
    fibrocyte
    finger clubbing
    finger counting
    flexion contracture
    flucytosine
    fluorocarbon
    fluorocytosine
    Foley catheter
    foramen cecum

FC — *(continued)*
> foster care
> fowl cholera
> free cholesterol
> frontal cortex
> functional capacity
> functional castration
> functional class

F/C — fever and chills

F + C — flare and cells

5-FC — 5-fluorocytosine

Fc′ — a fragment of an immuno-globulin molecule produced by papain digestion

Fc. —
> centroid frequency
> fragment, crystallizable [receptor, region]

fc. — foot candle

FCA —
> ferritin-conjugated antibodies
> fracture, complete, angulated
> Freund's complete adjuvant

FCAP — Fellow of the College of American Pathologists

F cath — Foley catheter

FCC —
> familial colonic cancer
> femoral cerebral catheter
> follicular center cells
> fracture complete and compound
> fracture compound and comminuted

fcc — face-centered-cubic

f/cc — fibers per cubic centimeter of air

FCCC — fracture complete, compound, and comminuted

FCCL — follicular center cell lymphoma

FCD —
> feces collection device
> fibrocystic disease
> fibrocystic dysplasia
> focal cytoplasmic degradation
> fracture complete and deviated

FCDB — fibrocystic disease of the breast

FCE — fibrocartilaginous embolism

FCF —
> fetal cardiac frequency
> fibroblast chemotactic factor

FCFC — fibroblast colony–forming cells

FCG — French catheter gauge

FCGP — Fellow of the College of General Practitioners

FCHL — familial combined hyper-lipidemia

FChS — Fellow of the Society of Chiropodists

FCI —
> fixed-cell immunofluorescence
> food chemical intolerance

fCi — femtocurie

FCIM — Federated Council for Internal Medicine

FCL — fibroblast cell line

fcly — face lying [position]

FCM —
> fetal cardiac motion
> flow cytometry

FCMC — family-centered maternity care

FCMD — Fukuyama-type congenital muscular dystrophy

FCMN — family-centered maternity nursing

FCMS —
> Fellow of the College of Medicine and Surgery
> Foix-Chavany-Marie syndrome

FCMW — Foundation for Child Mental Welfare

FCO — Fellow of the College of Osteopathy

FCP —
> fasting chemistry profile
> final common pathway
> Functional Communication Profile

FCPS — Fellow of the College of Physicians and Surgeons

FCR —
  flexor carpi radialis
  fractional catabolic rate
FcR — Fc receptor
FCRA —
  fecal collection receptacle assembly
  Fellow of the College of Radiologists of Australasia
FCRB — flexor carpi radialis brevis
FCRC — Frederick Cancer Research Center
FCS —
  fecal contaminant system
  feedback control system
  Fellow of the Chemical Society
  fetal calf serum
  foot compartment syndrome
FCSNVD — fever, chills, sweating, nausea, vomiting, and diarrhea
FCSP — Fellow of the Chartered Society of Physiotherapy
FCST — Fellow of the College of Speech Therapists
FCT — food composition table
FCU — flexor carpi ulnaris
FCV — forced vital capacity
FCVD — fracture complete and varus deformity
FCVDS — Framingham Cardiovascular Disease Survey
FCx — frontal cortex
FD —
  familial dysautonomia
  family doctor
  fan douche
  fatal dose
  fetal danger
  fetal demise
  fibrinogen derivative
  field desorption
  Filatov-Dukes [disease]
  fixed and dilated
  fluorescence depolarization
  fluphenazine decanoate
  focal disease

FD — (continued)
  focal distance
  Folin-Denis [assay]
  follicular diameter
  foot drape
  forceps delivery
  freeze dried
  frequency deviation
  full denture
F/D — fracture/dislocation
F & D — fixed and dilated
Fd —
  the heavy chain portion of a Fab fragment
  ferredoxin
  fundus
FD_{50} — median fatal dose
FDA —
  fluorescein diacetate
  Food and Drug Administration
  Frenchay Dysarthria Assessment
  fronto-dextra anterior (Lat.) right frontoanterior [position of fetus]
FDBL — fecal daily blood loss
FDC —
  follicular dendritic cell
  frequency dependence of compliance
FD&C —
  Food, Drug, and Cosmetic Act
  food, drugs, and cosmetics
FDCPA — Food, Drug, and Consumer Product Agency
FDCT — Franck Drawing Completion Test
FDD — Food and Drugs Directorate
FDDC — ferric dimethyldithiocarbonate
FDDQ — Freedom from Distractibility Deviation Quotient
FDDS — Family Drawing Depression Scale
FDE —
  female day-equivalent

FDE — *(continued)*
    final drug evaluation
FDF —
    fast death factor
    further differentiated fibroblast
FDFQ — Food/Drink Frequency Questionnaire
FDG — fluorodeoxyglucose
fdg — feeding
FDGF — fibroblast-derived growth factor
FDH —
    familial dysalbuminemic hyperthyroxinemia
    focal dermal hypoplasia
    formaldehyde dehydrogenase
FDI —
    Fédération Dentaire Internationale (Fr.) International Dental Federation
    first dorsal interosseus [muscle]
FDIU — fetal death in utero
FDL — flexor digitorum longus
FDLMP — first day of last menstrual period
FDLV — fer-de-lance virus
FDM —
    fetus of diabetic mother
    fibrous dysplasia of the mandible
FDNB —
    fluorodinitrobenzene
    1-fluoro-2,4-dinitrobenzene
FDO — Fleet Dental Officer
FDP —
    fibrin degradation products
    fibrinogen degradation products
    flexor digitorum profundus
    frontodextra posterior (Lat.) right frontoposterior [position of fetus]
    fructose-1,6-diphosphate
FDPase — fructose-1,6-diphosphatase
FDQB — flexor digiti quinti brevis

FDR —
    fractional disappearance rate
    frequency dependence of resistance
FDS —
    Fellow in Dental Surgery
    fiberduodenoscope
    flexor digitorum sublimis
    flexor digitorum superficialis
    for duration of stay
FDSRCSEng — Fellow in Dental Surgery of the Royal College of Surgeons of England
FDT — *frontodextra transversa* (Lat.) right frontotransverse [position of fetus]
F_3dTMP — trifluorothymidylate
F-dUMP — 5-fluorodeoxyuridine monophosphate
FDTVMP — Frostig Developmental Test of Visual Motor Perception
FDTVP — Frostig Developmental Test of Visual Perception
FDV — Friend disease virus
FDZ — fetal danger zone
FE —
    fatty ester
    fecal emesis
    fecal energy
    fetal erythroblastosis
    fetal erythrocyte
    fluid extract
    fluorescent erythrocyte
    forced expiration
    formaldehyde-ethanol
Fe —
    female
    ferret
    iron (Lat., *ferrum*)
Fe_2 — ferrous
Fe_3 — ferric
^{59}Fe — radioactive iron
fe — female
feb — febrile
feb. — *febris* (Lat.) fever
feb. dur. — *febre durante* (Lat.) while the fever lasts

FEBP — fetal estrogen-binding protein

FEBRIL — febrile agglutinins

FEBROA — febrile battery—acute

FEBS — Federation of European Biochemical Societies

FEC —
fecal
forced expiratory capacity
free erythrocyte coproporphyrin
Free-standing Emergency Center
Friend erythroleukemia cell

FECG — fetal electrocardiogram

$FeCO_3$ — ferrous carbonate

Fe_{CO_2} — fractional concentration of carbon dioxide in expired gas

FECP —
Factor VIII correctional time
free erythrocyte coproporphyrin

FECT — fibroelastic connective tissue

FECU — Factor VIII correctional unit

FECV —
feline enteric coronavirus
functional extracellular fluid volume

FeD — iron deficiency

FEDRIP — Federal Research in Progress [data base]

FEE — forced equilibrating expiration

FEEG — fetal electroencephalography

FEF —
Family Evaluation Form
forced expiratory flow [rate]

FEF_{50} — forced expiratory flow at 50% of forced vital capacity

FEF_{50}/FIF_{50} — ratio of expiratory flow to inspiratory flow at 50% of forced vital capacity

FEFV — forced expiratory flow volume

FEHBP — Federal Employee Health Benefits Program

FEIBA — Factor VIII inhibitor bypassing activity

FeINC — iron inclusion bodies

FEKG — fetal electrocardiogram

FEL — familial erythrophagocytic lymphohistiocytosis

FELC — Friend erythroleukemia cell

FeLV — feline leukemia virus

FEM —
finite element method
fluid-electrolyte malnutrition

fem —
female
feminine
femoral
femur

fem. — *femoris* (Lat.) thigh

fem. intern. — *femoribus internus* (Lat.) at inner side of the thighs

fem-pop — femoral-popliteal [bypass]

FEN — fluid, electrolytes, and nutrition

Fe_{NA} — excreted fraction of filtered sodium

FENF — fenfluramine

Fe_{O_2} — fractional concentration of oxygen in expired gas

Fe_2O_3 — ferric oxide

$Fe(OH)_3$ — ferric hydroxide

FEOM —
full extraocular motion
full extraocular movement

FEP —
fluorinated ethylene-propylene
free erythrocyte porphyrin
free erythrocyte protoporphyrin

FEPB — functional electronic peroneal brace

FEPP — free erythrocyte protoporphyrin

FER —
flexion, extension, rotation

FER — (*continued*)
  fractional esterification rate
fer. — *ferrum* (Lat.) iron
FERRIT — ferritin
fert —
  fertilized
  fertility
ferv. — *fervens* (Lat.) boiling
FES —
  Family Environment Scale
  fat embolism syndrome
  flame emission spectroscopy
  forced expiratory spirogram
  functional electrical stimulation
Fe/S — iron/sulfur [protein]
FESA — finite element stress analysis
FeSO$_4$ — ferrous sulfate
FeSV — feline sarcoma virus
FET —
  field-effect transistor
  Fisher exact test
  fixed erythrocyte turnover
  forced expiratory time
fet — fetus
FETE — Far Eastern tick-borne encephalitis
FETI — fluorescence excitation transfer immunoassay
FETs — forced expiratory time in seconds
FEUO — for external use only
FE-UR — iron in urine
FEV —
  familial exudative vitreoretinopathy
  forced expiratory volume
FEV$_1$ — forced expiratory volume in one second
fev — fever
FEVB — frequency ectopic ventricular beat
FEV$_t$ — forced expiratory volume timed
FEV$_1$/VC — forced expiratory volume in one second—vital capacity

FEVR — familial exudative vitreoretinopathy
FeZ — iron zone
FF —
  degree of fineness of abrasive particles
  fat free [diet]
  father factor
  fecal frequency
  fertility factor
  field of Forel
  F factor
  filtration factor
  filtration fraction
  fine fiber
  fine fraction
  finger flexion
  finger-to-finger [test]
  fixation fluid
  fixing fluid
  flat feet
  flip-flop
  fluorescent focus
  follicular fluid
  force fluid
  forearm flow
  forward flexion
  foster father
  Fox Fordyce [disease]
  free fat
  free fraction
  fresh frozen
  full field
  fundus firm
  further flexion
F factor — fertility factor
F & F —
  filiform and follower
  fixes and follows
fF —
  ultrafine fiber
  ultrafine fraction
ff —
  force fluids
  fundus firm
ff$^+$ — fertility inhibition positive
ff$^-$ — fertility inhibition negative
f→f — finger-to-finger

FFA —
> Fellow of the Faculty of Anaesthetists
> female-female adaptor
> free fatty acids

FFAP — free fatty acid phase

FFARCS — Fellow of the Faculty of Anaesthetists of the Royal College of Surgeons

FFB —
> fast feedback
> flexible fiberoptic bronchoscopy

FFC —
> fixed flexion contracture
> fluorescence flow cytometry
> free from chlorine

FFCM — Fellow of the Faculty of Community Medicine

FFCS — forearm flexion control strap

FFD —
> fat free diet
> Fellow in the Faculty of Dentistry
> focus-film distance

FFDCA — Federal Food, Drug, and Cosmetic Act

FFDSRCS — Fellow of the Faculty of Dental Surgery of the Royal College of Surgeons

FFDW — fat-free dry weight

FFE — fecal fat excretion

FFEM — freeze fracture electron microscopy

FFF —
> degree of fineness of abrasive particles
> field-flow fractionation
> flicker fusion frequency

FFG — free fat graft

FFHom — Fellow of the Faculty of Homeopathy

FFI —
> fast food intake
> free from infection
> fundamental frequency indicator

FFIT — fluorescent focus inhibition test

FFM —
> fat-free mass
> five-finger movement

FFOM — Fellow of the Faculty of Occupational Medicine

FFP —
> fistful of prisms
> fresh frozen plasma

FFR —
> Fellow of the Faculty of Radiologists
> frequency-following response

FFROM — full and free range of motion

FFS —
> failure of fixation suppression
> fat-free solids
> fat-free supper
> fee for services
> flexible fiberoptic sigmoidoscopy

FFT —
> fast Fourier transforms
> flicker fusion threshold

FFTP — first full-term pregnancy

FFU —
> femur-fibula-ulna [syndrome]
> focus forming unit

FFW — fat-free weight

FFWC — fractional free water clearance

FFWW — fat-free wet weight

FG —
> fasciculus gracilis
> fast-glycolytic [fiber]
> Feeley-Gorman [agar]
> fibrin glue
> fibrinogen
> field gain
> Flemish giant [rabbit]
> French gauge

fg — femtogram

FGAR — formylglycinamide ribonucleotide

FGB — fully granulated basophil

FGC — fibrinogen gel chromatography

FGD — fatal granulomatous disease

FgDP — fibrinogen degradation products

FGDS — fibrogastroduodenoscopy

FGF —
> father's grandfather
> fibroblast growth factor
> fresh gas flow

FGG —
> focal global glomerulosclerosis
> fowl gammaglobulin

FGL — fasting gastrin level

FGLU — fasting glucose

FGM — father's grandmother

FGN —
> fibrinogen
> focal glomerulonephritis

FGP — fundic gland polyp

FGRN — finely granular

FGS —
> fibrogastroscopy
> focal glomerular sclerosis

FGT —
> female genital tract
> fluorescent gonorrhea test

FGU — French gauge, urodynamic

FH —
> facial hemihyperplasia
> familial hypercholesterolemia
> family history
> Fanconi-Hegglin [syndrome]
> fasting hyperbilirubinemia
> favorable histology
> femoral hypoplasia
> fetal head
> fetal heart
> fibromuscular hyperplasia
> Ficoll-Hypaque [technique]
> floating hospital
> follicular hyperplasia
> Frankfort horizontal [plane]
> fundal height

FH$^+$ — family history positive

FH$^-$ — family history negative

FH$_4$ —
> folacin
> tetrahydrofolic acid

f.h. — *fiat haustus* (Lat.) let a draught be made

fh — fostered by hand [experimental animal]

FHA —
> familial hypoplastic anemia
> Fellow of the Institute of Hospital Administrators
> filamentous hemagglutinin
> filterable hemolytic anemia
> fimbrial hemagglutinin

FH/BC — frontal horn/bicaudate [ratio]

FHC —
> familial hypercholesterolemia
> family health center
> Ficoll-Hypaque centrifugation
> Fuchs' heterochromic cyclitis

FHCH — fortified hexachlorocyclohexane

FHD —
> familial histiocytic dermatoarthritis
> family history of diabetes

FHF —
> fetal heart frequency
> fulminating hepatic failure

fHg — free hemoglobin

FHH —
> familial hypocalciuric hypercalcemia
> family history of hirsutism
> fetal heart heard

FHI — Fuchs' heterochromic iridocyclitis

FHIP — Family Health Insurance Plan

FHL —
> flexor hallucis longus
> functional hearing loss

FHLDH — familial hypercholesterolemia, low density protein

FHM —
> fathead minnow [cells]
> fetal heart motion

FH-M — fumarate hydratase, mitochondrial

FHMI — family history of mental illness

FHN — family history negative
FHNH — fetal heart not heard
FHP — family history positive
FHR —
> familial hypophosphatemic
> rickets
> fetal heart rate
> fetal heart rhythm

FHRDC — family history, research
diagnostic criteria
FHRNST — fetal heart rate non-
stress test
FHR-NST — fetal heart rate non-
stress test
FHS —
> fetal heart sounds
> fetal hydantoin syndrome

FH-S — fumarate hydratase, soluble
FHT —
> fetal heart
> fetal heart tone

FHTG — familial hypertriglyceri-
demia
FH-UFS — femoral hypoplasia–
unusual facies syndrome
FHV — falcon herpesvirus
FHVP — free hepatic vein pressure
FHx — family history
FI —
> fasciculus interfascicularis
> fever caused by infection
> fibrinogen
> fiscal intermediary
> fixed interval [schedule]
> flame ionization
> follicular involution
> food intolerance
> forced inspiration
> frontoiliac
> functional inquiry

FIA —
> fluorescent immunoassay
> fluoroimmunoassay
> focal immunoassay
> Freund's incomplete adjuvant

FIAC —
> Fellow of the International
> Academy of Cytology

FIAC — (continued)
> 2′-fluoro-5-iodo-aracytosine

FIB —
> Fellow of the Institute of Biol-
> ogy
> fibrin
> fibrinogen
> fibrositis
> fibula

fib —
> fiber
> fibril
> fibrillation
> fibrin
> fibrinogen

fib. bronc. — fiberoptic bronchoscopy
fibrill — fibrillation
FIC —
> fasting intestinal contents
> Fellow of the Institute of
> Chemistry
> Fogarty International Center
> fractional inhibitory concen-
> tration

FICA — Federal Insurance Contri-
butions Act
FICD —
> Fellow of the Institute of Ca-
> nadian Dentists
> Fellow of the International
> College of Dentists

$FICO_2$, FI_{CO_2} — fractional concentration of carbon dioxide in
inspired gas
FICS — Fellow of the International College of Surgeons
FICSIT — Frailty and Injuries: Cooperative Studies of Intervention Techniques
FICU — fetal intensive care unit
FID —
> flame ionization detector
> free induction decay
> fungal immunodiffusion

field H_1 — fasciculus thalamicus
field H_2 — fasciculus lenticularis
FIF —
> feedback inhibition factor

FIF — *(continued)*
    fibroblast interferon
    forced inspiratory flow
    formaldehyde-induced fluo-
       rescence
FIFO — first in, first out
FIFR — fasting intestinal flow rate
fig. —
    figuratively
    figure
FIGD — familial idiopathic gonad-
    otropin deficiency
FIGE — Field inversion gel electro-
    phoresis
FIGLU — formiminoglutamic acid
FIGO — International Federation
    of Gynecology and Obstetrics
    [classification of tumor stag-
    ing]
FIH —
    familial isolated hypoparathy-
       roidism
    fat-induced hyperglycemia
fil —
    filament
    filamentous
    filial
FILAR — filariasis
filt. —
    filter
    filtration
FIM —
    field ion microscopy
    functional independence
       measure
FIMLT — Fellow of the Institute
    of Medical Laboratory Tech-
    nology
FIN — fine intestinal needle
FINCC — familial idiopathic non-
    arteriosclerotic cerebral calci-
    fication
F-insulin — fibrous insulin
FI_{O_2} —
    forced inspiratory oxygen
    fraction of inspired oxygen
    fractional concentration of
      oxygen in inspired gas

FI_{O_2} — *(continued)*
    fractional inspired oxygen
FIP — feline infectious peritonitis
FIPT — periarteriolar transudate
FIPV — feline infectious peritoni-
    tis virus
FIQ — full-scale intelligence quo-
    tient
FIR —
    far infrared
    fold increase in resistance
FIRDA — frontal intermittent
    rhythmic delta activity [elec-
    troencephalography]
FIRO-B — Fundamental Interper-
    sonal Relations
    Orientation—Behavior
FIRO-F — Fundamental Interper-
    sonal Relations Orientation-
    Feelings
FIS — forced inspiratory spirogram
FISP — fast imaging with steady-
    state precision
FISS — Flint Infant Security Scale
fist. — fistula
FIT —
    Flanagan Industrial Tests
    fluorescein isothiocyanate
    fusion inferred threshold [test]
FITC — fluorescein isothiocyanate
FITT — frequency, intensity, time,
    and conjugate type
FIUO — for internal use only
FIV —
    feline immunodeficiency
    forced inspiratory volume
FIV_1 — forced inspiratory volume
    in one second
FIVC — forced inspiratory vital ca-
    pacity
F-J — Fisher-John [melting point
    method]
FJN — familial juvenile
    nephrophthisis
FJN-MCD — familial juvenile
    nephrophthisis—medullary
    cystic disease
FJRM — full joint range of move-
    ment

FJS — finger joint size
FK —
> Feil-Klippel [syndrome]
> feline kidney
> functioning Kasai (Belgian Congo anemia)

FL —
> factor level
> fatty liver
> feline leukemia
> femur length
> fetal length
> fibers of Luschka
> fibroblast-like
> filtered load
> filtration leukapheresis
> flavomycin
> fluorescein
> flutamide and leuprolide acetate
> focal length
> Foster Kennedy [syndrome]
> Friend leukemia [cell]
> frontal lobe
> full liquid [diet]
> functional length

FL-2 — feline lung [cell]
Fl —
> florentium
> fluid
> fluorescence

fl —
> femtoliter
> filtered load
> flank
> flexible
> flexion
> flow
> fluid
> fluorescence
> flutter
> foot lambert

fl. — *fluidus* (Lat.) fluid
FLA —
> fluorescence-labeled antibody
> *frontolaeva anterior* (Lat.) left frontoanterior [position of the fetus]

f.l.a. — *fiat lege artis* (Lat.) let it be done according to rule
flac. —
> flaccid
> flaccidity

Fl Ang — fluorescein angiography
Fl Ant — fluorescent antibody
flav. — *flavus* (Lat.) yellow
FLC —
> fatty liver cell
> fetal liver cell
> Friend leukemia cell

FLD —
> fatty liver disease
> fibrotic lung disease
> flutamide and leuprolide acetate depot

fld. —
> field
> fluid

fl. dr. — fluid dram
fld. rest. — fluid restriction
fldxt. — *fluidextractum* (Lat.) fluid extract
FLES — Fairview Language Evaluation Scale
FLEX — Federation Licensing Examination
flex. —
> flexion
> flexor

flex. sig. — flexible sigmoidoscopy
FLGA — full term, large for gestational age
FLK — funny-looking kid
FLKS — fatty liver and kidney syndrome
FLM — fasciculus longitudinalis medialis
floc. — flocculation
flor. — *flores* (Lat.) flowers
fl. oz. — fluid ounce
FLP —
> few large platelets
> *frontolaeva posterior* (Lat.) left frontoposterior [position of the fetus]

FLPR — flurbiprofen

FLR — funny looking rash
FLS —
    fatty liver syndrome
    Fellow of the Linnean Society
    fibrous long-spacing [collagen]
    flashing lights and/or scotoma
    flow-limiting segment
    Functional Life Scale
FLSA — follicular lymphosarcoma
FLSP — fluorescein-labeled serum
    protein
FLT — *frontolaeva transversa* (Lat.)
    left frontotransverse [position
    of the fetus]
FLTA — Fullerton Language Test
    for Adolescents
FLTAC — Fisher-Logemann Test
    of Articulation Competence
FLU —
    flunitrazepam
    fluphenazine
flu — influenza
fluor —
    fluorescence
    fluorescent
    fluorometry
    fluoroscopy
fluores —
    fluorescence
    fluorescent
fluoro —
    fluoroscope
    fluoroscopy
fl up —
    flare-up
    follow-up
FLV —
    feline leukemia virus
    Friend leukemia virus
FLZ — flurazepam
FM —
    face mask
    facilities management
    family medicine
    Farnsworth-Munsell one hun-
    dred hue test
    feedback mechanism
    fetal movement

FM — *(continued)*
    fibrin monomer
    fibromuscular
    filtered mass
    flavin mononucleotide
    flowmeter
    fluid movement
    fluorescent microscopy
    foramen magnum
    forensic medicine
    formerly married
    foster mother
    frequency modulation
    Friend-Moloney [antigen]
    functional movement
    Fusobacterium micro-organ-
    isms
F.M. — *fiat mistura* (Lat.) make a
    mixture
F and M — firm and midline
Fm — fermium
f-M — free metanephrine
fm — femtometer
FMA — Frankfort mandibular
    plane angle
FMAT — fetal movement accelera-
    tion test
FMB — full maternal behavior
FMC —
    family medicine center
    fetal movement count
    Flight Medicine Clinic
    focal macular choroidopathy
    Foundation for Medical Care
FMCA — Forensic Medicine Con-
    sultant Advisor
FMD —
    family medical doctor
    fibromuscular dysplasia
    foot-and-mouth disease
    frontometaphyseal dysplasia
FMDV — foot and mouth disease
    virus
FME — full mouth extraction
Fmed — median frequency
FMEL — Friend murine erythroleu-
    kemia
FMEN — familial multiple endo-
    crine neoplasia

F-met — formylmethionine
FMF —
    familial Mediterranean fever
    fetal movement felt
    flow microfluorometry
    forced midexpiratory flow
FMFD1 — familial multiple factor
    deficiency 1
FMG —
    fine mesh gauze
    foreign medical graduate
FMGEMS — Foreign Medical
    Graduate Examination in
    Medical Sciences
FMH —
    family medical history
    fat-mobilizing hormone
    feto-maternal hemorrhage
    fibromuscular hyperplasia
FMI — Foods and Moods Inven-
    tory
FMIV — forced mandatory inter-
    mittent ventilation
FML —
    flail mitral leaflet
    fluorometholone
f-MLP — N-formyl-methionyl-
    leucyl-phenylalanine
FMN —
    first malignant neoplasm
    flavin mononucleotide (ribo-
    flavin 5'-phosphate)
    frontomaxillonasal [suture]
$FMNH_2$ — reduced form of flavin
    mononucleotide
FMO —
    Fleet Medical Officer
    Flight Medical Officer
fmol — femtomole
FMP —
    fasting metabolic panel
    first menstrual period
    fructose monophosphate
FMR —
    fetal movement record
    Friend-Moloney-Rauscher [an-
    tigen]
FMS —
    fat-mobilizing substance

FMS — (continued)
    Fellow of the Medical Society
    fibromyalgia syndrome
    full mouth series
FMSTB — Frostig Movement
    Skills Test Battery
FMU — first morning urine
FMULC — free monoclonal uri-
    nary light chain
F-MuLV — Friend murine leuke-
    mia virus
FMX — full mouth x-ray
FN —
    facial nerve
    false negative
    fastigial nucleus
    fibronectin
    final nitrogen
    fluoride number
F-N — finger-to-nose
FNA — fine-needle aspiration
FNa — filtered sodium
FNAB — fine-needle aspiration bi-
    opsy
FNAC — fine-needle aspiration cy-
    tology
FNC — fatty nutritional cirrhosis
FNCJ — fine needle catheter
    jejunostomy
FND —
    febrile neutrophilic dermatosis
    frontonasal dysplasia
f-NE — free norepinephrine
Fneg — false negative
FNF —
    false-negative fraction
    femoral neck fracture
    finger-nose-finger [test]
FNH — focal nodular hyperplasia
f-NM — free normetanephrine
FNP — Family Nurse Practitioner
FNR — false-negative rate
FNS — functional neuromuscular
    stimulation
FNT —
    false neurochemical transmit-
    ter
    finger-to-nose test

FNTC — fine-needle transhepatic cholangiography

FO —
　fiberoptic
　fish oil
　foot orthosis
　foramen ovale
　forced oscillation
　foreign object
　fronto-occipital

Fo —
　fomenting
　fomentation

FOA — Federation of Orthodontic Associations

FOAVF — failure of all vital forces

FOB —
　father of baby
　fecal occult blood
　feet out of bed
　fiberoptic bronchoscopy
　foot of bed
　functional observational battery

FOBT — fecal occult blood test

FOC —
　father of child
　fluid of choice
　frequency of contact scale
　fronto-occipital circumference

FOCAL — formula calculation

FOCMA — feline oncornavirus–associated cell membrane antigen

FOD — free of disease

FOG —
　Fluothane, oxygen, and gas
　fast oxidative glycolytic [fiber]

FOI — flight of ideas

fol — following

fol. — *folia* (Lat.) leaves

FOM —
　figure of merit
　floor of mouth

FOOB — fell out of bed

FOOSH — fell onto outstretched hand

FOP —
　fibrodysplasia ossificans progressiva
　forensic pathology

FOPR — full outpatient rate

FOR — forensic

for —
　foreign
　formula

form —
　formation
　formula

fort. — *fortis* (Lat.) strong

FORTRAN — *formula translation*

FOS —
　fiberoptic sigmoidoscopy
　fissura orbitalis superior
　fractional osteoid surface
　full of stool

found. — foundation

FOV — field of view

FOVI — field of vision intact

FOW — fenestration open window

FP —
　false positive
　family physician
　family planning
　family practice
　family practitioner
　Fanconi's Petrassi [syndrome]
　fibrinolytic potential
　fibrinopeptide
　filling pressure
　filter paper
　first pass
　fixation protein
　flash point
　flat plate
　flavin phosphate
　flavoprotein
　flexor profundus
　fluid pressure
　fluorescence polarization
　food poisoning
　forearm pronated
　freezing point
　frontoparietal
　frozen plasma

FP — *(continued)*
    full period
    fundal pressure
    fusion point
F-P — femoral popliteal
F/P —
    fluid-plasma [ratio]
    fluorescein-to-protein [ratio]
F-6-P — fructose-6-phosphate
Fp —
    filtered phosphate
    frontal polar electrode placement in electroencephalography
fp —
    flexor pollicis
    foot pound
    forearm pronated
    freezing point
f.p. —
    fiat potio (Lat.) let a potion be made
    fiat pulvis (Lat.) let a powder be made
FPA —
    Family Planning Association
    fibrinopeptide A
    filter paper activity
    fluorophenylalanine
fpA — fibrinopeptide A
FPAL — full-term deliveries, premature deliveries, abortions, and living children
FPB —
    femoral popliteal bypass
    fibrinopeptide B
    flexor pollicis brevis
FPC —
    familial polyposis coli
    Family Planning Clinic
    Family Practice Center
    Family Practitioner Center
    fish protein concentrate
    frozen packed cells
FpCA — 1-fluoromethyl-2-*p*-chlorophenyl-ethylamine
FPCL — fibroblast-populated collagen lattice

FPD —
    fetopelvic disproportion
    fixed partial denture
    flame photometric detector
FPDD — familial pure depressive disease
FPDVP — Frostig Program for the Development of Visual Perception
FPE —
    fatal pulmonary embolism
    first-pass effect
FPF —
    false-positive fraction
    fibroblast pneumocyte factor
FPG —
    fasting plasma glucose
    fluorescence plus Giemsa
    focal proliferative glomerulonephritis
FPGS — folylpolyglutamate synthetase
FPH_2 — flavin phosphate, reduced
FPHA — family planning health assistant
FPHE — formaldehyde-treated pyruvaldehyde-stabilized human erythrocytes
FPHx — family psychiatric history
FPI —
    femoral pulsatility index
    formula protein intolerance
    Freiburg Personality Identification Questionnaire
FPIA — fluorescence polarization immunoassay
f. pil. — *fiant pilulae* (Lat.) let pills be made
f. pil. xi — *fac pilulas xi* (Lat.) make eleven pills
FPK — fructose phosphokinase
FPL —
    fasting plasma lipids
    flexor pollicis longus
FPLA — fibrin plate lysis area
F(plasma) — plasma cortisol
FPM —
    filter paper microscopic [test]

FPM — *(continued)*
full passive movements

fpm. — feet per minute

FPN — ferric chloride, perchloric acid, and nitric acid [solution]

FPNA — first-pass nuclear angiocardiography

FPO —
Federation of Prosthodontic Organizations
freezing-point osmometer

FPP — free portal pressure

FPPH — familial primary pulmonary hypertension

FPR —
false-positive rate
finger peripheral resistance
fluorescence photobleaching recovery
fractional proximal resorption

FPRA — first-pass radionuclide angiogram

F/P ratio — fluid/plasma ratio

FPS —
Fellow of the Pathological Society
Fellow of the Pharmaceutical Society
fetal PCB (polychlorinated biphenyl) syndrome
footpad swelling

fps —
feet per second
foot-pound second
frames per second

FPSLT — Fluharty Preschool Speech and Language Screening Test

FPT — fixed parenchymal turnover

FPU — Family Participation Unit

FPV — fowl plague virus

FPVB — femoral popliteal vein bypass

FPZ — fluphenazine

FPZ-*D* — fluphenazine decanoate

FR —
failure rate
fasciculus retroflexus

FR — *(continued)*
father
Favre-Racouchot [disease]
febrile reaction
feedback regulation
fibrinogen-related
fibrin-related
Fischer-Race [notation]
fixed ratio
flocculation reaction
flow rate
fluid restriction
fluid retention
formatio reticularis (Lat.) reticular formation
fractional reabsorption
free radical
frequency of respiration
frequent relapses
Friend [virus]
full range
functional residual [capacity]

F&R — force and rhythm [pulse]

Fr — francium

fr —
fracture
franklin [unit charge]
French [catheter gauge]
from

Fr1 — first fraction

FRA —
fibrinogen-related antigen
fluorescent rabies antibody

fra — fragile [site]

FRAC — Food Research and Action Center

frac — fracture

FRACDS — Fellow of the Royal Australasian College of Dental Surgery

FRACGP — Fellow of the Royal Australasian College of General Practitioners

FRACO — Fellow of the Royal Australasian College of Ophthalmologists

FRACON — framycetin, colistin, and nystatin

FRACP — Fellow of the Royal Australasian College of Physicians

FRACR — Fellow of the Royal Australasian College of Radiologists

FRACS — Fellow of the Royal Australasian College of Surgeons

fract. — fracture

fract. dos. — *fracta dosi* (Lat.) in divided doses

frag. —
    fragile
    fragility
    fragment

FRANZCP — Fellow of the Royal Australian and New Zealand College of Psychiatrists

FRAP — fluorescence recovery after photobleaching

FRAT — free radical assay technique

FRAX — fragile [chromosome] X

fra(X) —
    fragile X [chromosome]
    fragile X [syndrome]

FRAX-MR — fragile X-mental retardation [syndrome]

Fr BB — fracture of both bones

FRC —
    Federal Radiation Council
    frozen red cells
    functional reserve capacity
    functional residual capacity

FRCD —
    Fellow of the Royal College of Dentists
    fixed ratio combination drug

FRCGP — Fellow of the Royal College of General Practitioners

FRCOG — Fellow of the Royal College of Obstetricians and Gynaecologists

FRCP — Fellow of the Royal College of Physicians

FRCPA — Fellow of the Royal College of Pathologists of Australia

FRCPath — Fellow of the Royal College of Pathologists

FRCP(C) — Fellow of the Royal College of Physicians of Canada

FRCPE — Fellow of the Royal College of Physicians of Edinburgh

FRCP(Glasg) — Fellow of the Royal College of Physicians and Surgeons of Glasgow

FRCPI — Fellow of the Royal College of Physicians of Ireland

FRCPsych — Fellow of the Royal College of Psychiatrists

FRCS — Fellow of the Royal College of Surgeons

FRCS(C) — Fellow of the Royal College of Surgeons of Canada

FRCSE — Fellow of the Royal College of Surgeons of Edinburgh

FRCSEng — Fellow of the Royal College of Surgeons of England

FRCS(Glasg) — Fellow of the Royal College of Physicians and Surgeons of Glasgow

FRCSI — Fellow of the Royal College of Surgeons of Ireland

FRCVS — Fellow of the Royal College of Veterinary Surgeons

FRE —
    Fischer rat embryo
    flow-related enhancement

FREIR — Federal Research on Biological and Health Effects of Ionizing Radiation

frem. — *fremitus vocalis* (Lat.) vocal fremitus

freq. — frequency

FRES — Fellow of the Royal Entomological Society

FRF —
    fasciculus retroflexus

FRF — *(continued)*
Fertility Research Foundation
filtration replacement fluid
follicle-stimulating hormone-
releasing factor
FRFC — functional renal failure of
cirrhosis
FRFPSG — Fellow of the Royal
Faculty of Physicians and Sur-
geons of Glasgow
FRH — follicle-stimulating hor-
mone–releasing hormone
FRh — fetal rhesus monkey kidney
[cell]
FRHS — fast-repeating high se-
quence
frict. — friction
Fried — Friedman [test]
frig. — *frigidus* (Lat.) cold
FRIPHH — Fellow of the Royal In-
stitute of Public Health and
Hygiene
FRJM —
full range of joint motion
full range of joint movement
FRMedSoc — Fellow of the Royal
Medical Society
FRMS — Fellow of the Royal Mi-
croscopical Society
FRN — fully resonant nucleus
FRNS — frequently relapsing ne-
phrotic syndrome
FROM —
full range of motion
full range of movement
FRP — functional refractory period
FRPS — functional resting posi-
tion splint
FRr — friction rub
FRS —
Fellow of the Royal Society
ferredoxin-reducing substance
first rank symptom
furosemide
FRSC — Fellow of the Royal Soci-
ety of Chemistry
FRSE — Fellow of the Royal Soci-
ety of Edinburgh

FRSH — Fellow of the Royal Society of Health
FRT —
Family Relations Test
full recovery time
fru. — fructose
frust. — *frustillatim* (Lat.) in small
pieces
FRV — functional residual volume
frx — fracture
FS —
factor of safety
Fanconi syndrome
Felty syndrome
female, spayed [animal]
fetoscope
fibromyalgia syndrome
field stimulation
finger stick
Fischer syndrome
flexible sigmoidoscopy
food service
forearm supination
foreskin [human cells]
Fourier series
fracture site
fragile site
Freeman-Sheldon [syndrome]
Friesinger score
frozen section
full scale [IQ]
full soft [diet]
full strength
function study
functional shortening
simple fracture
FSA —
fetal sialoglycoprotein antigen
fetal sulfoglycoprotein antigen
f.s.a. — *fiat secundum artem* (Lat.)
let it be made skillfully
f.s.a.r. — *fiat secundum artem reglas*
(Lat.) let it be made ac-
cording to the rules of the art
FSB —
fetal scalp blood
Fokes sentence builder
full spine blood

FSBA — fluorosulfonyl-
    benzoyladenosine
FSBG — finger-stick blood gas
FSBM — full-strength breast milk
FSBP — finger systolic blood pres-
    sure
FSBT — Fowler single breath test
FSC —
    Food Standards Committee
    Forer Sentence Completion
        [test]
    fracture simple and commi-
        nuted
    fracture simple and complete
    free secretory component
    free-standing clinic
FSCC — fracture simple, com-
    plete, and comminuted
FSD —
    focal skin distance
    fracture simple and depressed
    full-scale deflection
FSE —
    fetal scalp electrode
    filtered smoke exposure
FSF — fibrin stabilizing factor
FSG —
    fasting serum glucose
    focal and segmental glomeru-
        losclerosis
FSGA — full-term, small for gesta-
    tional age
FSGHS — focal segmental glomer-
    ular hyalinosis and sclerosis
FSGN — focal sclerosing glomeru-
    lonephritis
FSGO — floating spherical
    gaussian orbital
FSGS — focal segmental glomeru-
    losclerosis
FSH —
    fascioscapulohumeral
    focal and segmental hyalinosis
    follicle-stimulating hormone
FSHB — follicle-stimulating hor-
    mone, beta chain
FSHD — facioscapulohumeral dys-
    trophy

FSH/LH-RH — follicle-stimulating
    hormone and luteinizing hor-
    mone–releasing hormone
FSHMD — facioscapulohumeral
    muscular dystrophy
FSH-RF — follicle-stimulating hor-
    mone–releasing factor
FSH-RH — follicle-stimulating
    hormone–releasing hormone
FSI —
    foam stability index
    Food Sanitation Institute
    Function Status Index
FSIA — foot shock–induced anal-
    gesia
FSIQ — Full-Scale Intelligence
    Quotient
FSL —
    fasting serum level
    fixed slit light
FSM — furosemide
FSMB — Federation of State Medi-
    cal Boards
F-SM/C — fungus, smear, and cul-
    ture
FSP —
    familial spastic paraplegia
    fibrin split products
    fibrinogen split products
    fibrinolytic split products
    fine suspended particles
    free secretory piece
f. sp. — forma specialis (Lat.) spe-
    cial form
FSQ — Functional Status Ques-
    tionnaire
FSR —
    Fellow of the Society of Ra-
        diographers
    film screen radiography
    fragmented sarcoplasmic retic-
        ulum
    fusiform skin revision
FSR-3 — isoniazid
FSS —
    Familiar Sensory Stimulation
    Fear Survey Schedule
    focal segmental sclerosis

FSS — (*continued*)
    Freeman-Sheldon syndrome
    French steel sound
    front support strap
    full-scale score
    functional systems scale
FST — foam stability test
FSU —
    Family Service Unit
    functional spine unit
FSV — feline fibrosarcoma virus
FSW — Field Service Worker
FT —
    false transmitter
    family therapy
    fast twitch
    feeding tube
    ferritin
    ferromagnetic tamponade
    fetal tonsil
    fibrous tissue
    finger tapping
    fingertip
    follow through
    formol toxoid
    Fourier transform
    free testosterone
    free thyroxine
    full-term
    functional test
FT_3 — free triiodothyronine
FT_4 — free thyroxine [unbound]
F_t — ferritin
fT — free testosterone
ft —
    feet
    foot
ft. — *fiat* or *fiant* (Lat.) let there be made
FTA —
    fluorescein treponema
    fluorescent titer antibody
    fluorescent treponemal antibody
FTA-ABS — fluorescent treponemal antibody absorption [test]
FTAG — fast-binding target-attaching globulin

FTAT — fluorescent treponemal antibody test
FTB — fingertip blood
FTBD —
    fit to be detained
    full-term born dead
FTBE — focal tick-borne encephalitis
FTBS — Family Therapist Behavioral Scale
FTC —
    Federal Trade Commission
    frames to come [optometry]
    frequency threshold curve
ft-c — foot-candle
ft. cataplasm — *fiat cataplasma* (Lat.) let a poultice be made
ft. cerat. — *fiat ceratum* (Lat.) let a cerate be made
ft. chart. vi — *fiant chartulae vi* (Lat.) let six powders be made
ft. collyr. — *fiat collyrium* (Lat.) let an eyewash be made
FTD —
    failure to descend
    femoral total density
FTE — full-time equivalent
ft. emuls. — *fiat emulsio* (Lat.) let an emulsion be made
ft. enem. — *fiat enema* (Lat.) let an enema be made
FTF —
    finger-to-finger [test]
    free thyroxine fraction
FTFTN — finger-to-finger-to-nose [test]
FTG — full-thickness graft
ft. garg. — *fiat gargarisma* (Lat.) let a gargle be made
FTH — ferritin heavy chain
FTI — free thyroxine index
FT_3I — free triiodothyronine index
FT_4F — serum free thyroxine fraction
FT_4I — free thyroxine index
ft. infus. — *fiat infusum* (Lat.) let an infusion be made

ft. inject. — *fiat injectio* (Lat.) let an injection be made

FTIR — functional terminal innervation ratio

FTKA — failed to keep appointment

FTL — ferritin light chain

ftL — foot lambert

FTLB — full-term birth

ft-lb — foot-pound

FTLFC — full-term living female child

ft. linim. — *fiat linimentum* (Lat.) let a liniment be made

FTLMC — full-term living male child

FTLV — feline T-lymphotropic lentivirus

FTM —
fluid thioglycollate medium
fractional test meal

ft. mass. — *fiat massa* (Lat.) let a mass be made

ft. mas. div. in. pil. — *fiat massa dividenda in pilulae* (Lat.) let a mass be made, to be divided into pills

ft. mist. — *fiat mistura* (Lat.) let a mixture be made

FTN —
finger to nose [test]
full-term nursery

FTNB — full-term newborn

FTND — full-term normal delivery

FTNS — functional transcutaneous nerve stimulation

FTNSD — full-term normal spontaneous delivery

FTO — fructose-terminated oligosaccharide

F to N — finger-to-nose

FTP — failure to progress

FTPA — perfluorotripropylamine

ft. pil. — *fiant pilulae* (Lat.) let pills be made

ft. pulv. — *fiat pulvis* (Lat.) let a powder be made

FTR —
for the record

FTR — (*continued*)
fractional tubular reabsorption
fractional turnover rate

FTS —
facteur thymique sérique (Fr.) serum thymic factor
Family Tracking System
Feminizing testis syndrome
fetal tobacco syndrome
fingertips
fissured tongue syndrome
flexote synovitis
fractional turnover rate

FTSG — full-thickness skin graft

ft. solut. — *fiat solutio* (Lat.) let a solution be made

ft. suppos. — *fiat suppositorium* (Lat.) let a suppository be made

FTT —
failure to thrive
fat tolerance test
Fever Therapy Technician
fixed tissue turnover
fraternal twins raised together
fructose tolerance test

ft. troch. — *fiat trochisci* (Lat.) let lozenges be made

FTU — fluorescence thiourea

ft. ung. — *fiat unguentum* (Lat.) let an ointment be made

FTX — field training exercise

FU —
fecal urobilinogen
fetal urobilinogen
fluorouracil
follow-up
fractional urinalysis
fundus

F/U —
follow-up
fundus of umbilicus

F&U — flanks and upper quadrants

F ↑ U — fingers above umbilicus

F ↓ U — fingers below umbilicus

Fu — Finsen unit

5-FU — 5-fluorouracil

FUB — functional uterine bleeding
FUC — fucosidase
Fuc — fucose
FU$_{co}$ — functional uptake of carbon monoxide
FUDR, FUdR —
    floxuridine
    5-fluorouracildeoxyribonucleoside
FUE — fever of unknown etiology
FUFA — free volatile fatty acid
fulg. — fulguration
FUM —
    5-fluorouracil and methotrexate
    fumarase
    fumarate
    fumigation
FUMP — fluorouridine monophosphate
FUN — follow-up note
funct —
    function
    functional
FUNG-C — fungus culture
FUNG-S — fungus smear
FUO —
    fever of undetermined origin
    fever of unknown origin
FUOV — follow-up office visit
fu p — fusion point
FUR —
    fluorouracil riboside
    fluorouridine
    furosemide
FUS —
    feline urologic syndrome
    first-use syndrome
    fusion
FUT — fibrinogen uptake test
FUTP — fluorouridine triphosphate
FV —
    Fahr-Vochard [disease]
    femoral vein
    flow velocity
    flow volume

FV — (continued)
    fluid volume
    formaldehyde vapors
    Friend virus
FVA — Friend virus anemia
FVC —
    false vocal cord
    filled voiding flow rate
    forced vital capacity
FVD — fibrovascular tissue on disk
FVE — forced volume expiration
FVFR — filled voiding flow rate
FVH — focal vascular headache
FVIC — forced inspiratory vital capacity
FVL —
    femoral vein ligation
    flow volume loop
fvl — force, velocity, length
FVM — familial visceral myopathy
FVOP — finger venous opening pressure
FVP — Friend virus polycythemia
FVR —
    feline viral rhinotracheitis
    forearm vascular resistance
FVS — fetal valproate syndrome
f. vs. — *fiat venaesectio* (Lat.) let the patient be bled
FW —
    Falconer-Weddell [syndrome]
    Felix-Weil [reaction]
    Folin-Wu [method]
    forced whisper
    fracturing wall
    fragment wound
Fw — F wave
fw — fresh water
FWA — Family Welfare Association
FWB — full weight bearing
FWHM — full width at half maximum
FWM — Folin-Wu method
FWPCA — Federal Water Pollution Control Administration
FWR — Felix-Weil reaction

FWW — front wheel walker
FX —
   Factor X
   fluoroscopy
   fornix
   fractional
   fracture
   frozen section
Fx —
   fracture
   fractional urine
   friction
FxBB — fracture of both bones
Fx-dis — fracture-dislocation
FXN — function
FXR — fracture
FXS — fragile X syndrome
FY —
   fiscal year
   framycetin
   full year

FYA — Duffy A positive [blood type]
FYAN — Duffy A negative [blood type]
FYB — Duffy B positive [blood type]
FYBN — Duffy B negative [blood type]
FYI — for your information
F-Y test — fibrinogen qualitative test
FZ —
   focal zone
   frozen section
   furazolidone
Fz — frontal midline placement of electrodes in electroencephalography
FZRC — frozen red blood cells
FZS — Fellow of the Zoological Society

G

G —
   acceleration [force]
   conductance
   G force [pull of gravity]
   gallop
   ganglion
   gap
   gas
   gastrin
   gauge
   gauss
   geometric efficiency
   Gibbs free energy
   giga-
   gingiva
   gingival
   glabella
   globular
   globulin
   glucose
   glycine

G — (continued)
   glycogen
   goat
   gold inlay
   gonidial [colony]
   good
   goose
   grade
   Gräfenberg spot
   gram
   gravida
   gravitational constant
   gravity
   Greek
   green
   gross
   guanidine
   guanine
   guanosine
   gynecology
   unit of force of acceleration

G⁻ — gram-negative
G⁺ — gram-positive
G₀ — quiescent phase of cells leaving the mitotic cycle
G₁ — presynthetic gap [phase of cells prior to DNA synthesis]
G₂ — postsynthetic gap [phase of cells following DNA synthesis]
G₄ — dichlorophen
G₁₁ — hexachlorophene
GI — primigravida
GII — secundigravida
GIII — tertigravida
G⁰ — standard free energy
g —
    gender
    grain
    gram
    gravida
    gravity
    group
    ratio of magnetic moment of a particle to the Bohr magneton
    relative centrifugal force
g — standard acceleration due to gravity, 9.80665 m/s²
g% — gram percent
γ —
    a carbon separated from the carboxyl group by two other carbon atoms
    a constituent of the protein plasma fraction
    gamma (third letter of the Greek alphabet), lowercase
    heavy chain of immunoglobulins
    a monomer in fetal hemoglobin
    photon
GA —
    airway conductance
    Gamblers Anonymous
    gastric analysis
    gastric antrum
    general anesthesia

GA — (continued)
    general appearance
    gentisic acid
    gestational age
    ginger ale
    gingivoaxial
    glucoamylase
    glucose
    glucose/acetone
    glucuronic acid
    Golgi apparatus
    gramicidin A
    granulocyte adherence
    granuloma annulare
    guessed average
    gut-associated
    gyrate atrophy
G/A — globulin/albumin [ratio]
Ga —
    airway conductance
    gallium
    granulocyte agglutination
ga — gauge
GAA — gossypol acetic acid
GAAS — Goldberg Anorectic Attituder S
GABA — gamma-aminobutyric acid
GABAT — gamma-aminobutyric acid transaminase
GABHS — group A beta-hemolytic streptococcus
GABI — German Angioplasty Bypass Surgery Investigation
GABOA — gamma-amino-beta-hydroxybutyric acid
GABS — group A beta-hemolytic streptococcus
GAD —
    generalized anxiety disorder
    glutamic acid decarboxylase
GADH — gastric alcohol dehydrogenase
GADS — gonococcal arthritis/dermatitis syndrome
GAF —
    giant axon formation
    global assessment of functioning

GAG —
   glycosaminoglycan
   group-specific antigen gene
GAHS — galactorrhea-amenorrhea
   hyperprolactinemia syndrome
GAI — guided affective imagery
GAIPAS — General Audit Inpatient Psychiatric Assessment
   Scale
GAL —
   galactosemia
   galactosyl
   gallus adeno-like [virus]
   glucuronic acid lactone
gal —
   galactose
   gallon
G-ALB — globulin-albumin
GalC — galactocerebroside
GALK — galactokinase
gal/min — gallons per minute
GalN — galactosamine
GalNAc — N-acetylgalactosamine
gal-1-P — galactose-1-phosphate
GALT —
   galactose-1-phosphate-uridyl
      transferase
   gut-associated lymphoid tissue
GAL TT — galactose tolerance
   test
GaLV — gibbon ape lymphosarcoma virus
galv. —
   galvanic
   galvanized
GAMG — goat antimouse immunoglobulin G
gamma HCD — gamma heavy
   chain disease
GAN — giant axonal neuropathy
G and D — growth and development
gang — ganglion
gangl — ganglionic
GANS — granulomatous angiitis
   of the nervous system
GAP —
   Gardner Analysis of Personality

GAP — (continued)
   D-glyceraldehyde-3-phosphate
   Group for the Advancement
      of Psychiatry
   guanosine triphosphate acti-
      vating protein
GAPD — glyceraldehyde-3-
   phosphate dehydrogenase
GAPDH — reduced glyceralde-
   hyde-phosphate dehydrogenase
GAPO — growth retardation, alopecia, pseudoanodontia, and
   optic atrophy [syndrome]
GAR —
   genitoanorectal [syndrome]
   goat antirabbit [gamma globu-
      lin]
garg. — gargarisma (Lat.) gargle
GARP — Global Atmospheric Research Program
GARS — glycine amide phosphoribosyl synthetase
GAS —
   galactorrhea-amenorrhea syn-
      drome
   gastric acid secretion
   gastroenterology
   general adaptation syndrome
   generalized arteriosclerosis
   Glasgow Assessment Scale
   Global Assessment Score
   group A streptococcus
GASA — growth-adjusted sono-
   graphic age
GasAnal F&T — gastric analysis,
   free and total
GAST — gastric
GASTRN — gastrin
gastro —
   gastroenterology
   gastrointestinal
gastroc — gastrocnemius [muscle]
GAT —
   gas antitoxin
   gelatin agglutination test
   Gerontological Apperception
   Test

GAT — *(continued)*
    group adjustment therapy
GATase —
    6-alkyl guanine
    alkyl transferase
GATB — General Aptitude Test
    Battery
GAU — geriatric assessment unit
gav — gavage
GAW — airway conductance
GAZT — glucuronide derivative of
    azidothymidine
GB —
    gallbladder
    Gilbert-Behçet [syndrome]
    glial bundle
    goofball
    Gougerot-Blum [syndrome]
    Guillain-Barré [syndrome]
Gb — gilbert
GBA —
    ganglionic blocking agent
    gingivobuccoaxial
G banding — Giemsa banding
    [stain]
GBBHS — group B beta-hemo-
    cytic streptococcus
GBCE — Grassi Basic Cognitive
    Evaluation
GBD —
    gallbladder disease
    gender behavior disorder
    glassblower's disease
    granulomatous bowel disease
GBE — *Ginkgo biloba* extract
GBG —
    glycine-rich beta-glycoprotein
    gonadal steroid-binding globu-
    lin
GBGase — glycine-rich beta-glyco-
    proteinase
GBH —
    gamma-benzene hexachloride
    graphite, benzalkonium, hepa-
    rin
GBHA — glyoxal-*bis*-(2-
    hydroxyanil)
GBI — globulin-binding insulin

GBIA — Guthrie bacterial inhibi-
    tion assay
GBL —
    gamma-butyrolactone
    glomerular basal lamina
GBM —
    glioblastoma multiforme
    glomerular basement mem-
    brane
GBP —
    galactose-binding protein
    gastric bypass
    gated blood pool
GBPS — gallbladder pigment
    stones
GBq — gigabequerel
GBS —
    gallbladder series
    gastric bypass surgery
    glycerine-buffered saline [solu-
    tion]
    group B (beta-hemolytic)
    streptococcus
    Guillain-Barré syndrome
GBSS —
    Gey's balanced saline solution
    Guillain-Barré-Strohl syn-
    drome
GC —
    ganglion cell
    gas chromatography
    gel chromatography
    general circulation
    general closure
    general condition
    geriatric care
    geriatric chair
    germinal center
    glucocorticoid
    glycocholate
    goblet cell
    Golgi cell
    gonococcal
    gonococcus
    gonorrhea
    gonorrhea culture
    good condition
    Gougerot-Carteaud [syn-
    drome]

GC — (continued)
　　granular cast
　　granular cyst
　　granule cell
　　granulocyte cytotoxic
　　granulomatous colitis
　　granulosa cell
　　group-specific component
　　guanine cytosine
　　guanylcyclase
G^-C — gram-negative cocci
G^+C — gram-positive cocci
Gc —
　　gigacycle
　　gonococcus
　　group-specific component
GCA —
　　gastric cancer area
　　giant cell arteritis
g-cal — gram-calorie
GCB — gonococcal base
GCBM — glomerular capillary
　　basement
GCDFP — gross cystic disease fluid
　　protein
GCDP — gross cystic disease pro-
　　gram
GCF —
　　greatest common factor
　　growth-rate-controlling factor
GCFT — gonorrhea complement
　　fixation test
GCI — General Cognitive Index
GCIIS — glucose controlled insu-
　　lin infusion system
GCLO — gastric Campylobacter-
　　like organism
GCM — good control maintained
g-cm — gram-centimeter
GC-MS — gas chromatography–
　　mass spectrometry
GCN — giant cerebral neuron
g-coef — generalizability coeffi-
　　cient
GCR —
　　glucocorticoid receptor
　　Group Conformity Rating
GCRC — General Clinical Re-
　　search Centers

GCRS — gynecological chylous re-
　　flux syndrome
GCS —
　　general clinical service
　　Generalized Contentment
　　　Scale
　　Gianotti-Crosti syndrome
　　Glasgow Coma Scale
　　glucocorticosteroid
　　glutamylcysteine synthetase
Gc/s — gigacycles per second
GCSA — Gross cell surface anti-
　　gen
GCSF — granulocyte cell-stimulat-
　　ing factor
G-CSF — granulocyte colony–
　　stimulating factor
GCT —
　　general care and treatment
　　giant cell thyroiditis
　　giant cell tumor
GC type — guanine, cytosine type
GC(T)A — giant cell (temporal)
　　arteritis
GCU — gonococcal urethritis
GCV — great cardiac vein
GCVF — great cardiac vein flow
GCW — glomerular capillary wall
GCWM — General Conference
　　on Weights and Measures
GCY — gastroscopy
GD —
　　gastroduodenal
　　general diagnostics
　　general dispensary
　　gestational day
　　Gianotti's disease
　　gonadal dysgenesis
　　Graves' disease
　　growth and development
G&D — growth and development
Gd — gadolinium
GDA —
　　gastroduodenal artery
　　germine diacetate
GDB —
　　gas density balance
　　Guide Dogs for the Blind

GDC —
    General Dental Council
    giant dopamine-containing
      cell
    Guglielmi detachable coil
GDD — gay disaster disease
Gd-DTPA — gadolinium diethyl-
    enetriaminepentaacetic acid
GDF — gel diffusion precipitin
GDH —
    glucose dehydrogenase
    glutamate dehydrogenase
    glutamic acid dehydrogenase
    glycerophosphate dehydro-
      genase
    glycol dehydrogenase
    gonadotropin hormone
    growth and differential hor-
      mone
GDID — genetically determined
    immunodeficiency disease
g/dl — grams per deciliter
GDM — gestational diabetes melli-
    tus
GDMO — General Duties Medical
    Officer
gdn — guardian
GDNF — glial cell line–derived
    neurotrophic factor
GDP —
    gastroduodenal pylorus
    gel diffusion precipitin
    guanosine diphosphate
GDS —
    Gesell developmental sched-
      ule
    Global Deterioration Scale
    Gordon Diagnostic System
      [for attention disorders]
    gradual dosage schedule
GDT — gel development time
GDW — glass-distilled water
GDXY — XY gonadal dysgenesis
GE —
    gainfully employed
    Gänsslen-Erb [syndrome]
    gastric emptying
    gastroemotional

GE — (continued)
    gastroenteritis
    gastroenterology
    gastroenterostomy
    gastroesophageal
    gastrointestinal endoscopy
    gel electrophoresis
    generalized epilepsy
    generator of excitation
    gentamicin
    glandular epithelium
G/E — granulocyte-erythroid (ra-
    tio)
Ge —
    Gerbich red cell antigen
    germanium
g-e — gravity eliminated
GEC —
    galactose elimination capacity
    glomerular epithelial cell
GECC — Government Employee's
    Clinic Centre
GEE — glycine ethyl ester
GEF —
    gastroesophageal fundoplica-
      tion
    glossoepiglottic fold
    gonadotropin-enhancing fac-
      tor
GEFT — Group Embedded Figures
    Test
GEH — glycerol ester hydrolase
GEJ — gastroesophageal junction
gel. — gelatin
gel. quav. — *gelatina quavis* (Lat.)
    in any kind of jelly
GEMS — good emergency mother
    substitute
GEN —
    gender
    generation
    genetics
    genital
    genealogy
gen. —
    general
    genus
GEN-ENDO — general anesthesia
    with endotracheal intubation

genet —
>   genetic
>   genetics
GENETOX — Genetic Toxicology [data base]
gen. et sp. nov. — *genus et species nova* (Lat.) new genus and species
genit —
>   genital
>   genitalia
gen. nov. — *genus novum* (Lat.) new genus
GENOVA — generalized analysis of variance
gen proc — general procedure
GENPS — genital neoplasm-papilloma syndrome
GENT — gentamicin
GENTA/P — gentamicin peak
GENTA/T — gentamicin trough
GEP — gastroenteropancreatic
GEPG — gastroesophageal pressure gradient
GER —
>   gastroesophageal reflux
>   geriatrics
>   German
>   granular endoplasmic reticulum
Ger —
>   geriatric(s)
>   German
GERD — gastroesophageal reflux disease
geriat — geriatrics
GERL — Golgi-associated endoplasmic reticulum lysosome
Geront —
>   gerontologic
>   gerontologist
>   gerontology
GES —
>   glucose-electrolyte solution
>   Group Environment Scale
GEST — gestation
GET —
>   gastric emptying time

GET — *(continued)*
>   general endotracheal [anesthesia]
>   graded treadmill exercise test
GET½ — gastric emptying half-time
GETA — general endotrachael anesthesia
GEU — gestation extrauterine
GeV — giga electron volt
GEWS — Gianturco expandable wire stent
GEX — gas exchange
GF —
>   gastric fistula
>   gastric fluid
>   germ-free
>   glass factor
>   globule fibril
>   glomerular filtrate
>   glomerular filtration
>   gluten-free
>   grandfather
>   griseofulvin
>   growth factor
>   growth failure
>   growth fraction
gf — gram-force
G-F — globular-fibrous
GFA —
>   glial fibrillary acidic [protein]
>   global force applicator
G factor — general factor
GFAP — glial fibrillary acidic protein
GFD —
>   gluten-free diet
>   Goodenough Figure Drawing
GFFS — glycogen and fat-free solid
GFH — glucose-free Hanks [solution]
GFI —
>   glucagon-free insulin
>   ground-fault interrupter
GFL — giant follicular lymphoma
GFM — good fetal movement
G forces — acceleration forces

GFP —
> gamma-fetoprotein
> gel-filtered platelet
> glomerular-filtered phosphate

GFR —
> glomerular filtration rate
> grunting, flaring, and retracting

GFS —
> global focal sclerosis
> guaifenesin

GFTA — Goldman-Fristoe Test of Articulation

G-F-W Battery — Goldman-Fristoe-Woodcock Auditory Skills Test Battery

GG —
> gamma globulin
> genioglossus
> glyceryl guaiacolate
> glycylglycine
> guar gum

GGA — general gonadotropic activity

GGCS — gamma-glutamyl cysteine synthetase

GGCT — ground glass clotting time

GGE —
> generalized glandular enlargement
> gradient gel electrophoresis

GGFC — gamma globulin–free calf [serum]

GGG — glycine-rich gamma-glycoprotein

g.g.g. — *gummi guttae gambiae* (Lat.) gamboge

GGM — glucose-galactose malabsorption

GG or S — glands, goiter, or stiffness

GGPNA — gamma-glutamyl-*p*-nitroanilide

GGT — gamma-glutamyl-transferase

GGTP — gamma-glutamyl-transpeptidase

GGVB — gelatin, glucose, and veronal buffer

GH —
> Gee-Herter [disease]
> general health
> general hospital
> genetic hypertension
> genetically hypertensive [rat]
> geniohyoid
> Gilford-Hutchinson [syndrome]
> glenohumeral [joint]
> good health
> growth hormone

GHA —
> glucoheptanoic acid
> Group Health Association

GHAA — Group Health Association of America

GHB — gamma hydroxybutyrate

GHb — glycosylated hemoglobin

GHBA — gamma-hydroxybutyric acid

GHD — growth hormone deficiency

GHDT — Goodenough-Harris Drawing Test

GHK — Goldman-Hodgkin-Katz [equation]

GHPP — Genetically Handicapped Persons Program

GHPQ — General Health Perception Questionnaire

GHQ — General Health Questionnaire

GHR — granulomatous hypersensitivity reaction

GH-RF — growth hormone-releasing factor

GH-RH — growth hormone releasing hormone

GH-RIF — growth hormone-release-inhibiting factor

GH-RIH — growth hormone release–inhibiting hormone

GHV — goose hepatitis virus

GHz — gigahertz

GI —
> gastrointestinal

GI — (continued)
    gelatin infusion [medium]
    gingival index
    globin insulin
    glomerular index
    glucose intolerance
    granuloma inguinale
    gravida I
    growth-inhibiting
    growth inhibition
Gi — good impression
gi — gill
GIA — gastrointestinal anastomosis
GIB —
    gastric ileal bypass
    gastrointestinal bleeding
GIBF — gastrointestinal bacterial flora
GIC —
    gastric interdigestive contraction
    general immunocompetence
GICA —
    gastrointestinal cancer
    gastrointestinal cancer antigen
GID — gender identity disorder
GIDA — Gastrointestinal Diagnostic Area
GIF —
    gonadotropin-inhibitory factor
    growth hormone–inhibiting factor
GIFT —
    gamete intrafallopian transfer
    granulocyte immunofluorescence test
GIGO — garbage in, garbage out
GIH —
    gastric inhibitory hormone
    gastrointestinal hemorrhage
    growth-inhibiting hormone
GII —
    gastrointestinal infection
    gravida II
GIII — gravida III
GIK — glucose, insulin, and potassium [solution]

GIM — gonadotropin-inhibitory material
ging. — gingiva (Lat.) gum
g-ion — gram-ion
GIP —
    gastric inhibitory peptide
    gastric inhibitory polypeptide
    giant cell interstitial pneumonia
    giant cell interstitial pneumonitis
    glucose-dependent insulinotropic polypeptide
    glucose-dependent insulin-releasing peptide
    gonorrheal invasive peritonitis
GIR — global improvement rating
GIS —
    gas in stomach
    gastrointestinal series
    gastrointestinal system
    Gender Identity Service
GIT —
    gastrointestinal tract
    glutathione-insulin transhydrogenase
GITS — gastrointestinal therapeutic system
GITSG — Gastrointestinal Tumor Study Group
GITT —
    gastrointestinal transit time
    glucose-insulin tolerance test
GIV — gastrointestinal virus
GiV — gigavolt
GIWU — gastrointestinal work-up
GJ —
    gap junction
    gastric juice
    gastrojejunostomy
GJA-S — gastric juice aspiration syndrome
GK —
    galactokinase
    Gasser-Karrer [syndrome]
    glomerulocystic kidney
    glycerol kinase

GKA — guinea pig keratocyte

GKD — glycerol kinase deficiency

GKMDT — Graham-Kendall Memory for Designs Test

GL —
gastric lavage
Gilbert-Lereboullet [syndrome]
gland
glomerular layer
glycolipid
glycosphingolipid
glycyrrhiza
granular layer
greatest length
gustatory lacrimation

GL 54 — athomin

Gl —
beryllium (Lat., *glucinium*)
glabella

gl — gill

gl. — *glandula(e)* (Lat.) gland, glands

g/l — grams per liter

GLA —
alpha-galactosidase
gamma-linolenic acid
giant left atrium
gingivolinguoaxial
glucaric acid

glac — glacial

GLAD — gold-labeled antigen detection

GLAT — glutamic acid, lysine, alanine, and tyrosine

glau — glaucoma

GLC — gas-liquid chromatography

Glc — glucose

glc — glaucoma

GlcA — gluconic acid

GLC-MS — gas-liquid chromatography-mass spectrometry

GlcN — glucosamine

GlcNAc — *N*-acetylglucosamine

GlcUA — D-glucuronic acid

GLD —
globoid leukodystrophy
glutamate dehydrogenase

GLDH — glutamic dehydrogenase

GLH —
germinal layer hemorrhage
giant lymph node hyperplasia

GLI —
glicentin
glucagon-like immunoreactivity

GLIM — generalized linear interactive model

glio — glioma

GLL — glabellolambda line

GLM — general linear model

Gln —
glucagon
glutamine

GLNH — giant lymph node hyperplasia

GLNS — gay lymph node syndrome

GLO — glyoxalase

GLO1 — glyoxalase 1

glob —
globular
globulin

GLP —
Gambro Liendia Plate
glucose-L-phosphate
glycolipoprotein
good laboratory practice
group-living program

GL-PP — postprandial glucose

GLR — graphic level recorder

GLS —
generalized lymphadenopathy syndrome
guinea pig lung strip

GLTN — glomerulotubulonephritis

GLTT — glucose-lactate tolerance test

GLU —
glucose
glucuronidase
glutamic acid

Glu —
glucose
glucuronidase
glutamate

Glu — *(continued)*
  glutamic acid
  glutamine
GLuA — glucuronic acid
GLU-5 — five-hour glucose tolerance test
GLUC — glucosidase
Gluc — glucose
GLUC-S — urine glucose spot [test]
glucur — glucuronide
GLUD — glutamate dehydrogenase
glu ox — glucose oxidase
glut — glucose transporter
GLUTAM — glutamine
GLV — Gross leukemia virus
Glx — glutamic acid
Gly —
  glycerol
  glycine
  glycyl
glyc —
  glyceride
  glycerin
  glycerol
glyc. — *glyceritum* (Lat.) glycerite
GM —
  gastric mucosa
  Geiger-Müller [counter]
  general medical
  general medicine
  genetic manipulation
  genetic marker [monosialoganglioside]
  geometric mean
  giant melanosome
  grand mal [epilepsy]
  grandmother
  grand multiparity
  granulocyte-macrophage
  granulocyte-monocyte
  growth medium
G/M — granulocyte-macrophage
G-M — Geiger-Müller [counter]
GM$^+$ — gram-positive
GM$^-$ — gram-negative

Gm —
  an allotype marker on the heavy chains of immunoglobulins
  gamma
Gm% — gram percent
gm — gram
g-m — gram-meter
g/m — gallons per minute
GMA —
  glyceryl methacrylate
  glycol methacrylate
  gross motor activity
GMB —
  gastric mucosal barrier
  granulomembranous body
GMBF — gastric mucosal blood flow
GMC —
  general medical clinic
  General Medical Council (British)
  grivet monkey cell
gm cal — gram calorie
gm/cc — grams per cubic centimeter
GMCD — grand mal convulsive disorder
GM-CFU — granulocyte-macrophage colony-forming unit
GM-CSA — granulocyte-macrophage colony-stimulating activity
GM-CSF — granulocyte-macrophage colony-stimulating factor
GMD —
  geometric mean diameter
  glycopeptide moiety (modified) derivative
GME — graduate medical evaluation
GMENAC — Graduate Medical Education National Advisory Committee
GMEPP — giant miniature end-plate potential

GMH — germinal matrix hemorrhage
GMK — green monkey kidney
[cells]
GML —
glabellomeatal line
gut mucosal lymphocyte
gm/L — grams per liter
g/ml — grams per milliliter
GMM — Goldberg-Maxwell-
Morris [syndrome]
gm-m — gram-meter
GMO — General Medical Officer
g-mol — gram-molecule
GMP —
glucose monophosphate
guanosine-5-phosphate
guanosine monophosphate
G-MP — G-myeloma protein
3',5'-GMP — cyclic guanosine
monophosphate
GMR — gallops, murmurs, rubs
GMS —
General Medical Services
Gilbert-Meulengracht syn-
drome
glyceryl monostearate
Gomori's methenamine silver
[stain]
GM&S —
general medical and surgical
general medicine and surgery
GMSC — General Medical Services Committee
GMT —
geometric mean titer
gingival margin trimmer
Greenwich Mean Time
GMV — gram-molecular volume
GMW — gram-molecular weight
GN —
Gandy-Nanta [disease]
gaze nystagmus
glomerulonephritis
glucagon
glucose nitrogen [ratio]
gnotobiote
Graduate Nurse

GN — (continued)
gram-negative
G/N — glucose/nitrogen [ratio]
Gn. —
gnathion
gonadotropin
GNA — general nursing assistance
GNB —
ganglioneuroblastoma
gram-negative bacillus
GNBM — gram-negative bacillary
meningitis
GNC —
general nursing care
General Nursing Council
glandular neck cell
GNCA — gastric noncancerous
area
GND — gram-negative diplococ-
cus
GNID — gram-negative intracellu-
lar diplococci
GNP — Gerontologic Nurse Prac-
titioner
GNR — gram-negative rods
GnRF — gonadotropin-releasing
factor
GnRH — gonadotropin-releasing
hormone
GNS — gerontologic nurse-special-
ist
G/NS — glucose in normal saline
[solution]
GNTP — Graduate Nurse Transi-
tion Program
GO —
glucose oxidase
gonorrhea
Gordan-Overstreet [syndrome]
G&O — gas and oxygen
Go —
Golgi
gonion
GOAT — Galveston Orientation
and Amnesia Test
GOBAB — gamma-hydroxy-beta-
aminobutyric acid
GOD —
generation of diversity

GOD — (*continued*)
  glucose oxidase
GOE — gas, oxygen, and ether
GOG — Gynecologic Oncology
  Group
GOH — geroderma osteodysplas-
  tica hereditaria
GOL — glabello-opisthion line
GΩ — gigohm
GON — gonococcal ophthalmia
  neonatorum
GOND — glaucomatous optic
  nerve damage
Gonio —
  goniometric
  gonioscopy
GOO — gastric outlet obstruction
GOQ — glucose oxidation quotient
GOR —
  gastroesophageal reflux
  general operating room
GORT —
  Gilmore Oral Reading Test
  Gray Oral Reading Test
GOS — Glasgow Outcome Scale
GOT —
  aspartate aminotransferase
  glucose oxidase test
  glutamic-oxaloacetic transam-
    inase
  glutamine-oxaloacetic trans-
    aminase
  goal of treatment
GOTM — glutamic-oxaloacetic
  transaminase, mitochondrial
GOT-S — glutamic-oxaloacetic
  transaminase, soluble
GP —
  gangliocytic paraganglioma
  gastroplasty
  general paralysis
  general paresis
  general practice
  general practitioner
  general proprioception
  general purpose
  genetic prediabetes

GP — (*continued*)
  geometric progression
  globus pallidus
  glucose-6-phosphate
  glucose production
  glutathione peroxidase
  glycerophosphate
  glycopeptide
  glycoprotein
  Goodpasture's [syndrome]
  gram-positive
  group
  guinea pig
  gutta percha
G/P — gravida/para
G-1-P — glucose-1-phosphate
G3P —
  glyceraldehyde-3-phosphate
  glycerol-3-phosphate
G6PD — glucose-6-phosphate dehydrogenase
gp —
  gene product
  glycoprotein
  group
GPA —
  glutaraldehyde, pieric acid
  Goodpasture's antigen
  grade-point average
  gravida, para, abortus
  Group Practice Association
  guinea pig albumin
GP-A — glycophorin-A
GPAIS — guinea pig anti-insulin
  serum
G-6-Pase — glucose-6-phosphatase
GPB — glossopharyngeal breathing
GPBP — guinea pig myelin basic
  protein
GPC —
  gastric parietal cell
  gel permeation chromatogra-
    phy
  giant papillary conjunctivitis
  glycerylphosphorylcholine
  gram-positive cocci
  granular progenitor cell
  guinea pig complement

GP-C — glycophorin-C (glycoconnectin)

GPC/TP — glycerylphosphorylcholine to total phosphate [ratio]

GPD — glucose-6-phosphate dehydrogenase

G3PD — glyceraldehyde-3-phosphate dehydrogenase

G6PD — glucose-6-phosphate dehydrogenase

GPE —
  glycerylphosphorylethanolamine
  guinea pig embryo

GPEP — General Professional Education of the Physician

GPF —
  glomerular plasma flow
  granulocytosis-promoting factor

G6PDA — glucose-6-phosphate dehydrogenase coenzyme variant A

GPGG — guinea pig gamma globulin

GPh — Graduate in Pharmacy

GPHN — giant pigmented hairy nevus

GPHLV — guinea pig herpes-like virus

GPHV — guinea pig herpesvirus

GPI —
  general paralysis of the insane
  Gingival Periodontal Index
  glucose, potassium, and insulin
  glucose phosphate isomerase
  glycoprotein I
  Gordon Personal Inventory
  guinea pig ileum

GpIb — glycoprotein Ib

GPIMH — guinea pig intestinal mucosal homogenate

GPIPID — guinea pig intraperitoneal infectious dose

GPK — guinea pig kidney [antigen]

GPKA — guinea pig kidney absorption [test]

GPLV — guinea pig leukemia virus

Gply — gingivoplasty

GPM —
  general preventive medicine
  giant pigmented melanosome

GPMAL — gravida, para, multiple births, abortions, and live births

GPN — Graduate Practical Nurse

GPP — Gordon Personal Profile

GPPQ — General Purpose Psychiatric Questionnaire

GPR —
  good partial response
  gram-positive rod

GPRA — General Practice Reform Association

GPRBC — guinea pig red blood cell

GPS —
  Goodpasture's syndrome
  gray platelet syndrome
  guinea pig serum
  guinea pig spleen

GPT —
  glutamic-pyruvic transaminase
  guinea pig trachea

GpTh — group therapy

GPTSM — guinea pig tracheal smooth muscle

GPU — guinea pig unit

GPUT — galactose phosphate uridyl transferase

GPx — glutathione peroxidase

GQAP — general question-asking program

GR —
  gamma-ray
  gastric reaction
  gastric resection
  generalized rash
  general research
  glucocorticoid receptor
  glucose response
  glutathione reductase
  good recovery

G⁻R — gram-negative rod
G⁺R — gram-positive rod
gr —
  gamma roentgen
  grade
  graft
  grain
  gram
  gravida
  gravity
  gray
  gross
gr⁻ — gram-negative
gr⁺ — gram-positive
GRA —
  gated radionuclide angiography
  glucocorticoid-remedial aldosteronism
  Gombarts reducing agent
  gonadotropin-releasing agent
GRA⁺ — Gombarts reducing agent-positive
GRABS — group A beta-hemolytic streptococcal pharyngitis
grad —
  gradient
  gradually
  graduate
grad. — *gradatim* (Lat.) by degrees
GRAE — generally regarded as effective
gran —
  granulated
  granule
gran. — *granulatus* (Lat.) granulated
GRAS — generally recognized as safe
GRASS — gradient-recalled acquisition—the steady state
grav —
  gravid
  gravida
  gravity
grav I —
  pregnancy one
  primigravida

grav II — secundigravida—pregnancy two
GRD —
  gastroesophageal reflux disease
  gender role definition
grd — ground
GRE —
  gradient-recalled echo
  Graduate Record Examination
GREAT — Graduate Record Examination Aptitude Test
GRF —
  gastrin-releasing factor
  genetically related macrophage factor
  gonadotropin-releasing factor
  growth hormone-releasing factor
GR-FeSV — Gardner-Rasheed feline sarcoma virus
GRG — glycine-rich glycoprotein
GRH —
  gonadotropin-releasing hormone
  growth hormone-releasing hormone
GRID — gay-related immunodeficiency disease
GRIF — growth hormone release–inhibiting factor
GRL — granular layer
gr. m. p. — *grosso modo pulverisatum* (Lat.) ground in a coarse way
GRN —
  granules
  green
GrN — gram-negative
Grn —
  glycerone
  green
gros. — *grossus* (Lat.) coarse
GRP —
  gastrin-releasing peptide
  glucose-regulated protein
GrP — gram-positive
grp — group

Gr₁P₀AB₁ — gravida one, para none, abortus one (one pregnancy, no births, one abortion)

GRPS — glucose-Ringer-phosphate solution

GRS —
    beta-glucuronidase
    Golabi-Rosen syndrome

GRT —
    gastric residence time
    Graduate Respiratory Therapist

GRW — giant ragweed [test]

gr wt — gross weight

GS —
    gallstone
    Gardner syndrome
    gastric shield
    gastrocnemius soleus
    generalized seizure
    general surgery
    Gilbert's syndrome
    Glanzmann-Saland [syndrome]
    glomerular sclerosis
    glucagon secretion
    glutamine synthetase
    goat serum
    Goldenhar's syndrome
    Goodpasture's syndrome
    graft survival
    Gram stain
    granulocyte substance
    granulocytic sarcoma
    grip strength
    group section
    group-specific
    Guérin-Stern [syndrome]

G6S — glucosamine-6-sulfatase

G/S — glucose and saline

Gs — gauss

gs — group specific

g/s — gallons per second

GSA —
    general somatic afferent
    Gross (sarcoma) virus antigen
    group-specific antigen

GSA — (continued)
    guanidinosuccinic acid

GSB — graduated spinal block

GSBG — gonadal steroid–binding globulin

GSC —
    gas-solid chromatography
    gravity-settling culture

G-SC — guanosine-coupled spleen cell

GSCN — giant serotonin-containing neuron

GSD —
    genetically significant dose
    Gerstmann-Sträussler disease
    glutathione synthetase deficiency
    glycogen storage disease

GSE —
    general somatic efferent
    genital self-examination
    gluten-sensitive enteropathy
    grips strong and equal

GSEH — Governor's Committee on Employment of the Handicapped

GSF —
    galactosemic fibroblast
    genital skin fibroblast

GSH —
    glomerular-stimulating hormone
    golden Syrian hamster
    growth-stimulating hormone
    reduced glutathione

GSHP — reduced glutathione peroxidase

GSH-Px — glutathione synthetase, peroxidase

GSI —
    General Severity Index
    genuine stress incontinence

GSK — glycogen synthetase kinase

GSN — giant serotonin-containing neuron

GSoA — Gerontological Society of America

GSP —
    galvanic skin potential

GSP — (continued)
    general survey panel
    glycogen synthetase phos-
       phate
    glycosylated serum protein
GSPN — greater superficial petro-
    sal neurectomy
GSR —
    galvanic skin reflex
    galvanic skin resistance
    galvanic skin response
    generalized Shwartzman reac-
       tion
    glutathione reductase
GSS —
    gamete-shedding substance
    General Social Survey
    Gerstmann-Sträussler-
       Schenker [syndrome]
GSSG — oxidized glutathione
GSSG-R — glutathione reductase
GSSI — Global Sexual Satisfac-
    tion Index
GSSR — generalized Sanarelli-
    Shwartzman reaction
GST —
    glutathione-S-transferase
    gold salt therapy
    gold sodium thiomalate
    graphic stress telethermome-
       try
    graphic stress thermography
    group striction
GSTM — gold sodium thiomalate
GSW — gunshot wound
GSWA — gunshot wound, abdomi-
    nal
GT —
    gait training
    galactosyl transferase
    Gamow-Teller
    gastrostomy tube
    gastrotomy tube
    Gee-Thaysen [disease]
    generation time
    genetic therapy
    gingiva treatment
    Glanzmann's thrombasthenia

GT — (continued)
    glucagon test
    glucose therapy
    glucose tolerance
    glucose transport
    glucuronyl transferase
    glutamyl transpeptidase
    glycityrosine
    grand total
    granulation tissue
    great toe
    greater trochanter
    group tensions
    group therapy
G&T — gowns and towels
GT1 — glycogenosis type 1
GT1–GT10 — glycogen storage
    disease, types 1 to 10
GT II — galactosyl transferase iso-
    enzyme II
gt. — *gutta* (Lat.) drop
g/t —
    granulation time
    granulation tissue
GTA —
    gene transfer agent
    Glanzmann's thrombasthenia
    glycerol teichoic acid
GTB — gastrointestinal tract
    bleeding
GTCS — generalized tonic-clonic
    seizure
GTD — gestational trophoblastic
    disease
Gt^D — Duarte variant allele
GTF —
    gastrostomy tube feeding
    glucose tolerance factor
GTG — gold thioglucose
GTH — gonadotropic hormone
GTHR — generalized thyroid hor-
    mone resistance
GTII — galactosyl transferase iso-
    enzyme II
GTM — generalized tendomyopa-
    thy
GTN —
    gestational trophoblastic neo-
    plasia

GTN — *(continued)*
    gestational trophoblastic neoplasm
    glomerulotubulonephritis
    glyceryl trinitrate
GTO — Golgi tendon organ
GTP —
    glutamyl transpeptidase
    guanosine triphosphate
GTR —
    galvanic tetanus ratio
    generalized time reflex
    granulocyte turnover rate
GTS —
    Gilles de la Tourette syndrome
    glucose transport system
GTSTD — Grid Test of Schizophrenic Thought Disorder
GTT —
    gelatin-tellurite-taurocholate [agar]
    glucose tolerance test
gtt. — *guttae* (Lat.) drops
GU —
    gastric ulcer
    genitourinary
    glucose uptake
    glycogenic unit
    gonococcal urethritis
    gravitational ulcer
    guanethidine
GUA — group of units of analysis
Gua — guanine
guid — guidance
GUK — guanylate kinase
GULHEMP — general physique, upper extremity, lower extremity, hearing, eyesight, mentality, and personality
Guo — guanosine
GUS —
    genitourinary sphincter
    genitourinary system
Gus — conductance of upstream segment

GUSTO — Global Utilization of Streptokinase and Tissue Plasminogen Activator for Occluded Arteries
gutt. — *gutturi* (Lat.) to the throat
guttat. — *guttatim* (Lat.) drop by drop
gutt. quibusd. — *guttis quibusdam* (Lat.) with a few drops
GV —
    gastric volume
    gentian violet
    germinal vesicle
    gingivectomy
    granulosis virus
    griseoviridan
    Gross virus
GVA — general visceral afferent [nerve]
GVB — gelatin-veronal buffer
GVBD — germinal vesicle breakdown
GVE — general visceral efferent [nerve]
GVF —
    Goldman visual fields
    good visual fields
GVG — gamma-vinyl-gamma-aminobutyric acid
GVH — graft-versus-host [disease or reaction]
GVHD — graft-versus-host disease
GVHR — graft-versus-host reaction
GVL — graft-versus-leukemia [reaction]
Gvy — gingivectomy
GW —
    germ warfare
    gigawatt
    glycerin in water
    gradual withdrawal
    Gray-Wheelwright
    group work
G/W — glucose in water
G & W — glycerin and water
GWA — gunshot wound of the abdomen

GWBS — global ward behavior scale

GWE — glycerol and water enema

GWG — generalized Wegener's granulomatosis

GWT — gunshot wound of the throat

GX — glycinexylidide

GX EKG — graded exercise electrocardiogram

GXP — graded exercise program

GXT — graded exercise test

Gy — gray

GYN —
gynecologic
gynecologist
gynecology

GZ — Guilford-Zimmerman [personality test]

GZAS — Guilford-Zimmerman Aptitude Survey

GZTS — Guilford-Zimmerman Temperament Survey

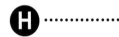

H —
bacterial antigen important in serological classification of enteric bacilli
deflection in the His bundle in electrogram [spike]
electrically induced spinal reflex
fucosal transferase–producing gene
Hancock
Hartnup's [disease]
Hauch (Ger.) breath; flagellum of motile microorganism
haustus (Lat.) a draft
head
heart
heart disease
heavy
heelstick
height
heller (Ger., lighter) region of sarcomere containing only myosin filaments
hemagglutination
hemisphere
hemolysis
henry
heparin
hernia

H — *(continued)*
heroin
hetacillin
high
histidine
histoplasmosis
history
Hoffmann [reflex]
Holzknecht unit
homosexual
hora (Lat.) hour
horizontal
hormone
horse
hospital
hospitalization
hot
Hounsfield unit
hour
human
husband
hydrogen
hydrolysis
hygiene
hyoscine
hypermetropia
hyperopia
hyperphoria
hyperplasia
hypodermic

H — (*continued*)
  hypothalamus
  magnetic field strength
  magnetization
  oersted (unit of magnetizing
    force)
  vectorcardiography electrode
    (at neck)
H. — *Histoplasma*
H^+ — hydrogen ion
$[H^+]$ — hydrogen ion concentration
H_0 — null hypothesis
^1H — protium
H_1 —
  alternative hypothesis
  histamine receptor type I
^2H — deuterium
H^2 — hiatal hernia
$H\text{-}2^b$ — mouse cells
^3H — tritium
H_3 — procaine hydrochloride
μH — microhenry
h —
  hand-rearing [of experimental
    animals]
  heat transfer coefficient
  hecto-
  height
  henry
  heteromorphic region
  high
  horizontal
  hour
  human
  human response
  hundred
  hypermetropia
  hyperopia
  hyperopic
  hypodermic
  negatively staining region of a
    chromosome
  Planck's constant
  quantum constant
  secondary constriction
  specific enthalpy
h —
  height

h — (*continued*)
  Planck's constant
h. —
  haustus (Lat.) a drink
  hora (Lat.) hour
HA —
  Hakim-Adams [syndrome]
  hallux abductus
  halothane anesthesia
  H antigen
  Hartley [guinea pig]
  headache
  hearing aid
  heated aerosol
  height age
  hemadsorbent
  hemadsorption [test]
  hemagglutinating activity
  hemagglutinating antibody
  hemagglutinating antigen
  hemagglutination
  hemagglutinin
  hemolytic anemia
  hemophilia with adenopathy
  hepatic adenoma
  hepatic artery
  hepatitis A
  hepatitis-associated [virus]
  herpangina
  heterophil antibody
  Heyden antibiotic
  high anxiety
  hippuric acid
  histamine
  histidine ammonia–lyase
  histocompatibility antigen
  Horton's arteritis
  hospital administration
  hospital admission
  hospital apprentice
  hospital-acquired
  human albumin
  hyaluronic acid
  hydroxyanisole
  hydroxyapatite
  hyperalimentation
  hyperandrogenism
  hypermetropic astigmatism

HA — *(continued)*
    hyperopia, absolute
    hypersensitivity alveolitis
    hypothalamic amenorrhea
H/A —
    headache
    head to abdomen
HA1 — hemadsorption virus 1
HA2 — hemadsorption virus 2
Ha —
    absolution hypermetropia
    hahnium
    hamster
    Hartmann number
H_a — alternative hypothesis
H/a — home with advice
ha — hectare
HAA —
    hearing aid amplifier
    hemolytic anemia antigen
    hepatitis A antibody
    hepatitis-associated antigen
    hospital activity analysis
HAAb — hepatitis A antibody
HAAg — hepatitis A antigen
HABA — hydroxybenzeneazobenzoic acid
HABF — hepatic artery blood flow
HAb/HAd — horizontal abduction/adduction
habt. — *habeatur* (Lat.) let [the patient] have
HAc — acetic acid
HAChT — high-affinity choline transport
HACR — hereditary adenomatosis of the colon and rectum
HACS — hyperactive child syndrome
hACSP — human adenylate cyclase–stimulating protein
HAD —
    hearing aid dispenser
    hemadsorption
    hospital administration
    hospital administrator
    human adjuvant disease
    hypophysectomized alloxan diabetic

HAd —
    hemadsorption
    hospital administrator
HADD — hydroxyapatite deposition disease
HADH — hydroxyacyl CoA dehydrogenase
HAd-I — hemadsorption-inhibition
HAE —
    health appraisal examination
    hearing aid evaluation
    hepatic artery embolism
    hereditary angioedema
HAF — hepatic arterial flow
HaF — Hageman factor
HAFP — human alpha-fetoprotein
HAG — heat-aggregated globulin
HAGG — hyperimmune antivariola gamma globulin
HAGH — hydroxyacyl-glutathione hydrolase
HAHTG — horse antihuman thymus globulin
HAI —
    hemagglutinating-inhibiting
    hemagglutination inhibition
    hemagglutinin inhibition
    hepatic arterial infusion
H&A Ins — health and accident insurance
HAIR-AN — hyperandrogenism, insulin resistance, and acanthosis nigricans [syndrome]
HaK — hamster kidney
HAL —
    haloperidol
    halothane
    hepatic artery ligation
    hyperalimentation
    hypoplastic acute leukemia
Hal — halogen
hal. —
    halogen
    halothane
HALC — high affinity–low capacity
halluc — hallucination

HALO —
   halothane
   hemorrhage, abruption, labor, placenta previa with mild bleeding
HALP — hyperalphalipoproteinemia
HALT — Heroin Antagonist and Learning Therapy
HaLV — hamster leukemia virus
HAM —
   hearing aid microphone
   helical axis of motion
   human albumin microsphere
   human alveolar macrophage
   hypoparathyroidism, Addison's disease, and mucocutaneous candidiasis [syndrome]
HAm — human amnion
HAMA —
   Hamilton Anxiety [scale]
   human anti-mouse antibody
   human anti-murine antibody
HAMD — Hamilton Depression (Scale)
HAMM — human albumin mini-microsphere
Hams — hamstrings
Ha-MSV — Harvey murine sarcoma virus
HAN —
   heroin-associated nephropathy
   hyperplastic alveolar nodule
HANA — hemagglutinin neuraminidase
H and E — hematoxylin and eosin [stain]
Handicp — handicapped
H and P — history and physical
H and V — hemigastrectomy and vagotomy
HANE — hereditary angioneurotic edema
HANES — Health and Nutrition Examination Survey
hANF — human atrial natriuretic factor

h-ANP — human atrial natriuretic polypeptide
H antigens — flagella antigens of motile bacteria
HAO —
   hearing aid follow-up and orientation
   hospitals, administrators, and organizations
HAP —
   Handicapped Aid Program
   held after positioning
   heredopathia atactica polyneuritiformis
   high-amplitude peristalsis
   histamine acid phosphate
   hospital-acquired pneumonia
   humoral antibody production
   hydrolyzed animal protein
   hydroxyapatite
HAPA — hemagglutinating anti-penicillin antibody
HAPC —
   high-amplitude peristaltic contraction
   hospital-acquired penetration contact
HAPE — high-altitude pulmonary edema
HAPO — high-altitude pulmonary (o)edema
HAPPHY — Heart Attack Primary Prevention in Hypertension
HAPS — hepatic arterial perfusion scintigraphy
HAPTO — haptoglobin
HAQ — Headache Assessment Questionnaire
HAR — high-altitude retinopathy
HAREM — heparin assay rapid easy method
HARH — high-altitude retinal hemorrhage
HARM — heparin assay rapid method
harm. — harmonic
HARPPS — heat, absence of use, redness, pain, pus, swelling [symptoms of infection]

HARS —
  Hamilton Anxiety Rating Scale
  histidyl-RNA synthetase
HART — Heparin-Aspirin Reinfarction Trial
HAS —
  Hamilton Anxiety Scale
  health advisory service
  highest asymptomatic [dose]
  hospital administrative service
  hospital advisory service
  human albumin solution
  hyperalimentation solution
  hypertensive arteriosclerosis
HASCHD — hypertensive arteriosclerotic heart disease
HASCVD — hypertensive arteriosclerotic cardiovascular disease
HASHD — hypertensive arteriosclerotic heart disease
HASP — Hospital Admission and Surveillance Program
HAsP — health aspects of pesticides
HAT —
  Halsted Aphasia Test
  harmonic attenuation table
  harmonic attenuation test
  head, arms, trunk
  heparin-associated thrombocytopenia
  heterophil antibody titer
  hospital arrival time
  hypoxanthine-aminopterin-thymidine
  hypoxanthine, azaserine, and thymidine
HATG — horse antihuman thymocyte globulin
HATH — Heterosexual Attitudes Toward Homosexuality [scale]
HATT —
  hemagglutination treponemal test
  heparin-associated thrombocytopenia and thrombosis

HATTS — hemagglutination treponemal test for syphilis
HAU — hemagglutinating unit
haust. — haustus (Lat.) a draft
HAV —
  hallux abducto valgus
  hemadsorption virus
  hepatitis A virus
HAWIC — Hamburg-Wechsler Intelligence Test for Children
HAZ MAT — hazardous material
HB —
  head backward
  health board
  heart block
  heel to buttock
  held back
  held backward
  hemoglobin
  hemolysis blocking
  hepatitis B
  His bundle
  hold breakfast
  hospital bed
  housebound
  Hutchinson-Boeck [disease]
  hybridoma bank
  hyoid body
HB1° — first-degree heart block
HB2° — second-degree heart block
HB3° — third-degree heart block
Hb — hemoglobin
hb — heart block
HbA —
  adult hemoglobin
  hemoglobin A
Hb A° — hemoglobin determination
HbA$_1$ —
  glycosylated hemoglobin
  major component of adult hemoglobin
HbA$_2$ — minor fraction of adult hemoglobin
HBAb — hepatitis B antibody
HbA$_{1b}$ — hemoglobin A$_{1b}$
HBABA — hydroxybenzeneazobenzoic acid

HBAC — hyperdynamic β-adrenergic circulatory
HBAg — hepatitis B antigen
HbAS — heterozygosity for hemaglobin A and hemaglobin S [sickle cell trait]
HBB —
  hemoglobin beta (chain)
  hospital blood bank
  hydroxybenzyl benzimidazole
Hb Barts — Bart's hemoglobin
HbBC — hemoglobin-binding capacity
HBBW — hold breakfast for blood work
HB$_c$ — hepatitis B core
HbC — hemoglobin C
HB$_c$Ab — hepatitis B core antibody
HB$_c$Ag — hepatitis B core antigen
HBCG — heat-aggregated Calmette-Guérin bacillus
HbCO —
  carbon monoxide hemoglobin
  carboxyhemoglobin
Hb CS — hemoglobin Constant Spring
HbCV — *Haemophilus influenzae* B conjugate vaccine
HBD —
  has been drinking
  hemoglobin δ [chain]
  hydroxybutyrate dehydrogenase
  hydroxybutyric acid dehydrogenase
  hypophosphatemic bone disease
HbD — hemoglobin D
HBDH — hydroxybutyrate dehydrogenase
HBDT — human basophil degranulation test
HBE —
  hemoglobin ε [chain]
  His bundle electrogram
HBE$_1$ — His bundle electrogram, distal

HBE$_2$ — His bundle electrogram, proximal
HbE — hemoglobin E
HB$_e$Ab — hepatitis B early antibody
HB$_e$Ag — hepatitis B early antigen
HBF —
  hand blood flow
  hemispheric blood flow
  hemoglobinuric bilious fever
  hepatic blood flow
  hypothalamic blood flow
HbF —
  fetal hemoglobin
  hemoglobin F
HBG1 — hemoglobin γ chain A
HBG2 — hemoglobin γ chain G
Hbg — hemoglobin
HBGA — had it before, got it again
HBGM — home blood glucose monitoring
HBGR — hemoglobin-gamma regulator
HBH — hindbrain hernia
HbH — hemoglobin H
HBHC — home-based hospital care
Hb-Hp — hemoglobin-haptoglobin [complex]
HBI —
  hemibody irradiation
  hepatobiliary imaging
  high (serum)-bound iron
HBID — hereditary benign intraepithelial dyskeratosis
HBIG — hepatitis B immunoglobulin
HBL — hepatoblastoma
HBLA — human B-cell lymphocyte antigen
HBLLSB — heard best at left lower sternal border
H$_2$ blockers — histamine blockers
HBLUSB — heard best at left upper sternal border
HBLV — human B-cell lymphotropic virus

HBM —
Health Belief Model
hypertonic buffered medium
HbM — hemoglobin Milwaukee
HbMet — methemoglobin
HBO —
hyperbaric oxygen
hyperbaric oxygenation
oxygenated hemoglobin
H_3BO_3 — boric acid
HbO — oxyhemoglobin
HbO_2 —
hyperbaric oxygen
oxygenated hemoglobin
oxyhemoglobin
HBOT — hyperbaric oxygen therapy
HBP —
hepatic binding protein
high blood pressure
HbP — primitive hemoglobin
HBPM — home blood pressure monitoring
Hb PV — *Haemophilus influenzae* b polysaccharide vaccine
HBr — hydrobromic acid
HbR — methemoglobin reductase
HBS —
Health Behavior Scale
hemoglobin S
hepatitis B surface [antigen]
hyperkinetic behavior syndrome
HB_S — hepatitis B surface
HbS —
hemoglobin S
sickle-cell hemoglobin
sulfhemoglobin
HB_SA — hepatitis B surface-associated
HB_sAb — hepatitis B surface antibody
HBsAG — hepatitis B surface antigen
HBsAg/adr — hepatitis B surface antigen manifesting group-specific determinant *a* and subtype-specific determinants *d* and *r*

HBSC — hematopoietic blood stem cell
HbSC — sickle cell hemoglobin C
HBSS — Hanks' balanced salt solution
HbSS —
hemoglobin SS
homozygosity for hemoglobin S
HBSSG — Hanks' balanced salt solution plus glucose
HBT —
human brain thromboplastin
human breast tumor
HBV —
hepatitis B vaccine
hepatitis B virus
honey bee venom
HBV-MN — membranous nephropathy associated with hepatitis B virus
HBW — high birth weight
H/BW —
heart-to-body weight
height-to-body weight
HbZ —
hemoglobin Z
hemoglobin Zürich
HC —
hair cell
hairy cell
handicapped
head check
head circumference
head compression
healthy control
heart cycle
heat conservation
heavy chain
heel cord
hemoglobin concentration
hemorrhage, cerebral
hemorrhagic colitis
heparin cofactor
hepatic catalase
hepatocellular
hepatocellular cancer
hereditary coproporphyria

HC — (continued)
    Hickman catheter
    high calorie
    hippocampus
    histamine challenge
    histochemistry
    home call
    home care
    homocystinuria
    hospital corps
    hospital course
    hospitalized controls
    house call
    Huntington's chorea
    hyaline casts
    hydranencephaly
    hydraulic concussion
    hydrocarbon
    hydrocodone
    hydrocortisone
    hydroxycorticoid
    hyoid cornu
    hypercholesterolemia
    hypertrophic cardiomyopathy
H&C — hot and cold
4-HC — 4-hydroperoxycyclo-
    phosphamide
Hc — hydrocolloid
HCA —
    health care aide
    heart cell aggregate
    hepatocellular adenoma
    home care aide
    Hospital Corporation of
        America
    hydrocortisone acetate
HCAP — handicapped
HCB — hexachlorobenzene
HCC —
    heat conservation center
    hepatitis contagiosa canis [vi-
        rus]
    hepatocellular carcinoma
    hepatoma carcinoma cell
    hexachlorocyclohexane (lin-
        dane)
    history of chief complaint
    hydroxycholecalciferol (vita-
        min D)

25-HCC — 25-hydroxycholecal-
    ciferol
HCD —
    health care delivery
    heavy-chain disease
    high calorie density
    high-calorie diet
    high-carbohydrate diet
    homologous canine distemper
    hydrocolloid dressing
γHCD — gamma-heavy chain dis-
    ease
HCE — hypoglossal carotid entrap-
    ment
HCF —
    hereditary capillary fragility
    high carbohydrate, high fiber
        [diet]
    highest common factor
    hypocaloric carbohydrate feed-
        ing
HCFA — Health Care Financing
    Administration
hCFSH — human chorionic folli-
    cle-stimulating hormone
hCG — human chorionic gonado-
    tropin
HCGN — hypocomplementemic
    glomerulonephritis
HCH — hexachlorocyclohexane
    (lindane)
Hch — hemochromatosis
HCHO — formaldehyde
HCHWA — hereditary cerebral
    hemorrhage with amyloidosis
HcImp — hydrocolloid impression
HCIS — Health Care Information
    System
HCL —
    hairy-cell leukemia
    hard contact lens
    hemocytology index
    human cultured lymphoblasts
HCl —
    hydrochloric acid
    hydrochloride
    hydrogen chloride
HCLF — high carbohydrate, low
    fiber [diet]

HCLs — hard contact lenses
HCM —
    health care maintenance
    health care management
    hypertrophic cardiomyopathy
HCMM — hereditary cutaneous
    malignant melanoma
HCMV — human cytomegalovirus
HCN —
    hereditary chronic nephritis
    human cortical neuron
    hydrocyanic acid
    hydrogen cyanide
HCO_3 — bicarbonate
H_2CO_3 — carbonic acid
HCP —
    handicapped
    hepatocatalase peroxidase
    hereditary coproporphyria
    hexachlorophene
    high cell passage
H&CP — hospital and community
    psychiatry
HCPCS — Health Care Financing
    Administrators Common Pro-
    cedure Coding System
HCQ — hydroxychloroquine
HCR —
    heme-controlled repressor
    host-cell reactivation
    human-controlled repressor
    hydrochloric acid
    hysterical conversion reaction
HCRE — Homeopathic Council
    for Research and Education
hCRH — human corticotropin-re-
    leasing hormone
Hcrit — hematocrit
HCS —
    Hajdu-Cheney syndrome
    Harvey Cushing Society
    Hazard Communication Stan-
        dard
    health care support
    hourglass contraction of the
        stomach
    human chorionic somatomam-
        motropin

HCS — (continued)
    human chorionic somato-
        tropin
    human cord serum
        hydroxycorticosteroid
17-HCS — 17-hydroxycortico-
    steroid
hCS — human chorionic somato-
    mammotropin
HCSD — Health Care Studies Di-
    vision
hCSM — human chorionic soma-
    tomammotropin
HCSS — hypersensitive carotid si-
    nus syndrome
HCT —
    health check test
    heart-circulation training
    hematocrit
    histamine challenge test
    historic control trial
    homocytotrophic
    human calcitonin
    human chorionic thyrotropin
    hydrochlorothiazide
    hydrocortisone
    hydroxycortisone
Hct. — hematocrit
hCT —
    human calcitonin
    human chorionic thyrotropin
hct — hundred count
HCTC — Health Care Technology
    Center
HCTD —
    hepatic computed tomography
        density
    high cholesterol and tocoph-
        erol deficient
HCTS — high cholesterol and to-
    copherol supplement
HCTU — home cervical traction
    unit
HCTZ — hydrochlorothiazide
HCU —
    homocystinuria
    hyperplasia cystica uteri
HCV —
    hepatitis C virus

HCV — *(continued)*
   human corona virus
HCVD — hypertensive cardiovascular disease
HCVR — hypercapnic ventilatory response
HCVS — human corona virus sensitivity
HCW — health care worker
Hcy —
   hemocyanin
   homocysteine
HD —
   Haab-Dimmer [syndrome]
   Hajna-Damon [broth]
   haloperidol decanoate
   Hanganatziu-Deicher
   Hansen's disease
   hearing distance
   heart disease
   helium dilution
   helix destabilizing [protein]
   heloma durum [hard corn]
   hemidiaphragm
   hemodialysis
   hemolytic disease
   hemolyzing dose
   herniated disc
   high density
   high dosage
   high dose
   hip disarticulation
   Hirschsprung's disease
   histidine decarboxylase
   Hodgkin's disease
   hormone-dependent
   hospital day
   house dust
   human diploid [cells]
   Huntington's disease
   hydatid disease
   hydroxydopamine
   hypnotic dosage
H&D — Hunter and Driffield [curve]
HD$_{50}$ — 50% hemolyzing dose of complement
hd — head

h.d. — *hora decubitus* (Lat.) at bedtime
HDA —
   Huntington's Disease Association
   hydroxydopamine
HDAg — hepatitis D antigen
HDARAC — high-dose cytarabine (ARAC)
HDBD — hydroxybutyric dehydrogenase
HDC —
   histidine decarboxylase
   human diploid cell
   hypodermoclysis
HDCS —
   human diploid cell strain
   human diploid cell system
HDCV — human diploid cell (rabies) vaccine
HDD —
   half-dose depth
   high-dosage depth
   Higher Dental Diploma
HDF —
   high dry field
   host defense factor
   human diploid fibroblast
HDFL — human development and family life
HDFP — Hypertension Detection and Follow-up Program
HDG — high-dose group
HDH —
   heart disease history
   Hostility and Direction of Hostility [questionnaire]
HDHQ — Hostility and Direction of Hostility Questionnaire
HDI —
   hemorrhagic disease of infants
   hexamethylene diisocyanate
HDL — high-density lipoprotein
HDL-C — high-density lipoprotein-cholesterol
HDL-c — high-density lipoprotein-cell surface
HDLP — high-density lipoprotein

HDLS — hereditary diffuse leukoencephalopathy with spheroids

HDLW — hearing distance, left, watch [distance from which a watch ticking is heard by left ear]

HDM — hexadimethrine

HDMP — high-dose methylprednisolone

HDMTX — high-dose methotrexate

HDMTX-CF — high-dose methotrexate and citrovorum factor

HDMTX-LV — high-dose methotrexate and leucovorin

HDN —
    hemolytic disease of the newborn
    high-density nebulizer

hDNA —
    deoxyribonucleic acid, histone
    hybrid deoxyribonucleic acid

HDP —
    hexose diphosphate
    high-density polyethylene
    hydroxydimethylpyrimidine

HDPAA — heparin-dependent platelet-associated antibody

HDRF — Heart Disease Research Foundation

HDRS — Hamilton Depression Rating Scale

HDRV — human diploid rabies vaccine

HDRW — hearing distance, right, watch [distance from which a watch ticking is heard by right ear]

HDS —
    Hamilton Depression Scale
    Health Data Services
    health delivery system
    Healthcare Data Systems
    herniated disc syndrome
    Hospital Discharge Survey

HDU —
    head-drop unit

HDU — (continued)
    hemodialysis unit

HDV —
    hepatitis delta virus
    hepatitis virus, type D

HDW —
    hearing distance (with) watch
    hemoglobin distribution width

HDZ — hydralazine

HE —
    hard exudate
    Hearing Examiner
    Hektoen enteric [agar]
    hemagglutinating encephalomyelitis
    hemoglobin electrophoresis
    hepatic encephalopathy
    hereditary elliptocytosis
    high exposure
    hollow enzyme
    human enteric [virus]
    hydroxyethyl [cellulose]
    hyperextension
    hypogonadotropic eunuchoidism
    hypophysectomy
    hypoxemic episode

H&E —
    hematoxylin and eosin [stain]
    hemorrhage and exudate
    heredity and environment

H-E — heat-exchanger

He —
    heart
    Hedstrom number
    helium

HEA —
    hexone-extracted acetone
    human erythrocyte antigen

HEADSS — home life, education level, activities, drug use, sexual activity, suicide ideation/attempts [adolescent medical history]

HEAL — Health Education Assistance Loan

HEART — Health Evaluation and Risk Tabulation

HEAT — human erythrocyte agglutination test

HEB — hemato-encephalic barrier

hebdom. — *hebdomada* (Lat.) a week

HEC —
 hamster embryo cell
 Health Education Council
 health evaluation center
 human endothelial cell
 hydroxyergocalciferol
 hydroxyethyl cellulose

HECTOR — heated experimental carbon thermal oscillator reactor

HED —
 Haut-Einheits-Dosis (Ger.) unit skin dose [of x-rays]
 Haut-Erythem-Dosis (Ger.) skin erythema dose
 hereditary ectodermal dysplasia
 hydrotropic electron donor
 hypohidrotic ectodermal dysplasia

HeD — helper determinant

HEDH — hypohidrotic ectodermal dysplasia with hypothyroidism

HEDIS — Health Plan Data and Information Set

HEDSPA — ^{99m}Tc-etidronate [bone-imaging agent]

HEENT — head, eyes, ears, nose, and throat

HEEP — health effects of environmental pollutants

HEF —
 hamster embryo fibroblast
 human embryo fibroblast

HEG — hemorrhagic erosive gastritis

HEHR — highest equivalent heart rate

HEI —
 Health Effects Institute
 high-energy intermediate
 homogeneous enzyme immunoassay

HEI — *(continued)*
 human embryonic intestine [cells]

HE inj — hyperextension injury

HEIR —
 health effects of ionizing radiation
 high-energy ionizing radiation

HEIS — high-energy ion scattering

HEK —
 human embryo kidney
 human embryonic kidney

HEL —
 hen's egg-white lysozyme
 human embryo lung
 human embryonic lung
 human erythroleukemia
 human erythroleukemia line

HeLa cells — from name of patient (Henrietta Lacks) whose carcinoma of the cervix uteri parent carcinoma cells were isolated

HELF — human embryo lung fibroblast

HELLIS — Health, Literature, Library, and Information Services

HELLP — *h*emolysis, *e*levated *l*iver enzymes and *l*ow *p*latelets

HELM — helmet cells

HELP —
 Health Education Library Program
 Health Emergency Loan Program
 Health Evaluation and Learning Program
 heat escape lessening posture
 Heroin Emergency Life Project
 Hospital Equipment Loan Project

HEM —
 hematology
 hematuria
 hemolysis
 hemolytic

HEM — *(continued)*
  hemorrhage
  hemorrhoids
HEMA — Health Education Media Association
hemat —
  hematocrit
  hematologist
  hematology
hematem — hematemesis
HEMB — hemophilia B
hemi —
  hemiparalysis
  hemiparesis
  hemiplegia
  hemisphere
hemo —
  hemoglobin
  hemolyzed
  hemophilia
hemocyt — hemocytometer
hemorr. — hemorrhage
HEMOSID — hemosiderin
HEMPAS — hereditary erythrocytic multinuclearity with positive acidified serum
HEMRI — hereditary multifocal relapsing inflammation
HEMS — helicopter emergency medical services
HEMSID — hemosiderin
HEN — hemorrhages, exudates, and/or nicking
HeNe — helium neon [laser]
HEP —
  hemolysis end point
  heparin
  hepatic
  hepatoerythropoietic porphyria
  hepatology
  high egg passage [virus]
  high-energy phosphate
  histamine equivalent prick
  human epithelial [cell]
Hep —
  hepatic
  hepatitis

hEP — human endorphin
HEp-1 — human cervical carcinoma cells
HEp-2 — human laryngeal tumor cells
HEPA —
  hamster egg penetration assay
  high-efficiency particulate air [filter]
HEP-AC — hepatitis battery—acute
Hep/Clav — hepatoclavicular
HEPES — *N*-2-hydroxyethyl-piperazine-*N*-2-ethane-sulfonic [acid]
HEPM — human embryonic palatal mesenchymal [cell]
HER —
  hemorrhagic encephalopathy of rats
  hernia
herb. recent. — *herbarium recentium* (Lat.) of fresh herbs
hered —
  hereditary
  heredity
hern —
  hernia
  herniated
  herniation
HERP — human exposure (dose)/rodent patency
HERS — Health Evaluation and Referral Service
HES —
  health examination survey
  hematoxylin-eosin stain
  human embryonic skin
  human embryonic spleen
  hydroxyethyl starch
  hypereosinophilic syndrome
  hyperprostaglandin E syndrome
HESCA — Health Sciences Communications Association
HET —
  Health Education Telecommunications

HET — (continued)
  helium equilibration time
  heterozygous
Het — heterophil
het — heterozygous
HET-BE — heterophile beef
HETE — hydroxyeicosatetraenoic
  [acid]
HET-GP — heterophile guinea pig
HETP —
  height equivalent to a theoretical plate [gas chromalography]
  hexaethyltetraphosphate
HET-PR — heterophile presumptive
HEV —
  health and environment
  hemagglutinating encephalomyelitis virus
  hepato-encephalomyelitis virus
  high endothelial venule
  human enteric virus
HEW — (Department of) Health, Education, and Welfare
HEX —
  hexaminidase
  hexosaminidase
HEx — hard exudate
Hex — hexamethylmelamine
HEX A — hexosaminidase A
HEX B — hexosaminidase B
HEX C — hexosaminidase C
HEXL — methohexital
HF —
  Hageman factor
  half
  haplotype frequency
  hard feces
  hard-filled [capsule]
  harvest fluid
  hay fever
  head forward
  head of fetus
  heart failure
  helper factor
  hemofiltration

HF — (continued)
  hemorrhagic factor
  hemorrhagic fever
  hepatocyte function
  Hertz frequency
  high flow
  high frequency
  high-fat [diet]
  hollow fiber
  hollow filter
  hot fomentation
  house formula
  human fibroblast
  hydrogen fluoride
  hyperflexion
H/F — HeLa/fibroblast [hybrid]
Hf — hafnium
hf —
  half
  high frequency
HFA — hypoglossal-facial anastomosis
HFAK — hollow-fiber artificial kidney
HFC —
  hand filled capsules
  hard-filled capsules
  high-frequency current
  histamine-forming capacity
HFCS — high-fructose corn syrup
HFCWC — high-frequency chest wall compression
HFD —
  hemorrhagic fever of deer
  high forceps delivery
  high-fiber diet
  hospital field director
HFDK — human fetal diploid kidney [cell]
HFDL — human fetal diploid lung [cell]
HFEC — human foreskin epithelial cell
HFF — human foreskin fibroblast
HFG — hand-foot-genital [syndrome]
HFH — hemifacial hyperplasia
HFHL — high-frequency hearing loss

HFHV — high frequency, high volume

HFI —
  hereditary fructose intolerance
  human fibroblast interferon

HFIF — human fibroblast interferon

HFJV — high-frequency jet ventilation

HFL — human fetal lung

HFM — hemifacial microsomia

HFMA — Healthcare Financial Management Association

HFO —
  hard food orientation
  high-frequency oscillation
  high-frequency oscillator
  high-frequency oscillatory [ventilation]

HFO-A — high-frequency oscillatory (ventilation)—active [expiratory phase]

HFOV — high-frequency oscillatory ventilation

HFP —
  hexafluoropropylene
  high-frequency pulsation
  hypofibrinogenic plasma

hFPA — human fibrinopeptide A

HFPPV — high-frequency positive-pressure ventilation

HFR — high frequency of recombination

Hfr —
  heart frequency
  high frequency
  high frequency of recombination

HFRS — hemorrhagic fever with renal syndrome

HFS —
  hemifacial spasm
  Hospital Financial Support

hfs — hyperfine structure

hFSH — human follicle-stimulating hormone

HFST — hearing-for-speech test

HFT —
  high-frequency transduction
  high-frequency transfer

Hft — high-frequency transfer

HFU — hand-foot-uterus [syndrome]

HFUPR — hourly fetal urine production rate

HFV — high-frequency ventilation

HG —
  hand grip
  hemoglobin
  herpes genitalis
  herpes gestationis
  Herter-Gee [syndrome]
  Heschl's gyrus
  high glucose
  human gonadotropin
  human growth [factor]
  Hutchinson-Gilford [syndrome]
  hypoglycemia

Hg —
  hemoglobin
  mercury (Lat., *hydrargyrum*)

hg. — hectogram

HGA — homogentisic acid

Hgb — hemoglobin

HGB EL — hemoglobin electrophoresis

Hgb F — hemoglobin F

HGB-PL — hemoglobin plasma

HGBS — methemoglobin-sulfhemoglobin

$HgCl_2$ — corrosive mercuric chloride

Hg_2Cl_2 — mild mercurous chloride

HGF —
  human growth factor
  hyperglycemic-glycogenolytic factor

Hg-F — fetal hemoglobin

HGG — herpetic geniculate ganglionitis

hGG — human gammaglobulin

HGH — high growth hormone

hGH — human growth hormone

hGHr — growth hormone recombinant

HGHRF — human growth hormone–releasing factor

HgI$_2$ — mercuric iodide

Hg$_2$I$_2$ — mercurous iodide

HGM —
hog gastric mucin
hog gastric mucosa
human gene mapping
human glucose monitoring

hgm — hectogram

HGMCR — human genetic mutant cell repository

Hg(NO$_3$)$_2$ — mercuric nitrate

HGO —
hepatic glucose output
hip guidance orthosis
human glucose output

HgO — mercuric oxide

Hg$_2$O — mercurous oxide

HGP —
hepatic glucose production
hyperglobulinemic purpura

HGPRT — hypoxanthine-guanine phosphoribosyltransferase

HG-PRTase — hypoxanthine-guanine phosphoribosyltransferase

HGPS —
hereditary giant platelet syndrome
Hutchinson-Gilford progeria syndrome

hGRH — human growth hormone-releasing hormone

HGRM — hemogram

HGSHS — Harvard Group Scale of Hypnotic Susceptibility

hgt — height

HH —
halothane hepatitis
hard-of-hearing
Head-Holms [syndrome]
healthy hemophiliac
healthy human
Henderson and Haggard [inhaler]
hiatal hernia
holistic health

HH — (continued)
home health
home help
Hunter-Hurler [syndrome]
hydroxyhexamide
hypergastrinemic hyperchlorhydria
hyperhidrosis
hypogonadotropic hypogonadism
hyporeninemic hypoaldosteronism

H&H — hematocrit and hemoglobin

Hh — hemopoietic histocompatibility

HHA —
Health Hazard Appraisal
hereditary hemolytic anemia
home health agency
home health aide
hypothalamic-hypophyseal-adrenal [system]

HHAA — hypothalamo-hypophyseal-adrenal axis

HHb —
hypohemoglobinemia
un-ionized hemoglobin

HHC — home health care

HHCS — high-altitude hypertrophic cardiomyopathy syndrome

HHD —
high heparin dose
home hemodialysis
hypertensive heart disease

HHE —
health hazard evaluation
hemiconvulsion-hemiplegia-epilepsy [syndrome]

HHFM — high-humidity face mask

HHG — hypertrophic hypersecretory gastropathy

HHH — hyperornithinemia, hyperammonemia, and homocitrullinemia [syndrome]

HHHO — hypotonia-hypomentia-hypogonadism-obesity [syndrome]

HHIE — Hearing Handicap Inventory for the Elderly

HHIE-S — Hearing Handicap Inventory for the Elderly—Screening Version

HHM —
  hemohydrometry
  humoral hypercalcemia of malignancy

H. and Hm. — compound hypermetropic astigmatism

HHN — hand-held nebulizer

HHNC — hyperosmolar hyperglycemic nonketotic (diabetic) coma

HHNK — hyperglycemic hyperosmolar nonketotic [coma]

HHNKS — hyperosmolar hyperglycemic nonketotic syndrome

HHPC — hyperoxic-hypercapnic

HHR — hydralazine, hydrochlorothiazide, and reserpine

HHRH —
  hereditary hypophosphatemic rickets with hypercalciuria
  hypothalamic hypophysiotropic-releasing hormone

HHS —
  (Department of) Health and Human Services
  Hearing Handicap Scale
  hereditary hemolytic syndrome
  human hypopituitary serum
  hyperglycemic hyperosmolar syndrome
  hyperkinetic heart syndrome

HHSSA — Home Health Services and Staffing Association

HHT —
  head halter traction
  hereditary hemolytic telangiectasia
  hereditary hemorrhagic telangiectasia

HHT — (continued)
  heterotopic heart transplantation
  hydroxyheptadecatrienoic acid

HHTA — hypothalamohypophyseothyroidal axis

HHTX — head halter traction

HHV — human herpes virus

HI —
  head injury
  health insurance
  hearing impaired
  heart infusion
  heat inactivated
  heat input
  hemagglutination inhibition
  hepatic insufficiency
  hepatobiliary imaging
  high impulsiveness
  histidine
  homicidal ideation
  hormone independent
  hormone insensitivity
  hospital induced
  hospital insurance
  humoral immunity
  hydriodic acid
  hydroxyindole
  hyperglycemic index
  hypomelanosis of Ito
  hypothermic ischemia

H-I — hemagglutination-inhibition

Hi —
  histamine
  histidine

HIA —
  Hearing Industries Association
  heart infusion agar
  hemagglutination inhibition antibody

HIAA — Health Insurance Association of America

5-HIAA — 5-hydroxyindole acetic acid

HIB —
  Haemophilus influenzae type B [vaccine]

HIB — *(continued)*
    heart infusion broth
    hemolytic immune body
HIBAC — Health Insurance Benefits Advisory Council
HIC —
    handling-induced convulsions
    Heart Information Center
HICA — hydroxyisocaproic acid
H-ICD-A — International Classification of Diseases, Adopted Code for Hospitals
HICHO — high carbohydrate [diet]
HiCn — cyanmethemoglobin
HID —
    headache, insomnia, depression [syndrome]
    herniated intervertebral disc
    human infectious dose
    hyperkinetic impulse disorder
HIDA —
    Health Industry Distributors Association
    hepatic 2,6-dimethyl-iminodiacetic acid
    hepato-iminodiacetic acid (lidofenin) [nuclear medicine scan]
HIE —
    human intestinal epithelium
    hyperimmunoglobulin E
    hypoxic-ischemic encephalopathy
HIES — hyper-IgE syndrome
HIF —
    higher integrative function
    higher intellectual function
    histoplasma inhibitory factor
    Historical Information Form
HIFBS — heat-inactivated fetal bovine serum
HIFC — hog intrinsic factor concentrate
HIFCS — heat-inactivated fetal calf serum
hIG — human immunoglobulin
HIg — hyperimmunoglobulin

HIH — hyperintensive intracerebral hemorrhage
HIHA — high impulsiveness, high anxiety
HiHb — hemiglobin (methemoglobin)
HII —
    Health Industries Institute
    Health Insurance Institute
    hemagglutination inhibitor immunoassay
HIL — hypoxic-ischemic lesion
HILA — high impulsiveness, low anxiety
HIM —
    hemopoietic inductive microenvironment
    hepatitis-infectious mononucleosis
    hexosephosphate isomerase
    Hill Interaction Matrix [psychological test]
HIMA — Health Industries Manufacturers Association
HIMC — hepatic intramitochondrial crystalloid
HIMP — high-dose intravenous methylprednisolone
HIMT — hemagglutination inhibition morphine test
H inf — hypodermoclysis infusion
Hint. — Hinton [test]
HIO —
    hypoiodism
    hypoiodite
HIO_3 — iodic acid
HIOMT — hydroxyindole-*o*-methyl transferase
HIOS — high index of suspicion
HIP —
    health illness profile
    health insurance plan
    homograft incus prosthesis
    hospital insurance program
    humoral immunocompetence profile
    hydrostatic indifference point
HIPA — heparin-induced platelet activation

HIPE — Hospital Inpatient Enquiry

HIPO —
   hemihypertrophy, intestinal web, preauricular skin tag, and congenital corneal opacity [syndrome]
   Hospital Indicator for Physicians Orders

Hi Prot — high protein

HIR —
   head injury routine
   high irradiance response

HIRF — histamine inhibitory-releasing factor

HIS —
   Hanover Intensive Score
   Haptic Intelligence Scale
   health information system
   Health Intention Scale
   Health Interview Survey
   histidine
   hospital information systems
   hyperimmune serum
   hyperimmunized suppressed

His — histidine

HISG — human immune serum globulin

HISMS — How I See Myself Scale [psychological test]

HISSG — Hospital Information Systems Sharing Group

HIST — Hospital In-Service Training

hist —
   histamine
   histidine
   histidinemia
   history

HISTLINE — History of Medicine On-Line

Histo —
   histology
   Histoplasma
   histoplasmin skin test
   histoplasmosis

Histol —
   histological

Histol — *(continued)*
   histologist
   histology

HIT —
   hemagglutination-inhibition test
   heparin-induced thrombocytopenia
   histamine inhalation test
   histamine ion transfer
   Holtzman Inkblot Technique
   hypertrophic infiltrative tendinitis
   hypertrophied inferior turbinate

HITB — *Haemophilus influenzae* type B

HITES — hydrocortisone, insulin, transferrin, estradiol, and selenium

HITT — heparin-induced thrombocytopenia and thrombosis

HITTS — heparin-induced thrombosis-thrombocytopenia syndrome

HIU —
   head injury unit
   hyperplasia interstitialis uteri

HIV — human immunodeficiency virus

HIV1 — human immunodeficiency virus type 1

HIV2 — human immunodeficiency virus type 2

HIV Ag — human immunodeficiency virus antigen

HIVAN — human immunodeficiency virus–associated nephropathy

HIVD — herniated intervertebral disc

HIV-G — human immunodeficiency virus–associated gingivitis

HIVIG — HIV immunoglobulin

HiVit — high vitamin

HJ — hepatojugular [reflux]

HJB — Howell-Jolly bodies

HJR — hepatojugular reflux

HK —
    hand to knee
    heat-killed
    heel-to-knee
    hexokinase
    Hoffa-Kastert [syndrome]
    human kidney [cell]

H-K —
    hand to knee [test]
    heel to knee [test]

H→K — hand to knee [coordination]

HK1 — hexokinase 1

HKAFO — hip-knee-ankle-foot orthosis

HKAO — hip-knee-ankle orthosis

HKC — human kidney cell

HKH — hyperkinetic heart [syndrome]

HKLM — heat-killed *Listeria monocytogenes*

HKO — hip-knee orthosis

HKS —
    heel-knee-shin [test]
    hyperkinesis syndrome

HL —
    hairline
    hairy leukoplakia
    half-life
    hallux limitus
    haloperidol
    harelip
    hearing level
    hearing loss
    heart and lungs
    heavy lifting
    hectoliter
    hemolysis
    heparin lock
    Hickman line
    histiocytic lymphoma
    histocompatibility locus
    Hodgkin's lymphoma
    human leukocyte
    human lymphocyte
    hydrophil/lipophil [number]
    hygienic laboratory

HL — *(continued)*
    hyperlipidemia
    hyperlipoproteinemia
    hypermetropia, latent
    hypertrichosis lanuginosa
    latent hypermetropia
    latent hyperopia
    lateral habenular [nucleus]

H/L — hydrophil/lipophil [ratio]

H&L — heart and lungs

hl — hectoliter

HLA —
    heart, lungs, and abdomen
    histocompatibility leukocyte antigen
    histocompatibility locus antigen
    homologous leukocyte antibody
    human leukocyte antigen
    human lymphocyte antibody
    human lymphocyte antigen
    hypoplastic left atrium

HL-A — human leukocyte antigen

HLAA — human leukocyte antigen A

HLAB — human leukocyte antigen B

HLAC — human leukocyte antigen C

HLAD — human leukocyte antigen D

HLALD — horse liver alcohol dehydrogenase

HLA-LD — human lymphocyte antigen—lymphocyte defined

HLA-SD — human lymphocyte antigen—serologically defined

HLB —
    hydrophilic-lipophilic balance
    hypotonic lysis buffer

HLBI — human lymphoblastoid interferon

HLC —
    heat loss center
    Human Lactation Center

HLCL — human lymphoblastoid cell line

HLD —
    haloperidol decanoate
    hepatolenticular degeneration
    herniated lumbar disk
    Hippel-Lindau disease
    hypersensitivity lung disease
HL-D — haloperidol decanoate
HLDH — heat-stable lactic dehy-
    drogenase
HLE — human leukocyte elastase
HLEG — hydrolysate lactalbumin
    Earle's glucose
HLF —
    heat-labile factor
    human lung field
    human lung fluid
HLFCB — horizontal laminar flow,
    clean benches
HLH —
    hemophagocytic lymphohis-
        tiocytosis
    hypoplastic left heart
hLH — human luteinizing hor-
    mone
HLHS — hypoplastic left heart
    syndrome
HLI —
    hemolysis inhibition
    human leukocyte interferon
    human lymphocyte interferon
HLK — heart, liver, and kidneys
HLL — hypoplastic left lung
HLN —
    hilar lymph node
    human Lesch-Nyhan [cell]
    hyperplastic liver nodules
HLP —
    hepatic lipoperoxidation
    hind leg paralysis
    hyperkeratosis lenticularis per-
        stans
    hyperlipoproteinemia
HLR —
    heart-lung resuscitation
    heart-lung resuscitator
HLS —
    Health Learning System
    Hippel-Lindau syndrome

HLT —
    heart-lung transplantation
    human lipotropin
hLT — human lymphocyte trans-
    formation
hlth. — health
HLV —
    herpes-like virus
    hypoplastic left ventricle
HLVS — hypoplastic left ventricu-
    lar syndrome
HM —
    hand motion
    hand movements
    harmonic mean
    health maintenance
    heart murmur
    heavily muscled
    Heine-Medin [disease]
    heloma molle (soft corn)
    hemifacial microsomia
    hepatic metabolism
    hexamethylmelamine
    Holter monitor
    Holter monitoring
    homosexual male
    hospital management
    human milk
    hydatidiform mole
    hyperimmune mouse
    hyperopia, manifest (hyperme-
        tropia)
    hypoxic-metabolic
Hm. —
    home
    manifest hypermetropia
    manifest hyperopia
hm — hectometer
HMA —
    hemorrhages and microaneu-
        rysms
    hydroxymethionine analogue
HMAC — Health Manpower Ad-
    visory Council
HMAS — hyperimmune mouse as-
    citic [fluid]
HMB — homatropine methylbro-
    mide

HMBA — hexamethylene bisacetamide

HMC —
    hand-mirror cell
    health maintenance cooperative
    heroin, morphine, and cocaine
    histocompatibility complex, major
    hospital management committee
    hydroxymethyl cytosine
    hyoscine-morphine-codeine
    hypertelorism-microtia-clefting [syndrome]

HMCCMP — human mammary carcinoma cell membrane proteinase

HMD — hyaline membrane disease

HMDP — hydroxymethylene diphosphonate

HME —
    Health Media Education
    heat and moisture exchanger
    heat, massage, and exercise

HMETSC — heavy metal screen

HMF — hydroxymethylfurfural

HMG —
    high-mobility group
    human menopausal gonadotropin
    3-hydroxy-3-methylglutaryl

hMG — human menopausal gonadotropin

HMG CoA — 3-hydroxy-3-methylglutaryl coenzyme A

HMI — healed myocardial infarct

HMIS —
    hazardous materials identification system
    hospital medical information system

HMK —
    high molecular weight kininogen
    homemaking

hML — human milk lysozyme

HM & LP — hand motion and light perception

HMM —
    heavy meromyosin
    hexamethylmelamine

HMMA — 4-hydroxy-3-methoxymandelic acid

HMO —
    Health Maintenance Organization
    heart minute output

HMP —
    hexose monophosphate
    hexose monophosphate pathway
    hot moist packs
    human menopausal
    hydromotive pressure

HMPA — hexamethylphosphoramide

HM-PAO — hexamethyl-propyleneamineoxime

HMPG — 4-hydroxy-3-methoxyphenyl-ethylene glycol

HMPS — hexose monophosphate shunt

HMPT — hexamethylphosphorotriamide

HMR — histiocytic medullary reticulosis

H-mRNA — H-chain messenger ribonucleic acid

HMRTE — human milk reverse transcriptase enzyme

HMS —
    hexose monophosphate shunt
    high methacholine sensitivity
    hypermobility syndrome

HMSA —
    Hawaii Medical Services Association
    health manpower shortage area

HMSAS — hypertrophic muscular subaortic stenosis

HMSN — hereditary motor and sensory neuropathy

HMSS — Hospital Management Systems Society

HMT —
- hematocrit
- hexamethylenetetramine
- histamine-*N*-methyl-transferase
- hospital management team

hMT — human molar thyrotropin

HMTA — hexamethylenetetramine

HMU — hydroxymethyl uracil

HMW — high-molecular-weight

HMWC — high-molecular-weight component

HMWGP — high-molecular-weight glycoprotein

HMWK — high-molecular-weight kininogen

HMWM — heavily muscled white male

HMW-NCF — high-molecular-weight neutrophil chemotactic factor

HMX — heat-massage-exercise

HN —
- head and neck
- head nurse
- Heller-Nelson [syndrome]
- hemagglutinin neuraminidase
- hematemesis neonatorum
- hemorrhage of newborn
- hereditary nephritis
- high necrosis
- high nitrogen
- hilar node
- histamine-containing neuron
- home nursing
- human nutrition
- hypertrophic neuropathy

H&N — head and neck

HN₂ — mechlorethamine

h.n. — *hoc nocte* (Lat.) tonight

HNA — heparin-neutralizing activity

HNB —
- human neuroblastoma
- hydroxynitrobenzylbromide

HNC —
- hypernephroma cell
- hyperosmolar nonketotic coma

HNC — *(continued)*
- hyperoxic normocapnic
- hypothalamoneurohypophyseal complex

HNKDC — hyperosmolar nonketotic diabetic coma

HNKDS — hyperosmolar nonketotic diabetic state

HNL — histiocytic necrotizing lymphadenitis

HNLN — hospitalization no longer necessary

H&N mot — head and neck motion

HNO₂ — nitrous acid

HNO₃ — nitric acid

HNP —
- hereditary nephritic protein
- herniated nucleus pulposus
- human neurophysin

HNPCC — hereditary nonpolyposis colorectal cancer

hnRNA — heterogeneous nuclear ribonucleic acid

hnRNP — heterogeneous nuclear ribonucleoprotein

HNS —
- head and neck surgery
- head, neck, and shaft [of bone]
- home nursing supervisor

HNSHA — hereditary nonspherocytic hemolytic anemia

HNTD — highest nontoxic dose

HNTLA — Hiskey-Nebraska Test of Learning Aptitude

HNV — has not voided

HO —
- hand orthosis
- hematology-oncology
- heterotopic ossification
- high oxygen
- hip orthosis
- Holt-Oram [syndrome]
- house officer
- hyperbaric oxygen
- hypertrophic ossification

H/O —
- hematology and oncology

H/O — *(continued)*
    history of
H₂O — water

H_2O — water
H_2O_2 — hydrogen peroxide
Ho —
    holmium
    horse [serum]
HOA —
    hip osteoarthritis
    hypertrophic osteoarthritis
    hypertrophic osteoarthropathy
    hypertrophic osteoarthroscopy
HoaRhLG — horse anti-rhesus
    lymphocyte globulin
HoaTTG — horse anti-tetanus tox-
    oid globulin
HOB — head of bed
HOB UPSOB — head of bed up
    for shortness of breath
HOC —
    Health Officer Certificate
    human ovarian cancer
    hydroxycorticoid
HOCM —
    high-osmolar contrast me-
        dium
    hypertrophic obstructive car-
        diomyopathy
hoc vesp. — *hoc vespere* (Lat.) this
    evening
HOD —
    hereditary opalescent dentin
    Hoffer-Osmond Diagnostic
    hyperbaric oxygen drenching
HoD — Hodgkin's disease
HOF — hepatic outflow
HofF — height of fundus
Hoff — Hoffmann [reflex]
HOG — halothane, oxygen, and
    gas (nitrous oxide)
HOGA — hyperornithinemia with
    gyrate atrophy
HOH — hard of hearing
HOI — hospital onset of infection
HoIg — horse immunoglobulin
HOLD — hemostatic occlusive le-
    verage device
HOM — high-osmolar (contrast)
    medium

HOME —
    Home Observation for Mea-
        surement of the Environ-
        ment
    Home-Oriented Maternity Ex-
        perience
Homeo. — homeopathy
HOMO —
    highest occupied molecular or-
        bital
    homosexual
homo. — homosexual
homolat — homolateral
$H_2O_5O_4$ — osmic acid
HOOD — hereditary osteo-ony-
    chodysplasia
HOODS — hereditary onycho-
    osteodysplasia syndrome
HOOI — Hall Occupational Ori-
    entation Inventory
HOP — high oxygen pressure
HOPD — hospital outpatient de-
    partment
HOPE —
    Healthcare Options Plan Enti-
        tlement
    health-oriented physical edu-
        cation
    holistic orthogonal parameter
        estimation
HOPI — history of present illness
HOPP — hepatic occluded portal
    pressure
hor — horizontal
hor. decub. — *hora decubitus* (Lat.)
    at bedtime
hor. interm. — *horis intermediis*
    (Lat.) at the intermediate
    hours
hor. som. — *hora somni* (Lat.) at
    bedtime
hor. un. spatio — *horae unius spatio*
    (Lat.) at the end of one hour
HOS —
    Holt-Oram syndrome
    human osteogenic sarcoma
    human osteosarcoma
HoS — horse serum

hosp — hospital
HOST — hypo-osmotic shock
    treatment
HOT —
    human old tuberculin
    hyperbaric oxygen therapy
HOTS — hypercalcemia-osteolysis-
    T-cell syndrome
HP —
    Haemophilus pleuropneumonia
    halogen phosphorus
    handicapped person
    haptoglobin
    hard palate
    Harding-Passey [melanoma]
    Harvard pump
    hastening phenomenon
    health profession(al)
    heater probe
    heat production
    heel to patella
    hemiparesis
    hemiparkinsonism
    hemipelvectomy
    hemiplegia
    hemoperfusion
    heparin
    high potency
    high power
    high pressure
    high protein
    highly purified
    Hodgen and Pearson [suspen-
        sion traction]
    horizontal plane
    horsepower
    hospital participation
    hot pack
    hot pad
    house physician
    human pituitary
    hybridoma product
    hydrocollator pack
    hydrogen peroxide
    hydrophilic petrolatum
    hydrophobic protein
    hydrostatic pressure
    hydroxyproline

HP — (*continued*)
    hydroxypyruvate
    hyperparathyroidism
    hyperphoria
    hypersensitivity pneumonitis
    hypertension plus proteinuria
    hypoparathyroidism
    hypopharynx
    hypophoria
H&P —
    history and physical
    Hodgen and Pearson [suspen-
        sion traction]
H→P — heel-to-patella
Hp —
    haptoglobin
    hematoporphyrin
    hemiplegia
hp —
    heaping
    horsepower
HPA —
    Helix pomatia agglutinin
    hemagglutinating penicillin
        antibody
    Histoplasma capsulatum poly-
        saccharide antigen
    human papilloma [virus]
    humeroscapular periarthritis
    hypothalamic-pituitary-
        adrenal [axis]
    hypothalamo-pituitary-
        adrenocortical [system]
HPAA —
    hydroperoxyarachidonic acid
    hydroxyphenylacetic acid
    hypothalamo-pituitary-
        adrenal axis
HPAC — hypothalamo-pituitary-
    adrenocortical
HPBC — hyperpolarizing bipolar
    cell
HPBF — hepatotrophic portal
    blood factor
HPBL — human peripheral blood
    leukocyte
HPC —
    hemangiopericytoma

HPC — (continued)
    hippocampal pyramidal cell
    history of present complaint
    holoprosencephaly
    hydroxyphenyl-cinchoninic
      [acid]
    hydroxypropylcellulose
HPCA — human progenitor cell
    antigen
HPCHA — high (red-cell) phos-
    phatidylcholine hemolytic
    anemia
HPD —
    dialysate of hydropenic
      plasma
    hearing protective device
    hematoporphyrin derivative
    highly probably drunk
    high-protein diet
    home peritoneal dialysis
HP-D — Hough-Powell digitizer
HPE —
    hepatic portoenterostomy
    high permeability edema
    history and physical examina-
      tion
    hydrostatic pulmonary edema
HPETE — hydroperoxy eicosa-
    tetraenoic [acid]
HPF —
    heparin-precipitable fraction
    hepatic plasma flow
    high-pass filter
    high-power field
    hypocaloric protein feeding
HPFH — hereditary persistence of
    fetal hemoglobin
hPFSH — human pituitary follicle-
    stimulating hormone
hPG — human pituitary gonado-
    tropin
HPGe — high-purity germanium
HPH — halothane-percent-hour
HPI —
    hepatic perfusion index
    Heston Personality Inventory
    history of present illness
HPL —
    human parotid lysozyme

HPL — (continued)
    human peripheral lymphocyte
hPL —
    human placental lactogen
    human platelet lactogen
HPLA — hydroxyphenyllactic acid
HPLAC — high-pressure liquid-
    affinity chromatography
HPLC —
    high-performance liquid chro-
      matography
    high-power liquid chromatog-
      raphy
    high-pressure liquid chroma-
      tography
HPLE — hereditary polymorphic
    light eruption
HPM —
    Harding-Passey melanoma
    hemiplegic migraine
    high-performance membrane
HPMC — human peripheral mono-
    nuclear cell
HPN —
    home parenteral nutrition
    hypertension
hpn — hypertension
h.p.n. — *haustus purgans noster*
    (Lat.) our own purgative draft
HPNS — high pressure neurologi-
    cal syndrome
HPO —
    high-pressure oxygen
    hydroperoxide
    hydrophilic ointment
    hypertrophic pulmonary osteo-
      arthritis
    hypertrophic pulmonary os-
      teoarthropathy
HPO_3 — metaphosphoric acid
H_3PO_2 — hypophosphorous acid
H_3PO_3 — phosphorous acid
H_3PO_4 —
    orthophosphoric acid
    phosphoric acid
$H_4P_2O_6$ — hypophosphoric acid
$H_4P_2O_7$ — pyrophosphoric acid
HPP —
    hereditary pyropoikilocytosis

HPP — (continued)
    history and presenting prob-
        lems
    hydroxyphenylpyruvate
    hydroxypyrazolopyrimidine
    human pancreatic polypeptide
2 HPP — two hours postprandial
    [blood sugar]
HPPA — hydroxyphenylpyruvic
    acid
HPPH — hydroxyphenyl-
    phenylhydantoin
HPPO —
    high partial pressure of oxy-
        gen
    hydroxyphenyl pyruvate oxi-
        dase
HPR — hospital peer review
hPr — human prolactin
HPRP — human platelet-rich
    plasma
HPRT —
    hot plate reaction time
    hypoxanthine phosphoribosyl-
        transferase
HPS —
    hematoxylin-phloxine-saffron
    Hermansky-Pudlak syndrome
    high-protein supplement
    His-Purkinje system
    human platelet suspension
    hypertrophic pyloric stenosis
    hypothalamic pubertal syn-
        drome
HPSC — hippocampal sclerosis
HPSL — Health Professions Stu-
    dent Loan
HPT —
    histamine provocation test
    hot plate test
    hyperparathyroidism
    hypothalamo-pituitary-
        thyroid [system]
hPT — human placental thyrotro-
    pin
HPTH —
    hyperparathyroid hormone
    hyperparathyroidism

hPTH — human parathyroid hor-
    mone
HPTIN — human pancreatic tryp-
    sin inhibitor
HPTM — home prothrombin time
    monitoring
HPU — heater probe unit
HPV —
    Haemophilus pertussis vaccine
    hepatic portal vein
    human papillomavirus
    human parvovirus
    human pulmonary vasocon-
        striction
    hypoxic pulmonary vasocon-
        striction
HPVD — hypertensive pulmonary
    vascular disease
HPV-DE — high-passage
    virus—duck embryo [cell]
HPV-DK — high-passage
    virus—dog kidney [cell]
HPVG — hepatic portal venous
    gas
HPW — hypergammaglobulinemic
    purpura of Waldenström
HPX —
    high peroxide-containing
        [cell]
    hypophysectomized
Hpx — hemopexin
HPZ — high-pressure zone
HQC — hydroquinone cream
HR —
    hallux rigidus
    Halstead-Reitan [battery]
    Hamman-Rich [syndrome]
    Harrington rod
    heart rate
    hemirectococcygeus
    hemorrhagic retinopathy
    heterosexual relations [scale]
    high resolution
    higher rate
    hormonal response
    hospital record
    hospital report
    hour

HR — *(continued)*
Howship-Romberg syndrome
human resources
hydroxyethylrutinosides
hyperimmune reaction
hypophosphatemic rickets
hypoxic responder
H&R — hysterectomy and radiation
2HR — two-hour pregnancy test
Hr. — blood type factor
hr. —
hairless [mouse]
host-range [mutant]
hour
HRA —
Health Resources Administration
health risk appraisal
heart rate audiometry
high right atrial
high right atrium
histamine-releasing activity
Human Resources Administration
HRAE — high right atrium electrogram
HRANA — histone-reactive antinuclear antibody
HRB —
Halstead-Reitan Battery
histamine release (from) basophils
HRBC — horse red blood cells
HRC —
help-rejecting complainer
high-resolution chromatography
horse red cells
human rights committee
HRCT — high-resolution computed tomography
HRE —
hepatic reticuloendothelial [cell]
high-resolution electrocardiogram
high-resolution electrocardiography

HRE — *(continued)*
hormone-receptor enzyme
HREC — hepatic reticuloendothelial cell
HREH — high-renin essential hypertension
HREM — high-resolution electron microscopy
HRF —
Harris return flow
histamine-releasing factor
HRH — hypothalamic-releasing hormone
HRI — Harrington rod instrumentation
HRIG — human rabies immunoglobulin
HRL — head rotation to the left
HRLA — human reovirus-like agent
HRLM — high-resolution light microscopy
hRNA — heterogeneous ribonucleic acid
HRNB — Halstead-Reitan Neuropsychological Battery
HRP —
high right parasternal [view]
high-risk patient
high-risk pregnancy
histidine-rich protein
horseradish peroxidase
HRPD — Hamburg Rating Scale for Psychiatric Disorders
HRR —
Hardy-Rand-Ritter [color vision test kit]
head rotation to the right
heart rate range
HRRI — heart rate retardation index
HRS —
Hamilton Rating Scale
hepatorenal syndrome
high rate of stimulation
hormone receptor site
humeroradial synostosis
HRSA — Health Resources and Services Administration

HRS-D —
  Hamilton Rating Scale for Depression
  Hirschsprung's disease
HRT —
  half relaxation time
  heart rate
  hormone replacement therapy
HRTE — human reverse transcriptase enzyme
HRTEM — high-resolution transmission electron microscopy
HRV —
  heart rate variability
  human reovirus
  human rotavirus
HRVL — human reovirus-like
HS —
  Haber syndrome
  half strength
  Hallervorden-Spatz [syndrome]
  hamstrings
  hand surgery
  Hartmann's solution
  head sign
  head sling
  healthy subject
  heart sounds
  heat-stable
  heavy smoker
  heel spur
  heelstick
  Hegglin's syndrome
  heme synthetase
  Henoch-Schönlein [purpura]
  heparan sulfate
  hereditary spherocytosis
  herpes simplex
  hidradenitis suppurativa
  hippocampal sclerosis
  homologous serum
  Hopelessness Scale
  hora somni (Lat.) at bedtime
  horizontally selective
  Horner's syndrome
  horse serum
  hospital ship

HS — *(continued)*
  hospital staff
  hospital stay
  hour of sleep
  house surgeon
  human serum
  Hurler's syndrome
  hypereosinophilic syndrome
  hypersensitivity
  hypertonic saline
H/S — helper-suppressor [ratio]
H&S —
  hemorrhage and shock
  hysterectomy and sterilization
H→S — heel-to-shin
H_2S — hydrogen sulfide
Hs — hypochondriasis
h.s. — *hora somni* (Lat.) at bedtime
HSA —
  Hazardous Substances Act
  health service area
  Health Services Administration
  Health Systems Agency
  hereditary sideroblastic anemia
  horse serum albumin
  human serum albumin
  hypersomnia-sleep apnea [syndrome]
HSAG — *N*-2-hydroxyethylpiperazine-*N*-2-ethanesulfonate-saline-albumin-gelatin
HSAN — hereditary sensory and autonomic neuropathy
HSAP — heat-stable alkaline phosphatase
HSAS — hypertrophic subaortic stenosis
HSBG — heelstick blood gas
HSC —
  Hand-Schüller-Christian [syndrome]
  Health and Safety Commission
  health sciences center
  health screening center
  hematopoietic stem cell

HSC — (*continued*)
  horizontal semicircular canal
  human skin collagenase
HSCD — Hand-Schüller-
  Christian disease
HSCL — Hopkins Symptom
  Check List
HS-CoA — reduced coenzyme A
HSD —
  honest significant difference
  hydroxysteroid dehydrogenase
H(SD) — Holtzman Sprauge-Daw-
  ley [ratio]
HSDA — high single dose alternate day
HSDB — Hazardous Substances
  Data Bank
HSDI — Health Self-Determina-
  tion Index
HSE —
  herpes simplex encephalitis
  hemorrhagic shock and en-
    cephalopathy
  human serum esterase
Hse — homoserine
HSES — hemorrhagic shock–
  encephalopathy syndrome
HSF —
  histamine-induced suppressor
    factor
  histamine-sensitizing factor
  human serum esterase
  hydrazine-sensitive factor
  hypothalamic secretory factor
HSG —
  herpes simplex genitalis
  hysterosalpingogram
  hysterosalpingography
hSGF — human skeletal growth
  factor
HSGP — human sialoglycoprotein
HSHC — hemisuccinate (of) hydrocortisone
HSI —
  heat stress index
  herpes simplex I
  human seminal (plasma) in-
    hibitor

H_2SiO_3 — metasilicic acid
H_4SiO_4 — orthosilicic acid
HSK — herpes simplex keratitis
HSL — herpes simplex labialis
HSLC — high-speed liquid chromatography
HSM —
  hepatosplenomegaly
  holosystolic murmur
HSMHA — Health Services and
  Mental Health Administration
HSN —
  Hanson-Street nail
  hereditary sensory neuropathy
  herpes simplex neonatorum
H_2SO_3 — sulfurous acid
H_2SO_4 — sulfuric acid
hSOD — human superoxide dismutase
h. som. — *hora somni* (Lat.) at bedtime
HSP —
  Health Systems Plan
  hemostatic screening profile
  Henoch-Schönlein purpura
  hereditary spastic paraparesis
  Hospital Service Plan
  human serum prealbumin
  human serum protein
  hysterosalpingography
hsp — heat shock protein [gene]
HS-PG — heparan sulfate-proteo-
  glycan
HSPM — hippocampal synaptic
  plasma membrane
HSPN — Henoch-Schönlein purpura nephritis
HSQB — Health Standards and
  Quality Bureau
HSR —
  Harleco synthetic resin
  heated serum reagent
  homogeneously staining re-
    gions [of chromosome]
HSRA — Health Services and Resources Administration
HSRC —
  Health Services Research
    Center

HSRC — *(continued)*
    Human Subjects Review
        Committee
HSRD — hypertension secondary
    to renal disease
HSRI — Health Systems Research
    Institute
HSRS —
    Health-Sickness Rating Scale
    Hess School Readiness Scale
HSRV — human spuma retrovirus
HSS —
    Hallerman-Streiff syndrome
    Hallervorden-Spatz syndrome
    Henoch-Schönlein syndrome
    hepatic stimulator substance
    high-speed supernatant
    hyperstimulation syndrome
    hypertrophic subaortic steno-
        sis
HSSCC — hereditary site-specific
    colon cancer
HSSE — high soapsuds enema
HST —
    health screening test(s)
    Hemoccult slide test
    horseshoe tear
HSTF — human serum thymus fac-
    tor
HSTK — herpes simplex thymi-
    dine kinase
HSTS — human-specific thyroid
    stimulator
HSV —
    herpes simplex virus
    highly selective vagotomy
    hop stunt viroid
    hyperviscosity syndrome
HSV-1 — herpes simplex virus 1
HSV-2 — herpes simplex virus 2
HSVE — herpes simplex virus en-
    cephalitis
HSVtk — herpes simplex virus thy-
    midine kinase
HSyn — heme synthase
HT —
    hammertoe
    Hashimoto's thyroiditis

HT — *(continued)*
    hearing test
    hearing threshold
    heart
    heart transplant
    heart transplantation
    height
    hemagglutination titer
    hereditary tyrosinemia
    high temperature
    high tension
    high-frequency transduction
    histologic technician
    histologic technologist
    home treatment
    hospital treatment
    Hubbard tank
    Huhner test
    human thrombin
    hydrocortisone test
    hydrotherapy
    hydroxytryptamine
    hypermetropia, total
    hyperopia, total
    hypertension
    hyperthyroidism
    hypertransfusion
    hypertropia
    hypothalamus
    hypothyroidism
H&T — hospitalization and treat-
    ment
3-HT — 3-hydroxytyramine (dopa-
    mine)
^{3}HT — tritiated thymidine
5-HT — 5-hydroxytryptamine
    (serotonin)
Ht —
    heart
    height
    height of heart
    heterozygote
    hyperopia
    hypothalamus
    total
ht —
    heart
    heart tone

ht — (continued)
  heat
  height
  high tension
ht. — *haustus* (Lat.) a draft, drink
HTA —
  heterophil transplantation antigen
  human thymocyte antigen
  5-hydroxytryptamine
  hypophysiotropic area
HTACS — human thyroid adenylate cyclase stimulators
ht. aer. — heated aerosol
HT(ASCP) — Histologic Technician certified by the American Society of Clinical Pathologists
HTAT — human tetanus antitoxin
HTB —
  hot tub bath
  house tube [feeding]
  human tumor bank
HTC —
  hepatoma cell
  hepatoma tissue culture
  homozygous typing cells
  hypertensive crisis
HTCA — human tumor clonogenic assay
HTCFA — human tumor colony–forming assay
HTCVD — hypertensive cardiovascular disease
HTD — human therapeutic dose
³H-TdR — tritium-labeled thymidine
HTDW — heterosexual development of women
HTF —
  heterothyrotropic factor
  house tube feeding
HTG — hypertriglyceridemia
HTH — homeostatic thymus hormone
Hth — hypothalamus
HTHD — hypertensive heart disease

HTI —
  hemispheric thrombotic infarction
  human tetanus immunoglobulin
HTIG — homologous tetanus immune globulin
hTIG — human tetanus immunoglobulin
HTK — heel-to-knee
HTL —
  hamster tumor line
  hearing threshold level
  histologic technologist
  histotechnologist
  human T-cell leukemia
  human T-cell lymphoma
  human thymic leukemia
  hypermetropia, left
HTLA —
  high titer, low acidity
  human thymus-lymphocyte antigen
HTL(ASCP) — Histotechnologist certified by the American Society of Clinical Pathologists
HTLV —
  human T-cell leukemia/lymphoma virus
  human T-cell lymphotropic virus
HTLV-MA — human T-cell leukemia virus–associated membrane antigen
HTLV-I-MA — human T-cell leukemia virus-I–associated membrane antigen
HTN —
  Hantaan-[like virus]
  hypertension
  hypertensive
  hypertensive nephropathy
HTO —
  heterotropic ossification
  high tibial osteotomy
  hospital transfer order
  tritiated water
HTOH — hydroxytryptophol

HTOR — 5-hydroxytryptamine oxygenase regulator
HTP —
House-Tree-Person [test]
hydroxytryptophan
hypothromboplastinemia
5-HTP — 5-hydroxy-L-tryptophan
HtPA — hexahydrophthalic anhydride
HTPN — home total parenteral nutrition
HTR — hypermetropia, right
hTR-beta — human thyroid receptor-beta
HTS —
head traumatic syndrome
heel-to-shin [test]
hemangioma-thrombocytopenia syndrome
human thyroid-stimulating hormone
human thyroid stimulator
hTSAB — human thyroid-stimulating antibody
HTSCA — human tumor stem cell assay
hTSH — human thyroid-stimulating hormone
HTST — high temperature, short time
HTT — hand thrust test
HTV — herpes-type virus
HTVD — hypertensive vascular disease
HTX —
hemothorax
histrionicotoxin
HU —
head unit
heat unit
hemagglutinating unit
hemagglutinin unit
hemolytic unit
Hounsfield unit
human urinary
human urine
hydroxyurea
hyperemia unit

Hu — human
HUC — hypouricemia
HuEPO — human erythropoietin
HU-FSH — human urinary follicle-stimulating hormone
HUI — headache unit index
HUIFM — human leukocyte interferon milieu
HuIFN — human interferon
HUIS — high-dose urea in invert sugar
HUK — human urinary kallikrein
HUM —
heat or hot packs, ultrasound, and massage
hematourimetry
Hum — humerus
HUP — Hospital Utilization Project
HUR — hydroxyurea
HURA — health in underserved rural areas
HURT — hospital utilization review team
HUS —
hemolytic-uremic syndrome
hyaluronidase unit for semen
HuSA — human serum albumin
husb — husband
hut — histidine utilization [gene]
HUTHAS — human thymus antiserum
HUV — human umbilical vein
HV —
hallux valgus
Hantaan virus
has voided
heart volume
Hemovac
hepatic vein
hepatic venous
herpesvirus
high voltage
high volume
home visit
hospital visit
hyperventilation
H&V — hemigastrectomy and vagotomy

h.v. — *hoc vespere* (Lat.) this evening

HVA — homovanillic acid

HVAC — heating, ventilating, and air conditioning

HVC — Health Visitor's Certificate

HVc — hyperstriatum ventrale, pars caudale

HVD —
hypertensive vascular disease
hypoxic ventilatory drive

HVE —
hepatic venous effluence
high-voltage electrophoresis

HUVEC — human umbilical vein endothelial cell

HVEM — high-voltage electron microscope

HVF — hepatocycle volume fraction

HVFP — hepatic vein free pressure

HVG —
hematoxylin and van Gieson [stain]
host versus graft

HVGS — high-voltage galvanic stimulation

HVH — Herpesvirus hominis

HVHMA — Herpesvirus hominis membrane antigen

HVID — horizontal visible iris diameter

HVJ — hemagglutinating virus of Japan

HVL — half-value layer

HVLP — high volume, low pressure

HVLT — high-velocity lead therapy

HVM —
high-velocity missile
hypothalamic ventromedial [nucleus]

HVPC — high-voltage pulsed current

HVPE — high-voltage paper electrophoresis

HVPG — hepatic venous pressure gradient

HVR — hypoxic ventilation response

HVS —
herpesvirus of Saimiri
herpesvirus sensitivity
hyperventilation syndrome
hyperviscosity syndrome

H vs A — home versus (against) advice

HVSD — hydrogen-detected ventricular septal defect

HVT —
half-value thickness
herpesvirus of turkeys

HVTEM — high-voltage transmission electron microscopy

HVUS — hypocomplementemic vasculitis-urticaria syndrome

HW —
Hayrem-Widal [syndrome]
healing well
heart weight
hemisphere width
heparin well
Hertwig-Weyers [syndrome]
housewife

HWB — hot water bottle

HWC — Health and Welfare, Canada

HWD — heartworm disease

HWE —
healthy worker effect
hot water extract

HWOK — heel walking normal (OK)

HWP —
hepatic wedge pressure
hot wet pack
Hutchinson-Weber-Pentz [syndrome]

HWRS — Habits of Work and Recreation Survey

HWS — hot water–soluble

HWY — hundred woman years [of exposure]

HX —
histiocytosis X

HX — *(continued)*
    history
    hospitalization
    hydrogen exchange
    hypophysectomized
    hypoxanthine
Hx. —
    history
    hypoxanthine
2-HxG — di(hydroxyethyl)glycine
HXIS — hard x-ray imaging spectrometry
HXM — hexamethylmelamine
HXR — hypoxanthine riboside
HXV — herpes simplex virus
HY — hypophysis
Hy —
    history
    hydraulics
    hydrostatics
    hypermetropia
    hyperopia
    hypophysis
    hypothenar
    hysteria
hy — hysteria
HYD —
    hydralazine
    hydrated
    hydration
    hydrocortisone
    hydroxyurea
Hyd —
    hydrocortisone
    hydrostatics
hyd and tur — hydration and turgor
HYD-PR — hydroxyproline
hydr — hydraulic
hydrarg. — *hydrargyrum* (Lat.) "liquid silver" (mercury)
hydro — hydrotherapy
hydrox — hydroxyline
hyg. —
    hygiene
    hygienic
    hygienist
HYL — hydroxylysine

HYP —
    hydroxyproline
    hypnosis
Hyp. —
    hydroxyproline
    hyperresonance
    hypertrophy
    hypothalamus
    hypoxanthine
hyp. —
    hypalgesia
    hypophysectomy
    hypophysis
hyper A — hyperactive
hyperal — hyperalimentation
hyper-IgE — hyperimmunoglobulinemia E
hyperpara — hyperparathyroidism
hyper T&A — hypertrophy of tonsils and adenoids
hypes — hypesthesia
hypn. — hypertension
hypno. —
    hypnosis
    hypnotism
Hypo. —
    hypochromasia
    hypochromia
    hypodermic
hypo A — hypoactive
hypox. — hypophysectomized
HYPP — hypersegmented neutrophil
HypRF — hypothalamic-releasing factor
hypro — hydroxyproline
hyst —
    hysterectomy
    hysteria
    hysterical
HZ — herpes zoster
Hz — hertz
HZFO — hamster zona-free ovum [test]
HZO — herpes zoster ophthalmicus
HZV — herpes zoster virus

I — (continued)

electric current
implantation
impression
inactive
incisal
incisor
increased
independent
index
indicated
induction
inertia
inhalation
inhibition
inhibitor
initial
inosine
insoluble
inspiration
inspired
insulin
intact
intake
intensity of magnetism
intercalary
intermediate
intermittent
internal medicine
internist
intestine
iodide
iodine
ionic strength
iota (ninth letter of the
   Greek alphabet), uppercase
iris
isochromosome
isoleucine
isotope
isotropic
luminous intensity
moment of inertia
permanent incisor

I — (continued)
   region of a sarcomere that
      contains only actin fila-
      ments
^{123}I — radioactive iodine
^{125}I — radioactive iodine
^{130}I — radioactive iodine
^{131}I — radioactive iodine
^{132}I — radioactive iodine
i —
   incisor [deciduous]
   insoluble
   isochromosome
   optically inactive
ι — iota (ninth letter of the Greek
   alphabet), lowercase
IA —
   ibotenic acid
   image amplification
   immune adherence
   immunoadsorbent
   immunobiologic activity
   impedance angle
   inactive alcoholic
   incidental appendectomy
   incurred accidentally
   indolaminergic accumulation
   indolic acid
   indulin agar
   infantile apnea
   infected area
   inferior angle
   inhibitory antigen
   internal auditory
   intra-alveolar
   intra-amniotic
   intra-aortic
   intra-arterial
   intra-articular
   intra-atrial
   intra-auricular
   intrinsic activity
   isonicotinic acid
I&A — irrigation and aspiration

Ia — immune (response gene)-associated antigen

IAA —
imidazoleacetic acid
indoleacetic acid
infectious agent, arthritis
insulin autoantibody
International Antituberculosis
    Association
interruption of the aortic arch
iodoacetic acid

I-3-AA — indole-3-acetic acid

IAAR — imidazoleacetic acid ribonucleotide

IAB —
Industrial Accident Board
intra-abdominal
intra-aortic balloon

IABA — intra-aortic balloon assistance

IABC — intra-aortic balloon catheter

IABCP — intra-aortic balloon counterpulsation

IABM — idiopathic aplastic bone marrow

IABP — intra-aortic balloon pump

IABPA — intra-aortic balloon pumping assistance

IAC —
ineffective airway clearance
internal auditory canal
interposed abdominal compression
intra-arterial catheter
intra-arterial chemotherapy
isolated adrenal cell

IACB — intra-aortic counterpulsation balloon

IAC-CPR — interposed abdominal compressions—cardiopulmonary resuscitation

IACD —
implantable automatic cardioverter-defibrillator
intra-atrial conduction defect

IACP — intra-aortic counterpulsation

IACPA — Inter-American Council of Psychiatric Associations

IACS — International Academy of Cosmetic Surgery

IACVF — International Association of Cancer Victims and Friends

IAD —
inactivating dose
inhibiting antibiotic dose
internal absorbed dose

IADH — inappropriate antidiuretic hormone

IADHS — inappropriate antidiuretic hormone syndrome

IADL — instrumental activities of daily living

IADR — International Association for Dental Research

IAds — immunoadsorption

IA-DSA — intra-arterial digital subtraction arteriography

IAE —
intra-arterial electrocardiogram
intra-atrial electrocardiogram

IAEA — International Atomic Energy Agency

IAFI — infantile amaurotic familial idiocy

IAG —
International Association of Gerontology
International Academy of Gnathology

IAGP — International Association of Geographic Pathology

IAGT — indirect antiglobulin test

IAGUS — International Association of Genito-Urinary Surgeons

IAH —
idiopathic adrenal hyperplasia
implantable artificial heart

IAHA —
idiopathic autoimmune hemolytic anemia
immune adherence hemagglutination assay

IAHD — idiopathic acquired hemolytic disease

IAHP — International Association of Heart Patients

IAHS —
- infection-associated hemophagocytic syndrome
- International Association of Hospital Security

IAI — intra-abdominal infection

IAIMS — Integrated Academic Information Management System

IAIS — insulin autoimmune syndrome

IAL — International Association of Laryngectomees

IAM —
- Institute of Applied Microbiology [Japan]
- Institute of Aviation Medicine
- internal acoustic meatus
- internal auditory meatus
- intercellular adhesion molecules

iam — intra-amniotic

IAMM — International Association of Medical Museums

IAN —
- idiopathic aseptic necrosis
- indole acetonitrile
- interim admission note
- intern admission note

IANP — immunoreactive atrial natriuretic peptide

IAO —
- immediately after onset
- intermittent aortic occlusion
- International Association of Orthodontists

I and O — intake and output

IAOM — International Association of Oral Myology

IAP —
- immunosuppressive acidic protein
- innervated antral pouch

IAP — (continued)
- inosinic acid pyrophosphorylase
- Institute of Animal Physiology
- intermittent acute porphyria
- International Academy of Pathology
- International Academy of Proctology
- intra-abdominal pressure
- intracisternal A-type particle
- islet-activating protein

IAPB — International Association for Prevention of Blindness

IAPG — interatrial pressure gradient

IAPM — International Academy of Preventive Medicine

IAPP —
- International Association for Preventive Pediatrics
- islet amyloid polypeptide

IAR —
- immediate asthmatic reaction
- inhibitory anal reflex
- iodine-azide reaction

IARC — International Agency for Research on Cancer

IARF — ischemic acute renal failure

IARSA — idiopathic acquired refractory sideroblastic anemia

IAS —
- idiopathic ankylosing spondylitis
- immunosuppressive acidic substance
- infant apnea syndrome
- insulin autoimmune syndrome
- interatrial septum
- interatrial shunting
- internal anal sphincter
- intra-amniotic saline [infusion]

IASA — interatrial septal aneurysm

IASD —
- interatrial septal defect

IASD — (continued)
   interauricular septal defect
IASH — isolated asymmetric septal hypertrophy
IASHS — Institute for Advanced Study in Human Sexuality
IASL — International Association for Study of the Liver
IASP — International Association for Study of Pain
IAT —
   immunoaugmentative therapy
   indirect antiglobulin test
   instillation abortion time
   invasive activity test
   iodine-azide test
   Iowa Achievement Test
IAV —
   interactive video
   intermittent assisted ventilation
   intra-arterial vasopressin
IAVM — intramedullary arteriovenous malformation
IB —
   Ibrahim-Beck [disease]
   idiopathic blepharospasm
   ileal bypass
   immune balance
   immune body
   inclusion body
   index of body build
   infectious bronchitis
   Institute of Biology
   isolation bed
ib. — ibidem (Lat.) in the same place
IBA —
   isobutyric acid
   Industrial Biotechnology Association
I band — isotropic band
IBAT — intravascular bronchoalveolar tumor
IBB — intestinal brush border
IBBB — intrablood-brain barrier
IBBBB — incomplete bilateral bundle branch block

IBC —
   Institutional Biosafety Committee
   iodine-binding capacity
   iron-binding capacity
IBCA — isobutyl-2-cyanoacrylate
IBD —
   infectious bowel disease
   inflammatory bowel disease
   irritable bowel disease
   ischemic bowel disease
IBE — International Bureau for Epilepsy
IBED — Inter-African Bureau for Epizootic Diseases
iB-EP — immunoreactive beta-endomorphin
IBF —
   immature brown fat [cells]
   immunoglobulin-binding factor
   Insall-Burstein-Freeman [total knee instrumentation]
IBG — insoluble bone gelatin
IBI —
   intermittent bladder irrigation
   ischemic brain infarction
ibid. — ibidem (Lat.) in the same place
ibili — indirect bilirubin
IBK — infectious bovine keratoconjunctivitis
IBL — immunoblastic lymphadenopathy
IBM —
   inclusion body myositis
   isotonic-isometric brief maximum
IBMP — International Board of Medicine and Psychology
IBMX — 3-isobutyl-L-methylxanthine
IBNR — incurred but not reported
IBO — ibotenic acid
IBOW — intact bag of waters
IBP —
   International Biological Program

IBP — *(continued)*
    intra-aortic balloon pumping
    iron-binding protein
IBPMS — indirect blood pressure measuring system
IBQ — Illness Behavior Questionnaire
IBR — infectious bovine rhinotracheitis
IBRO — International Brain Research Organization
IBRS — Inpatient Behavior Rating Scale
IBRV — infectious bovine rhinotracheitis virus
IBS —
    imidazole buffered saline
    immunoblastic sarcoma
    Interpersonal Behavior Survey
    irritable bowel syndrome
    isobaric solution
IBSA —
    immunoreactive bovine serum albumin
    iodinated bovine serum albumin
IBSN — infantile bilateral striated necrosis
IBT —
    ink blot test
    isatin-beta-thiosemicarbasone
IBTR — ipsilateral breast tumor recurrence
IBU —
    ibuprofen
    international benzoate unit
i-Bu — isobutyl
IBV —
    infectious bronchitis vaccine
    infectious bronchitis virus
IBW — ideal body weight
IC —
    icteric
    icterus
    ileocecal
    iliococcygeal
    iliocostal
    immune complex

IC — *(continued)*
    immunocompromised
    immunoconjugate
    immunocytochemistry
    immunocytotoxicity
    impedance cardiogram
    incomplete
    indirect calorimetry
    indirect Coombs' [test]
    individual counseling
    infection control
    inferior colliculus
    inhibitory concentration
    inner canthal [distance]
    inorganic carbon
    inspiratory capacity
    inspiratory center
    Institutional Care
    integrated circuit
    integrated concentration
    intensive care
    intercarpal
    intercostal
    intermediate care
    intermittent catheterization
    intermittent claudication
    internal capsule
    internal carotid
    internal cerebral
    internal cholecystectomy
    internal conjugate [diameter]
    International Classification
    interstitial cells
    interstitial change
    intracapsular
    intracardiac
    intracarotid
    intra cavitary
    intracellular
    intracellular concentration
    intracerebral
    intracisternal
    intracoronary
    intracranial
    intracutaneous
    intrapleural catheter
    irritable colon
    islet cells

IC — (continued)
　isovolumic contraction
IC$_{50}$ — inhibitory concentration of
　50%
i.c. — inter cibos (Lat.) between
　meals
ICA —
　Institute of Clinical Analysis
　intercountry adoption
　intermediate care area
　internal carotid artery
　intracranial aneurysm
　islet cell antibody
iCa — ionized calcium
ICAA —
　International Council on Al-
　　cohol and Addictions
　Invalid Children's Aid Associ-
　　ation
ICAb — islet cell antibody
ICAF — internal carotid artery
　flow
ICAM-1 — intercellular adhesion
　molecule 1
ICAM-2 — intercellular adhesion
　molecule 2
ICAMI — International Commit-
　tee Against Mental Illness
ICAO — internal carotid artery oc-
　clusion
ICAP — intracisternal A particle
ICAV — intracavitary
ICB — intracranial bleeding
ICBF — inner cortical blood flow
ICBP — intracellular binding pro-
　tein
ICBR — increased chromosomal
　breakage rate
ICBT — intercostobronchial trunk
ICC —
　immunocompetent cells
　immunocytochemistry
　Indian childhood cirrhosis
　intensive coronary care
　intercanthal distance
　interchromosomal crossing
　　over
　interclass correlation coeffi-
　　cient

ICC — (continued)
　intermediate cell column
　intermittent clean catheteriza-
　　tion
　Internal Conversion Coeffi-
　　cient
　International Certification
　　Commission
　intracervical device
　intraclass correlation coeffi-
　　cient
　islet cell carcinoma
ICCE — intracapsular cataract ex-
　traction
iCCK — immunoreactive cholecys-
　tokinin
ICCM — idiopathic congestive
　cardiomyopathy
ICCR — International Committee
　for Contraceptive Research
ICCU —
　intensive coronary care unit
　intermediate coronary care
　　unit
ICD —
　I-cell disease
　immune complex disease
　implantable cardioverter-de-
　　fibrillator
　inclusion cell disease
　induced circular dichroism
　instantaneous cardiac death
　Institute for Crippled and Dis-
　　abled
　intercanthal distance
　internal cervical device
　International Center for the
　　Disabled
　International Classification of
　　Diseases of the World
　　Health Organization
　International College of Den-
　　tists
　intracervical device
　intrauterine contraceptive de-
　　vice
　ischemic coronary disease
　isocitrate dehydrogenase

ICD — *(continued)*
isolated conduction defect
ICDA — International Classification of Diseases, Adapted
ICDC — implantable cardioverter-defibrillator catheter
ICDCD — International Classification of Diseases and Causes of Death
ICD-9-CM — International Classification of Diseases-Ninth Revision, Clinical Modification
ICDH —
isocitrate dehydrogenase
isocitric dehydrogenase
ICD-O — International Classification of Diseases-Oncology
ICDRC — International Contact Dermatitis Research Center
ICDS — Integrated Child Development Scheme
ICE —
ice, compression and elevation
ichthyosis-cheek-eyebrow [syndrome]
iridocorneal endothelial [syndrome]
ICEA — International Childbirth Education Association
ICES —
ice, compression, elevation, and support
information collection and evaluation system
ICET — Item Counseling Evaluation Test
ICF —
indirect centrifugal flotation
intensive care facility
intercellular fluorescence
interciliary fluid
intermediate-care facility
International Cardiology Foundation
intracellular fluid
intravascular coagulation and fibrinolysis

ICFA —
incomplete Freund's adjuvant
induced complement-fixing antigen
ICF(M)A — International Cystic Fibrosis (Mucoviscidosis) Association
ICFMR — Intermediate-Care Facility for the Mentally Retarded
Icfx — intracapsular fracture
ICG —
indocyanine green
isotope cisternography
ICGC — indocyanine-green clearance
ICGN — immune-complex glomerulonephritis
ICH —
idiopathic cortical hyperostosis
immunocompromised host
infectious canine hepatitis
intracerebral hematoma
intracerebral hemorrhage
intracerebral hypertension
intracranial hemorrhage
intracranial hypertension
ICHD —
Inter-Society Commission for Heart Disease Resources
ischemic coronary heart disease
ICHPPC —
International Classification of Health Problems in Primary Care
interpersonal communication inventory
ICI — intracardiac injection
ICIC —
International Cancer Information Center
intracisternal
ICIDH — International Classification of Impairments, Disabilities, and Handicaps
ICJ — ileocecal junction

ICL —
   idiopathic CD4 T-cell lymphocytopenia
   intracorneal lens
   iris-clip lens
   isocitrate lyase
ICLA — International Committee on Laboratory Animals
ICLE — intracapsular lens extraction
ICLH — Imperial College, London Hospital
ICM —
   infracostal margin
   inner cell mass
   intercostal margin
   International Confederation of Midwives
   intracytoplasmic membrane
   ion conductance modulator
   ipsilateral competing message
   isolated cardiovascular malformation
ICMI — Inventory of Childhood Memories and Imaginings
ICMSF — International Commission on Microbiological Specifications for Foods
ICN —
   infection control nurse
   intensive care neonatal
   intensive care nursery
   intermediate care nursery
   International Council of Nurses
ICNa — intracellular concentration of sodium
ICNC — intracerebral nuclear cell
ICNND — Interdepartmental Committee on Nutrition in National Defense
ICNV — International Committee on Nomenclature of Viruses
ICO —
   idiopathic cyclic oedema
   impedance cardiac output
ICP —
   incubation period

ICP — (continued)
   inductively coupled plasma
   indwelling catheter program
   Infection-Control Practitioner
   infectious cell protein
   inflammatory cloacogenic polyp
   intermittent catheterization protocol
   intracranial pressure
   intracytoplasmic
ICPA — International Commission for the Prevention of Alcoholism
ICPB — International Collection of Phytopathogenic Bacteria
ICPC — intracranial pressure catheter
ICPEMC — International Commission for Protection against Environmental Mutagens and Carcinogens
ICPI — Intersociety Committee on Pathology Information
ICPMM — incisors, canines, premolars, and molars
ICPP —
   intubated continuous positive-pressure
   Isochromic Color Perception Plates
ICPS — Interpersonal Cognitive Problem Solving
ICR —
   (distance between) iliac crests
   Institute for Cancer Research
   Institute for Cancer Research [mouse]
   intermittent catheter routine
   international calibrated ratio
   International Congress of Radiology
   intracardiac catheter recording
   intracavitary radium
   intracranial reinforcement
   ion cyclotron resonance
ICRC — International Committee of the Red Cross

ICRD — Index of Codes for Research Drugs
ICRETT — International Cancer Research Technology Transfer
ICREW — International Cancer Research Workshop
ICRF — Imperial Cancer Research Fund (British)
I-CRF — immunoreactive corticotropin-releasing factor
ICRF-159 — razoxane
ICRFSDD — Independent Citizens Research Foundation for the Study of Degenerative Diseases
ICRP — International Commission on Radiological Protection
ICRS — Index Chemicus Registry System
ICRU — International Commission on Radiological Units and Measurements
ICS —
    ileocecal sphincter
    immotile cilia syndrome
    Imperial College of Science (British)
    impulse-conducting system
    intensive care, surgical
    intercellular space
    intercostal space
    International Cardiovascular Study
    International College of Surgeons
    International Craniopathic Society
    intracellular-like solution
    intracranial stimulation
    irritable colon syndrome
ICSA — islet cell surface antibody
ICSC — idiopathic central serous chorioretinopathy
ICSH —
    International Committee for Standardization in Hematology
    interstitial cell-stimulating hormone

ICSI — intracytoplasmic sperm injection
ICSO — intermittent coronary sinus occlusion
ICSP — International Council of Societies of Pathology
ICSS — intracranial self-stimulation
ICSU — International Council of Scientific Unions
ICT —
    icteric
    icterus
    immunoglobulin consumption test
    indirect Coombs' test
    inflammation of connective tissue
    insulin coma therapy
    insulin convulsive therapy
    intensive conventional therapy
    intermittent cervical traction
    interstitial cell tumor
    intracardiac thrombus
    intracranial tumor
    intradermal cancer test
    intraoral cariogenicity test
    isometric contraction time
    isovolumic contraction time
Ict — icterus
iCT — immunoreactive calcitonin
ICTH — International Committee on Thrombosis and Homeostasis
ict. ind. — icterus index
ICTMM — International Congress on Tropical Medicine and Malaria
ICTS — idiopathic carpal tunnel syndrome
ICTV — International Committee on Taxonomy of Viruses
ICTX — intermittent cervical traction
ICU —
    immunologic contact urticaria
    infant care unit

ICU — (continued)
    intensive care unit
    intermediate care unit
ICV —
    intracellular volume
    intracerebroventricular
ICVH — ischemic cerebrovascular
    headache
ICVS — International Cardiovas-
    cular Society
ICW —
    intact canal wall
    intensive care ward
    intracellular water
ICx — immune complex
ID —
    identification
    identify
    iditol dehydrogenase
    ill-defined
    immunodeficiency
    immunodiffusion
    immunoglobulin deficiency
    inappropriate disability
    inclusion disease
    index of discrimination
    individual dose
    induction delivery
    infant death
    infectious disease
    infective dose
    inferior division
    inhibitory dose
    inhomogeneous deposition
    initial diagnosis
    initial dose
    initial dyskinesia
    injected dose
    inside diameter
    insufficient data
    interdigitating [cells]
    interhemispheric discon-
      nection
    internal diameter
    interstitial disease
    intradermal
    intraduodenal
    isosorbide dinitrate

I&D —
    incision and drainage
    irrigation and débridement
    irrigation and drainage
I-D — intensity-duration
ID_{50} —
    median infectious dose
    median infective dose
Id —
    idiotypic
    infradentale
    interdentale
id. — idem (Lat.) the same
i.d. —
    in diem (Lat.) during the day
    intradermal
IDA —
    image display and analysis
    iminodiacetic acid
    insulin-degrading activity
    iron deficiency anemia
id. ac — idem ac (Lat.) the same as
IDAMIS — Integrated Dose Abuse
    Management Informational
    Systems
IDARP — Integrated Drug Abuse
    Reporting Process
IDAT — indirect antiglobulin test
IDAV — immunodeficiency-
    associated virus
IDBR — indirect bilirubin
IDBS — infantile diffuse brain scle-
    rosis
IDC —
    idiopathic dilated cardiomyop-
      athy
    interdigitating cells
IDCF — immunodiffusion comple-
    ment fixation
IDCI — intradiplochromatid inter-
    change
IDD —
    insulin-dependent diabetes
    intraluminal duodenal diver-
      ticulum
    Inventory to Diagnose Depres-
      sion
IDDF — investigational drug data
    form

IDDM — insulin-dependent diabetes mellitus

IDDS —
> implantable drug delivery system
> investigational drug data sheet

IDDT — immune double diffusion test

IDE —
> inner dental epithelium
> Investigational Device Exemption

ID/ED — internal diameter to external diameter

IDEM — ischemic, drug, electrolyte, metabolic [effect]

IDFC — immature dead female child

IDG —
> interdisciplinary group
> intermediate dose group

IDH — isocitric dehydrogenase

IDH-M — isocitric dehydrogenase, mitochondrial

IDH-S — isocitric dehydrogenase, soluble

IDI —
> immunologically detectable insulin
> induction-delivery interval
> interdentale inferius
> Instant Drug Index

IDIC — Internal Dose Information Center

idic — isodicentric

IDISA — intraoperative digital subtraction angiography

IDK — internal derangement of knee

IDL —
> Index to Dental Literature
> intermediate-density lipoprotein

IDLH — immediate danger to life and health

IDM —
> idiopathic disease of the myocardium

IDM — (continued)
> immune defense mechanism
> indirect method
> infant of diabetic mother
> intermediate-dose methotrexate

IDMC —
> immature dead male child
> interdigestive motility complex

IDMEC — interdigestive myoelectric complex

IDMS — isotope dilution-mass spectrometry

IDNA — intercalary deoxyribonucleic acid

idon. vehic. — *idoneo vehiculo* (Lat.) in a suitable vehicle

IDP —
> imidoliphosphonate
> immunodiffusion procedure
> initial dose period
> inosine diphosphate
> instantaneous diastolic pressure

IDPase — inosine diphosphatase

IDPH — idiopathic pulmonary hemosiderosis

IDPN — beta-iminodipropionitrile

IDR — intradermal reaction

IDS —
> immunity deficiency state
> incremented dynamic scanning
> Infectious Disease Service
> inhibitor of DNA synthesis
> intraduodenal stimulation
> investigational drug service
> Investigative Dermatological Society

IdS — interdentale superius

IDSA —
> Infectious Disease Society of America
> intraoperative digital subtraction angiography

IDSAN — International Drug Safety Advisory Network

IDT —
  immune diffusion test
  instillation delivery time
  interdivision time
  International Diagnostic
    Technology
  intradermal typhoid [vaccine]
IDU —
  idoxuridine
  injection or intravenous drug
    user
  iododeoxyuridine
IdUA — iduronic acid
IDUR — idoxuridine
IdUrd — idoxuridine
IDV — intermittent demand ventilation
IDVC — indwelling venous catheter
Idx — cross-reactive idiotype
IE —
  immunitäts Einheit (Ger.) im-
    munizing unit
  immunoelectrophoresis
  induced emesis
  infectious endocarditis
  inner ear
  intake energy
  internal ear
  internal elastica
  intraepithelial
  Introversion-Extraversion
    [scale]
I/E — inspiratory/expiratory [ratio]
I&E — internal/external
i.e. — *id est* (Lat.) that is
IEA —
  immediate early antigen
  immunoelectroadsorption
  immunoelectrophoretic analy-
    sis
  immunoenzyme assay
  infectious equine anemia
  International Epidemiological
    Association
  intravascular erythrocyte ag-
    gregation
IEC —
  injection electrode catheter

IEC — *(continued)*
  inpatient exercise center
  intraepithelial carcinoma
  ion-exchange chromatography
IECa — intraepithelial carcinoma
IED — inherited epidermal dysplasia
IEE — inner enamel epithelium
IEEE — Institute of Electrical and
  Electronics Engineers
IEF —
  International Eye Foundation
  isoelectric focusing
IEI — isoelectric interval
IEL —
  internal elastic lamina
  intimal elastic lamina
  intraepithelial lymphocyte
IEM —
  immunoelectron microscopy
  inborn error of metabolism
IEMA — immunoenzymometric
  assay
IEMG — integrated electromyogram
IEOP — immunoelectro-
  osmophoresis
IEP —
  immunoelectrophoresis
  individualized education pro-
    gram
  isoelectric point
IER — Institute of Educational Research
IES — ingressive-egressive sequence
IF —
  idiopathic fibroplasia
  idiopathic flushing
  ifosfamide
  immersion foot
  immunofluorescence
  indirect fluorescence
  indirect immunofluoresence
  inferior facet
  infrared
  inhibiting factor
  initiation factor

IF — (continued)
    inspiratory force
    interferon
    interior facet
    intermaxillary fixation
    intermediate filament
    intermediate frequency
    internal fixation
    internal friction
    interstitial fluid
    intracellular fluid
    intrinsic factor
    involved field [radiotherapy]
IFA —
    idiopathic fibrosing alveolitis
    immunofluorescence assay
    immunofluorescent antibody
    incomplete Freund's adjuvant
    indirect fluorescent antibody
    indirect fluorescent assay
    International Fertility Association
    International Filariasis Association
IFAT — indirect fluorescent antibody test
IFC —
    inspiratory flow cartridge
    intermittent flow centrifugation
    intrinsic factor concentrate
IFCC — International Federation of Clinical Chemistry
IFCL — intermittent flow centrifugation leukapheresis
IFCR — International Foundation for Cancer Research
IFCS — inactivated fetal calf serum
IFDS —
    immunofixation electrophoresis
    isolated follicle-stimulating hormone deficiency syndrome
IFE — interfollicular epidermis
IFF — inner fracture of face
IFFH — International Foundation for Family Health

IFGO — International Federation of Gynecology and Obstetrics
IFGS — interstitial fluids and ground substance
IFHP — International Federation of Health Professionals
IFHPMSM — International Federation for Hygiene, Preventive Medicine, and Social Medicine
IFI — Institutional Functioning Inventory
IFIX — immunofixation
IFL — immunofluorescence
IFLrA — recombinant human leukocyte interferon A
IFM —
    internal fetal monitor
    intrafusal muscle
IFMBE — International Federation for Medical and Biological Engineering
IFME — International Federation for Medical Electronics
IFMP — International Federation for Medical Psychotherapy
IFMSA — International Federation of Medical Student Associations
IFMSS — International Federation of Multiple Sclerosis Societies
IFN —
    immunoreactive fibronectin
    interferon
if nec — if necessary
IFO — Institute for Fermentation (Japan)
IFOS — ifosfamide
IFP —
    inflammatory fibroid polyp
    insulin, compound F (hydrocortisone), prolactin
    intermediate filament protein
    intrapatellar fat pad
IFPM — International Federation of Physical Medicine
IFR —
    infrared

IFR — (continued)
  inspiratory flow rate
IFRA — indirect fluorescent rabies antibody [test]
IFRP — International Fertility Research Program
IFRT — involved field radiotherapy
IFS — interstitial fluid space
IFSM — International Federation of Sports Medicine
IFSSH — International Federation of Societies for Surgery of the Hand
IFT —
  immunofluorescence test
  International Frequency Tables
IFU — interferon unit
IFV —
  interstitial fluid volume
  intracellular fluid volume
IFX — ifosfamide
IG —
  immature granule
  immune globulin
  immunoglobulin
  intragastric
  irritable gut
I-G — insulin-glucagon
Ig — immunoglobulin
iG — immunoreactive human gastrin
IGA — infantile genetic agranulocytosis
IgA — immunoglobulin A
IgA1, IgA2 — subclasses of immunoglobulin A
IgAGN — immunoglobulin A glomerulonephritis
IGC —
  immature germ cell
  intragastric cannula
IGD —
  idiopathic growth hormone deficiency
  interglobal distance
  isolated gonadotropin deficiency

IgD — immunoglobulin D
IgD1, IgD2 — subclasses of immunoglobulin D
IGDE — idiopathic gait disorders of elderly
IGDM — infant of gestational diabetic mother
IGE — impaired gas exchange
IgE — immunoglobulin E
IgE1 — subclass of immunoglobulin E
IGF — insulin-like growth factor
IGFET — insulated gate field effect transistor
IgG — immunoglobulin G
IgG1, IgG2, IgG3, IgG4 — subclasses of immunoglobulin G
IGH —
  idiopathic growth hormone
  immunoreactive growth hormone
IGHD — isolated growth hormone deficiency
IGI — Institutional Goals Inventory
IGIM — immune globulin, intramuscular
IGIV — immune globulin, intravenous
IgM — immunoglobulin M
IgM1 — subclass of immunoglobulin M
IgMN — immunoglobulin M nephropathy
IGP — intestinal glycoprotein
IGQ — immunoglobulin quantitation
IGR —
  immediate generalized reaction
  integrated gastrin response
  intrauterine growth retardation
IGS —
  inappropriate gonadotropin secretion
  internal guide sequence
Igs — immunoglobulins

IgSC — immunoglobulin-secreting
  cell
IGT —
  impaired glucose tolerance
  interpersonal group therapy
  intragastric titration
IGTT — intravenous glucose tolerance test
IGV — intrathoracic gas volume
IgY — immunoglobulin Y
IH —
  ichthyosis hystrix
  idiopathic hirsutism
  idiopathic hypercalciuria
  immediate hypersensitivity
  incompletely healed
  indirect hemagglutination
  industrial hygiene
  infantile hydrocephalus
  infectious hepatitis
  inguinal hernia
  inhibiting hormone
  in hospital
  inner half
  inpatient hospital
  intermittent heparinization
  intracerebral hematoma
  intracranial hematoma
  iron hematoxylin
IHA —
  idiopathic hyperaldosteronism
  immune hemolytic anemia
  indirect hemagglutination
  indirect hemagglutination an-
    tibody
  infusion hepatic arteriography
IHAC — Industrial Health and
  Advisory Committee
IHAS — idiopathic hypertrophic
  aortic stenosis
IHB — incomplete heart block
IHBT — incompatible hemolytic
  blood transfusion
IHC —
  idiopathic hemochromatosis
  idiopathic hypercalciuria
  immobilization hypercalcemia
  inner hair cell

IHC — (continued)
  intrahepatic cholestasis
IHCA — isocapnic hyperventilation with cold air
IHCP — Institute of Hospital and
  Community Psychiatry
IHD —
  in-center hemodialysis
  intrahepatic duct
  intrahepatic ductulus
  ischemic heart disease
IHES — idiopathic hypereosinophilic syndrome
IHF —
  Industrial Health Foundation
  integration host factor
  International Hospital Foun-
    dation
IHGD — isolateral human growth
  deficiency
IHH —
  idiopathic hypogonadotropic
    hypogonadism
  idiopathic hypothalamic hypo-
    gonadism
  infectious human hepatitis
IHHS — idiopathic hyperkinetic
  heart syndrome
IHL — International Homeopathic
  League
IHMS — isonicotinylhydrazide
  methanesulfonate
IHO — idiopathic hypertrophic os-
  teoarthropathy
IHP —
  idiopathic hypoparathyroidism
  idiopathic hypopituitarism
  interhospitalization period
  inverted hand position
IHPC — intrahepatic cholestasis
IHPH — intrahepatic portal hypertension
IHPP — Intergovernmental Health
  Project Policy
IHR —
  intrahepatic resistance
  intrinsic heart rate
IHRA — isocapnic hyperventilation with room air

IHRB — Industrial Health Research Board
IHS —
    Idiopathic Headache Score
    idiopathic hypereosinophilic syndrome
    inactivated horse serum
    Indian Health Service
    infrahyoid strap
    International Health Society
IHs — iris hamartomas
IHSA — iodinated human serum albumin
IHSC — immunoreactive human skin collagenase
IHSS — idiopathic hypertrophic subaortic stenosis
IHT —
    insulin hypoglycemia test
    intravenous histamine test
    ipsilateral head turning
15HT — intraplatelet serotonin
IHW — inner heel wedge
Ii — incision inferius
II —
    icterus index
    image intensifier
    irradiated iodine
I&I — illness and injuries
IIA — internal iliac artery
IIC — integrated ion current
IICP — increased intracranial pressure
IICU — infant intensive care unit
IID — insulin-independent diabetes
IIDM — insulin-independent diabetes mellitus
IIE — idiopathic ineffective erythropoiesis
IIF —
    immune interferon
    indirect immunofluorescence
    indirect immunofluorescent
IIFT — intraoperative intra-arterial fibrinolytic therapy
IIGR — ipsilateral instinctive grasp reaction

II-para — secundipara
III-para — tertipara
IIIVC — infrahepatic interruption of inferior vena cava
IIME — Institute of International Medical Education
IIP —
    idiopathic interstitial pneumonia
    idiopathic intestinal pseudoobstruction
    increased intracranial pressure
    indirect immunoperoxidase
IIS —
    intensive immunosuppression
    intermittent infusion sets
    International Institute of Stress
IIT —
    ineffective iron turnover
    integrated isometric tension
IJ —
    ileojejunal
    internal jugular
    intrajejunal
    intrajugular
IJC — internal jugular catheter
IJD — inflammatory joint disease
IJP —
    inhibitory junction potential
    internal jugular pressure
IJR — idiojunctional rhythm
IJT — idiojunctional tachycardia
IJV — internal jugular vein
IK —
    immobilized knee
    Immunekörper (Ger.) immune body
    immunoconglutinin
    Infusoria killing [unit]
    interstitial keratitis
IKE — ion kinetic energy
IKI — iodine potassium iodide
IKU — *Infusoria* killing unit
IL —
    ileum
    incisolingual

IL — (continued)
  independent laboratory
  iliolumbar
  immature lung
  inciso-lingual
  independent laboratory
  inspiratory load
  intensity load
  interleukin
  intralipid
  intralumbar
  intraocular lens
I-L — intensity-latency
IL-1 — interleukin-1
IL-2 — interleukin-2
IL-3 — interleukin-3
Il — illinium (promethium)
il — intralesional
ILA —
  insulin-like activity
  International Leprosy Association
ILa — incisolabial
ILB —
  infant, low birth [weight]
  initial lung burden
ILBBB — incomplete left bundle branch block
ILBW — infant, low birth weight
ILC —
  ichthyosis linearis circumflex
  incipient lethal concentration
ILD —
  interstitial lung disease
  ischemic leg disease
  ischemic limb disease
  isolated lactase deficiency
ILE — infantile lobar emphysema
Ile — isoleucine
ILFC — immature living female child
ILGF — insulin-like growth factor
ILH — immunoreactive luteinizing hormone
ILL — intermediate lymphocytic lymphoma
ill. — illusion
ILM —
  insulin-like material

ILM — (continued)
  internal limiting membrane
ILMC — immature living male child
ILMI — inferolateral myocardial infarction
ILMN — incomplete lower motor neuron
ILNR — intralobar nephrogenic rest
ILo — iodine lotion
ILP —
  inadequate luteal phase
  insufficiency of luteal phase
  interstitial lymphocytic pneumonia
ILR — irreversible loss rate
ILS —
  idiopathic leucine sensitivity
  idiopathic lymphadenopathy syndrome
  increase in life span
  infrared liver scanner
  intermittent light stimulation
  intralobal sequestration
ILSI — International Life Sciences Institute
ILSS —
  Integrated Life Support System
  intraluminal somatostatin
ILT — iliotibial tract
ILVEN — inflammatory linear verrucal epidermal nevus
IM —
  idiopathic myelofibrosis
  immunosuppression method
  Index Medicus
  indomethacin
  Industrial Medicine
  infection medium
  infectious mononucleosis
  inner membrane
  innocent murmur
  inspiratory muscle
  Institute of Medicine
  intermediate
  intermediate megaloblast

IM — (continued)
  intermetatarsal
  intermuscular
  internal malleolus
  internal mammary [artery]
  Internal Medicine
  internal monitor
  intestinal mesenchyme
  intramedullary
  intramuscularly
  invasive mole
IMA —
  Industrial Medical Association
  inferior mesenteric artery
  Interchurch Medical Assistance
  internal mammary artery
  Irish Medical Association
IMAA — iodinated macroaggregated albumin
[131]IMAA — radioiodinated macroaggregated albumin
IMAB — internal mammary artery bypass
IMAG — internal mammary artery graft
IMAI — internal mammary artery implant
IMB —
  Institute of Microbiology
  intermenstrual bleeding
IMBC — indirect maximum breathing capacity
IMBI — Institute of Medical and Biological Illustrators
IMC —
  interdigestive migrating contractions
  interdigestive myoelectric complex
  internal mammary chain
  intestinal mast cell
  intramedullary catheter
IMCT — Information-Memory-Concentration Test
IMCU — intermediate medical care unit

IMD —
  immunologically mediated disease
  inherited metabolic disorder
ImD_{50} — median immunizing dose
IMDC — intramedullary metatarsal decompression
IMDD — idiopathic midline destructive disease
IMDG — International Maritime Dangerous Goods [code]
IMDM — Iscove's modified Dulbecco's medium
IMDP — imidocarb dipropionate
IME — independent medical examination
IMEM — improved minimum essential medium
IMET — isometric endurance test
IMF —
  idiopathic myelofibrosis
  immunofluorescence
  intermaxillary fixation
  intermediate filament
IMG —
  inferior mesenteric ganglion
  internal medicine group [practice]
  international medical graduate
IMGG — intramuscular gamma-globulin
IMH —
  idiopathic myocardial hypertrophy
  indirect microhemagglutination [test]
IMHP — 1-iodomercuri-2-hydroxypropane
IMHT — indirect microhemagglutination test
IMI —
  imipramine
  immunologically measurable insulin
  impending myocardial infarction
  Imperial Mycological Institute (Great Britain)

IMI — (*continued*)
    indirect membrane immuno-
        fluorescence
    inferior myocardial infarction
    intermeal interval
    intramuscular injection
Imi — imipramine
IMIC — International Medical In-
    formation Center
IMIG — intramuscular immuno-
    globulin
IML —
    inner molecular layer
    internal mammary lympho-
        scintigraphy
IMLA — intramural left anterior
    [artery]
IMLAD — intramural left anterior
    descending [artery]
IMLC — incomplete mitral leaflet
    closure
IMLNS — idiopathic minimal le-
    sion nephrotic syndrome
IML/SG — inner molecular layer/
    stratum granulosum
ImLy — immune lysis
IMM —
    inhibitor-containing minimal
        medium
    internal medial malleolus
immat —
    immature
    immaturity
IMMC — interdigestive migrating
    motor complex
immed. — immediately
immobil. —
    immobilization
    immobilize
immun. —
    immune
    immunity
    immunization
Immuno — immunoglobulin
Immunol — immunology
IMN — internal mammary node
IMNS — Imperial Military Nurs-
    ing Service

IMP —
    idiopathic myeloid prolifera-
        tion
    impacted
    impaction
    important
    impression
    improved
    incomplete male pseudoher-
        maphroditism
    individual Medicaid prac-
        titioner
    inosine 5'-monophosphate
    Inpatient Multidimensional
        Psychiatric [scale]
    intramembranous particle
    intramuscular (compartment)
        pressure
imp. —
    impacted
    impaction
    imperfect
    impression
    improved
IMPA — incisal mandibular plane
    angle
IMPAC —
    Immediate Psychiatric Aid
        and Referral Center
    Information for Management,
        Planning, Analysis and Co-
        ordination
IMPC — International Myopia
    Prevention Center
IMPEX — immediate postexercise
IMPL — impulse
IMPRV — improvement
IMPS —
    Inpatient Multidimensional
        Psychiatric Scale
    intact months of patient sur-
        vival
Impx —
    impacted
    impaction
IMR —
    individual medical record
    infant mortality rate

IMR — (continued)
    infant mortality risk
    Institute for Medical Research
    institution for mentally re-
        tarded
    International Medical Re-
        search
IMRAD — introduction, methods,
    results, and discussion
IMS —
    incurred in military service
    Indian Medical Service
    industrial methylated spirit
    Integrated Medical Services
    International Medication Sys-
        tems
    International Metric System
IMSS — In-Flight Medical Sup-
    port System
IMT —
    indomethacin
    induced muscular tension
    inspiratory muscle training
IMTLYM — immature lymphocytes
IMU — Index of Medical Under-
    writers
ImU — international milliunit
IMV —
    inferior mesenteric vein
    intermittent mandatory venti-
        lation
    intermittent mechanical ven-
        tilation
IMVP — idiopathic mitral valve
    prolapse
IMVPC — indole, methyl red,
    Voges-Proskauer, and citrate
    [test]
IMVS — Institute of Medical and
    Veterinary Science
IN —
    icterus neonatorum
    impetigo neonatorum
    incidence
    incompatibility number
    infantile nephrotic [syndrome]
    infundibular nucleus
    insulin

IN — (continued)
    intermediate nucleus
    interneuron
    interstitial nephritis
    intranasal
    irritation of nociceptors
In —
    index
    indium
    inion
    insulin
    inulin
in — inch
in. — inch
in^2 — square inch
in^3 — cubic inch
INA —
    infectious nucleic acid
    inferior nasal artery
    International Neurological
        Association
INAA — instrumental neutron ac-
    tivation analysis
INAD —
    infantile neuroaxonal dystro-
        phy
    investigational new animal
        drug
INAH — isonicotinic acid hydra-
    zide
INB —
    internuclear bridging
    ischemic necrosis of bone
inbr. — inbreeding
INC —
    internodular cortex
    inside needle catheter
inc. —
    incisal
    incision
    including
    inclusion
    incompatibility
    incomplete
    inconclusive
    incontinent
    increase(d)
    increment

inc. — (continued)
    incurred
Inc-Ab —
    inside-the-needle catheter
    incomplete abortion
IncB — inclusion body
INCD — infantile nuclear cerebral
    degeneration
incid. — incide (Lat.) cut
incl. —
    including
    inclusion
incomp. — incomplete
incont. — incontinent
incr. —
    increase
    increased
    increment
INCS — incomplete resolution
    scan to follow
incur. — incurable
IND —
    indapamide
    indomethacin
    industrial medicine
    Investigational New Drug
ind. —
    independent
    index
    indirect
    induction
in d. — in dies (Lat.) daily
Indep — independent
indic. —
    indicated
    indication
indig. — indigestion
indiv. — individual
INDM — infant of nondiabetic
    mother
Ind. Med. — Index Medicus
INDO — indomethacin
INDOR — internuclear double res-
    onance
indust. — industrial
INE — infantile necrotizing en-
    cephalomyelopathy
INEX — inexperienced

in extrem. — in extremis (Lat.) in
    the last hours of life
INF —
    infant
    infantile
    infarction
    infected
    infection
    infective
    infectious
    inferior
    infirmary
    infundibulum
    interferon
inf. —
    infunde (Lat.) pour in
    infusum (Lat.) infusion
INFH — ischemic necrosis of femo-
    ral head
INFL —
    inflammation
    influence
    influx
Inflam. —
    inflammation
    inflammatory
inf. mono. — infectious mononu-
    cleosis
info. — information
ING — isotope nephrogram
ing. — inguinal
InGP — indolglycerophosphate
INH —
    inhalation
    isoniazid
    isonicotinic hydrazide
inhal. — inhalation
inhib. —
    inhibiting
    inhibition
    inhibitory
INI —
    intranasal insulin
    intranuclear inclusion
inj. —
    injection
    injurious
    injury

inject. — injection
inj. enem. — *injiciatur enema* (Lat.) let an enema be injected
INK — injury not known
inl. — inlay
INLSD — ichthyosis and neutral lipid storage disease
INN — International Nonpropri-etary Names
innerv. —
    innervated
    innervation
innom. — innominate
INO —
    internuclear ophthalmoplegia
    inosine
Ino. — inosine
INOC — isonicotinoloxycarbonyl
inoc. —
    inoculate
    inoculation
inop. —
    inoperable
    inoperative
inorg. — inorganic
Inox — inosine, oxidized
INP — idiopathic neutropenia
INPAV — intermittent negative pressure-assisted ventilation
INPEA — isopropyl nitrophenyl-ethanolamine
INPH — iproniazid phosphate
INPRONS — information pro-cessing in the central nervous system
IN-PT — inpatient
in pulm. — *in pulmento* (Lat.) in gruel
INPV — intermittent negative pressure-assisted ventilation
INQ — interior nasal quadrant
INR — International Normalized Ratio
INREM — internal roentgen-equivalent, man
INS —
    idiopathic nephrotic syn-drome

INS — (*continued*)
    insurance
ins. —
    insertion
    insulin
    insurance
    insured
INS AB — insulin antibody
insem. — insemination
insol. — insoluble
Insp. —
    inspection
    inspiration
    inspiratory
$InsP_3$ — inositol 1,4,5-triphosphate
INSR — insulin receptor
Inst. —
    institute
    institution
    instrument
instab. — instability
instill. — instillation
INSU — intensive neurosurgery unit
insuf. —
    insufficiency
    insufficient
insuff. — insufflation
INT —
    intact
    integral
    intermediate
    intermittent
    intern
    internal
    internist
    internship
    interval
    intestinal
    intima
    p-iodonitrotetrazolium
Int. —
    international
    intestinal
int. cib. — *inter cibos* (Lat.) be-tween meals
INTEG — integument
intern. — internal

Internat. — international

Intest —
    intestinal
    intestine

Int/Ext — internal/external

INTH — intrathecal

Int hist — interval history

Intmd. — intermediate

Int. Med. — internal medicine

int. noct. — *inter noctem* (Lat.) during the night

int. obst. — intestinal obstruction

INTOX — intoxication

INTR — intermittent

intracal — intracalvarium

int rot — internal rotation

Int trx — intermittent traction

intub — intubation

INV — inferior nasal vein

inv. —
    invalid
    inverse
    inversion
    involuntary

Inv/Ev — inversion/eversion

invest. — investigation

invol. — involuntary

involv. —
    involvement
    involved

inv(p + q −) — pericentric inversion

inv(p − sq +) — pericentric inversion

inv ins — inverted insertion

IO —
    incisal opening
    inferior oblique
    inferior olive
    initial opening
    inside-out
    intensive observation
    internal os
    interorbital
    intestinal obstruction
    intraocular
    intraoperative

I/O — input/output

I&O —
    in and out
    intake and output

Io — ionium

IOA —
    inner optic anlage
    International Osteopathic Association

IOC —
    in our culture
    International Organizing Committee on Medical Librarianship
    intern on call

IOCG — intraoperative cholangiogram

IOD —
    injured on duty
    integrated optical density
    interorbital distance

IODA — Iron Overload Diseases Association

IODM — infant of diabetic mother

IOEBT — intraoperative electron beam therapy

IOF — intraocular fluid

IOFB — intraocular foreign body

I of L — Institute of Living

IOFNA — intraoperative fine needle aspiration

IOH — idiopathic orthostatic hypotension

IOI — intraosseous infusion

IOL — intraocular lens

IOLI — intraocular lens implantation

IOM — Institute of Medicine

IOML — infraorbitomeatal line

IOMP — International Organization for Medical Physics

ION — ischemic optic neuropathy

IOP — intraocular pressure

IOR —
    index of response
    information outflow rate

IORT — intraoperative (electron beam) radiation therapy

IOS —
    International Organization for
        Standardization
    intraoperative sonography
IOT —
    intraocular tension
    intraocular transfer
    ipsilateral optic tectum
IOTA — information overload test-
    ing aid
IOU —
    intensive care observation
        unit
    international opacity unit
IOV — initial office visit
IP —
    icterus praecox
    iliopsoas [muscle]
    immune precipitate
    immunoblastic plasma
    immunoperoxidase technique
    implantation
    inactivated pepsin
    incisoproximal
    incisopulpal
    incontinentia pigmenti
    incubation period
    index of pathology
    individualized plan
    induced potential
    induced protein
    induction period
    infection prevention
    infundibular process
    infundibulopelvic [ligament]
    infusion pump
    initial pressure
    inorganic phosphate
    inosine phosphorylase
    inpatient
    in plaster
    instantaneous pressure
    International Pharmacopoeia
    interpeduncular [nucleus]
    interphalangeal [joint]
    interpositus [nucleus]
    interpupillary
    intestinal pseudo-obstruction

IP — (continued)
    intracellular proteolysis
    intraperitoneally
    intrapulmonary
    ionization potential
    isoelectric point
    isoproterenol
    L'Institut Pasteur
IP_3 — inositol 1,4,5-triphosphate
IPA —
    immunoperoxidase assay
    incontinentia pigmenti
        achromians
    independent practice associa-
        tion
    Individual Practice Associa-
        tion
    indole, pyruvic acid
    infantile papular acroderma-
        titis
    International Pediatric Associ-
        ation
    International Pharmaceutical
        Association
    International Psychoanalytical
        Association
    intrapulmonary artery
    invasive pulmonary aspergillo-
        sis
    isopropyl alcohol
IPAA — International Psychoana-
    lytical Association
IPAO — insulin-induced peak acid
    output
IPAR — Institute of Personality
    Assessment and Research
I-para — primipara
IPAT —
    Institute for Personality and
        Ability Testing
    Iowa Pressure Articulation
        Test
IPB — infrapopliteal bypass
IPC —
    intermittent pneumatic com-
        pression
    International Poliomyelitis
        Congress

IPC — (continued)
  interpeduncular cistern
  ion pair chromatography
  isopropyl phenyl carbamate
  isopropyl chlorophenyl
IPCD — infantile polycystic disease
IPCS — intrauterine progesterone contraception system
IPD —
  idiopathic Parkinson's disease
  idiopathic protracted diarrhea
  immediate pigment darkening
  increase in pupillary diameter
  incurable problem drinker
  inflammatory pelvic disease
  intermittent peritoneal dialysis
  intermittent pigment darkening
  interpupillary distance
  Inventory of Psychosocial Development
IPE —
  infectious porcine encephalomyelitis
  initial psychiatric evaluation
  interstitial pulmonary emphysema
IPEH — intravascular papillary endothelial hyperplasia
IPF —
  idiopathic pulmonary fibrosis
  infection-potentiating factor
  interstitial pulmonary fibrosis
IPFD — intrapartum fetal distress
IPG —
  impedance plethysmograph
  impedance plethysmography
  inspiratory phase gas
iPGE — immunoreactive prostaglandin E
IPH —
  idiopathic portal hypertension
  idiopathic pulmonary hemosiderosis
  inflammatory papillary hyperplasia

IPH — (continued)
  interphalangeal [joint]
  intraparenchymal hemorrhage
IPHR — inverted polypoid hamartoma of the rectum
IPI —
  Imagined Process Inventory
  interphonemic interval
  interpulse interval
IPIA — immunoperoxidase infectivity assay
IPJ — interphalangeal joint
IPK —
  interphalangeal keratosis
  intractable plantar keratosis
IPKD — infantile polycystic kidney disease
IPL —
  inner plexiform layer
  interpupillary line
  intrapleural
IPM —
  impulses per minute
  inches per minute
  infant passive mitt
IPMI — inferoposterior myocardial infarction
IPMS — inhibited power motive syndrome
IPN —
  infantile periarteritis nodosa
  infectious pancreatic necrosis [of trout]
  intern progress note
  interpeduncular nucleus
  interpenetrating polymer network
  interstitial pneumonitis
IPNA — isopropyl noradrenaline
IPO —
  improved pregnancy outcome
  initial planning option
IPOF — immediate postoperative fitting
IPOP — immediate postoperative prosthesis
IPP —
  independent practice plan

IPP — *(continued)*
    inferior point of pubic [bone]
    inflatable penile prosthesis
    inorganic pyrophosphate
    inosine, pyruvate, and phosphate
    intermittent positive pressure
    intrahepatic portal pressure
    intrapleural pressure
    L' Institut Pasteur Productions
IPPA — inspection, palpation, percussion, and auscultation
IPPB — intermittent positive-pressure breathing
IPPB-I — intermittent positive-pressure breathing-inspiration
IPPF —
    International Planned Parenthood Federation
    immediate postoperative prosthetic fitting
IPPI — interruption of pregnancy for psychiatric indication
IPPO — intermittent positive-pressure inflation with oxygen
IPPR —
    integrated pancreatic polypeptide response
    intermittent positive-pressure respiration
IPPT — Inter-Person Perception Test
IPPUAD — immediate postprandial upper abdominal distress
IPPV — intermittent positive-pressure ventilation
IPQ — intimacy potential quotient
IPR —
    insulin production rate
    interval patency rate
    intraparenchymal resistance
    iproniazid
i-Pr — isopropyl
IPRL —
    isolated perfused rabbit lung
    isolated perfused rat liver
IPRT — interpersonal reaction test

IPS —
    idiopathic postprandial syndrome
    impulses per second
    inches per second
    infundibular pulmonary stenosis
    initial prognostic score
    intermittent photic stimulation
    Interpersonal Perception Scale
    intrapartum stillbirth
    intraperitoneal shock
    ischiopubic synchondrosis
ips — inches per second
IPSB — intrapartum stillbirth
IPSC — inhibitory postsynaptic current
IPSC-E — Inventory of Psychic and Somatic Complaints in the Elderly
IPSF — immediate postsurgical fitting [prosthesis]
IPSID — immunoproliferative small intestinal disease
IPSP — inhibitory postsynaptic potential
IPT —
    immunoperoxidase technique
    immunoprecipitation
    intermittent pelvic traction
    interpersonal psychotherapy
    ipratropium
    isoproterenol
IPTG — isopropyl thiogalactoside
iPTH — immunoreactive parathyroid hormone
IPTX — intermittent pelvic traction
IPU — inpatient unit
IPV —
    inactivated poliomyelitis vaccine
    inactivated polio vaccine
    incompetent perforator vein
    infectious pustular vaginitis
    infectious pustular vulvovaginitis [of cattle]

IPV — (*continued*)
  intrapulmonary vein
IPVC — interpolated premature
  ventricular contraction
IPVD — index of pulmonary vascular disease
IPW — interphalangeal width
IPZ — insulin protamine zinc
IQ — intelligence quotient
i.q. — *idem quod* (Lat.) the same as
IQB — individual quick blanch
IQ&S — iron, quinine, and strych-
  nine
IR —
  drop of voltage across a resis-
    tor produced by a current
  ileal resection
  immune response
  immunization rate
  immunologic response
  immunoreactive
  immunoreagent
  index of response
  individual reaction
  inferior rectus [muscle]
  inflow resistance
  information retrieval
  infrared
  infrarenal
  inside radius
  insoluble residue
  inspiratory reserve
  inspiratory resistance
  insulin receptor
  insulin resistance
  intelligence ratio
  internal reduction
  internal resistance
  internal rotation
  intrarectal
  intrarenal
  inversion recovery
  inverted repeat
  irritant reaction
  isovolumic relaxation
I&R — insertion and removal
I-R — Ito-Reenstierna [reaction]
Ir —
  immune response

Ir — (*continued*)
  iridium
ir —
  immunoreactive
  intrarectal
  intrarenal
IRA —
  immunoradioassay
  immunoregulatory alpha-glob-
    ulin
  inactive renin activity
IR-ACTH — immunoreactive
  adrenocorticotropic hormone
IRA-EEA — ileorectal anastomosis
  with end-to-end anastomosis
IrANP — immunoreactive atrial
  natriuretic peptide
IR-AVP — immunoreactive argi-
  nine-vasopressin
IRB — Institutional Review Board
IRBBB — incomplete right bundle
  branch block
IRBC —
  immature red blood cell
  infected red blood cell
IRBP — interphotoreceptor reti-
  noid-binding protein
IRC —
  indirect radionuclide cystogra-
    phy
  infrared coagulator
  inspiratory reserve capacity
  instantaneous resonance
    curve
  International Red Cross
  International Research Com-
    munications System
IRCA — intravascular red cell ag-
  gregation
IRCC — International Red Cross
  Committee
IRCS — International Research
  Communications System
IRCU — intensive respiratory care
  unit
IRD —
  infantile Refsum's syndrome
  isorhythmic dissociation

IRDP — insulin-related DNA polymorphism

IRDS —
idiopathic respiratory distress syndrome
infant respiratory distress syndrome

IRE — internal rotation in extension

IRF —
idiopathic retroperitoneal fibrosis
internal rotation in flexion

IRG —
immunoreactive gastrin
immunoreactive glucagon
immunoreactive glucose

IRGH — immunoreactive growth hormone

IRGL — immunoreactive glucagon

IRH —
Institute for Research in Hypnosis
Institute of Religion and Health
intrarenal hemorrhage

IRhCG — immunoreactive human chorionic gonadotropin

IRHCS — immunoradioassayable human chorionic somatomammotropin

IRhGH — immunoreactive human growth hormone

IRhPL — immunoreactive human placental lactogen

IRI —
immunoreactive insulin
insulin radioimmunoassay
insulin resistance index

IRIA — indirect radioimmunoassay

IRICU — Intermountain Respiratory Intensive Care Unit

irid. — iridescent

IRIg — insulin-reactive immunoglobulin

IRIS —
Integrated Risk Information System

IRIS — *(continued)*
interleukin regulation of immune system
International Research Information Service

IRM —
innate releasing mechanism
Institute of Rehabilitation Medicine

IRMA —
immunoradiometric assay
intraretinal microangiopathy
intraretinal microvascular abnormalities

IRMP — Intermountain Regional Medical Program

iRNA —
immune ribonucleic acid
informational ribonucleic acid

IRO — International Refugee Organization

IROS — ipsilateral routing of signal

IRP —
immunoreactive plasma
immunoreactive proinsulin
incus replacement prosthesis
insulin-releasing polypeptide
International Reference Preparation
interstitial radiation pneumonitis

IRR — intrarenal reflux

irr. —
irradiation
irrigate
irritation

IRRD — Institute for Research in Rheumatic Diseases

irreg. —
irregular
irregularity

irrig. —
irrigate
irrigation

IRS —
immunoreactive secretin
infrared spectrophotometry

IRS — *(continued)*
    instrument retrieval system
    insulin receptor species
    internal resolution site
    International Rhinologic Society
IRSA —
    idiopathic refractory sideroblastic anemia
    iodinated rat serum albumin
IRSE — inversion-recovery spin-echo
IRT —
    immunoreactive trypsin
    immunoreactive trypsinogen
    instrument retrieval [container]
    inter-response time
    isometric relaxation time
    item response theory
IRTO — immunoreactive trypsin output
IRTU — integrating regulatory transcription unit
IRU —
    Industrial Rehabilitation Unit
    interferon reference unit
IRV —
    inferior radicular vein
    inspiratory reserve volume
    inverse ratio ventilation
IS —
    ileal segment
    immediate sensitivity
    immune serum
    immunosuppressive
    impingement syndrome
    incentive spirometer
    index of saponification
    index of sexuality
    induced sputum
    infant size
    infantile spasms
    information system
    infrahyoid strap
    initial segment
    insertion sequence
    in situ

IS — *(continued)*
    insulin secretion
    intercellular space
    intercostal space
    interictal spike
    internal standard
    interspace
    interstitial space
    interventricular septum
    intracardial shunt
    intraspinal
    intrasplenic
    intrastriatal
    intraventricular septum
    invalided from service
    inventory of systems
    Ionescu-Shiley [cardiac valve]
    ipecac syrup
    ischemic score
    isoproterenol
I-10-S — invert sugar (10%) in saline
Is — incision superius
is —
    in situ
    island
    islet
    isolated
ISA —
    Instrument Society of America
    intracarotid sodium amytal
    intrinsic stimulating activity
    intrinsic sympathomimetic activity
    iodinated serum albumin
    irregular spiking activity
ISA_5 — internal surface area of lung at volume of 5 liters
ISADH — inappropriate secretion of antidiuretic hormone
IS and R — information storage and retrieval
ISB — incentive spirometry breathing
ISBI — International Society for Burn Injuries
ISBP — International Society for Biochemical Pharmacology

ISBT — International Society for Blood Transfusion

ISC —
    immunoglobulin-secreting cell
    insoluble collagen
    intensive supportive care
    International Society of Cardiology
    International Society of Chemotherapy
    International Statistical Classification
    intershift coordination
    interstitial cell
    intersystem crossing
    irreversibly sickled cell
    Isolette servo control

ISCCO — intersternocostoclavicular ossification

ISCF — interstitial cell fluid

ISCLT — International Society for Clinical Laboratory Technology

ISCM — International Society of Cybernetic Medicine

ISCN — International System for Human Cytogenetic Nomenclature

ISCO — immunostimulating complex [vaccine]

ISCP —
    infection surveillance and control program
    International Society of Comparative Pathology

ISCS — International Society for Cardiovascular Surgery

ISCs — irreversible sickle cells

ISD —
    immunosuppressive drug
    Information Services Division
    inhibited sexual desire
    initial sleep disturbance
    interatrial septal defect
    interventricular septal defect
    isosorbide dinitrate

ISDB — indirect self-destructive behavior

ISDN — isosorbide dinitrate

ISE —
    inhibited sexual excitement
    International Society of Endocrinology
    International Society of Endoscopy
    ion-selective electrode

ISEK — International Society of Electromyographic Kinesiology

ISEM — immunosorbent electron microscopy

ISF — interstitial fluid

ISFET — ion-specific field effect transducer

ISFV — interstitial fluid volume

ISG — immune serum globulin

ISGE — International Society of Gastroenterology

ISH —
    icteric serum hepatitis
    inner self helper
    International Society of Hematology
    isolated systolic hypertension

ISI —
    infarct size index
    initial slope index
    injury severity index
    Institute for Scientific Information
    insulin sensitivity index
    International Sensitivity Index
    interstimulus interval

ISIH — interspike interval histogram

ISIS — International Study of Infarct Survival

ISKDC — International Study of Kidney Diseases in Childhood

ISL —
    interscapular line
    interspinous ligament
    isoleucine

ISM —
    International Society of Microbiologists

ISM — (continued)
    intersegmental muscles
ISMA — infantile spinal muscular
    atrophy
ISMED — International Society of
    Metabolic Eye Disorders
ISMH — International Society of
    Medical Hydrology
ISMHC — International Society
    of Medical Hydrology and Cli-
    matology
ISN —
    interactive surgical navigation
      [detector system]
    International Society of Ne-
      phrology
    International Society of Neu-
      rochemistry
ISO — International Standards Or-
    ganization
iso. —
    isoproterenol
    isotropic
Is of Lang — islands of Langerhans
Isol — Isolette
isol. —
    isolated
    isolation
isom. —
    isometric
    isometrophic
isox — isoxsuprine
ISP —
    distance between iliac spines
    interspace
    interspinal
    intraspinal
    isoproterenol
ISPO — International Society for
    Prosthetics and Orthotics
ISPT — interspecies (ovum) pene-
    tration test
ISPX — Ionescu-Shiley pericardial
    xenograft
i.s.q. — in status quo (Lat.) un-
    changed
ISR —
    information storage and re-
    trieval

ISR — (continued)
    Institute for Sex Research
    Institute of Surgical Research
    insulin secretion rate
    integrated secretory response
ISRM — International Society of
    Reproductive Medicine
ISS —
    Index-Injury Severity Score
    International Society of Sur-
      gery
    ion-scattering spectroscopy
    ion surface scattering
ISSN — International Standard
    Serial Number
ISSVD — International Society for
    the Study of Vulvar Disease
IST —
    inappropriate sinus tachycar-
      dia
    insulin sensitivity test
    insulin shock therapy
    International Society on Toxi-
      cology
    isometric systolic tension
ISTD — International Society of
    Tropical Dermatology
ISU — International Society of
    Urology
I-sub — inhibitor substance
ISW — interstitial water
ISWI — incisional surgical wound
    infection
ISY — intrasynovial
IT —
    iliotibial
    immunity test
    immunological test
    immunotherapy
    implantation test
    individual therapy
    inferior temporal
    inferior turbinate
    inhalation test
    Inhalation Therapist
    inhalation therapy
    inspiratory time
    insulin therapy

IT — (continued)
  intensive therapy
  intentional tremor
  intermittent traction
  internal thoracic
  interstitial tissue
  intertrochanteric
  intertuberous
  intimal thickening
  intradermal test
  intratesticular
  intrathecal
  intrathoracic
  intratracheal
  intratracheal tube
  intratumoral
  ischial tuberosity
  isomeric transition
I/T — intensity/time
I&T — intolerance and toxicity
ITA —
  individual treatment assessment
  inferior temporal artery
  internal thoracic artery
  International Tuberculosis Association
ITAG — internal thoracic artery graft
ITB — iliotibial band
ITC —
  imidazolyl-thioguanine chemotherapy
  incontinence treatment center
  Interagency Testing Committee
ITc — International Table calorie
ITCP — idiopathic thrombocytopenic purpura
ITCU — intensive thoracic cardiovascular unit
ITCVD — ischemic thrombotic cerebrovascular disease
ITD —
  insulin-treated diabetic
  intensely transfused dialysis
ITE —
  insufficient therapeutic effect

ITE — (continued)
  in the ear
  in-training examination
  intrapulmonary interstitial emphysema
ITET — isotonic endurance test
ITF — interferon
ITFF — intertrochanteric femoral fracture
ITFS —
  iliotibial tract friction syndrome
  incomplete testicular feminization syndrome
ITGV — intrathoracic gas volume
ITh — intrathecal
IThP — intrathyroidal parathyroid
ITI — intertrial interval
ITLC — instant thin-layer chromatography
ITM —
  improved Thayer-Martin [medium]
  intrathecal methotrexate
  Israel turkey meningoencephalitis
ITOU — intensive therapy observation unit
ITP —
  idiopathic thrombocytopenic purpura
  immune thrombocytopenia
  immunogenic thrombocytopenic purpura
  inosine triphosphate
  interim treatment plan
  islet-cell tumor of the pancreas
  isotachophoresis
ITPA —
  Illinois Test of Psycholinguistic Abilities
  Independent Telephone Pioneer Association
  inosine triphosphatase
ITQ —
  Infant Temperament Questionnaire

ITQ — (continued)
  inferior temporal quadrant
ITR —
  intraocular tension recorder
  intratracheal
ITS — infective toxic shock
ITSHD — isolated thyroid-stimulating hormone deficiency
ITT —
  iliotibial tract
  insulin tolerance test
  internal tibial torsion
  iron tolerance test
ITU — intensive therapy unit
ITV — inferior temporal vein
ITVAD — indwelling transcutaneous vascular access device
ITX — intertriginous xanthoma
IU —
  immunizing unit
  in utero
  International Unit
  intrauterine
iu — infectious unit
μIU — micro-International Unit
IUA — intrauterine adhesions
IUB — International Union of Biochemistry
IUBS — International Union of Biological Sciences
IUC —
  idiopathic ulcerative colitis
  intrauterine catheter
IUCD — intrauterine contraceptive device
IUD —
  intrauterine death
  intrauterine device
IUDR —
  idoxuridine
  iododeoxyuridine
IUF — isolated ultrafiltration
IUFB — intrauterine foreign body
IUFD —
  intrauterine fetal death
  intrauterine fetal distress
IUFGR — intrauterine fetal growth retardation

IUG —
  infusion urogram
  intrauterine gestation
  intrauterine growth
IUGR —
  intrauterine growth rate
  intrauterine growth retardation
IUI — intrauterine insemination
IU/l — International Units per liter
IUM —
  internal urethral meatus
  intrauterine (fetally) malnourished
  intrauterine malnourishment
  intrauterine membrane
IU/min — International Units per minute
IUP —
  intrauterine pregnancy
  intrauterine pressure
IUPAC — International Union of Pure and Applied Chemistry
IUPAP — International Union of Pure and Applied Physics
IUPC — intrauterine pressure catheter
IUPD — intrauterine pregnancy delivered
IUPHAR — International Union of Pharmacology
IUPS — International Union of Physiological Sciences
IUPTB — intrauterine pregnancy, term birth
IUR — intrauterine retardation
IURES — International Union of Reticuloendothelial Societies
IUT — intrauterine transfusion
IUTM — International Union Against Tuberculosis
IUVDT — International Union Against Venereal Diseases and the Treponematoses
IV —
  ichthyosis vulgaris
  in vitro

IV — (*continued*)
   in vivo
   initial visit
   interventricular
   intervertebral
   intravaginal
   intravascular
   intravenous(ly)
   intraventricular
   intravertebral
   invasive

i.v. —
   iodine value
   symbol for class-4 controlled
      substances

IVAC — intravenous accurate control [device]

IVAD — implantable vascular access device

IVag — intravaginal

IVAP — in vivo adhesive platelet

IVAR — insulin variable

IVB —
   intraventricular block
   intravitreal blood

IVBAT — intravascular bronchioalveolar tumor

IVBC — intravascular blood coagulation

IVC —
   individually viable cells
   inferior vena cava
   inferior vena cavogram
   inferior vena cavography
   inspiratory vital capacity
   inspired vital capacity
   integrated vector control
   intravascular coagulation
   intravenous cholangiogram
   intravenous cholangiography
   intraventricular catheter
   isovolumic contraction

IVCC — intravascular consumption coagulopathy

IVCD —
   interventricular conduction
      delay
   intraventricular conduction
      defect

IVCD — (*continued*)
   intraventricular conduction
      delay

IVCH —
   intravenous cholangiogram
   intravenous cholangiography

IVCP — inferior vena cava pressure

IVCR — inferior vena cava reconstruction

IVCT —
   inferior vena cava thrombosis
   intravenously enhanced computed tomography
   isovolumic contraction time

IVCU — isotope-voiding cystourethrogram

IVCV —
   inferior venacavogram
   inferior venacavography

IVD —
   intervertebral disc
   intravenous drip

IVDA — intravenous drug abuse

IVDSA — intravenous digital subtraction angiography

IVDU — intravenous drug use

IVF —
   in vitro fertilization
   in vivo fertilization
   interventricular foramen
   intervertebral foramen
   intravascular fluid
   intravenous fluid

IVFE — intravenous fat emulsion

IVFT — intravenous fetal transfusion

IVG — isotopic ventriculogram

IVGG — intravenous gammaglobulin

IVGTT — intravenous glucose tolerance test

IVH —
   in vitro hyperploidy
   intravenous hyperalimentation
   intraventricular hemorrhage

IVIgG — intravenous immune globulin G

IVJC — intervertebral joint complex

IVL — intravenous lock

IVLBW — infant of very low birth weight

IVM — intravascular mass

IVMP — intravenous methylprednisolone

IVN — intravenous nutrition

IVOTTS — Irvine viable organ-tissue transport system

IVOX — intravascular oxygenator

IVP —
    intravenous Pitocin
    intravenous pyelogram
    intravenous pyelography
    intraventricular pressure
    intravesical pressure

IVp — intravenous push

IVPB — intravenous piggyback

IVPD — in vitro protein digestibility

IVPF — isovolume pressure flow [curve]

IVPU — intravenous push

IVR —
    idioventricular rhythm
    internal visual reference
    intravaginal ring
    isolated volume responder

IVRD — in vitro rumen digestibility

IVROBA — intraventricular rupture of brain abscess

IVRT — isovolumic relaxation time

IVS —
    inappropriate vasopressin secretion
    intact ventricular septum
    intervening sequence
    interventricular septum
    intervillous space
    irritable voiding syndrome

IVSA — International Veterinary Students Association

IVSD — interventricular septal defect

IVSE — interventricular septal excursion

IVSS — intravenous Soluset

IVT —
    in vitro tetraploidy
    index of vertical transmission
    intravenous transfusion
    intraventricular
    isovolumic time

IVTTT — intravenous tolbutamide tolerance test

IVU —
    intravenous urogram
    intravenous urography

IVUS — intravascular ultrasound

IVV —
    influenza virus vaccine
    intravenous vasopressin

IV vol — intravenous volume

I-5-W — invert sugar (5%) in water

IW — inner wall

IWGMT — International Working Group on Mycobacterial Taxonomy

IWI —
    inferior wall infarction
    interwave interval

IWL — insensible water loss

IWMI — inferior wall myocardial infarction

IWML — idiopathic white matter lesion

IWS — Index of Work Satisfaction

i(Xq) — long arm isochromosome

IYDP — International Year of Disabled Persons

IYS — inverted Y suspensor

IZ — infarction zone

IZS — insulin zinc suspension

J

J —
dynamic movement of inertia
electric current density
flux (density)
joint
joule
journal
juvenile
juxtapulmonary-capillary receptor
magnetic polarization
polypeptide chain in polymeric immunoglobulins
sound intensity
J-1,2,3 — Jaeger test, type number 1, 2 and 3
j —
flux [density]
jaundice
joint
journal
juice
mechanical equivalent
JA —
judgment analysis
juvenile arthritis
juvenile atrophy
juxta-articular
JAI — juvenile amaurotic idiocy
JAMA — Journal of the American Medical Association
JAMG — juvenile autoimmune myasthenia gravis
JAR — junior admitting resident
JAS —
Jenkins Activity Survey
Job Attitude Scale
jaund. — jaundice
JBC — Jesness' Behavior Checklist
JBE — Japanese B encephalitis
JC —
joint contracture
junior clinician

J/C — joule per coulomb
jc — juice
JCA — juvenile chronic arthritis
JCAE — Joint Committee on Atomic Energy
JCAH — Joint Commission on Accreditation of Hospitals
JCAHO — Joint Commission on Accreditation of Healthcare Organizations
JCAHPO — Joint Commission on Allied Health Personnel in Ophthalmology
JCAI — Joint Council of Allergy and Immunology
JCAST — Joint Commission on Archives of Science and Technology
JCC — Joint Committee on Contraception
JCF — juvenile calcaneal fracture
JCM — Japanese Collection of Microorganisms
JCMHC — Joint Commission on Mental Health of Children
JCMIH — Joint Commission on Mental Illness and Health
JCML —
juvenile chronic myelocytic leukemia
juvenile chronic myelogenous leukemia
JCP — juvenile chronic polyarthritis
JCPA — Joint Commission on Public Affairs
jct. — junction
JCV —
Jamestown Canyon virus
JC virus
JD —
Janet's disease
jejunal diverticulitis
jugulodigastric [node]

JD — *(continued)*
    juvenile delinquent
    juvenile diabetes
JDC — Joslin Diabetes Center
JDF — Juvenile Diabetes Foundation
JDM — juvenile-onset diabetes mellitus
JDMS — juvenile dermatomyositis
JE —
    Japanese encephalitis
    junctional escape
JEBL — junctional epidermolysis bullosa letalis
JEE — Japanese equine encephalitis
JEJ — jejunum
JEMBEC — agar plates for transporting cultures of gonococci
JEN — Journal of Emergency Nursing
jentac. — *jentaculum* (Lat.) breakfast
JEPI — Junior Eysenck Personality Inventory
JER —
    Japanese erection ring
    junctional escape rhythm
JEV — Japanese encephalitis virus
JF —
    joint fluid
    jugular foramen
    junctional fold
JFET — junction field effect transistor
JFS — jugular foramen syndrome
J.F.S. — Jewish Family Service
JG —
    June grass [test]
    juxtaglomerular
JGA — juxtaglomerular apparatus
JGC — juxtaglomerular cell
j-g complex — juxtaglomerular complex
JGCT —
    juvenile granulosa cell tumor
    juxtaglomerular cell tumor
JGI —
    jejunogastric intussusception

JGI — *(continued)*
    juxtaglomerular granulation index
JGP —
    juvenile general paralysis
    juvenile general paresis
JH — juvenile hormone
J_H — heat transfer factor
JHA — juvenile hormone analogue
JHMO — Junior Hospital Medical Officer
JHMV — J. Howard Mueller virus
JHR — Jarisch-Herxheimer reaction
JHU — Johns Hopkins University
JI —
    jejunoileal
    jejunoileitis
    jejunoileostomy
JIB — jejunoileal bypass
JIH — joint interval histogram
JIS — juvenile idiopathic scoliosis
JJ —
    jaw jerk
    jejunojejunostomy
J/kg — joules per kilogram
JKST — Johnson-Kenney screening test
JL —
    Jadassohn-Lewandowski [syndrome]
    Jaffee-Lichtenstein [syndrome]
JLP — juvenile laryngeal papilloma
JM —
    josamycin
    jugomaxillary
Jm — mass transfer factor
JMD — juvenile macular degeneration
JMH — John Milton Hagen [antibody]
JMR — Jones-Mote reactivity
JMS — junior medical student
JMSB — John Milton Society for the Blind
JN — Jamaican neuropathy
JNA — Jena Nomina Anatomica

JND — just noticeable difference
jnt. — joint
JOD — juvenile-onset diabetes
JODM — juvenile-onset diabetes
  mellitus
JOMAC — judgment, orientation,
  memory, abstraction, and cal-
  culation
JOMACI — judgment, orientation,
  memory, abstraction, and cal-
  culation intact
jour — journal
JP —
  Jackson-Pratt [drain]
  Jobst's pump
  joining peptide
  joint protection
  juvenile periodontitis
JPB — junctional premature beat
JPC — junctional premature con-
  traction
JPD — juvenile plantar dermatosis
JPI — Jackson Personality Inven-
  tory
JPS — joint position sense
JPSA — Joint Program for the
  Study of Abortions
JR —
  Jolly reaction
  junctional rhythm
JRA — juvenile rheumatoid arthritis
JRAN — junior resident admission
  note
JRC —
  joint replacement center
  Junior Red Cross
JRC-CVT — Joint Review Committee on Education in Car-
  diovascular Technology
JRC-DMS — Joint Review Com-
  mittee on Education in Diag-
  nostic Medical Sonography
JRC-EEG — Joint Review Com-
  mittee on Education in Electroencephalographic Technology

JRC-EMT-P — Joint Review Committee on Educational Programs for the Emergency Medical Technician-Paramedic
JRCERT — Joint Review Committee on Education in Radiologic Technology
JRC-NMT — Joint Review Committee on Educational Programs in Nuclear Medicine
  Technology
JRC-OMA — Joint Review Committee on Educational Programs for the Ophthalamic
  Medical Assistant
JRC-PA — Joint Review Committee on Educational Programs
  for Physician Assistants
JRCPE — Joint Review Commit-
  tee for Perfusion Education
JRCRTE — Joint Review Commit-
  tee for Respiratory Therapy
  Education
JRC-ST — Joint Review Commit-
  tee on Education for the Sur-
  gical Technologist
J-receptor — juxtapulmonary-
  capillary receptor
JRN — junior resident note
JrNAD — Junior National Associa-
  tion for the Deaf
JROM — joint range of motion
JRT — junctional recovery time
JS —
  jejunal segment
  Job's syndrome
  junctional slowing
J/s — joules per second
JSI — Jansky's screening index
JS unit — Junkman-Schoeller unit
JSV — Jerry-Slough virus
JT — jejunostomy tube
J/T — joules per tesla
jt — joint
jt. asp. — joint aspiration
JTF — jejunostomy tube feeding
JTPS — juvenile tropical pancre-
  atitis syndrome

JU — jugale
JUA — Joint Underwriting Association
jucund. — *jucunde* (Lat.) pleasantly
jug. — jugular
jug. comp. — jugular compression [test]
junct. — junction
juscul. — *jusculum* (Lat.) broth, soup
juv. — juvenile
juxt. — *juxta* (Lat.) near
JV —
 jugular vein
 jugular venous

JV — *(continued)*
 Junin virus
JVC — jugular venous catheter
JVD — jugular venous distension
JVIS — Jackson Vocational Interest Survey
JVP —
 jugular vein pulse
 jugular venous pressure
 jugular venous pulse
JVPT — jugular venous pulse tracing
JW — jump walker
Jx — junction
JXG — juvenile xanthogranuloma

K

K —
 absolute zero
 calix
 capsular antigen
 carrying capacity
 cathode
 coefficient of heat transfer
 coefficient of scleral rigidity
 cretaceous
 dissociation constant
 electron capture
 electrostatic capacity
 equilibrium constant
 ionization constant
 kallikrein-inhibiting unit
 kanamycin
 kappa (tenth letter of the Greek alphabet), uppercase
 Kapsel (Ger.) capsule
 kathode (cathode)
 Kell blood system
 Kell factor
 kelvin
 Kerley [lines]
 kerma
 kidney
 killer [cell]

K — *(continued)*
 kilo-
 kinetic energy
 Klebsiella
 knee
 Küntscher [nail]
 lowest level [of x-ray]
 lysine
 modulus of compression
 motor coordination
 potassium (Lat., *kalium*)
 1024 in computer core memory
 vitamin K
°K — degree on the Kelvin scale
K^+ — potassium ion
K_a —
 acid dissociation constant
 acid ionization constant
K_b —
 base dissociation constant
 base ionization constant
K_d —
 dissociation constant
 distribution coefficient
 partition coefficient
K_e — exchangeable body potassium

K_{eq} — equilibrium constant
K_i —
   dissociation of enzyme-inhibitor complex
   inhibition constant
K_m —
   Michaelis constant
   Michaelis-Menten dissociation constant
K_{sp} —
   potassium solubility product
   solubility product constant
K_w — ion product of water
K_1 — phylloquinone
K_3 — vitamin K_3 (menadione)
K_4 — vitamin K_4 (menadiol sodium diphosphate)
K-10 — gastric tube
17-K — 17-ketosteroids
^{40}K — radioactive potassium isotope
^{42}K — radioactive potassium isotope
^{43}K — radioactive potassium isotope
k —
   Boltzmann's constant
   kilo-
   magnetic susceptibility
   rate of velocity constant
κ —
   kappa (tenth letter of the Greek alphabet), lowercase
   magnetic susceptibility
   one of the two immunoglobulin light chains
KA —
   alkaline phosphatase
   kainic acid
   kathode (cathode)
   keratoacanthoma
   keto acid
   ketoacidosis
   King-Armstrong [unit]
   kynurenic acid
K/A — ketogenic/antiketogenic [ratio]
K_a —
   acid dissociation constant

K_a — (continued)
   acid ionization constant
kA — kiloampere
KAAD — kerosene, alcohol, acetic acid, and dioxane
KAB — knowledge, attitude, and behavior
KABC — Kaufman Assessment Battery for Children
KAF —
   conglutinogen-activating factor
   killer-assisting factor
   kinase-activating factor
KAFO — knee-ankle-foot orthosis
KAL — Kallmann's syndrome
kal. — kalium (Lat.) potassium
KAO — knee-ankle orthosis
KAP — knowledge, attitude, and practice
kappa — a light chain of human immunoglobulins
KAS — Katz's Adjustment Scales
KAST — Kindergarten Auditory Screening Test
KAT — kanamycin acetyltransferase
kat — katal
kat/l — katals per liter
KAU — King-Armstrong unit
KB —
   Kashin-(Beck)Bek [disease]
   ketone body
   kilobyte
   Kleihauer-Betke [test]
   knee brace
K/B — knee-bearing [prosthesis]
K_b —
   base ionization constant
   dissociation constant of a base
kb — kilobase (1000 bases)
kbp — kilobase pairs (1000 base pairs)
KBr — potassium bromide
KB splint — knuckle-bender splint
KBS — Klüver-Bucy syndrome
KC —
   kathodal (cathodal) closing

KC — *(continued)*
    keratoconjunctivitis
    keratoconus
    keratoma climacterium
    knee-to-chest
    knuckle cracking
    Kupffer cell
kC — kilocoulomb
kc — kilocycle
KCC —
    kathodal (cathodal)-closing
      contraction
    Kulchitsky cell carcinoma
KCCT — kaolin-cephalin clotting
    time
K cell — killer cell
KCG — kinetocardiogram
$KC_2H_3O_2$ — potassium acetate
kCi — kilocurie
KCl — potassium chloride
$KClO_3$ — potassium chlorate
KCN — potassium cyanide [broth
    base]
KCNS — potassium thiocyanate
K_2CO_3 — potassium carbonate
kcps — kilocycles per second
KCS — keratoconjunctivitis sicca
KCT — kathodal (cathodal)-clos-
    ing tetanus
KD —
    kathodal (cathodal)-duration
    Kawasaki disease
    Keto-Diastix
    kidney donor
    killed
    knee disarticulation
    knitted Dacron
K_d —
    dissociation constant
    distribution coefficient
    partition coefficient
kD, kDa — kilodalton
KDA — known drug allergies
KDC —
    kathodal (cathodal)-duration
      contraction
    kidney disease treatment cen-
    ter

KDNA — kinetoplast deoxyribo-
    nucleic acid
KDO —
    ketodeoxyoctonate
    ketodeoxyoctonic [acid]
KDP — potassium dihydrogen
    phosphate
KDS —
    Kaufman's Developmental
      Scale
    King-Denborough syndrome
    Kocher-Debré-Sémélaigne
      [syndrome]
KDSM — keratinizing desquama-
    tive squamous metaplasia
KDT — kathodal (cathodal)-dura-
    tion tetanus
kdyn — kilodyne
KE —
    Kendall's compound E
    kinetic energy
Ke — Kern
K_e — exchangeable body potassium
KEC — *Klebsiella, Enterobacter,*
    Citrobacter
KED — Kendrick's extrication de-
    vice
Ke/kg — exchangeable potassium
    per kilogram of body weight
Keln — Kell negative
KemoTx — chemical therapy [che-
    motherapy]
K_{eq} — equilibrium constant
Kera — keratitis
KERV — Kentucky equine respira-
    tory virus
17-keto — 17-ketosteroid [test]
keV — kilo electron volt
KF —
    Kayser-Fleischer [ring]
    kidney function
    Klippel-Feil [syndrome]
kf. — flocculation speed in anti-
    gen-antibody reaction
KFAB — kidney-fixing antibody
K factor — gamma ray dose
KFAO — knee-foot-ankle orthosis
KFD —
    Kinetic Family Drawing

KFD — *(continued)*
  Kyasanur Forest disease
KFR — Kayser-Fleischer ring
KFS — Klippel-Feil syndrome
KG — ketoglutarate
αKG — alpha-ketoglutarate
KG-1 — Koeffler Golde-1 [cell line]
kG — kilogauss
kg — kilogram
KGC — Keflin, gentamicin, and carbenicillin
kg-cal — kilogram-calorie
kg/cm^2 — kilograms per square centimeter
KGDHC — ketoglutarate dehydrogenase complex
kgf — kilogram-force
KGHT — kidney Goldblatt hypertension
kg/l — kilograms per liter
kg/m — kilograms per meter
kg-m — kilogram-meter
kg-m/s^2 — kilogram-meter per second squared
Kgn — kininogen
kgps — kilograms per second
KGS — ketogenic steroid
17-KGS — 17-ketogenic steroid
KH — Krebs-Henseleit [cycle]
K24H — potassium, urine 24-hour
KHB — Krebs-Henseleit (bicarbonate) buffer
KHb — potassium hemoglobinate
KHC — kinetic hemolysis curve
KHCO$_3$ — potassium bicarbonate
KHD — kinky hair disease
KHF — Korean hemorrhagic fever
Khgb — potassium hemoglobinate
KHM — keratoderma hereditaria mutilans
KHN — Knoop hardness number
KHP — King's Honorary Physician
KHS —
  King's Honorary Surgeon
  kinky hair syndrome
  Krebs-Henseleit solution
kHz — kilohertz

KI —
  karyopyknotic index
  knee immobilizer
  Krönig's isthmus
  potassium iodide
K$_i$ —
  dissociation of enzyme-inhibitor complex
  inhibition constant
KIA — Kligler iron agar
KIC —
  ketoisocaproate
  ketoisocaproic [acid]
KICB — killed intracellular bacteria
KID —
  keratitis, ichthyosis, and deafness [syndrome]
  kidney
KIDS — Kent Infant Development Scale
kilo. — one thousand
KIMSA — Kirsten murine sarcoma
KIMSV — Kirsten murine sarcoma virus
KIP — key intermediary protein
KIS — Krankenhaus' Information System
KISS —
  key integrative social system
  kidney internal splint/stent
  saturated solution of potassium iodide
KIT — Kahn Intelligence Test
KIU —
  kallikrein inactivation unit
  kallikrein-inhibiting unit
KIVA — ketoisovaleric acid
kJ — kilojoule
kj — knee jerk
k.k. — knee kick
kkat — kilokatal
KKK — Kolmer, Kline, Kahn [test]
KKS — kallikrein-kinin system
KL —
  kidney lobe
  Klebs-Löffler [bacillus]
  Kleine-Levin [syndrome]

kl —
> kiloliter
> *Klanag* (Ger.) musical over-tone

KL bac. — Klebs-Löffler bacillus

KL-BET — Kleihauer-Betke [test]

Kleb. — *Klebsiella*

KLH — keyhole-limpet hemocyanin

KLS —
> kidney, liver, spleen
> Kreuzbein's lipomatous syndrome

KLST — Kindergarten Language Screening Test

KM —
> kanamycin
> kappa immunoglobulin light chain
> Kraepelin-Morel [disease]

K_m —
> Michaelis constant
> Michaelis-Menten dissociation constant

km — kilometer

km^2 — square kilometer

kMc — kilomegacycle

K-MCM — potassium-containing minimal capacitation medium

KMDAT — Key Math Diagnostic Arithmetic Test

KMEF — keratin, myosin, epidermin, and fibrin

$KMnO_4$ — potassium permanganate

km.p.s. — kilometers per second

KMS — kwashiorkor-marasmus syndrome

KMV — killed measles virus vaccine

Kn — knee

KN — Knudsen number

kN — kilonewton

KNO — keep needle open

KNO_3 — potassium nitrate

KNRK — Kirsten sarcoma virus in normal rat kidney

KO —
> killed organism

KO — (*continued*)
> knee orthosis
> knocked out

K/O —
> keep on
> keep open

$K\Omega$ — kilohm

KOC — kathodal (cathodal)-opening contraction

KO'd — knocked out

KOH — potassium hydroxide

KOIS — Kuder Occupational Interest Survey

KOT — Knowledge of Occupations Test

KP —
> Kaufmann-Peterson [base]
> keratitic precipitates
> keratitis punctata
> keratoprecipitates
> keratotic patch
> kidney protein
> kidney punch [test]
> killed parenteral [vaccine]
> *Klebsiella pneumoniae*

K-P — Kaiser-Permanente [diet]

Kp — solubility product constant

kPa — kilopascal

K-pad — Aqua-K module with pad

kPa.s./l. — kilopascal seconds per liter

KPB —
> kalium (potassium) phosphate buffer
> ketophenylbutazone

KPE — Kelman pharmacoemulsification

KPI —
> kallikrein-protease inhibitor
> karyopyknotic index

K-PL — potassium-plasma

KPM — kilo/pound/meter

K_3PO_3 — normal ortho- or tribasic potassium phosphate

KPR —
> key pulse rate
> Kuder Preference Record

KPR-V — Kuder Preference Record—Vocational

KPS — Karnofsky performance score

KPT —
kidney punch test
Kuder Performance Test

KPTI — Kunitz pancreatic trypsin inhibitor

KPTT — kaolin partial thromboplastin time

KPV —
key process variable
killed parenteral vaccine
killed polio vaccine

KR —
key ridge
knowledge of results
Kopper-Reppart [medium]

Kr — krypton

kR — kiloroentgen

KRA — Klinefelter-Reifenstein-Albright [syndrome]

KRB — Krebs-Ringer buffer

KRBB — Krebs-Ringer bicarbonate buffer

KRBG — Krebs-Ringer bicarbonate buffer with glucose

KRBS — Krebs-Ringer bicarbonate solution

KRP —
Kolmer's test with Reiter protein [antigen]
Krebs-Ringer phosphate

KRPS — Krebs-Ringer phosphate buffer solution

KRRS — kinetic resonance Raman spectroscopy

KS —
Kallmann syndrome
Kaposi's sarcoma
Kartagener syndrome
Kawasaki syndrome
keratan sulfate
ketosteroid
Klinefelter's syndrome
Kochleffel syndrome
Korsakoff syndrome
Kugel-Stoloff [syndrome]
Kveim-Siltzbach [test]

17-KS — 17-ketosteroid

K_2SO_4 — potassium sulfate

ks — kilosecond

KSA — knowledge, skills, and abilities

KSC — kathodal (cathodal) closing contraction

KSCN — potassium thiocyanate

KS/OI — Kaposi's sarcoma with opportunistic infection

KSP —
Karolinska Scale of Personality
kidney-specific protein

K_{sp} —
potassium solubility product
solubility product constant

K-SPT — potassium-urine spot

KSS —
Kearns-Sayre syndrome
Kearns-Sayre-Shy [syndrome]

KST — kathodal (cathodal) closing tetanus

K stoff — chloromethyl chloroformate

KSU — Kent State University [speech discrimination test]

KT —
kidney transplant
kidney transplantation
Klippel-Trenaunay [syndrome]
Kuder's test

KTI — kallikrein-trypsin inhibitor

KTS —
kethoxal thiosemicarbazone
Kiersley Temperament Sorter

KTSA — Kahn Test of Symbol Arrangement

KTU — kidney transplant unit

KTVS — Keystone Telebinocular Visual Survey

KTWS — Klippel-Trenaunay-Weber syndrome

KU —
kallikrein unit
Karmen's unit

Ku — kurchatovium

KUB —
kidney and upper bladder

KUB — (continued)
    kidney, ureter, and bladder
KUF — kidney ultrafiltration rate
KUS — kidney, ureter, and spleen
KV —
    kanamycin-vancomycin
    killed vaccine
kV — kilovolt
kVa — kilovolt-ampere
kvar — kilovar
KVBA — kanamycin-vancomycin blood agar
kVcp — kilovolt constant potential
KVE — Kaposi's varicelliform eruption
KVLBA — kanamycin-vancomycin laked blood agar
KVO — keep vein open

KVO C D5W — keep vein open cum 5% dextrose in water
kVp — kilovolts peak
K wire — Kirschner wire
KW —
    Keith-Wagener [classification]
    Kimmelstiel-Wilson [syndrome]
    Kugelberg-Welander [disease]
Kw — weighted kappa
K_w — ion product of water
kW — kilowatt
KWB — Keith, Wagener, Barker [classification]
KWE — Keith-Welti-Ernst [method]
kW-hr — kilowatt-hour
kyph — kyphosis
KZ —
    Kaplan-Zuelzer [syndrome]
    ketoconazole

L —
    angular momentum
    Avogadro's constant
    Avogadro's number
    coefficient of induction
    diffusion length
    inductance
    lambda
    lambert
    latent heat
    latex
    Latin
    leader sequence
    left
    length
    Lente insulin
    lesser
    lethal
    leucine
    lewisite
    liber (Lat.) book

L — (continued)
    libra (Lat.) pound
    licensed (to practice)
    lidocaine
    ligament
    light chain
    light sense
    lilac
    limen (Lat.) threshold
    limes (Lat.) boundary
    lincomycin
    lingual
    liquor
    liter
    liver
    living
    longitudinal
    low
    lower
    lowest
    lues (Lat.) pestilence (syphilis)

L — (continued)
    lumbar
    lumen
    luminance
    lung
    lymph
    lymphocyte
    lymphogranuloma
    lysosome
    outer membrane layer of cell
        wall of gram-negative bacte-
        ria
    radiance
    self-inductance
L. —
    Lactobacillus
    Legionella
    Leishmania
    Leptospira
    Leptotrichia
    Listeria
L_0 — limes nul (limes [Lat.] zero)
    [neutralized toxin-antitoxin
    mixture]
L_+ — limes tod [fatal dose toxin-
    antitoxin mixture]
L1, L2, L3, L4, L5 — first, second,
    third, fourth, and fifth lumbar
    vertebrae
LI, LII, LIII — first, second, and
    third stages of syphilis (lues)
L/3 — lower third
L —
    chemical prefix
    stereochemical structure
    sterically related to L-glyceral-
        dehyde
l —
    azimuthal quantum number
    left eye
    length
    lethal
    levo-
    levorotatory
    line
    liter
    long
    longitudinal

l — (continued)
    lumen
    radioactive constant
    specific latent heat
l. —
    liber (Lat.) book
    libra (Lat.) pound
    limen (Lat.) threshold
    limes (Lat.) boundary
    lues (Lat.) pestilence (syphi-
        lis)
l — levorotatory
λ —
    craniometric point
    decay constant
    immunoglobulin light chain
    junction of lambdoid and
        sagittal sutures
    lambda (eleventh letter of the
        Greek alphabet), lowercase
    mean free path
    microliter
    thermal conductivity
    wavelength
LA —
    lactic acid
    language age
    large amount
    late abortion
    late antigen
    latex agglutination
    left angle
    left angulation
    left arm
    left atrial
    left atrium
    left auricle
    left auricular
    leucine aminopeptidase
    leukemia antigen
    leukoagglutination
    leuprolide acetate
    levator ani
    lichen amyloidosis
    Lightwood-Albright [syn-
        drome]
    linguoaxial
    linoleic acid

LA — (continued)
    lobuloalveolar
    local anesthesia
    long-acting [drug]
    long-arm [cast]
    low anxiety
    Ludwig's angina
    lupus anticoagulant
    lymphocyte antibody
L&A —
    light and accommodation
    living and active
LA50 — total body surface area of burn that will kill 50% of patients (lethal area)
La —
    labial
    lambert
    lanthanum
l.a. — *lege artis* (Lat.) according to the art
LAA —
    left atrial abnormality
    left atrial appendage
    left auricular appendage
    leukemia-associated antigen
    leukocyte ascorbic acid
LAAM — *l*-acetyl-α-methadol
LAAO — L-amino acid oxidase
LA/Ao — left atrial/aortic [ratio]
LAARD — long-acting antirheumatic drug
lab. — laboratory
LABS — Laboratory Admission Baseline Studies
LABV — left atrial ball valve
LABVT — left atrial ball valve thrombus
LAC —
    La Crosse subtype encephalitis [virus]
    laceration
    lactose
    left atrial contraction
    linguoaxiocervical
    long-arm cast
    low-amplitude contraction

LAC — (continued)
    lung adenocarcinoma cells
    lupus anticoagulant
LaC — labiocervical
lac. —
    laceration
    lactate
    lactation
lac. & cont. — lacerations and contusions
LACN — local area communications network
lacr. — lacrimal
LACT —
    lactic acid
    Lindamood Auditory Conceptualization Test
LAC T — lactose tolerance
lact. —
    lactate
    lactating
    lactation
    lactic
LACT-ART — lactate, arterial
lact. hyd. — lactalbumin hydrolysate
LAD —
    lactic acid dehydrogenase
    language acquisition device
    left anterior descending [artery]
    left axis deviation
    leukocyte adhesion deficiency
    ligament augmentation device
    linoleic acid depression
    lipoamide dehydrogenase
    lymphocyte-activating determinant
LADA —
    laboratory animal dander allergy
    left acromiodorsoanterior [position]
    left anterior descending artery
LADCA — left anterior descending coronary artery
LADD —
    lacrimoauriculodentodigital [syndrome]

LADD — *(continued)*
   left anterior descending diagonal [coronary artery]
LADH —
   lactic acid dehydrogenase
   liver alcohol dehydrogenase
LADME — liberation, absorption, distribution, metabolism, excretion
LAD-MIN — left axis deviation, minimal
LADP — left acromiodorsoposterior [position]
LADu — lobuloalveolar-ductal
LAE —
   left atrial enlargement
   long above-elbow [cast]
LAEDV — left atrial end-diastolic volume
LAEI — left atrial emptying index
LAESV — left atrial end-systolic volume
laev. — *laevus* (Lat.) left
LAF —
   laminar airflow
   Latin American female
   leukocyte-activating factor
   low animal fat
   lymphocyte-activating factor
LAFB — left anterior fascicular block
LAFR — laminar airflow room
LAFU — laminar airflow unit
LAG —
   labiogingival
   linguoaxiogingival
   lymphangiogram
   lymphangiography
LaG — labiogingival
lag. — *lagena* (Lat.) flask
LAH —
   lactalbumin hydrolysate
   left anterior hemiblock
   left atrial hypertrophy
   Licentiate of Apothecaries Hall
   lithium aluminum hydride
LAHB — left anterior hemiblock
LAHC — low affinity–high capacity

LAHV — leukocyte-associated herpesvirus
LAI —
   labioincisal
   latex (particle) agglutination inhibition
   left atrial involvement
   leukocyte adherence inhibition
LaI — labioincisal
LAIF — leukocyte adherence inhibition factor
LAIT — latex agglutination inhibition test
LAK — lymphokine-activated killer [cells]
LAL —
   left axillary line
   Limulus amebocyte lysate
   low air loss
   lysosomal acid lipase
LaL — labiolingual
L-Ala — L-alanine
LALB — low air-loss bed
LALI — lymphocyte antibody–lymphocytolytic interaction
LAM —
   lactation amenorrhea method
   lamina
   laminar airflow
   laminectomy
   late ambulatory monitoring
   Latin American male
   left anterior measurement
   left atrial myxoma
   lymphangioleiomyomatosis
lam. —
   lamina
   laminectomy
   laminogram
lam & fus — laminectomy and fusion
LA-MAX — maximal left atrial [dimension]
LAMB — lentigines, atrial myxoma, mucocutaneous myxomas, and blue nevi [syndrome]
lami — laminotomy

LAMMA — laser microprobe mass analyzer

LAN —
  local area network
  long-acting neuroleptic
  lymphadenopathy

LANC — long-arm navicular cast

L ANT — left anterior

LANV — left atrial neovascularization

LAO —
  left anterior oblique
  left anterior occipital
  left atrial overload
  Licentiate of the Art of Obstetrics

LAP —
  laparoscopy
  laparotomy
  left arterial pressure
  left atrial pressure
  leucine aminopeptidase
  leukocyte adhesion protein
  leukocyte alkaline phosphatase
  low atmospheric pressure
  lyophilized anterior pituitary

lap —
  laparoscopy
  laparotomy

LAPA — leukocyte alkaline phosphatase activity

LAPF — low-affinity platelet factor

lapid. — *lapideum* (Lat.) stony

LAPMS — long-arm posterior-molded splint

LAPSE — long-term ambulatory physiological surveillance

LAPW — left atrial posterior wall

LAR —
  laryngology
  late asthmatic response
  late reaction
  left arm, reclining
  left arm, recumbent

lar — larynx

LARC — leukocyte automatic recognition computer

LARD — lacrimoauriculoradiodental [syndrome]

LARS — Language-Structured Auditory Retention Span [test]

laryn —
  laryngeal
  laryngitis
  laryngoscopy

Laryngol. —
  laryngologist
  laryngology

LAS —
  Laboratory Automation System
  lateral amyotrophic sclerosis
  laxative abuse syndrome
  left anterior-superior
  left arm, sitting
  leucine acetylsalicylate
  linear alkylate sulfonate
  local adaptation syndrome
  long-arm splint
  lower abdominal surgery
  lymphadenopathy syndrome
  lymphangioscintigraphy

LASA — left anterior spinal artery

LASER — light amplification by stimulated emission of radiation

LASFB — left anterior-superior fascicular block

LASH — left anterior-superior hemiblock

L-ASP — L-asparaginase

LASS —
  labile aggregation-stimulating substance
  Linguistic Analysis of Speech Samples

LAST — leukocyte-antigen sensitivity testing

LAT —
  latent
  lateral
  latex agglutination test
  left anterior thigh
  left atrial thrombus
  lysolecithin acyltransferase

Lat. — Latin
lat —
    latent
    lateral
    latissimus (dorsi)
    latitude
LAT-A — latrunculin A
lat. admov. — *lateri admoveatur*
    (Lat.) let it be applied to the
    side
LAT-B — latrunculin B
lat bend — lateral bending
LATCH — literature attached to
    charts
lat. dol. — *lateri dolenti* (Lat.) to
    the painful side
lat & loc — lateralizing and localiz-
    ing
l-atm — liter-atmosphere
lat. men. — lateral meniscectomy
LATP — left atrial transmural pres-
    sure
LATPT — left atrial transesopha-
    geal pacing test
lat Rin — lactated Ringer's [solu-
    tion]
LATS —
    long-acting thyroid-stimulat-
      ing [hormone]
    long-acting thyroid stimulator
    long-acting transmural stimu-
      lator
LATS-P — long-acting thyroid
    stimulator-protector
LATu — lobuloalveolar tumor
LAV —
    leafhopper A virus
    lymphadenopathy-associated
      virus
lav. — lavatory
LAW — left atrial wall
lax. —
    laxative
    laxity
LB —
    laboratory [data]
    lamellar body
    large bowel

LB — *(continued)*
    lateral binding
    Lederer-Brill [syndrome]
    left breast
    left bundle
    left buttock
    leiomyoblastoma
    lipid body
    live birth
    liver biopsy
    Living Bank
    loose body
    low back [pain]
    low breakage
    lung biopsy
L&B — left and below
L-B — Liebermann-Burchard [test]
Lb — pound force
lb. — *libra* (Lat.) pound
LBA — left basal artery
lb ap — libra apothecary (apothe-
    cary pound)
lb av — libra avoirdupois (avoirdu-
    pois pound)
LBB —
    left breast biopsy
    left bundle branch
    low back bending
LBBB — left bundle branch block
LBBsB — left bundle branch sys-
    tem block
LBBX — left breast biopsy exami-
    nation
LBC —
    lidocaine blood concentration
    lymphadenosis benigna cutis
LBCD — left border cardiac dull-
    ness
LBCF — Laboratory Branch Com-
    plement Fixation [test]
LBD —
    large bile duct
    left border dullness
LBDQ — Leader Behavior Descrip-
    tion Questionnaire
LBE — long below-elbow [cast]
LBF —
    Lactobacillus bulgaricus factor

LBF — (continued)
    limb blood flow
    liver blood flow
lbf — pound force
lb-ft — pound-feet
lbf-ft — pound force foot
LBH — length, breadth, height
LBI —
    low back injury
    low serum-bound iron
lb/in² — pounds per square inch
LBL —
    labeled lymphoblast
    lymphoblastic lymphoma
LBM —
    last bowel movement
    lean body mass
    loose bowel movement
    lung basement membrane
LBNP — lower-body negative pressure
LBO — large bowel obstruction
LBP —
    low back pain
    low blood pressure
LBPF — long bone or pelvic fracture
LBPQ — Low Back Pain Questionnaire
LBRF — louse-borne relapsing fever
LBS —
    lactobacillus selector
    low back strain
    low back syndrome
lbs. — librae (Lat.) pounds
LBSA — lipid-bound sialic acid
LBT —
    low back tenderness
    low back trouble
    lupus band test
lb t — pound troy
LBTI — lima bean trypsin inhibitor
lb tr — pound troy
LBV —
    left brachial vein
    lung blood volume

LBW —
    lean body weight
    low birth weight
LBWI — low-birth-weight infant
LBWR — lung-body weight ratio
LC —
    lactation consultant
    Laënnec's cirrhosis
    lamina cortex
    Langerhans' cell
    laparoscopic cholecystectomy
    large chromophobe
    large cleaved [cell]
    late clamped
    lecithin cholesterol (acyl-transferase)
    left [ear], cold [stimulus]
    left circumflex [artery]
    leisure counseling
    lethal concentration
    Library of Congress
    life care
    light chain
    light coagulation
    linguocervical
    lining cell
    lipid cytosomes
    liquid chromatography
    liquid crystal
    lithocolic [acid]
    liver cirrhosis
    liver clinic
    living children
    locus caeruleus
    long-chain [triglycerides]
    longus capitis
    low calorie
    lung cancer
    lung cell
    lymph capillary
    lymphocyte count
    lymphocytotoxin
    lymphoma culture
LC₅₀ — median lethal concentration
l.c. — loco citato (Lat.) in the place cited
LCA —
    Leber's congenital amaurosis

LCA — *(continued)*
    left carotid artery
    left circumflex artery
    left coronary artery
    leukocyte common antigen
    light contact assist
    lithocholic acid
    lymphocyte chemoattractant activity
    lymphocyte chemotactic activity
    lymphocytotoxic antibody
LCAD — long-chain acyl-CoA dehydrogenase
LCAO — linear combination of atomic orbitals
LCAO-MO — linear combination of atomic orbital–molecular orbital
LCAR — late cutaneous anaphylactic reaction
LCAT — lecithin-cholesterol acyltransferase
LCB —
    Laboratory of Cancer Biology
    left costal border
    lymphomatosis cutis benigna
LCBF — local cerebral blood flow
LCC —
    lactose coliform count
    left circumflex coronary [artery]
    left common carotid
    left coronary cusp
    lipid-containing cell
    liver cell carcinoma
LCCA —
    late cortical cerebellar atrophy
    left circumflex coronary artery
    left common carotid artery
    leukoclastic angiitis
    leukocytoclastic angiitis
LCCME — Liaison Committee on Continuing Medical Education
LCCP — limited channel-capacity process

LCCS — lower cervical cesarean section
LCCSCT — large-cell calcifying Sertoli cell tumor
LCD —
    liquid crystal diode
    liquor carbonis detergens (coal tar solution)
    localized collagen dystrophy
    low-calcium diet
LCDD — light-chain deposition disease
LCED — liquid chromatography with electrochemical detection
LCF —
    least common factor
    left circumflex [artery]
    left common femoral [artery]
    linear correction factor
    low-frequency (current) field
    lymphocyte culture fluid
LCFA — long-chain fatty acid
LCFAO — long-chain fatty acid oxidation
LCFC — linear combination of fragment configuration
LCFM — left circumflex marginal
LCFU — leukocyte colony-forming unit
LCG — Langerhans cell granule
LCGL — large-cell granulocytic leukemia
LCGME — Liaison Committee on Graduate Medical Education
LCGU — local cerebral glucose utilization
LCH —
    Langerhans cell histiocytosis
    local city hospital
L.Ch. — Licentiate in Surgery
L chain — light chain
LCI —
    length complexity index
    lung clearance index
LCIS — lobular carcinoma in situ
LCL —
    lateral collateral ligament

LCL — (continued)
    Levinthal-Coles-Lillie [body]
    lower confidence limit
    lymphoblastoid cell line
    lymphocytic leukemia
    lymphocytic lymphosarcoma
    lymphoid cell line
LCLC — large cell lung carcinoma
LCM —
    latent cardiomyopathy
    left costal margin
    leukocyte-conditioned medium
    lower costal margin
    lowest common multiple
    lymphatic choriomeningitis
    lymphocytic choriomeningitis
LCME — Liaison Committee on Medical Education
LCMG — long-chain monoglyceride
L/cm H_2O — liters per centimeter of water
LCMV — lymphocytic choriomeningitis virus
LCN —
    lateral cervical nucleus
    left caudate nucleus
LCO — low cardiac output
LCOS — low cardiac output syndrome
LCP —
    Legg-Calvé-Perthes [disease]
    long-chain polysaturated [fatty acids]
LCPD — Legg-Calvé-Perthes disease
LCPS — Licentiate of the College of Physicians and Surgeons
LCQG — left caudal quarter ganglion
LCR —
    late cortical response
    late cutaneous reaction
LCS —
    left coronary sinus
    Leydig cell stimulation
    lichen chronicus simplex

LCS — (continued)
    Life Care Services
    liquor cerebrospinalis (Lat.) cerebrospinal fluid
    low constant suction
    low continuous suction
    lymphocyte culture supernatants
LCSB — Liaison Committee for Specialty Boards
LCSW — Licensed Clinical Social Worker
LCT —
    liver cell tumor
    long-chain triglyceride
    low cervical transverse
    lung capillary time
    Luscher Color Test
    lymphocytotoxicity test
    lymphocytotoxin
LCTA — lymphocytotoxic antibody
LCTD — low-calcium test diet
LCU — life change unit
LCV —
    lecithovitellin
    leucovorin
    low cervical vertical [incision]
LCx — left circumflex [coronary artery]
LD —
    labor and delivery
    laboratory data
    labyrinthine defect
    lactate dehydrogenase
    lactic (acid) dehydrogenase
    laser Doppler
    last dose
    L-dopa
    learning disability
    learning-disabled
    learning disorder
    left deltoid
    legionnaires' disease
    Leishman-Donovan [body]
    lethal dose
    levodopa
    light difference

LD — *(continued)*
    light differentiation
    light-dark
    limited disease
    limited duty
    linear dichroism
    linguodistal
    lipodystrophy
    lithium diluent
    lithium discontinuation
    liver disease
    living donor
    loading dose
    Lombard-Dowell [agar]
    long (time) dialysis
    longitudinal diameter [of heart]
    low density
    low dosage
    low dose
    lung destruction
    lymphocyte depletion
    lymphocyte-defined
    lymphocytically determined
L/D — light/darkness [ratio]
L-D — Leishman-Donovan [bodies]
L&D —
    labor and delivery
    light and distance
LD_1 — isoenzyme of lactate dehydrogenase found in the heart, erythrocytes, and kidneys
LD_2 — isoenzyme of lactate dehydrogenase found in the lungs
LD_3 — isoenzyme of lactate dehydrogenase found in the lungs
LD_4 — isoenzyme of lactate dehydrogenase found in the liver
LD_5 — isoenzyme of lactate dehydrogenase found in the liver and muscles
LD_{50} — median lethal dose
$LD_{50/30}$ — a dose that is lethal for 50% of test subjects within 30 days
LD_{100} — lethal dose in all exposed subjects

Ld — *Leishmania donovani*
LDA —
    laser Doppler anemometry
    left dorsoanterior [fetal position]
    linear displacement analysis
    lymphocyte-dependent antibody
LDAR — latex direct agglutination reaction
LDB —
    lamb dysentery bacillus
    legionnaires' disease bacillus
LDC —
    leukocyte differential count
    lymphoid dendritic cell
    lysine decarboxylase
LDCA — low dose cytosine arabinoside
LDCC — lectin-dependent cellular cytotoxicity
LDCI — low-dose continuous infusion
LDCT — late distal cortical tubule
LDD —
    late dedifferentiation
    light-dark discrimination
LDE — lauric diethamide
LDER — lateral-view dual-energy radiography
LD-EYA — Lombard-Dowell egg yolk agar
LDF —
    laser Doppler flowmetry
    laser Doppler flux
    limit dilution factor
LDG —
    lactic (acid) dehydrogenase
    lingual developmental groove
    long-distance group
    low-dose group
LDH —
    lactate dehydrogenase
    lactic (acid) dehydrogenase
    low-dose heparin
LDH_1–LDH_5 — lactate dehydrogenase fractions 1 through 5
LDHA — lactate dehydrogenase A

LDHB — lactate dehydrogenase B
LDHC — lactate dehydrogenase C
LDHI — lactate dehydrogenase iso-
enzymes
LDHK — lactate dehydrogenase K
LDIH — left direct inguinal hernia
LDISO — lactate dehydrogenase
isoenzyme
LDL —
loudness discomfort level
low-density lipoprotein
low-density lymphocyte
LDLA — low-density lipoprotein
apheresis
LDLC — low-density lipoprotein
cholesterol
LDLP — low-density lipoprotein
LDM — lactate dehydrogenase,
muscle
LDMF — latissimus dorsi myocuta-
neous flap
LD-NEYA — Lombard-Dowell
neomycin egg yolk agar
L-dopa — levodopa
L doses — limes doses [toxin/anti-
toxin combining power]
LDP —
left dorsoposterior [fetal posi-
tion]
lumbodorsal pain
LDRP — labor, delivery, recovery,
postpartum
LDS —
Licentiate in Dental Surgery
ligating and dividing stapler
LDSc — Licentiate in Dental Science
LDT — left dorsotransverse [fetal
position]
LDU — long double upright
[brace]
LDUB — long double upright
brace
LDV —
lactic dehydrogenase virus
large dense-cored vesicle
laser Doppler velocimetry
lateral distant view

LE —
left ear
left eye
lens extraction
leukocyte elastase
leukocyte esterase
leukoerythrogenic
live embryo
Long Evans [rat]
low exposure
lower extremity
lupus erythematosus
Le —
Leonard [unit for cathode
rays]
Lewis (number, diffusivity: diffusion coefficient of a fluid)
LEA —
lower extremity amputation
lower extremity arterial
lumbar epidural anesthesia
LEADS — Leadership Evaluation
and Development Scale
LEB — lupus erythematosus body
LEC —
leukoencephalitis
low-energy charged [particle]
lower esophageal contractility
LECP — low-energy charged particle
LED —
light-emitting diode
lowest effective dose
lupus erythematosus disseminatus
LEED — low-energy electron diffraction
LEEDS — low-energy electron diffraction spectroscopy
LEEP —
left end-expiratory pressure
loop electrocautery excision
procedure
LEER — lower extremity equipment related
LEF —
leukokinesis-enhancing factor
lupus erythematosus factor

leg. —
    legal
    legally
    legislation
    legislative
leg com —
    legal commitment
    legally committed
LEHPZ — lower esophageal high-pressure zone
LeIF — leukocyte interferon
leio — leiomyoma
LEIS — low-energy ion scattering
LEJ — ligation of esophagogastric junction
LEL —
    lower explosive limit
    lowest effect level
LEM —
    lateral eye movement
    Leibovitz-Emory medium
    leukocyte endogenous mediator
    light electron microscope
    light emission microscopy
LEMO — lowest empty molecular orbital
LEMS — Lambert-Eaton myasthenic syndrome
lenit — lenitive
lenit. — *leniter* (Lat.) gently
LEOD — lens extraction, oculus dexter
LEOPARD — lentigines, electrocardiogram abnormalities, ocular hypertelorism, pulmonary stenosis, abnormal genitalia, retardation of growth, and deafness [syndrome]
LEOS — lens extraction, oculus sinister
LEP —
    leptospirosis
    lethal effective phase
    lipoprotein electrophoresis
    low egg passage
    lower esophageal pressure
    lower esophagus

LEP — (*continued*)
    lupus erythematosus preparation
L_{EPN} — effective perceived noise level
LE_{prep} — lupus erythematosus preparation
LEPT — leptocyte
LEPTOS — leptospirosis agglutinins
Leq — loudness equivalent
LER — lysosomal enzyme release
LERG — local electroretinogram
L-ERX — leukoerythroblastic reaction
LES —
    Lambert-Eaton syndrome
    lateral epithelial space
    Lawrence Experimental Station [agar]
    Life Experience Survey
    local excitatory state
    Locke egg serum
    lower esophageal segment
    lower esophageal sphincter
    lower esophageal stricture
    lupus erythematosus, systemic
les —
    lesion
    local excitatory state
    low excitatory state
LESA — liposomally entrapped second antibody
LESP — lower esophageal sphincter pressure
LESS — lateral electrical spine stimulation
LET —
    language enrichment therapy
    linear energy transfer
    low energy transfer
LETD — lowest effective toxic dose
LETS — large external transformation-sensitive (protein)
LEU —
    leucovorin
    leukocyte equivalent unit

Leu — leucine
leuc — leucocyte
leuk —
  leukocyte
  leukemia
LEUKAP — leukocyte alkaline
  phosphatase
LEV — lower extremity venous
lev — levator [muscle]
lev. — *levis* (Lat.) light
levit. — *leviter* (Lat.) lightly
LEVT — lower extremity venous
  tracing
LEW — Lewis [rat]
LEX — lactate extraction
l/ext — lower extremity
LF —
  labile factor
  lactoferrin
  laryngofissure
  Lassa fever
  latex fixation
  lavage fluid
  left foot
  left forearm
  lethal factor
  leucine flux
  leukotactic factor
  ligamentum flavum
  limes flocculation [unit, dose
    of toxin per ml]
  limit of flocculation
  low-fat [diet]
  low-forceps [delivery]
  low-frequency
Lf — limit of flocculation
lf —
  lactoferrin
  left
  low-frequency
LFA —
  left femoral artery
  left forearm
  left frontal craniotomy
  left frontoanterior [fetal posi-
    tion]
  leukocyte function-associated
    anticoagulation

LFA — (*continued*)
  leukotactic factor activity
  low-friction arthroplasty
LFA-1 — leukocyte function-associated antigen 1
LFA-2 — leukocyte function-associated antigen 2
LFA-3 — leukocyte function-associated antigen 3
LFB —
  lingual-facial-buccal
  liver, iron, and B complex
LFC —
  left frontal craniotomy
  living female child
  low fat and cholesterol [diet]
LFD —
  lactose-free diet
  large for date [fetus]
  late fetal death
  lateral facial dysplasia
  least fatal dose
  low-fat diet
  low-fiber diet
  low-forceps delivery
LFECT — loose fibroelastic connective tissue
LFER — linear free-energy relationship
LFH — left femoral hernia
LFL —
  left frontolateral
  leukocyte feeder layer
  lower flammable limit
LFN — lactoferrin
L-[form] — a defective bacterial
  variant that can multiply on
  hypertonic medium
LFoV — large field of view
LFP — left frontoposterior [fetal
  position]
LFPPV — low-frequency positive
  pressure ventilation
LFPS — Licentiate of the Faculty
  of Physicians and Surgeons
LFR — lymphoid follicular reticulosis

LF-RF — local-regional failure

LFS —
    lateral facet syndrome
    limbic forebrain structure
    liver function series

LFT —
    latex fixation test
    latex flocculation test
    left frontotransverse [fetal position]
    liver function test
    low-frequency tetanic [stimulation]
    low-frequency tetanus
    low-frequency transduction
    low-frequency transfer

LFTSW — left foot switch

LFU —
    limit flocculation unit
    lipid fluidity unit

LFV —
    large field of view
    Lassa fever virus
    low-frequency ventilation

LFx — linear fracture

LG —
    lactoglobulin
    lamellar granule
    large
    laryngectomy
    left gluteal
    left gluteus
    Lennox-Gastaut [syndrome]
    leucylglycine
    linguogingival
    lipoglycopeptide
    liver graft
    low glucose
    lymph gland
    lymphatic gland

lg —
    large
    left gluteus
    leg
    long

LGA —
    large for gestational age
    left gastric artery

LGB —
    Landry-Guillain-Barré [syndrome]
    lateral geniculate body

LGBS — Landry-Guillain-Barré syndrome

LGC — left giant cell

LGD — Leaderless Group Discussion [situational test]

LGd — dorsal lateral geniculate [nucleus]

LGE — Langat encephalitis

lge — large

LGF — lateral giant fiber

LGH —
    lactogenic hormone
    little growth hormone

LGI —
    large glucagon immunoreactivity
    lower gastrointestinal

LGL —
    labioglossolaryngeal
    large granular leukocyte
    large granular lymphocyte
    lobular glomerulonephritis
    Lown-Ganong-Levine [syndrome]

LGL-NK — large granular lymphocyte—natural killer

LGMD — limb-girdle muscular dystrophy

LGN —
    lateral geniculate nucleus
    lateral glomerulonephritis
    lobular glomerulonephritis

LGP — labioglossopharyngeal

LGS —
    large green soft [stool]
    Lennox-Gastaut syndrome
    limb girdle syndrome

LGT —
    Langat encephalitis
    late generalized tuberculosis

lgt —
    ligament
    ligamentum

LGV —
    large granular vesicle

LGV — (continued)
  lymphogranuloma venereum
LGVHD — lethal graft-versus-host disease
LgX — lymphogranulomatosis X
LH —
  late healing
  lateral hypothalamic [syndrome]
  lateral hypothalamus
  left hand
  left heart
  left hemisphere
  left hyperphoria
  liver homogenate
  lower half
  lues hereditaria
  lung homogenate
  luteinizing hormone
  luteotropic hormone
LHA —
  lateral hypothalamic area
  left hepatic artery
LHb — lateral habenulate
LHBV — left heart blood volume
LHC —
  Langerhans cell histiocytosis
  left heart catheterization
  left hypochondrium
  light-harvesting complex
LHCG — luteinizing hormone–chorionic gonadotropin [hormone]
LHF —
  left heart failure
  ligament of head of femur
LHFA — lung Hageman factor activator
LH/FSH-RF — luteinizing hormone/follicle-stimulating hormone–releasing factor
LHG —
  left hand grip
  localized hemolysis in gel
LHH — left homonymous hemianopia
LHI — lipid hydrocarbon inclusion
LHL —
  left hemisphere lesion

LHL — (continued)
  left hepatic lobe
LHMP — Life Health Monitoring Program
LHN — lateral hypothalamic nucleus
LHP —
  left hemiparesis
  left hemiplegia
LHPZ — lower (esophageal) high-pressure zone
LHQ — Life History Questionnaire
LHR —
  leukocyte histamine release
  liquid holding recovery
l-hr — lumen-hour
LH-RF —
  luteinizing hormone–releasing factor
  luteotropic hormone–releasing factor
LH-RH — luteinizing hormone–releasing hormone
LHS —
  left hand side
  left heart strain
  left heelstrike
  lymphatic and hematopoietic system
LHT — left hypertropia
L-5HTP — L-5-hydroxytryptophan
LI —
  labeling index
  lactose intolerance
  lacunar infarct
  lamellar ichthyosis
  large intestine
  learning impaired
  left iliac [artery]
  left injured
  left involved
  Leptospira icterohaemorrhagiae
  life island
  linguoincisal
  lithogenic index
  low impulsiveness
L&I — liver and iron

Li —
    a blood group system
    labrale inferius
    lithium
LIA —
    Laser Institute of America
    left iliac artery
    leukemia-associated inhibitory
        activity
    lock-in amplifier
    lymphocyte-induced angiogen-
        esis
    lysine-iron agar
LIAC — light-induced absorbance
    change
LIAF — lymphocyte-induced an-
    giogenesis factor
LIAFI — late infantile amaurotic
    familial idiocy
LIB — left in bottle
lib. — *libra* (Lat.) a pound
LIBC — latent iron-binding capac-
    ity
LIBR — Librium
LiBr — lithium bromide
LIC —
    least incompatible
    left iliac crest
    left internal carotid [artery]
    leisure-interest class
    limiting isorrheic concentra-
        tion
    local intravascular coagula-
        tion
Lic — licentiate
LICA — left internal carotid ar-
    tery
LICC — lectin-induced cellular cy-
    totoxicity
LICD — lower intestinal Crohn's
    disease
LICM — left intercostal mar-
    gin
Lic.-Med. — Licentiate in Medi-
    cine
Li_2CO_3 — lithium carbonate
LICS — left intercostal space

LID —
    late immunoglobulin defi-
        ciency
    lymphocytic infiltrative dis-
        ease
LIDC — low-intensity direct cur-
    rent
LIDO — lidocaine
LIF —
    laser-induced fluorescence
    left iliac fossa
    left index finger
    leukemia-inhibiting factor
    leukocyte infiltration factor
    leukocyte inhibitory factor
    leukocytosis-inducing factor
    liver (migration) inhibitory
        factor
LIFE —
    Longitudinal Interval Follow-
        up Evaluation
    lung imaging fluorescence en-
        doscope
LIFO — last in, first out
LIFT — lymphocyte immunofluo-
    rescence test
lig. —
    ligament
    ligamentum
    ligate
    ligation
    ligature
ligg. —
    ligamenta
    ligaments
    ligatures
LIH — left inguinal hernia
LIHA — low impulsiveness, high
    anxiety
LII — Leisure Interest Inventory
LIJ — left internal jugular
LILA — low impulsiveness, low
    anxiety
LIM —
    limes (Lat.) boundary
    line isolation monitor
lim. —
    limit

lim. — *(continued)*
limitation
limited
LIMA — left internal mammary artery [graft]
LIMIT — The Leicester Intravenous Magnesium Intervention Trial
lin —
linear
liniment
LINAC — linear accelerator
ling —
lingual
lingular
Linim — liniment
LIO — left inferior oblique
Li₂O — lithium oxide
LiOH — lithium hydroxide
LIP —
lithium-induced polydipsia
lymphocytic interstitial pneumonitis
Lip — lipoate
lip — lipemic
LIPA — lysosomal acid lipase A
LIPB — liposomal acid lipase B
LIPHE — Life Interpersonal History Enquiry
lipoMM — lipomyelomeningocele
LIP-P — lipid profile
LIPS — Leiter International Performance Scale
LIPT — Leiter International Performance Test
LIQ — lower inner quadrant
liq. — *liquor* (Lat.) liquid, liquor
liq. dr. — liquid dram
liq. oz. — liquid ounce
liq. pt. — liquid pint
liq. qt. — liquid quart
LIR —
left iliac region
left inferior rectus
LIRBM — liver, iron, red bone marrow
LIS —
laboratory information system

LIS — *(continued)*
lateral intercellular space
left intercostal space
lithium salicylate
lobular *in situ* [carcinoma]
locked-in syndrome
low intermittent suction
low ionic strength
LISA — Library and Information Science Abstracts
LISP — List Processing Language
LISS —
low-ionic-strength saline
low-ionic-strength solution
lit. —
literal
literally
LITH — lithium
litho — lithotripsy
LIV —
law of initial value
left innominate vein
liver [battery test]
liv —
live
living
LIV-BP — leucine, isoleucine, and valine-binding protein
LIVC — left inferior vena cava
LIVEN — linear inflammatory verrucous epidermal nevus
LIVER S RB — liver scan rose bengal
LIVER S TECHN — liver scan technetium
LIVER S W FLOW — liver scan with flow
LIVIM — lethal intestinal virus of infant mice
LIVPRO — liver profile
LJ —
Larsen-Johansson [syndrome]
Löwenstein-Jensen [medium]
LJI — List of Journals Indexed
LJL — lateral joint line
LJM —
limited joint mobility
Löwenstein-Jensen medium

LK —
  lamellar keratoplasty
  Landry-Kussmaul [syndrome]
  left kidney
  lichenoid keratosis
  Löhr-Kindberg [syndrome]
  lymphokine
LK⁺ — low potassium ion
LKA — Lazare-Klerman-Armour
  (Personality Inventory)
LKESTR — leukocyte esterase
LKID — left kidney
LKM — liver-kidney microsomal
  [antibody]
LKP — lamellar keratoplasty
LKPD — Lillehei-Kaster pivoting
  disk
LKS —
  Landau-Kleffner syndrome
  liver, kidneys, and spleen
LKSB — liver, kidneys, spleen,
  bladder
LKS non pal — liver, kidneys, and
  spleen not palpable
LKV — laked kanamycin-vancomycin [agar]
LL —
  large local
  large lymphocyte
  lateral lemniscus
  left lateral
  left leg
  left lower
  left lung
  lepromatous leprosy
  Lewandowski-Lutz [syndrome]
  lid lag
  limb lead
  lines
  lingual lipase
  lipoprotein lipase
  long leg
  loudness level
  lower leg
  lower lid
  lower [eye]lid
  lower limb
  lower lip

LL — (continued)
  lower lobe
  lumbar length
  lung length
  lymphoblastic lymphoma
  lymphocytic leukemia
  lymphocytic lymphoma
  lymphoid leukemia
  lysolecithin
L&L — lids and lashes
LLA —
  lids, lashes, and adnexa
  limulus lysate assay
  lupus-like anticoagulant
L lam — lumbar laminectomy
LLAT —
  left lateral
  lysolecithin acyltransferase
L lat — left lateral
LLB —
  left lateral bending
  left lateral border
  left lower border
  long-leg brace
  lower lobe bronchus
LLBCD — left lower border of cardiac dullness
LLBP — long-leg brace with pelvic
  (band)
LLC —
  Lewis lung carcinoma
  liquid-liquid chromatography
  long-leg cast
  lower level of care
  lymphocytic leukemia,
    chronic
LLCC — long-leg cylinder cast
LLC-MK1 — rhesus monkey kidney cells
LLC-MK2 — rhesus monkey kidney cells
LLC-MK3 — Cercopithecus monkey
  kidney cells
LLC-RK1 — rabbit kidney cells
LLD —
  Lactobacillus lactis Dorner [fac-
    tor]
  left lateral decubitus [posi-
    tion]

LLD — *(continued)*
    leg length discrepancy
    liquid-liquid distribution
    long-lasting depolarization
LLDF — *Lactobacillus lactis* Dorner factor (vitamin B_{12})
LLDH — liver lactate dehydrogenase
LLE — left lower extremity
LLF —
    Laki-Lorand factor
    left lateral femoral [injection site]
    left lateral flexion
LL-GXT — low-level graded exercise test
LLL —
    left liver lobe
    left lower leg
    left lower [eye]lid
    left lower limb
    left lower lobe
    left lower lung
LLL brace — left long-leg brace
LLLE — lower lid, left eye
LLLM — low liquid level monitor
LLLNR — left lower lobe, no rales
LLM —
    localized leukocyte mobilization
    lysis, lavage and manipulation [of disk and capsule]
LLN — lower limit of normal
LLO — *Legionella*-like organism
LLOD — lower lid, oculus dexter
LLOS — lower lid, oculus sinister
LLP —
    late luteal phase
    long-lasting potentiation
    long-leg plaster [cast]
LLPMS — long-leg posterior molded splint
LLQ — left lower quadrant
LLR —
    large local reaction
    left lateral rectus [muscle]
    left lumbar region
LLRE — lower lid, right eye

LLS —
    lateral loop suspensor
    lazy leukocyte syndrome
    long-leg splint
LLSB —
    left lower scapular border
    left lower sternal border
LLT —
    left lateral thigh
    lysolecithin
LLV —
    lymphatic leukemia virus
    lymphoid leukosis virus
LLVAH — Loma Linda Veterans Administration Hospital
LLV-F — lymphatic leukemia virus, Friend-associated
LLVP — left lateral ventricular pre-excitation
LLW — low-level waste
LLWC — long-leg walking cast
LLX — left lower extremity
LM —
    labiomental
    lactic (acid) mineral [medium]
    lactose malabsorption
    laryngeal muscle
    lateral malleolus
    left main
    left median
    legal medicine
    lemniscus medialis
    Licentiate in Medicine
    Licentiate in Midwifery
    light microscope
    light microscopy
    light minimum
    lincomycin
    lingual margin
    linguomesial
    lipid-mobilizing [hormone]
    liquid membrane
    Listeria monocytogenes
    localized movement
    longitudinal muscle
    Looser-Milkman [syndrome]
    lower motor [neuron]

L/M — liters per minute
Lm — *Listeria monocytogenes*
lm. — lumen
l/m — liters per minute
LMA —
> left mentoanterior [fetal position]
> limbic midbrain area
> liver membrane antibody
> liver [cell] membrane autoantibody

LMB —
> Laurence-Moon-Biedl [syndrome]
> left main-stem bronchus
> leiomyoblastoma

LMBB — Laurence-Moon-Bardet-Biedl [syndrome]
LMBS — Laurence-Moon-Biedl syndrome
LMC —
> large motile cell
> lateral motor column
> left main coronary [artery]
> left middle cerebral [artery]
> living male child
> lymphocyte-mediated cytolysis
> lymphocyte-mediated cytotoxicity
> lymphocyte microcytotoxicity
> lymphomyeloid complex

LMCA —
> left main coronary artery
> left middle cerebral artery

LMCAD — left main coronary artery disease
LMCAT — left middle cerebral artery thrombosis
LMCC — Licentiate of the Medical Council of Canada
LMCL — left midclavicular line
LMCT — ligand-to-metal charge transfer
LMD —
> left main disease
> lipid-moiety modified derivative
> local medical doctor

LMD — (*continued*)
> low molecular (weight) dextran

LMDF — lupus miliaris disseminatus faciei
LMDX — low molecular weight dextran
LME —
> left mediolateral episiotomy
> leukocyte migration enhancement

LMed&Ch — Licentiate in Medicine and Surgery
LMEE — left middle ear exploration
LMF —
> left middle finger
> leukocyte mitogenic factor
> lymphocyte mitogenic factor

lm/ft^2 — lumens per square foot
LMG —
> lethal midline granuloma
> low mobility group

LMH — lipid-mobilizing hormone
lmh — lumen hour
LMI — leukocyte migration inhibition [assay]
LMIF — leukocyte migration inhibition factor
l/min — liters per minute
l/min/m^2 — liters per minute per square meter
LMIR — leukocyte migration inhibition reaction
LMIT — leukocyte migration inhibition test
LML —
> large and medium lymphocytes
> left mediolateral [episiotomy]
> left middle lobe
> lower midline

LMLE — left mediolateral episiotomy
LML scar w/h — lower midline scar with hernia
LMM —
> *Lactobacillus* maintenance medium

LMM — (continued)
  lentigo maligna melanoma
  light (molecular weight)
    meromyosin
lm/m² — lumens per square meter
LMN — lower motor neuron
LMNL — lower motor neuron lesion
LMO — localized molecular orbital
LMP —
  last menstrual period
  latent membrane potential
  left mentoposterior [fetal position]
  lumbar puncture
LMR —
  left medial rectus [muscle]
  linguomandibular reflex
  localized magnetic resonance
  log magnitude ratio
  lymphocytic meningoradiculitis
LMRCP — Licentiate in Midwifery of the Royal College of Physicians
LMS —
  lateral medullary syndrome
  leiomyosarcoma
  Licentiate in Medicine and Surgery
lms — lumen-second
LMSSA — Licentiate in Medicine and Surgery of the Society of Apothecaries
LMSV — left maximal spatial voltage
LMT —
  left main trunk
  left mentotransverse [fetal position]
  leukocyte migration technique
  luteomammotrophic [hormone]
Lmt. — limited
LMTA — Language Modalities Test for Aphasia
LMV — larva migrans visceralis

LMW — low molecular weight
lm/W — lumens per watt
LMWD — low molecular weight dextran
LMWH — low molecular weight heparin
LN —
  labionasal
  later (onset) nephrotic [syndrome]
  Lesch-Nyhan [syndrome]
  lipoid nephrosis
  lobular neoplasia
  low necrosis
  lupus nephritis
  lymph node
L/N — letter/numerical [system]
LN₂ — liquid nitrogen
ln — logarithm, natural
LNAA — large neutral amino acid
LNB — lymph node biopsy
LNC — lymph node cell
LND —
  Lesch-Nyhan disease
  light-near dissociation
  lymph node dissection
LNE — lymph node enlargement
LNG — liquefied natural gas
LNGFR — low affinity nerve growth factor-receptor
LNH — large number hypothesis
LNI — logarithm neutralization index
LNKS — low natural killer syndrome
LNL —
  lower normal limit
  lymph node lymphocyte
LNLS — linear-nonlinear least squares
LNMP — last normal menstrual period
LNNB — Luria-Nebraska Neuropsychological Battery
LNP — large neuronal polypeptide
LNPF — lymph node permeability factor
LNR — lymph node region

LNS —
 lateral nuclear stratum
 Lesch-Nyhan syndrome
 lymph node seeking [equiva-
  lent]
LO —
 lateral oblique
 lenticular opacity
 leucine oxidation
 linguo-occlusal
 low lumbar orthosis
LOA —
 leave of absence
 Leber's optic atrophy
 left anterior oblique
 left occipitoanterior [fetal po-
  sition]
 looseness of associations
 lysis of adhesions
LOC —
 laxative of choice
 level of care
 level of consciousness
 liquid organic compound
 locus of control
 loss of consciousness
Loc. —
 local
 localized
 location
lo. cal. — low calorie
lo. calc. — low calcium
LOC-C — Locus of Control–
  Chance
loc. cit. — *loco citato* (Lat.) in the
  place cited
loc. dol. — *loco dolenti* (Lat.) to
  the painful spot
LOC-E — Locus of Control–
  External
lo. CHO. — low carbohydrate
lo. chol. — low cholesterol
LOC-I — Locus of Control–
  Internal
LOCM — low osmolar contrast
  medium
LOC-PO — Locus of Control–
  Powerful Others

LOD —
 line of duty
 logarithm of the odds
  [score]
LOF —
 lofexidine
 low outlet forceps
log. — logarithm
LOH —
 loop of Henle
 loss of heterozygosity
LOI —
 level of incompetence
 level of injury
 Leyton Obsessive Inventory
 limit of impurities
LOIH — left oblique inguinal hernia
lo K — low kalium (potassium)
LOL — left occipitolateral [fetal
  position]
LOM —
 left otitis media
 limitation of motion
 limitation of movement
 loss of motion
 loss of movement
 low osmolar (contrast) medium
LOMPT — Lincoln-Oseretsky Motor Performance Test
LOMSA — left otitis media, suppurative, acute
LOMSCh — left otitis media, suppurative, chronic
lo. Na. — low sodium
long — longitudinal
long. — *longus* (Lat.) long
LOP —
 leave on pass
 left occipitoposterior [fetal po-
  sition]
LOPRO — low protein
LOPS — length of patient stay
LOQ —
 Leadership Opinion Questionnaire
 lower outer quadrant

LOR —
    long open reading [frame]
    lorazepam
    lorcainide
    loss of righting [reflex]
lord —
    lordosis
    lordotic
LORS 1 — Level of Rehabilitation
    Scale-1
LOS —
    length of stay
    Licentiate in Obstetrical Sci-
        ence
    lipo-oligosaccharide
    lower (o)esophageal sphincter
    low output syndrome
LOS(P) — lower (o)esophageal
    sphincter [pressure]
LOT —
    lateral olfactory tract
    left occipitotransverse [fetal
        position]
    lengthened off time
lot. — *lotio* (Lat.) lotion
LOV —
    large opaque vesicle
    loss of vision
LOWBI — low-birth-weight infant
lox — liquid oxygen
LOZ — lozenge
LP —
    labile peptide
    labile protein
    laboratory procedure
    lactic peroxidase
    lamina propria
    laryngopharyngeal
    latency period
    latent period
    lateral plantar
    lateral posterior
    lateral pylorus
    [nucleus] lateralis posterior
    latex particle
    leading pole
    Legionella pneumophila
    leukocyte-poor

LP — *(continued)*
    leukocytic pyrogen
    levator palati
    lichen planus
    ligamentum patellae
    light perception
    lightly padded
    linear programming
    lingua plicata
    linguopulpal
    lipoprotein
    liver plasma [concentration]
    loss of privileges
    low potency
    low power
    low pressure
    low protein
    lower power
    lumbar puncture
    lumboperitoneal
    lung parenchyma
    lymphocyte predominant
    lymphoid plasma
    lymphoid predominance
    lymphomatoid papulosis
L/P —
    lactate/pyruvate [ratio]
    liver to plasma (concentra-
        tion) [ratio]
    lymphocyte/polymorph [ratio]
    lymph/plasma [ratio]
alpha-LP — alpha-lipoprotein
beta-LP — beta-lipoprotein
LPA —
    larval photoreceptor axon
    latex particle agglutination
    left pulmonary artery
    lysophosphatidic acid
LPAM — L-phenylalanine mustard
    (melphalan)
LPB — lipoprotein B
LPBP — low-profile bioprosthesis
LPC —
    laser photocoagulation
    late positive component
    leukocyte-poor cell
    lysophosphatidylcholine
LPCM — low-placed conus medul-
    laris

LPc̄P — light perception with projection
LPCT — late proximal cortical tubule
LPD —
  low-protein diet
  luteal phase defect
LPDF — lipoprotein-deficient fraction
LPE —
  lipoprotein electrophoresis
  lysophosphatidylethanolamine
LPerc — light perception
LPF —
  leukocytosis-promoting factor
  leukopenia factor
  lipopolysaccharide factor
  liver plasma flow
  localized plaque formation
  lymphocytosis-promoting factor
lpf —
  low-power field
  low-powered field
LPFB — left posterior fascicular block
LPFN — low-pass filtered noise
LPFS — low-pass filtered signal
LPG — liquefied petroleum gas
LPH —
  left posterior hemiblock
  lipotropic pituitary hormone
LPI —
  laser peripheral iridectomy
  left posterior-inferior
  long process of incus
  lysinuric protein intolerance
LPICA — left posterior internal carotid artery
LPIFB — left posteroinferior fascicular block
LPIH — left posteroinferior hemiblock
LPK — liver pyruvate kinase
LPL —
  lamina propria lymphocyte
  lichen planus–like lesion
  lipoprotein lipase

LPLA — lipoprotein lipase activity
LPLIS — lipoprotein lipase inactivation system
LPM —
  lateral pterygoid muscle
  left posterior measurement
  liver plasma membrane
  localized pretibial myxedema
  lymphoproliferative malignancy
lpm —
  lines per minute
  liters per minute
LPN — Licensed Practical Nurse
LPO —
  lateral preoptic [area]
  left posterior oblique
  left posterior occipital
  light perception only
  lipid peroxidation
LPOA — lateral preoptic area
LpOH — lysopine dehydrogenase
L POST — left posterior
LPP — lateral pterygoid plate
LP&P — light perception and projection
LPPH — late postpartum hemorrhage
LPR —
  lactate-pyruvate ratio
  late-phase response
L/P ratio —
  liver to plasma concentration ratio
  lymph plasma ratio
LPRBC — leukocyte-poor red blood cell
LProj — light projection
LPS —
  Lanterman-Petris-Short [Act]
  last Papanicolaou smear
  levator palpebrae superioris [muscle]
  linear profile scan
  lipase
  lipopolysaccharide
  London Psychogeriatric Scale
lps — liters per second

LP shunt — lumbar-peritoneal shunt

LPSR — lipopolysaccharide receptor

LPT —
  lateral position test
  lipotropin

LPV —
  left portal view
  left pulmonary vein
  lymphopathia venereum
  lymphotropic papovavirus

LPVP — left posterior ventricular pre-excitation

LPW — lateral pharyngeal wall

lpw — lumens per watt

Lp.-X — lipoprotein-X

LQ —
  longevity quotient
  lordosis quotient
  lower quadrant
  lowest quadrant

lq. — liquid

LQTS — long QT syndrome

LR —
  labeled release
  labor room
  laboratory reference
  laboratory report
  lactated Ringer's [solution]
  large reticulocyte
  latency reaction
  latency relaxation
  lateral rectus [muscle]
  lateral retinaculum
  left rotation
  ligand receptor
  light reaction
  light reflex
  limb reduction [defect]
  limit of reaction
  logistic regression
  low renin
  lymphocyte recruitment

L/R — left-to-right [ratio]

L&R — left and right

L→R — left to right

Lr —
  lawrencium

Lr — (continued)
  limes-reacting dose of diphtheria toxin

LRA —
  left renal artery
  low right atrium

LRC —
  locomotor-respiratory coupling
  lower rib cage

LRCP — Licentiate of the Royal College of Physicians

LRCS — Licentiate of the Royal College of Surgeons

LRCSE — Licentiate of the Royal College of Surgeons, Edinburgh

LRD —
  living related donor
  living renal donor

LRDT — living related donor transplant

LRE —
  lamina rara externa
  least restrictive environment
  leukemic reticuloendotheliosis
  lymphoreticuloendothelial

LREH — low renin essential hypertension

LRF —
  latex and resorcinol formaldehyde
  left rectus femoris
  liver residue factor
  luteinizing [hormone]–releasing factor

LRH — luteinizing [hormone]–releasing hormone

LRI —
  lamina rara interna
  lower respiratory (tract) illness
  lower respiratory (tract) infection
  lymphocyte reactivity index

LRL — Lunar Research Laboratory

LRM — left radical mastectomy

LRMP — last regular menstrual period

LRN — lateral reticular nucleus

LRNA — low renin, normal aldosterone

LRND — left radical neck dissection

LROP — lower radicular obstetrical paralysis

LRP —
  lichen ruber planus
  long-range planning

LRQ — lower right quadrant

LRQG — left rostral quarter ganglion

LRR —
  labyrinthine righting reflex
  lymph return rate
  lymphatic return rate

LRS —
  lactated Ringer's solution
  lateral recess syndrome
  Lights Retention Scale
  low rate of stimulation
  lumboradicular syndrome

LRSF —
  lactating rat serum factor
  liver regenerating serum factor

LR-SH — left-right shunt

LRSP — long-range systems planning

LRSS — late respiratory systemic syndrome

LRT —
  local radiation therapy
  long terminal repeat
  lower respiratory tract

LRTI —
  lower respiratory tract illness
  lower respiratory tract infection

LRV — left renal vein

LRZ — lorazepam

LS —
  lateral septal
  lateral suspensor
  left sacrum
  left septum
  left side

LS — (continued)
  legally separated
  leiomyosarcoma
  length of stay
  Leriche syndrome
  lesser sac
  Letterer-Siwe [disease]
  Libman-Sacks [disease]
  Licentiate in Surgery
  Life Science
  light sensitive
  light sensitivity
  light sleep
  liminal sensation
  liminal sensitivity
  linear scleroderma
  lipid synthesis
  liver and spleen
  liver scan
  long sleep
  lower segment
  lower strength
  low-sodium [diet]
  lumbar spine
  lumbosacral
  lung strip
  lung surfactant
  lymphosarcoma

L/S —
  lactase/sucrase [ratio]
  lecithin/sphingomyelin [ratio]
  lipid/saccharide [ratio]
  liver/spleen [ratio]
  lumbosacral

L-S — lipid-saccharide

L&S — liver and spleen

LSA —
  Language Sampling Analysis
  left sacroanterior [fetal position]
  left subclavian artery
  leukocyte-specific activity
  Licentiate of Society of Apothecaries
  lichen sclerosus et atrophicus
  lipid-bound sialic acid
  lymphosarcoma

LS&A — lichen sclerosus et atrophicus

LSANA — leukocyte-specific anti-nuclear antibody

LSAR — lymphosarcoma cell

LSA/RCS — lymphosarcoma-reticulum cell sarcoma

LSB —
   least significant bit
   left scapular border
   left sternal border
   local standby
   long spike burst
   lumbar sympathetic block

LS-BMD — lumbar spine bone mineral density

LS-BPS — laparoscopic bilateral partial salpingectomies

LSC —
   late systolic click
   left subclavian [artery]
   left-sided colon [cancer]
   lichen simplex chronicus
   lid, sclera, conjunctiva
   liquid scintillation counting
   liquid-solid chromatography
   lower segment cesarean [section]

LSc — local scleroderma

LSCA — left subclavian artery

LScA — left scapuloanterior [fetal position]

LSCL — lymphosarcoma cell leukemia

LScP — left scapuloposterior [fetal position]

LSCS — lower segment cesarean section

LSCV — left subclavian vein

LSD —
   least significant difference
   least significant digit
   low-salt diet
   low-sodium diet
   lysergic acid diethylamide

LSD-25 — D-lysergic acid diethylamide tartrate 25

LSE —
   left sternal edge
   local side effects

l/sec — liters per second

LSEP —
   left somatosensory evoked potential
   lumbosacral somatosensory evoked potential

LSF —
   low saturated fat
   lymphocyte-stimulating factor

LSG — labial salivary gland

LSH —
   lutein-stimulating hormone
   lymphocyte-stimulating hormone

LSHTM — London School of Hygiene and Tropical Medicine

LSI —
   large-scale integration
   Life Satisfaction Index
   light-scattering index
   lumbar spine index

LSK — liver, spleen, and kidneys

LSKM — liver-spleen-kidney-megaly

LSL —
   left sacrolateral [fetal position]
   left short-leg [brace]
   lymphosarcoma (cell) leukemia

LSM —
   late systolic murmur
   lymphocyte separation medium
   lysergic acid morpholide

LSN —
   left substantia nigra
   left sympathetic nerve

LSO —
   lateral superior olive
   left salpingo-oophorectomy
   left superior oblique
   lumbosacral orthosis

LSP —
   left sacroposterior [fetal position]
   liver-specific protein

L-sp — lumbar spine

LSp — life span
L-Spar — Elspar (asparaginase)
L-spine — lumbar spine
LSQ — least square
LSSA — lipid-soluble secondary
    antioxidant
LSR —
    lanthanide shift reagent
    lecithin-sphingomyelin ratio
    left superior rectus [muscle]
LSRA — low septal right atrium
L/S ratio — lecithin-sphingomyelin
    ratio
LSS —
    Life Span Study
    Life Study Sample
    life support station
    liver-spleen scan
    lumbosacral spine
LSSA — lipid-soluble secondary
    antioxidant
LST —
    lateral sinus thrombophlebitis
    lateral spinothalamic tract
    left sacrotransverse [fetal posi-
        tion]
    life-sustaining treatment
LSTC —
    laparoscopic tubal cautery
    laparoscopic tubal coagulation
LSTL — laparoscopic tubal liga-
    tion
Ls & Ts — lines and tubes
LSU —
    lactose-saccharose-urea [agar]
    life support unit
LSV —
    lateral sacral vein
    left subclavian vein
LSVC — left superior vena cava
LSW — left-sided weakness
LSWA — large amplitude, slow
    wave activity
LSX — Labstix
LT —
    [heat-]labile toxin
    laminar tomography

LT — (continued)
    left
    left thigh
    less than
    lethal time
    leukotriene
    Levin tube
    levothyroxine
    light
    light touch
    long-term
    low temperature
    low transverse
    lues test [syphilis]
    lumbar traction
    lymphocyte transformation
    lymphocyte transitional
    lymphocytic thyroiditis
    lymphocytotoxin
    lymphotoxin
L-T3 — L-triiodothyronine
L-T4 — L-thyroxine
lt. —
    left
    light
    low tension
LTA —
    leukotriene A
    lipoate transacetylase
    lipotechoic acid
    local tracheal anesthesia
    lymphocyte-transforming
        activity
LTAF — local tissue-advancement
    flap
LTAS — lead tetra-acetate Schiff
LTB —
    laparoscopic tubal banding
    laryngotracheobronchitis
    leukotriene B
LTC —
    large transformed cell
    left to count
    leukotriene C
    lidocaine tissue concentration
    long-term care
    lysed tumor cell

LTCF — long-term care facility
LTCP — L-tryptophan–containing
    product
LTCS — low transverse cesarean
    section
LTD —
    largest tumor dimension
    Laron-type dwarfism
    leukotriene D
    limited
    long-term disability
ltd. — limited
LTDA — limited amount
LTDQ — limited quantity
LTE —
    laryngotracheoesophageal
    leukotriene E
LT-ECG — long-term electrocardi-
    ography
LTF —
    lactotransferrin
    lipotropic factor
    lymphocyte-transforming fac-
        tor
LTG — long-term goal
LTGA — left transposition of the
    great arteries
LTH —
    lactogenic hormone
    local tumor hyperthermia
    low-temperature holding
    luteotropic hormone
LtH — left-handed
LTHM — low temperature holding
    method
LTI —
    low temperature isotropic
    lupus-type inclusions
LTL — laparoscopic tubal ligation
lt. lat. — left lateral
LTM — long-term memory
LTOT — long-term oxygen ther-
    apy
LTP —
    leukocyte thromboplastin
    long-term potentiation
    L-tryptophan

LTPP — lipothiamide pyrophos-
    phate
LTR —
    long terminal repeat
    lymphocyte transfer reaction
LTS —
    laparoscopic tubal sterilization
    light tactile stimulation
    long-term storage
    long-term survival
    long tract sign
LTT —
    lactose tolerance test
    leucine tolerance test
    limited treadmill test
    lymphoblastic transformation
        test
    lymphocyte transformation
        test
LTUI — low transverse uterine in-
    cision
LTV —
    Lucké tumor virus
    lung thermal volume
lt vent BBB — left ventricular bun-
    dle branch block
LTW — Leydig-cell tumor in
    Wistar [rat]
LU —
    left uninjured
    left uninvolved
    left upper
    living unit
    loudness unit
    lung
    lytic unit
L&U — lower and upper
Lu —
    lumbar
    lung
    lutetium
LUA — left upper arm
LUC — large unstained cell
luc. prim. — luce prima (Lat.) at
    daybreak
LUE — left upper extremity
lues 1 — primary syphilis

lues 2 — secondary syphilis
lues 3 — tertiary syphilis
LUF — luteinized unruptured follicle
LUFS — luteinized unruptured follicle syndrome
LUIS — low-dose urea in invert sugar
LUL —
    left upper [eye]lid
    left upper limb
    left upper lobe
    left upper lung
lumb. — lumbar
LUMD — lowest usual maintenance dose
LUMO — lowest unoccupied molecular orbital
LUO — left ureteral orifice
LUOB — left upper outer buttock
LUOQ — left upper outer quadrant
LUP — left ureteropelvic [junction]
LUQ — left upper quadrant
LURD — living unrelated donor
LUS — lower uterine segment
LUSB —
    left upper scapular border
    left upper sternal border
lut. — *luteum* (Lat.) yellow
LUTT — lower urinary tract tumor
LUV — large unilamellar vesicle
LUX — left upper extremity
LV —
    Lactobacillus viridescens
    lacto-ovo-vegetarian
    laryngeal vestibule
    lateral ventricle
    lecithovitellin
    left ventricle
    left ventricular
    leucovorin
    leukemia virus
    live vaccine
    live virus

LV — *(continued)*
    low vertical
    low volume
    lumbar vertebra
    lung volume
Lv — brightness or luminance
lv — leave
LVA —
    left ventricular aneurysm
    left ventricular aneurysmectomy
    left vertebral artery
    low vision aid
LVAD — left ventricular assist device
L-variant — a defective bacterial variant that can multiply on hypertonic medium
LVAS — left ventricular assist system
LVAT — left ventricular activation time
LVBP — left ventricular bypass pump
LVC — low-viscosity cement
LVCS — low vertical cesarean section
LVD —
    left ventricular dimension
    left ventricular dysfunction
LV_D — left ventricular end-diastolic pressure
LVDd — left ventricular dimension (in end-)diastole
LVDI — left ventricular dimension
LVDP — left ventricular diastolic pressure
LVDT — linear variable differential transformer
LVDV — left ventricular diastolic volume
LVE —
    left ventricular ejection
    left ventricular enlargement
LVED — left ventricular end-diastole
LVEDC — left ventricular end-diastolic circumference

LVEDD —
    left ventricular end-diastolic
      diameter
    left ventricular end-diastolic
      dimension

LVEDP — left ventricular end-diastolic pressure

LVEDV — left ventricular end-diastolic volume

LVEF — left ventricular ejection fraction

LVEndo — left ventricular endocardial [half]

LVEP — left ventricular end-diastolic pressure

LVESD — left ventricular end-systolic dimension

LVESV — left ventricular end-systolic volume

LVESVI — left ventricular end-systolic volume index

LVET — left ventricular ejection time

LVETI — left ventricular ejection time index

LVF —
    left ventricular failure
    left ventricular function
    left visual field
    low-voltage fast
    low-voltage foci

LVFP — left ventricular filling pressure

$LVFT_2$ — left ventricular slow filling time

LVG — left ventrogluteal

LVH —
    large vessel hemotocrit
    left ventricular hypertrophy

LVI —
    left ventricular insufficiency
    left ventricular ischemia

LVID —
    left ventricular internal diastolic
    left ventricular internal dimension

LVIDd — left ventricular internal dimension diastole

LVID(ed) — left ventricular internal diameter (end-diastole)

LVID(es) — left ventricular internal diameter (end-systole)

LVIDP — left ventricular initial diastolic pressure

LVIDs — left ventricular internal dimension systole

LVIV — left ventricular infarct volume

LVL — left vastus lateralis

LVLG — left ventrolateral gluteal

LVM —
    lateral ventromedial [nucleus]
    left ventricular mass

LVMF — left ventricular minute flow

LVMM — left ventricular muscle mass

LVN —
    lateral ventricular nerve
    lateral vestibular nucleus
    Licensed Visiting Nurse
    Licensed Vocational Nurse
    limiting viscosity number

LVO —
    left ventricular outflow
    left ventricular overactivity

LVOA — left ventricular overactivity

LVOT — left ventricular outflow tract

LVP —
    large volume parenteral [infusion]
    left ventricular pressure
    levator veli palatini
    lysine-vasopressin

LVPEP — left ventricular pre-ejection period

LVPFR — left ventricular peak filling rate

LVPSP — left ventricular peak systolic pressure

LVPW — left ventricular posterior wall

LVPWT — left ventricular posterior wall thickness

LVR —
leucovorin
limb vascular resistance

LVS — left ventricular strain

LV_s — (mean) left ventricular systolic [pressure]

LVSEMI — left ventricular subendocardial myocardial ischemia

LVSI — left ventricular systolic index

LVSO — left ventricular systolic output

LVSP — left ventricular systolic pressure

LVST — lateral vestibulospinal tract

LVSV — left ventricular stroke volume

LVSW —
left ventricular septal wall
left ventricular stroke work

LVSWI — left ventricular stroke work index

LVT —
left ventricular tension
lysine vasotonin

LVT_1 — left ventricular fast filling time

LVV —
left ventricular volume
LeVeen valve
live varicella vaccine
live varicella virus

LVW —
lateral vaginal wall
lateral ventricular width
left ventricular wall
left ventricular work

LVW/HW — lateral ventricular width to hemispheric width

LVWI — left ventricular work index

LVWM — left ventricular wall motion

LVWMA — left ventricular wall motion abnormality

LVWMI — left ventricular wall motion index

LVWT — left ventricular wall thickness

LW —
lacerating wound
lateral wall
Lee-White [method]
left (ear), warm [stimulus]
Léri-Weill [syndrome]
lung weight
lung width

L/W — living and well

L&W —
Lee and White [clotting time]
living and well

L-10-W — levulose 10% in water

Lw — lawrencium

LWBS — left without being seen

LWC — leave without consent

LWCT — Lee-White clotting time

LWD — living with disease

LWK — large white kidney

LWP —
large whirlpool
lateral wall pressure

LX —
local irradiation
lower extremity

lx —
larynx
latex
lower extremity
lux

LXC — laxative of choice

LXT — left exotopia

LY —
lactoalbumin and yeastolate [medium]
lymphocyte
lyophilization

Ly — a T-cell antigen used for grouping T-lymphocytes into different classes

LYDMA — lymphocyte-detected membrane antigen
LYEL — last years of expected life
LYES — liver yang exuberance syndrome
LYG — lymphomatoid granulomatosis
LYM — lymph
lymph —
    lymphocyte
    lymphocytic
LyNeF — lytic nephritic factor

lyo — lyophilized
LYP —
    lactose, yeast, and peptone [agar]
    lower yield point
Lys —
    lysine
    lysosome
LySLk — lymphoma syndrome leukemia
lytes — electrolytes
Lzm — lysozyme

M —
    blood factor in the MNS blood group system
    concentration in moles per liter
    macroglobulin
    macroglobulinemia [component]
    magnetization
    male
    malignant
    manipulus (Lat.) handful
    manual
    marital
    married
    masculine
    massage
    maternal contribution
    matrix
    mature
    maximal
    maximum
    meatus
    media
    medial
    median
    mediator
    medical
    medicine
    medium

M — *(continued)*
    mega-
    megohm
    melts at
    membrane
    memory
    mental
    mentum
    mesial
    meta-
    metabolite
    metal
    metanephrine
    metastasis
    meter
    methionine
    method
    methotrexate
    mexiletine
    mild
    million
    minim
    minimal
    minimum
    minute
    mitochondria
    mitosis
    mitral
    mix
    mixed

M — (continued)

  mixture
  molar [permanent tooth]
  molar [solution]
  molarity
  mole
  molecular [weight]
  moment of force
  monkey
  monocyte
  month
  morgan
  morphine
  mother
  motile
  mouse
  mouth
  mu (twelfth letter of the
    Greek alphabet), uppercase
  mucoid [colony]
  mucous [adjective]
  mucus [noun]
  multipara
  murmur [cardiac]
  muscle
  muscular response to an elec-
    trical stimulation of its mo-
    tor nerve [wave]
  myeloma [component]
  myopia
  myopic
  myosin
  strength of pole

M —

  molar mass
  mutual inductance

M. —

  Micrococcus
  Microsporum
  Mycobacterium
  Mycoplasma

M0 — no evidence of distant metastases

M1 — left mastoid

M-I — first meiotic metaphase

M_1 —

  mitral first heart sound
  mitral valve closure

M_1 — (continued)

  myeloblast
  slight dullness [on ausculta-
    tion]
  sphenoidal segment of middle
    cerebral artery

M-II — second meiotic metaphase

M2 — right mastoid

M^2 — square meter [body surface]

M_2 —

  insular segment of middle
    cerebral artery
  marked dullness [on ausculta-
    tion]
  mitral second heart sound
  promyelocyte

$\alpha_2 M$ — alpha$_2$-macroglobulin

3-M [syndrome] — initials for
  Miller, McKusick, and Mal-
  vaux, who first described the
  syndrome

M/3 — middle third [long bones]

M_3 —

  absolute dullness [on ausculta-
    tion]
  mitral third heart sound
  myelocyte at the 3rd stage of
    maturation
  opercular segment of middle
    cerebral artery

M_4 —

  cortical segment of middle
    cerebral artery
  myelocyte at the 4th stage of
    maturation

M_5 — metamyelocyte

M_6 — band form at the 6th stage
  of myelocyte maturation

M_7 — polymorphonuclear neutrophil

M/10 — one-tenth molar solution

M/100 — one-hundredth molar solution

$M\Omega$ — megohm

m —

  electromagnetic moment
  electron rest mass
  magnetic moment

m — (*continued*)

    magnetic quantum number

    mass

    mean

    median

    medium

    melts at [temperature]

    mentum

    mesial

    meter

    milli-

    minim

    minimum

    minute

    modulus

    molal

    molality

    molar [deciduous tooth]

    morphine

    motile

    mucoid

    murmur

    sample mean

μ —

    chemical potential

    dynamic viscosity

    electrophoretic mobility

    heavy chain of immunoglobulin M

    linear attenuation coefficient

    magnetic moment

    mean

    micro-

    micrometer

    micron

    milliunit

    mu (twelfth letter of the Greek alphabet), lowercase

    mutation rate

    permeability

    population mean

μ_0 — permeability of vacuum

m- — meta-

m. —

    macerare (Lat.) macerate, macerated

    mane (Lat.) in the morning

    manipulus (Lat.) a handful

    meridies (Lat.) noon

m. — (*continued*)

    mille (Lat.) thousand

    misce (Lat.) mix

    mistura (Lat.) mixture

    mitte (Lat.) send

    mors (Lat.) death

    musculus

    mutitas (Lat.) dullness of sound

(m) — by mouth

m^2 — square meter [body surface]

m^3 — cubic meter

m_8 — spin quantum number

MA —

    machine

    mafenide acetate

    malignant arrhythmia

    mandelic acid

    Martin-Albright [syndrome]

    masseter

    Master of Arts

    maternal aunt

    mean arterial [blood pressure]

    medical abbreviation

    medical assistance

    medical assistant

    medical audit

    medical authorization

    mega-ampere

    megaloblastic anemia

    megestrol acetate

    membrane antigen

    menstrual age

    mental age

    mentum anterior [fetal position]

    metatarsus adductus

    meter angle

    microadenoma

    microagglutination

    microaneurysm

    microcytotoxicity assay

    microscopic agglutination

    Miller-Abbott [tube]

    mitochondrial antibody

    mitogen activation

    mitotic apparatus

    mitral annulus

    mixed agglutination

MA — *(continued)*
  moderately advanced
  monoamine
  monoclonal antibody
  motorcycle accident
  multiple action
  muscle activity
  mutagenic activity
  myelinated axon
M/A —
  male, altered [animal]
  mood and/or affect
MA-104 — embryonic rhesus monkey kidney cells
MA-111 — embryonic rabbit kidney cells
MA-163 — human embryonic thymus cells
MA-184 — newborn human foreskin cells
Ma —
  male
  mass of atom
  masurium (technetium)
mA —
  milliamperage
  milliampere
μA — microampere
mÅ — milliangstrom
ma — meter angle
MAA —
  macroaggregated albumin
  macroaggregates of albumin
  medical administrative assistant
  Medical Assistance to the Aged
  melanoma-associated antigen
  moderate aplastic anemia
  monoarticular arthritis
MAAAP — macroaggregated albumin arterial perfusion
MAAC — Medical Assistants Advisory Council
MAACL — Multiple Affect Adjective Check List
MAAGB — Medical Artists Association of Great Britain

MAB — monoclonal antibody
m-AB — m-aminobenzamide
MABI — Mother's Assessment of the Behavior of [her] Infant
MABP — mean arterial blood pressure
Mabs — monoclonal antibodies
MAC —
  MacConkey's [broth]
  MacIntosh [blade]
  macrocytic erythrocyte
  macule
  major ambulatory categories
  malignancy-associated changes
  maximal acid concentration
  maximum allowable concentration
  maximum allowable cost
  Medical Alert Center
  membrane attack complex
  midarm circumference
  minimal alveolar concentration
  minimal anesthetic concentration
  minimum antibiotic concentration
  mitral anular calcium
  modulator of adenylate cyclase
  monitored anesthesia care
  multidimensional actuarial classification
  Mycobacterium avium complex
Mac — macula
mac. — *macerare* (Lat.) macerate
MACC — macro-ovalocyte
m. accur. — *misce accuratissime* (Lat.) mix very accurately
MACDP — Metropolitan Atlanta Congenital Defects Program
MACE — Mayo Asymptomatic Carotid Endarterectomy [trial]
Mace — methylchloroform chloroacetophenone
macer — maceration
mAChR — muscarinic acetylcholine receptor

MAC INH — membrane attack complex inhibitor

MACR —
macrocytosis
mean axillary count rate

macro —
macrocyte
macrocytic
macroscopic

MAD —
maximum allowable dose
methandriol
methylandrostenediol
mind-altering drugs
minimum average dose
myoadenylate deaminase

MADA — muscle adenylate deaminase

MADD —
Mothers Against Drunk Driving
multiple acyl CoA dehydrogenation deficiency

MADRS — Montgomery-Asberg Depression Rating Scale

MADU — methylaminodeoxyuridine

MAE —
Medical Air Evacuation
moves all extremities
Multilingual Aphasia Examination

MAEEW — moves all extremities equally well

MAEW — moves all extremities well

MAF —
macrophage-activating factor
macrophage-agglutinating factor
maximum atrial fragmentation
minimum audible field
mouse amniotic fluid
movement aftereffect

MAFA — midarm fat area

MAFAs — movement-associated fetal (heart rate) accelerations

MAFH — macroaggregated ferrous hydroxide

MAG — myelin-associated glycoprotein

Mag — magnesium

Mag. —
magnification
magnify

mag. — *magnus* (Lat.) large

mag cit — magnesium citrate

MAGE — mean amplitude of glycerine excursion

MAGF — male accessory gland fluid

MAggF — macrophage agglutination factor

MAGIC — microprobe analysis generalized intensity correction

magn. — *magnus* (Lat.) large

MAGS — Multidimensional Assessment of Gains in School

mag sulf — magnesium sulfate

mA-h — milliampere-hours

MAHA —
microangiopathic hemolytic anemia
microangiopathic hemolytic aneurysm

MAHH — malignancy-associated humoral hypercalcemia

MAI —
maximal aggregation index
microscopic aggregation index
minor acute illness
morbid anxiety inventory
movement assessment of infants
Mycobacterium avium-intracellulare

MAIDS — mouse acquired immunodeficiency syndrome

MAIS — *Mycobacterium avium-intracellulare-scrofulaceum*

MAKA — major karyotypic abnormality

MAL —
malfunction
malignant
midaxillary line

Mal —
   malate
   malfunction
   malignancy
mal —
   malaise
   malignant
   malposition
mal. —
   malanandro (Lat.) by blistering
   malum (Lat.) ill
MALA — malarial parasites
MALAR — malaria
Mal-BSA — maleated bovine serum albumin
MALG — Minnesota anti-lymphoblast globulin
malig. — malignant
MALIMET — Master List of Medical Indexing Terms
MALT —
   male, altered [animal]
   mucosa-associated lymphoid tissue
   Munich Alcoholism Test
MAM — methylazoxymethanol
M&Am—myopic astigmatism [compound]
mAm — milliampere-minute
MAMA —
   midarm muscle area
   monoclonal anti-malignin antibody
MAM Ac — methylazoxymethanol acetate
MAMC —
   mean arm muscle circumference
   midarm muscle circumference
MAmg — medial amygdaloid [nucleus]
mA-min — milliampere-minute
m-AMSA — amsacrine
MAN —
   magnocellular nucleus
   mannose
Man. — manipulate

mand —
   mandible
   mandibular
manifest — manifestation
Manip. — manipulation
manip. — *manipulus* (Lat.) handful
MANOVA — multivariate analysis of variance
MAN-6-P — mannose-6-phosphate
man. pr. — *mane primo* (Lat.) early in the morning
MAO —
   Master of the Art of Obstetrics
   maximal acid output
   medical ankle orthosis
   monoamine oxidase
MAOA — monoamine oxidase A
MAOB — monoamine oxidase B
MAOI — monoamine oxidase inhibitor
MAOT — Member of the Association of Occupational Therapists
MAP —
   malignant atrophic papulosis
   maximal aerobic power
   mean airway pressure
   mean aortic pressure
   mean arterial pressure
   Medical Audit Program
   megaloblastic anemia of pregnancy
   mercapturic acid pathway
   methyl acceptor protein
   methylacetoxyprogesterone
   methylaminopurine
   microlithiasis alveolarum pulmonum
   microtubule-associated protein
   minimum audible pressure
   monophasic action potential
   motor (nerve) action potential
   mouse antibody production [test]
   muscle-action potential

MAP — *(continued)*
    Musical Aptitude Profile
MAPA — muscle adenosine phosphoric acid
MAPC — migrating action potential complex
MAPF — microatomized protein food
MAPI —
    microbial alkaline protease inhibitor
    Millon Adolescent Personality Inventory
MAPS — Make a Picture Story [test]
MAR —
    main admissions room
    marasmus
    margin
    marrow
    maximal aggregation ratio
    medication administration record
    microanalytical reagent
    minimal angle resolution
    mixed antiglobulin reaction
mar —
    margin
    marker [chromosome]
MARC — multifocal and recurrent choroidopathy
marg — margin
MARIA — macroaggregated radioiodinated albumin
MARS —
    Mathematics Anxiety Rating Scale
    mouse antirat serum
MARS-A — Mathematics Anxiety Rating Scale—Adolescents
MARTI — mobile advanced real-time image
MAS —
    Management Appraisal Survey
    Manifest Anxiety Scale
    McCune-Albright syndrome
    meconium aspiration syndrome

MAS — *(continued)*
    Medical Administrative Service
    Medical Advisory Service
    mesoatrial shunt
    milk-alkali syndrome
    milliampere-second
    minor axis shortening [of left ventricle]
    mobile arm support
    monoclonal antibodies
    Morgagni-Adams-Stokes [syndrome]
    motion analysis system
mAs — milliampere-second
MASA — Medical Association of South Africa
masc. —
    masculine
    mass concentration
MASER —
    microwave amplification by stimulated emission of radiation
    molecular amplication by stimulated emission of radiation
MASF — Melcher acid-soluble fraction
MASH —
    Mobile Army Surgical Hospital
    multiple automated sample harvester
MASP — microaerophilus stationary phase
mas. pil. — *massa pilularum* (Lat.) pill mass
MASQ — Multiple Ability Self-report Questionnaire
mass —
    massage
    massive
massc — mass concentration
MAST —
    medical antishock trousers
    Michigan Alcoholism Screening Test

MAST — (*continued*)
    Military Antishock Trousers
mAST — mitochondrial aspartate
    aminotransferase
mast. —
    mastectomy
    mastoid
MASU — Mobile Army Surgical
    Unit
MAT —
    Manipulative Aptitude Test
    manual arts therapist
    maternal
    maternity
    mature
    mean absorption time
    medical assistance team [emer-
      gency medicine]
    medication administration
      team
    methionine adenosyltransfer-
      ase
    Metropolitan Achievement
      Tests
    microagglutination test
    Miller-Abbott tube
    Miller Analogies Test
    motivation analysis test
    multifocal atrial tachycardia
    multiple agent therapy
Mat —
    maternal [origin]
    maternity
    mature
MATE — Maternal Attitudes Eval-
    uation
mat gf — maternal grandfather
mat gm — maternal grandmother
MATRIS — Medical Manpower
    and Training Information Ser-
    vice (British)
MATSA — Marek-associated tu-
    mor-specific antigen
matut. — *matutinus* (Lat.) in the
    morning
MAU — Meyenburg-Altherr-
    Uehlinger [syndrome]

MAV —
    mechanical auxiliary ventricle
    minimum apparent viscosity
    minute alveolar volume
    movement arm vector
    myeloblastosis-associated virus
    transmembrane activation
      voltage
MAVA — multiple abstract vari-
    ance analysis
MAVIS — mobile artery and vein
    imaging system
MAVR — mitral and aortic valve
    replacement
max —
    maxilla
    maxillary
    maximal
    maximum
MaxEP — maximum esophageal
    pressure
MB —
    buccal margin
    isoenzyme of creatine kinase
      containing M and B sub-
      units
    Mallory body
    mammillary body
    Marsh-Bendall [factor]
    maximum breathing
    Medicinae Baccalaureus (Lat.)
      Bachelor of Medicine
    medulloblastoma
    megabyte
    mercury bougie
    mesiobuccal
    methyl bromide
    methylene blue
    microbiological assay
    muscle balance
    myocardial band
6MB — six-meal bland [diet]
Mb —
    mandible body
    mouse brain
    myoglobin
mb — millibar

m.b. — *misce bene* (Lat.) mix well

MBA —
> methylbenzyl alcohol
> methylbischloroethylamine (nitrogen mustard)
> methylbovine albumin

MBAC — Member of the British Association of Chemists

MBAR — myocardial beta-adrenergic receptor

mbar. — millibar

μbar — microbar

MBAS — methylene blue active substance

MBB — modified barbital buffer

MBC —
> male breast cancer
> maximal bladder capacity
> maximal breathing capacity
> metastatic breast cancer
> methylthymol blue complex
> microcrystalline bovine collagen
> minimal bactericidal concentration

MB-CK — creatine kinase isoenzyme containing M and B subunits

MBCL — monocytoid B-cell lymphoma

MbCO — myoglobin combination with carbon monoxide

MBCU — metallic bead-chain urethrocystograph

MBD —
> Marchiafava-Bignami disease
> maximal bactericidal dilution
> methylene blue dye
> minimal brain damage
> minimal brain dysfunction
> Morquio-Brailsford disease

MBDG — mesiobuccal developmental groove

MBE —
> may be elevated
> medium below-elbow [cast]

MBEST — modulus blipped echoplanar single-pulse technique

MBF —
> meat base formula
> medullary blood flow
> muscle blood flow
> myocardial blood flow

MBFC — medial brachial fascial compartment

MBFLB — monoaural bifrequency loudness balance

MBG —
> mean blood glucose
> morphine-benzedrine group [scale]

MBGS — morphine-benzedrine group scale

MBH —
> maximal benefit from hospitalization
> medial basal hypothalamus

MBH₂ — reduced methylene blue

MBHI — Millon Behavioral Health Inventory

MBI —
> Maslach Burnout Inventory
> maximum blink index
> methylene blue instillation

MBK — methyl butyl ketone

MBL —
> Marine Biological Laboratory
> medium brown loose [stool]
> menstrual blood loss
> minimal bactericidal level

MBl — methylene blue

MBLA —
> methylbenzyl linoleic acid
> mouse-specific bone marrow–derived lymphocyte antigen

MBM —
> mineral basal medium
> mother's breast milk

MBNOA — Member of the British Naturopathic and Osteopathic Association

MBNW — multiple-breath nitrogen washout

MBO — mesiobucco-occlusal

MbO₂ — myoglobin combination with oxygen

MBP —
> major basic protein
> maltose-binding protein
> mean blood pressure
> melitensis, bovine, porcine [antigen from *Brucella bovis*, *B. melitensis*, and *B. suis*]
> mesiobuccopulpal
> myelin basic protein

MBPS — multigated blood pool scanning

MBq — megabecquerel

MBR — methylene blue, reduced

MBRT — methylene blue reduction time

MBS — Martin-Bell syndrome

MBSA — methylated bovine serum albumin

MBSD — maple bark stripper disease

MBT —
> mercaptobenzothiazole
> mixed bacterial toxin

MBTH — 3-methyl-2-benzothiazoline hydrazone

MBTI — Myers-Briggs Type Indicator [psychologic test]

MC —
> *Magister Chirurgiae* (Lat.) Master of Surgery
> mass casualties
> mast cell
> maximum cell
> maximum concentration
> mean corpuscular
> Medical Corps
> medium-chain [triglycerides]
> medullary cavity
> medullary cyst
> megacoulomb
> megacurie
> megacycle
> melanoma cell
> meningeal carcinomatosis
> menstrual cycle
> Merkel's cell
> mesenteric collateral

MC — *(continued)*
> mesiocervical
> mesocaval
> metacarpal
> metatarsocuneiform
> methyl cellulose
> methylcholanthrene
> microcephaly
> microcirculation
> midcapillary
> midcarpal
> mineralocorticoid
> minimal change
> Minkowski-Chauffard [syndrome]
> miscarriage
> mitochondrial complementation
> mitomycin C
> mitotic cycle
> mitral commissurotomy
> mixed cellularity
> mixed cryoglobulinemia
> molluscum contagiosum
> monkey cells
> mononuclear cell
> mouth care
> mucociliary clearance
> mucous cell
> mycelial phase [of fungi]
> myocarditis

M/C — male, castrated [animal]

M-C —
> Magovern-Cromie [prosthesis]
> medico-chirurgical
> mineralocorticoid

M&C — morphine and cocaine

Mc. —
> mandible coronoid
> megacycle

mC — millicoulomb

μC — microcoulomb

MCA —
> main coronary artery
> major coronary artery
> Maternity Center Association
> medical care administration

MCA — (continued)
  3-methylcholanthrene
  middle cerebral aneurysm
  middle cerebral artery
  monocarboxylic acid
  monoclonal antibody
  motorcycle accident
  multichannel analyzer
  multiple congenital abnormal-
    ities
  multiple congenital anomalies
MCAB — monoclonal antibody
MCAD — medium-chain acyl-
  CoA dehydrogenase [defi-
  ciency]
MCA/MR — multiple congenital
  anomalies/mental retardation
  [syndrome]
MCAR — mixed cell agglutination
  reaction
MCAS — middle cerebral artery
  syndrome
MCAT —
  Medical College Admission
    Test
  middle cerebral artery throm-
    bosis
m. caute — misce caute (Lat.) mix
  with caution
MCB —
  membranous cytoplasmic
    body
  monochlorobenzidine
McB — McBurney's [point]
mCBF — mean cerebral blood flow
MCBM — muscle capillary basement membrane
MCBMT — muscle capillary basement membrane thickening
MCBR — minimum concentration
  of bilirubin
MCC —
  marked cocontraction
  mean corpuscular [hemoglo-
    bin] concentration
  medial cell column
  metacarpal-carpal [joints]
  metacerebral cell

MCC — (continued)
  metastatic cord compression
  microcrystalline collagen
  midstream clean catch
  minimum complete-killing
    concentration
  mucocutaneous candidiasis
McC —
  McCarthy [panendoscope]
  McCoy [antibody]
MCCD — minimum cumulative
  cardiotoxic dose
MCCU — Mobile Coronary Care
  Unit
MCD —
  magnetic circular dichroism
  margin crease distance
  mast-cell degranulation
  mean cell diameter
  mean corpuscular diameter
  mean of consecutive differ-
    ences
  medium corpuscular density
  medullary collecting duct
  medullary cystic disease
  metabolic coronary dilation
  metacarpal cortical density
  millicuries destroyed
  minimal cerebral dysfunction
  minimal change disease
  multicystic disease
  multiple carboxylase defi-
    ciency
  muscle carnitine deficiency
MCDI — Minnesota Child Development Inventory
MCDK — multicystic dysplastic
  kidney
MCDP — mast cell degranulating
  peptide
MCDT —
  mast cell degranulation test
  multiple choice discrimina-
    tion test
MCE —
  medical care evaluation
  Medicare Code Editor
  multicystic encephalopathy

MCE — *(continued)*
>   multiple cartilaginous exostosis

MCES — multiple cholesterol emboli syndrome

MCF —
>   macrophage chemotactic factor
>   macrophage cytotoxicity factor
>   median cleft face
>   medium corpuscular fragility
>   microcomplement fixation
>   monocyte [leukotactic] factor
>   mononuclear cell factor
>   most comfortable frequency
>   myocardial contractile force

MCFA —
>   medium-chain fatty acid
>   miniature centrifugal fast analyzer

MCFP — mean circulating filling pressure

MCG —
>   magnetocardiogram
>   membrane-coating granule
>   mesencephalic central gray
>   monoclonal gammopathy

mcg — microgram

MCGC — metacerebral giant cell

MCGF — mast cell growth factor

MCGN —
>   mesangiocapillary glomerulonephritis
>   minimal-change glomerulonephritis
>   mixed cryoglobulinemia with glomerulonephritis

MCH —
>   Maternal and Child Health
>   mean cell hemoglobin
>   mean corpuscular hemoglobin
>   methacholine
>   microfibrillar collagen hemostat
>   muscle contraction headache

M.Ch. — *Magister Chirurgiae* (Lat.) Master of Surgery

MCHB — Maternal and Child Health Bureau

MCHb — mean corpuscular hemoglobin

MCHbC —
>   mean cell hemoglobin concentration
>   mean corpuscular hemoglobin concentration
>   mean corpuscular hemoglobin count

MCHC —
>   maternal/child health care
>   mean cell hemoglobin concentration
>   mean corpuscular hemoglobin concentration
>   mean corpuscular hemoglobin count

MChD — Master of Dental Surgery

MCHg — mean corpuscular hemoglobin

MChOrth — Master of Orthopaedic Surgery

MChOtol — Master of Otology

MCHR — Medical Committee for Human Rights

mc-hr — millicurie-hour

MCHS — Maternal and Child Health Service

MChS — Member of the Society of Chiropodists

MCI —
>   mean cardiac index
>   methicillin
>   mucociliary insufficiency

MCi — megacurie

mCi — millicurie

μCi — microcurie

MCICU — medical coronary intensive care unit

mCid — millicuries destroyed

mCi-hr — millicurie-hour

μCi-hr — microcurie-hour

MCI/MI — mixture of methylchloroisothiazolinone and methylisothiazolinone

MCINS — minimal change idiopathic nephrotic syndrome

MCK — multicystic kidney

MCKD — multicystic kidney disease

MCL —
  maximal comfort level
  maximum containment laboratory
  medial collateral ligament
  midclavian line
  midclavicular line
  midcostal line
  minimal change lesion
  mixed culture, leukocyte
  modified chest lead
  most comfortable listening [level]
  most comfortable loudness [level]

MCLD — *Mycobacterium chelonei*–like disease

MCLL —
  most comfortable listening level
  most comfortable loudness level

MCLNS — mucocutaneous lymph node syndrome

MClSci — Master of Clinical Science

MCM — minimum capacitation medium

MCMAI — Millon Clinical Multiaxial Inventory

MCMV —
  mouse cytomegalovirus
  murine cytomegalovirus

MCN —
  minimal change nephropathy
  mixed cell nodular [lymphoma]

MCNS — minimal change nephrotic syndrome

MCO —
  medical care organization
  multicystic ovary

M colony — mucoid colony

MCommH — Master of Community Health

mcoul — millicoulomb

μcoul — microcoulomb

MCP —
  maximum closure pressure
  maximum contraction pattern
  melanosis circumscripta precancerosa
  metacarpal
  metacarpophalangeal
  metaclopramide
  methyl-accepting chemotaxis protein
  mitotic-control protein
  mucin clot prevention [test]

MCPA — Member of the College of Pathologists, Australasia

MCPH — metacarpophalangeal

MCPJ — metacarpal phalangeal joint

MCPP —
  metacarpophalangeal pattern profile
  meta-chlorophenylpiperazine

MCPPP — metacarpophalangeal pattern profile plot

MCPS —
  Member of the College of Physicians and Surgeons
  Missouri Children's Picture Series [psychological test]

mcps — megacycles per second

MCQ — multiple choice question

MCR —
  Medical Corps Reserve
  message competition ratio
  metabolic clearance rate

MCRA — Member of the College of Radiologists, Australasia

MCRE — mother-child relationship evaluation

MCRI — Multifactorial Cardiac Risk Index

MCS —
  malignant carcinoid syndrome
  Marlowe-Crown (Social Desirability) Scale

MCS — *(continued)*
>massage of the carotid sinus
>mesocaval shunt
>methylcholanthrene (-induced) sarcoma
>microculture and sensitivity
>moisture-control system
>multiple chemical sensitivity
>multiple combined sclerosis
>myocardial contractile state

mc/s — megacycles per second

MCSA —
>minimal cross-sectional area
>Moloney cell surface antigen

MCSDS — Marlowe-Crowne Social Desirability Scale

M-CSF — macrophage colony-stimulating factor

MCSP — Member of the Chartered Society of Physiotherapists (British)

MCT —
>manual cervical traction
>mean cell thickness
>mean cell threshold
>mean circulation time
>mean corpuscular thickness
>medium-chain triglyceride
>medullary carcinoma of thyroid
>medullary collecting tubule
>microtoxicity test
>monocrotaline
>multiple compressed tablet

MCTC — metrizamide computed tomographic cisternography

MCTD — mixed connective tissue disease

MCTF — mononuclear cell tissue factor

MCU —
>Malaria Control Unit [Army]
>maximum care unit
>micturating cystourethrography
>Mobile Care Unit
>motor cortex unit

MCUG — micturating urogram

MCV —
>mean cell volume
>mean clinical value
>mean corpuscular volume
>median cell volume
>motor conduction velocity

MCZ — miconazole

MD —
>macula densa
>macular degeneration
>magnesium deficiency
>main duct
>maintenance dialysis
>maintenance dose
>major depression
>malate dehydrogenase
>malic acid dehydrogenase
>malignant disease
>malrotation of duodenum
>mammary dysplasia
>mandibular
>manic-depression
>manic-depressive
>Mantoux diameter
>Marek's disease
>maternal deprivation
>maximum dose
>mean deviation
>mean diastolic
>measurable disease
>Meckel's diverticulum
>(nucleus) medialis dorsalis
>mediastinal disease
>medical department
>Medical Design [brace]
>medical doctor
>*Medicinae Doctor* (Lat.) Doctor of Medicine
>mediodorsal
>medium dosage
>Meniere's disease
>mental deficiency
>mental depression
>mentally deficient
>mesiodistal
>Minamata disease
>minimal dosage
>minimum dose

MD — *(continued)*
  mitral disease
  mixed diet
  moderate disability
  monocular deprivation
  movement disorder
  multiple deficiency
  muscular dystrophy
  myelodysplasia
  myeloproliferative disease
  myocardial damage
  myocardial disease
  myotonic dystrophy
Md — mendelevium
md —
  mean diastolic
  median
m.d. — *more dicto* (Lat.) as directed
MDA —
  malondialdehyde
  manual dilation of anus
  mentodextro-anterior (Lat.)
    right mentoanterior [fetal position]
  methylene dianiline
  methylenedioxyamphetamine
  minimal deviation adenocarcinoma
  monodehydroascorbate
  motor discriminative acuity
  multivariate discriminant analysis
MDa — megadalton
MDAC — multiplying digital-to-analog converter
MDAD — mineral dust airway disease
MDAP — Machover Draw-A-Person [test]
MDB — Mental Deterioration Battery
MDBDF — March of Dimes Birth Defect Foundation
MDBK — Madin-Darby bovine kidney [cell]
MDBSS — Mischell-Dutton balanced salt solution

MDC —
  major diagnostic categories
  medial dorsal cutaneous [nerve]
  minimum detectable concentration
  monocyte-depleted (mononuclear) cell
MDCK — Madin-Darby canine kidney [cell]
MDCR — Miller-Dieker chromosome region
MDD —
  Doctor of Dental Medicine
  major depressive disorder
  manic-depressive disorder
  mean daily dose
MDDA — Minnesota Differential Diagnosis of Aphasia
MDE — major depressive episode
MDEBP — mean daily erect blood pressure
MDentSc — Master of Dental Science
MDF —
  mean dominant frequency
  myocardial depressant factor
MDG — mean diastolic gradient
MDGF — macrophage-derived growth factor
MDH —
  malate dehydrogenase
  malic acid dehydrogenase
  medullary dorsal horn
MDHM — malate dehydrogenase, mitochondrial
MDHR — maximum determined heart rate
MDHS — malate dehydrogenase, soluble
MDHV — Marek's disease herpesvirus
MDI —
  manic-depressive illness
  metered-dose inhaler
  multiple daily injection
  multiple-dosage insulin
  Multiscore Depression Inventory

MDIA — Mental Development Index, Adjusted

m. dict. — *more dicto* (Lat.) as directed

MDII — multiple daily insulin injections

MDIT — mean disintegration time

MDL — Master Drug List

MDLVP — mean diastolic left ventricular pressure

MDM —
  medical decision making
  mid-diastolic murmur
  minor determinant mixture [penicillin]

MDMA — methylenedioxymethamphetamine

mdn — median

MDNB —
  mean daily nitrogen balance
  metadinitrobenzene

MDOPA — methyldopa

MDP —
  mandibular dysostosis and peromelia
  manic-depressive psychosis
  maximum deliverable pressure
  maximum digital pulse
  ^{99m}Tc medronate methylene diphosphonate
  mentodextra posterior (Lat.) right mentoposterior [fetal position]
  methylene diphosphonate
  muramyl-dipeptide
  muscular dystrophy, progressive

MDPD — maximum daily permissible dose

MDPI — maximal daily permissible intake

MDPIT — Multicenter Diltiazem Postinfarction Trial

MDQ —
  memory deviation quotient
  Menstrual Distress Questionnaire
  minimum detectable quantity

MDR —
  mammalian diving response
  median duration of response
  medical device reporting
  minimum daily requirement
  multidrug resistance

MDRH — multidisciplinary rehabilitation hospital

MDRS — Mattis Dementia Rating Scale

MDR TB — multidrug-resistant tuberculosis

MDS —
  Master of Dental Surgery
  maternal deprivation syndrome
  medical data screening
  medical data system
  mesonephric duct system
  microdilution system
  microsurgical drill system
  milk drinker's syndrome
  Miller-Dieker syndrome
  multidimensional scaling
  myelodysplasia
  myelodysplastic syndrome
  myocardial depressant substance

MDSBP — mean daily supine blood pressure

MDSO —
  mentally disordered sex offender
  mentally disturbed sex offender

MDT —
  mast (cell) degeneration test
  mean dissolution time
  median detection threshold
  mentodextra transversa (Lat.) right mentotransverse [fetal position]
  multidisciplinary team

MDTA — McDonald Deep Test of Articulation

MDTP — multidisciplinary treatment plan

MDTR — mean diameter-thickness ratio

MDUO — myocardial disease of unknown origin

MDV —
Marek's disease virus
mean dye (bolus) velocity
mucosal disease virus
multiple dose vial

MDY — month, date, year

Mdyn — megadyne

ME —
macular edema
magnitude estimation
male equivalent
malic enzyme
manic episode
maximum effort
medial episiotomy
median eminence
medical education
Medical Examiner
meningoencephalitis
mercaptoethanol
metabolic and electrolyte [disorder]
metabolic energy
metabolism
metabolizable energy
metamyelocyte
methyleugenol
microembolism
microembolization
middle ear
mouse embryo
mouse epithelial [cell]
muscle examination
myoepithelial

2-ME — 2-mercaptoethanol

ME_{50} — 50% maximal effect

Me —
menton
methyl

MEA —
Medical Exhibition Association
mercaptoethylamine
monoethanolamine
multiple endocrine abnormalities

MEA — (continued)
multiple endocrine adenomata
multiple endocrine adenomatosis
multiple endocrine adenopathy

MEA-I — multiple endocrine adenomatosis type I

mEAD — monophasic action potential early afterdepolarization

meas —
measure
measurement

MEB —
Medical Evaluation Board
methylene blue
muscle-eye-brain [disease]

MeB — methylene blue

ME-BH — medial eminence of basal hypothalamus

MeBSA — methylated bovine serum albumin

MEC —
mecillinam
meconium
median effective concentration
middle ear canal
middle ear cells
minimum effective concentration
myoepithelial cell

mec. — meconium

Mecano — mechanotherapy

MeCbl — methylcobalamin

MECG —
maternal electrocardiogram
mixed essential cryoglobulinemia

MECT — maximal extrapolated clotting time

MECTA — mobile electroconvulsive therapy apparatus

MED —
medial
median erythrocyte diameter

MED — (*continued*)
    medical
    medication
    medicine
    medium
    minimal effective dose
    minimal erythema dose
    multiple epiphyseal dysplasia
med. —
    medial
    median
    medical
    medication
    medicine
    medium
MEDAC —
    multiple endocrine deficiency,
        Addison's disease, and can-
        didiasis [syndrome]
    multiple endocrine defi-
        ciency–autoimmune-can-
        didiasis
MED-ART — Medical Automated
    Records Technology
MEDEX — *médecin extension* (Fr.)
    extension of physician
MEDF — midexpiratory dynamic
    flow [rate]
medic. — *medicus* (Lat.) military
    medical corpsman
MEDICO —
    Medical Information Coopera-
        tion
    Medical International Cooper-
        ation
MEDIHC — Military Experience
    Directed into Health Careers
MEDLARS — Medical Literature
    Analysis and Retrieval Sys-
    tem
MEDLINE — MEDLARS On-Line
med men —
    medial meniscectomy
    medial meniscus
MEDPAR — Medical Provider
    Analysis and Review
MEdREP — Medical Education Re-
    inforcement and Enrichment
    Program

MEDs —
    medications
    medicines
MedScD — Doctor of Medical Sci-
    ence
med-surg — medicine and surgery
Med Tech —
    medical technician
    medical technologist
    medical technology
MEE —
    measured energy expenditure
    methylethyl ether
    middle ear effusion
MEET — Multistage Exercise Elec-
    trocardiographic Test
MEF —
    maximal expiratory flow
    maximum expired flow [rate]
    middle ear fluid
    midexpiratory flow
    migration enhancement factor
    mouse embryo fibroblast
MEF_{50} — mean maximal expiratory
    flow
MEFR — maximal expiratory flow
    rate
MEFSR — maximal expiratory
    flow–static recoil curve
MEFV — maximal expiratory flow
    volume
MEFVC —
    maximal expiratory flow vol-
        ume curve
    mechanical expiratory flow
        volume curve
MEG —
    magnetoencephalograph
    magnetoencephalography
    megakaryocyte
    mercaptoethylguanidine
    multifocal eosinophilic granu-
        loma
meg. —
    megacycle
    megakaryocyte
    megaloblast
Meg-CSA — megakaryocyte col-
    ony–stimulating activity

MEGD — minimal euthyroid Graves' disease
mEGF — mouse epidermal growth factor
MEGX — monoethylglycinexylidide
MEK — methylethylketone
MEL —
    metabolic equivalent level
    mouse erythroleukemia
    murine erythroleukemia
mel —
    melanoma
    melena
MELAN — melanin
MELAS — mitochondrial encephalomyopathy–lactic acidosis–and stroke-like symptoms [syndrome]
MEL B — brand name for melarsoprol
MELC — murine erythroleukemia cell
MELDOS — melioidosis
MELI — met-enkephalin-like immunoreactivity
MEM —
    macrophage electrophoretic mobility [test]
    malic enzyme, mitochondrial
    minimum essential medium
MEMA — methyl methacrylate
memb —
    membrane
    membranous
MEMR —
    multiple exostoses–mental retardation [syndrome]
MEN —
    methylethylnitrosamine
    multiple endocrine neoplasia
men —
    meningeal
    meninges
    meningitis
    meniscus
    menstruation
MEND — Medical Education for National Defense

MEN-I, II — multiple endocrine neoplasia, type I, II
menst —
    menstrual
    menstruate
    menstruating
ment —
    mental
    mentality
MEO —
    malignant external otitis [media]
    Medical Emergency Officer
MeOH — methyl alcohol
MEOS — microsomal ethanol-oxidizing system
MEP —
    maximum expiratory pressure
    mean effective pressure
    mitochondrial encephalopathy
    motor end-plate
    multimodality evoked potential
mep. — meperidine
MEPC — miniature end-plate current
MEPH — mephobarbital
MEPP — miniature end-plate potential
MePr — methylprednisolone
MEPROB — meprobamate
mEq — milliequivalent
mEq/L — milliequivalents per liter
MER —
    mean ejection rate
    mersalyl [acid]
    methanol-extruded residue
    molar esterification rate
    multimodality evoked response
    myeloid-erythrocyte ratio
    myeloid-erythroid ratio
MER-29 — triparanol
M/E ratio — myeloid/erythroid ratio
MERB —
    Medical Examination and Review Board

MERB — *(continued)*
  met-enkephalin receptor binding
MERG — macular electroretinogram
MERRF — myoclonus epilepsy with ragged red fibers [syndrome]
MES —
  maintenance electrolyte solution
  maximal electroshock
  maximal electroshock seizures
  mesial
  Metrazol-electroshock seizure
  morpholinoethanesulfonic acid
  multiple endocrine syndrome
  muscle in elongated state
  myoelectric signal
Mes —
  mesencephalic
  mesencephalon
MESA — myoepithelial sialadenitis
Mesc. — mescaline
MESCH — Multi-Environment Scheme
MESGN — mesangial glomerulonephritis
MeSH — Medical Subject Headings [in MEDLARS]
MesPGN — mesangial proliferative glomerulonephritis
MET —
  medical emergency treatment
  metabolic
  metabolic equivalent of the task
  metabolic equivalent test
  metamyelocyte
  metastasis
  metastatic
  methionine
  metoprolol
  microsurgical endoscopic technique
  midexpiratory time

MET — *(continued)*
  multistage exercise test
Met. — methionine
met —
  metallic [chest sounds]
  metastasis
  metastasize
  metastasizing
META — metamyelocyte
META1 — Metabolic Profile 1
meta —
  metacarpal
  metatarsal
metab —
  metabolic
  metabolism
metaph — metaphysics
Met-Enk — methionine-enkephalin
METH — methicillin
Meth. — methedrine
meth — methyl
MetHb — methemoglobin
MeTHF — methyltetrahydrofolic acid
MetMb — metmyoglobin
m. et n. — *mane et nocte* (Lat.) morning and night
METS — metabolic equivalents [of oxygen consumption]
Mets. — metastases
m. et sig. — *misce et signa* (Lat.) mix and write a label
METT — maximum exercise tolerance test
m. et v. — *mane et vespere* (Lat.) morning and evening
MEU — maximum expected utility
MEV —
  maximum exercise ventilation
  million electron volts
  murine erythroblastosis virus
MeV, Mev —
  megaelectron volt
  megavolt
  megavoltage
mev — million electron volts
MEWD — multiple evanescent white dot [syndrome]

MEX — mexiletine

MF —
    masculinity/femininity
    mass fragmentography
    meat free
    medium frequency
    megafarad
    melamine formaldehyde
    membrane filter
    Merthiolate-formaldehyde [solution]
    methanol formaldehyde
    methoxyflurane
    5-methyltetrahydrofolate
    microfibril
    microfilament
    microflocculation
    microscopic factor
    midcavity forceps
    mitochondrial fragments
    mitogenic factor
    mitotic figure
    mossy fiber
    mucosal fluid
    multifactorial
    multiplying factor
    mutation frequency
    mycosis fungoides
    myelin figure
    myelofibrosis
    myocardial fibrosis
    myofibrillar

M/F — male/female [ratio]

M&F —
    male and female
    mother and father

Mf —
    maxillofrontal
    microfilaria

mF — millifarad

μF — microfarad

mf —
    microfilaria
    millifarad

MFA —
    methyl fluoracetate
    monofluoroacetate
    multifocal functional autonomy

MFA — (continued)
    multifunctional acrylic
    multiple factor analysis

MFAT — multifocal atrial tachycardia

MFB —
    medial forebrain bundle
    metallic foreign body

MFC —
    mean frequency of compensation
    minimal fungicidal concentration

m-FC — membrane focal coli [broth]

MFCC — Marriage, Family, and Child Counselor

MFCM — Master, Faculty of Community Medicine

MFCV — muscle fiber conduction velocity

MFD —
    mandibulofacial dysostosis
    midforceps delivery
    milk-free diet
    minimal fatal dose

mfd — microfarad

MFEM — maximal forced expiratory maneuver

MFG — modified heat-degraded gelatin

MFH —
    malignant fibrous histiocytoma
    membrane-free hemolysate

MFHom — Member of the Faculty of Homeopathy

MFID — multielectrode flame ionization detector

m. flac. — *membrana flaccida* (Lat.) flaccid membrane (pars flaccida membranae tympani; Shrapnell's membrane)

MFM — Millipore filter method

MFO — mixed-function oxidase

MFOM — Master, Faculty of Occupational Medicine

MFP —
    monofluorophosphate

MFP — (continued)
    myofascial pain
MFPVC — multifocal premature
    ventricular contraction
MFR —
    mean flow rate
    midforceps rotation
    mucus flow rate
MFRL — maximal force at rest
    length
MFS —
    medical fee schedule
    Merthiolate-formaldehyde so-
        lution
    Minnesota Follow-up Study
MF sol — Merthiolate-formalde-
    hyde solution
MFSS — Medical Field Service
    School
MFST — Medical Field Service
    Technician
MFT —
    multifocal atrial tachycardia
    muscle function test
m. ft. — *mistura fiat* (Lat.) let a
    mixture be made
MFTVP — Motor-Free Test of Vi-
    sual Perception
MFU — medical follow-up
MFVD — midforceps vaginal deliv-
    ery
MFVNS — middle fossa vestibular
    nerve section
MFVPT — Motor-Free Visual Per-
    ception Test
MFW — multiple fragment
    wounds
MG —
    Marcus Gunn [pupil]
    margin
    medial gastrocnemius [muscle]
    membranous glomerulonephri-
        tis
    membranous glomerulopathy
    menopausal gonadotropin
    mesiogingival
    methylglucoside
    methyl-guanidine

MG — (continued)
    Michaelis-Gutmann [bod-
        ies]
    minigastrin
    monoclonal gammopathy
    monoglyceride
    mucigen granule
    mucous granule
    muscle group
    myasthenia gravis
    myoglobin
M3G — morphine-3-glucuronide
Mg — magnesium
m⁷G — 7-methylguanosine
mg — milligram
mγ — milligamma (millimicro-
    gram, micromilligram, or
    nanogram)
μg — microgram
μγ — microgamma (micromicro-
    gram or picogram)
mg% —
    milligrams percent
    milligrams per 100 cubic cen-
        timeters or per 100 grams
    milligrams per deciliter
    milligrams per 100 milliliters
MGA —
    medical gas analyzer
    melengestrol acetate
MgATP — magnesium adenosine
    triphosphate
MGB — medial geniculate body
MGBG — methylglyoxal-*bis*-
    guanylhydrazone
MGC —
    minimal glomerular change
    minimum gelling concentra-
        tion
    multinucleated giant cell
MgC — magnocellular (neuroen-
    docrine) cell
MGCE — multifocal giant cell en-
    cephalitis
MgCl₂ — magnesium chloride
MGD —
    maximal glucose disposal
    mixed gonadal dysgenesis

mgd — million gallons per day
mg/dl — milligrams per deciliter
MGDS — Member in General Dental Surgery
mg-el — milligram-element
MGES — multiple gated equilibrium scintigraphy
MGF —
    macrophage growth factor
    maternal grandfather
    mother's grandfather
MGG —
    May-Grünwald-Giemsa [staining]
    molecular and general genetics
    mouse gamma globulin
MGGH — methylglyoxal guanylhydrazone
MGH — monoglyceride hydrolase
mgh — milligram-hour
MGI — macrophage and granulocyte inducer
mg/kg — milligrams per kilogram
MGL — minor glomerular lesion
Mgl — myoglobin
mg/L — milligrams per liter
MGM —
    maternal grandmother
    mother's grandmother
mgm — milligram [former symbol]
MGMA — Medical Group Management Association
MGN —
    medial geniculate nucleus
    membranous glomerulonephritis
MgO — magnesium oxide
MGP —
    Marcus Gunn pupil
    marginal granulocyte pool
    marginated granulocyte pool
    membranous glomerulonephropathy
    methyl green–pyronin [dye]
    mucin glycoprotein
    mucous glycoprotein
MGR —
    modified gain ratio

MGR — (continued)
    multiple gas rebreathing
    murmurs, gallops, or rubs
MGS — metric gravitational system
MGSA — melanoma growth-stimulating activity
MGSD — mean gestational sac diameter
MgSO$_4$ — magnesium sulfate
MGT — multiple glomus tumors
mgtis — meningitis
MGUS — monoclonal gammopathy of undetermined significance
MGW — magnesium sulfate, glycerin, and water
MGXT — multistage graded exercise test
mGy — milligray
MH —
    maleic hydrazide
    malignant histiocytosis
    malignant hyperpyrexia
    malignant hypertension
    malignant hyperthermia
    mammotropic hormone
    mannoheptulose
    marital history
    Master Herbalist
    medial hypothalamus
    medical history
    melanophore(-stimulating) hormone
    menstrual history
    mental health
    mental hygiene
    moist heat
    monosymptomatic hypochondriasis
    multiply handicapped
    murine hepatitis
    mutant hybrid
    myohyoid
M/H — microcytic hypochromic [anemia]
M-H — Mueller-Hinton [agar]
Mh — mandible head

mH — millihenry
μH — microhenry
MHA —
>   major histocompatibility antigen
>   May-Hegglin anomaly
>   Mental Health Association
>   methemalbumin
>   microangiopathic hemolytic anemia
>   microhemagglutination
>   middle hepatic artery
>   mixed hemadsorption
>   Mueller-Hinton agar
MHA-TP — microhemagglutination assay—*Treponema pallidum*
MHB —
>   maximum hospital benefit
>   mental health (assistance) benefit
>   Mueller-Hinton base
MHb. —
>   medial habenular
>   methemoglobin
>   myohemoglobin
MHBSS — modified Hank's balanced salt solution
MHC —
>   major histocompatibility complex
>   mental health care
>   mental health center
>   mental health clinic
>   mental health counselor
>   multiphasic health check-up
mhcp — mean horizontal candlepower
MHCS — Mental Hygiene Consultation Service
m/hct — microhematocrit
MHCU — Mental Health Care Unit
MHD —
>   magnetohydrodynamics
>   maintenance hemodialysis
>   maximal human dose
>   mean hemolytic dose

MHD — *(continued)*
>   Medical Holding Detachment
>   Mental Health Department
>   minimum hemolytic dilution
>   minimum hemolytic dose
MHDPS — Mental Health Demographic Profile System
MHDU — medical hemodialysis unit
MHI —
>   malignant histiocytosis of intestine
>   Mental Health Index
>   Mental Health Institute
MHL — medial hypothalamic lesion
MHLC — Multidimensional Health Locus of Control
MHLS — metabolic heat load stimulator
MH/MR — mental health/mental retardation
MHN —
>   massive hepatic necrosis
>   Mohs hardness number
>   morbus hemolyticus neonatorum
MHNTG — multiheteronodular toxic goiter
MHO — microsomal heme oxygenase
mho — reciprocal ohm (ohm spelled backward): siemens unit
MHP —
>   maternal health program
>   Mental Health Project
>   1-mercuri-2-hydroxypropane
>   methoxyhydroxypropane
>   monosymptomatic hypochondriacal psychosis
MHPA —
>   mild hyperphenylalaninemia
>   Minnesota-Hartford Personality Assay
MHPE — 3-methoxy-4-hydroxyphenylethanol
MHPE Conj — 3-methoxy-4-hydroxyphenylethanol conjugate

MHPG — 3-methoxy-4-hydroxyphenylglycol
MHPG Conj — 3-methoxy-4-hydroxyphenylglycol conjugate
MHR —
    major histocompatibility region
    malignant hyperthermia resistance
    maternal heart rate
    maximal heart rate
    methemoglobin reductase
MHRI — Mental Health Research Institute
MHS —
    major histocompatibility system
    malignant hyperthermia in swine
    malignant hyperthermia syndrome
    malignant hypothermia susceptibility
    maximum Histalog stimulation
    multiple health screening
MHSA — microaggregated human serum albumin
MHST — multiphasic health screen test
MHT —
    mixed hemagglutination test
    multiphasic health testing
MHTI — minor hypertensive infant
MHTS — Multiphasic Health Testing Services
MHV —
    magnetic heart vector
    minimal height velocity
    mouse hepatitis virus
MHVD — Marek's herpesvirus disease
MH virus — murine hepatitis virus
MHW —
    medial heel wedge
    mental health worker

M.Hx. — medical history
MHyg — Master of Hygiene
MHz — megahertz
MI —
    maturation index
    medical illustration
    medical illustrator
    medical inspection
    melanophore index
    membrane intact
    menstruation induction
    mental illness
    mental institution
    mercaptoimidazole
    mesioincisal
    metabolic index
    metaproterenol inhaler
    methyl indole
    migration index
    migration inhibition
    mild irritant
    mitotic index
    mitral incompetence
    mitral insufficiency
    mononucleosis infectiosa
    morphology index
    motility index
    myocardial infarction
    myocardial ischemia
    myo-inositol
M&I — maternal and infant [care]
Mi — mitomycin
mi — mile
MIA —
    medically indigent adult
    missing in action
    multi-institutional arrangement
MIAA — microaggregated albumin
MIAP — modified innervated antral pouch
MIAs — multiple intracranial aneurysms
MIB — Medical Impairment Bureau
mIBG — metaiodobenzylguanidine
MIBiol — Member of the Institute of Biology

MIBK — methylisobutyl ketone
MIBT — methyl isatin-beta-thio-semicarbazone
MIC —
    Maternity and Infant Care
    medical intensive care
    Medical Interfraternity Conference
    methacholine inhalation challenge
    microcytic erythrocyte
    microcytosis
    microscope
    microscopic
    microscopy
    minimal inhibitory concentration
    minimal isorrheic concentration
    minocycline
    mobile intensive care
    model immune complex
    mononuclear inflammatory cell
MICC — mitogen-induced cellular cytotoxicity
MICG — macromolecular insoluble cold globulin
MICN —
    medical intensive care nurse
    mobile intensive care nurse
mic. pan. — *mica panis* (Lat.) bread crumb
MICR — methacholine inhalation challenge response
MIC-RN — Mobile Intensive Care Registered Nurse
micro —
    microcyte
    microcytic
    microscopic
    microscopy
microbiol. —
    microbiological
    microbiology
MICU —
    Medical Intensive Care Unit
    Mobile Intensive Care Unit

MID —
    maximum inhibiting dilution
    maximum inhibiting duration
    mesioincisodistal
    midazolam
    minimal infective dose
    minimal inhibiting dose
    minimal inhibitory dilution
    minimal inhibitory dose
    minimal irradiation dose
    multi-infarct dementia
    multiple ion detection
mid — middle
MIDAS — Multicenter Isradipine Diuretic Arteriosclerosis [study]
MIDS — Management Information Decision System
midsag — midsagittal
MIE —
    medical improvement expected
    methylisoeugenol
MIF —
    macrophage-inhibiting factor
    melanocyte-inhibiting factor
    melanocyte(-stimulating hormone)-inhibiting factor
    maximum inspiratory flow
    Merthiolate-iodine-formaldehyde [method, solution]
    methylene-iodine-formalin
    microimmunofluorescence
    midinspiratory flow
    migration-inhibiting factor
    mixed immunofluorescence
    müllerian inhibiting factor
MIFC — Merthiolate-iodine-formaldehyde concentration
MIFR —
    maximal inspiratory flow rate
    midinspiratory flow rate
MIFT — Merthiolate-iodine-formaldehyde technique
MIG —
    measles immune globulin
    Medicare Insured Groups

MIg —
    malaria immunoglobulin
    measles immunoglobulin
    membrane immunoglobulin
MIGT — multiple inert gas elimi-
    nation technique
MIGW — maximal increment in
    growth and weight
MIH —
    Master of Industrial Health
    melanocyte-stimulating hor-
        mone–inhibitory hormone
    migraine with interparoxys-
        mal headache
    migraine with interval head-
        ache
    minimal intermittent heparin
        [dose]
    monoiodohistidine
MIHA — minor histocompatibility
    antigen
MI insuf — mitral insufficiency
MIKA — minor karyotype abnor-
    malities
MIKE — mass-analyzed ion kinetic
    energy
MIL — mother-in-law
mil —
    military
    milliliter
MILP — mitogen-induced lympho-
    cyte proliferation
MILS — medication information
    leaflet for seniors
MIME — mean indices of meal ex-
    cursions
MIMR — minimal inhibitor mole
    ratio
MIMS —
    Medical Information Manage-
        ment System
    Medical Inventory Manage-
        ment System
    Monthly Index of Medical
        Specialties
MIN —
    medial interlaminar nucleus
    mineral

MIN — *(continued)*
    minimum
    minor
    minute
min —
    mineral
    minim
    minimal
    minimum
    minor
    minute
min. — *minimum* (Lat.) a minim
MINA — monoisonitrosoacetone
MINE — medical improvement
    not expected
MINIA — monkey intranuclear
    inclusion agent
MIO —
    minimal identifiable odor
    motility indol ornithine
        [medium]
MiO — microorchidism
MIP —
    maximal intensity projection
    maximum inspiratory pressure
    mean incubation period
    mean intravascular pressure
    medical improvement possible
    metacarpointerphalangeal
    middle interphalangeal [joint]
    minimal inspiratory pressure
MIPS — myocardial isotopic perfu-
    sion scan
MIR — multiple isomorphous re-
    placement
MIRC — microtubuloreticular
    complex
MIRD — Medical Internal Radia-
    tion Dose
MIRF — macrophage immuno-
    genic antigen-recruiting factor
MIRP — myocardial infarction re-
    habilitation program
MIRU — myocardial infarction re-
    search unit
MIS —
    management information sys-
        tem

MIS — *(continued)*
　　medical information service
　　meiosis-inducing substance
　　mitral insufficiency
　　müllerian-inhibiting substance
misc. —
　　miscarriage
　　miscellaneous
MISG — modified immune serum
　　globulin
MISHAP — microcephalus–imper-
　　forate anus–syndactyly–
　　hamartoblastoma–abnormal
　　lung lobulation–polydac-
　　tyly [syndrome]
MISO — misonidazole
MISS — Modified Injury Severity
　　Scale
MISSGP — mercury in Silastic
　　strain gauge plethysmography
MIST — Medical Information Ser-
　　vice by Telephone
mist. — *mistura* (Lat.) mixture
MIT —
　　male impotence test
　　marrow iron turnover
　　meconium in trachea
　　melodic intonation therapy
　　metabolism inhibition test
　　migration inhibition test
　　miracidial immobilization test
　　mitomycin
　　monoiodotyrosine
mit — mitral
mit. — *mitte* (Lat.) send, give
Mit-C — mitomycin C
Mith — mithramycin
mit insuf — mitral insufficiency
Mito-C — mitomycin C
mit. sang. — *mitte sanguinem* (Lat.)
　　bleed
mit. tal. — *mitte tales* (Lat.) send
　　such
mIU — milli-International unit
μIU — micro-International unit
Mix Astig — mixed astigmatism
mix mon — mixed monitor
mixt. — mixture

MJ —
　　Machado-Joseph [disease]
　　marijuana
　　megajoule
mJ — millijoule
MJA — mechanical joint appara-
　　tus
MJAD — Machado-Joseph Azor-
　　ean disease
MJD — Machado-Joseph dis-
　　ease
MJL — medial joint line
MJRT — maximum junctional
　　recovery time
MJT —
　　Mead Johnson tube
　　Mowlem-Jackson technique
MK —
　　main kitchen
　　marked
　　megakaryocyte
　　menaquinone
　　monkey kidney
　　myokinase
MK-6 — vitamin K_2
Mk — monkey
MKAB — may keep at bedside
mkat — millikatal
μkat — microkatal
mkat/L — millikatal per liter
MKB — megakaryoblast
MKC — monkey kidney cell
MK-CSF — megakaryocyte colony-
　　stimulating factor
mkg — meter-kilogram
MKHS — Menkes' kinky hair syn-
　　drome
MkL — megakaryoblastic leukemia
MKP — monobasic potassium
　　phosphate
mks — meter-kilogram-second
MKSAP — Medical Knowledge
　　Self-Assessment Program
MKTC — monkey kidney tissue
　　culture
ML —
　　Licentiate in Medicine
　　Licentiate in Midwifery

ML — *(continued)*
    lingual margin
    malignant lymphoma
    marked latency
    maximal left
    maximum likelihood
    medial leminiscus
    meningeal leukemia
    mesiolingual
    middle lobe
    midlife
    midline
    molecular layer
    motor latency
    mucolipidosis
    multiple lentiginosis
    muscular layer
    myeloid leukemia
M/L —
    maltase/lactase [ratio]
    monocyte/lymphocyte [ratio]
    mother-in-law
M-L — Martin-Lewis [medium]
ML I, II, III, IV — mucolipidosis I, II, III, IV
mL — milliliter
ml —
    midline
    milliliter
μl — microliter
MLA —
    Medical Library Association
    medium long-acting
    mentolaeva anterior (Lat.) left mentoanterior [fetal position]
    mesiolabial
    monocytic leukemia, acute
    multilanguage aphasia
MLa — mesiolabial
mLa — millilambert
MLAB — Multilingual Aphasia Battery
MLaI — mesiolabioincisal
MLAP — mean left atrial pressure
MLaP — mesiolabiopulpal
MLB — monaural loudness balance

MLb — macrolymphoblast
MLBP — mechanical low back pain
MLBW — moderately low birth weight
MLC —
    minimal lethal concentration
    mixed leukocyte concentration
    mixed leukocyte culture
    mixed ligand chelate
    mixed lymphocyte concentration
    mixed lymphocyte culture
    morphine-like compound
    multilamellar cytosome
    multilevel care
    multilumen catheter
    myelomonocytic leukemia, chronic
    myosin light chain
MLCK — myosin light-chain kinase
MLCN — multilocular cystic nephroma
MLCO — Member of the London College of Osteopathy
MLCP — myosin light-chain phosphatase
MLCR — mixed lymphocyte culture reaction
MLCT — metal-to-ligand charge transfer
ML-CVP — multilumen central venous pressure
MLCW — mixed lymphocyte culture, weak
MLD —
    masking level difference
    median lethal dose
    metachromatic leukodystrophy
    minimal lesion disease
    minimum lethal dose
ml/dl — milliliters per deciliter
MLE —
    maximum likelihood estimation

MLE — (continued)
  midline episiotomy
MLF —
  medial longitudinal fasciculus
  median longitudinal fasciculus
  morphine-like factor
MLG —
  mesiolingual groove
  mitochondrial lipid glycogen
MLGN — minimal lesion glomerulonephritis
ML-H — malignant lymphoma,
  histiocytic
MLI —
  mesiolinguoincisal
  mixed lymphocyte interaction
  motilin-like immunoreactivity
MLL — malignant lymphoma,
  lymphoblastic [type]
ml/L — milliliters per liter
MLN —
  manifest latent nystagmus
  membranous lupus nephropa-
    thy
  mesenteric lymph node
MLNS —
  minimal lesion nephrotic syn-
    drome
  mucocutaneous lymph node
    syndrome
MLO —
  mesiolinguo-occlusal
  Mycoplasma-like organism
MLP —
  mentolaeva posterior (Lat.) left
    mentoposterior [fetal posi-
    tion]
  mesiolinguopulpal
  microsomal lipoprotein
ML-PDL — malignant lymphoma,
  poorly differentiated lymphocytic [type]
MLR —
  mean length response
  middle latency response
  mixed leukocyte reaction
  mixed leukocyte response
  mixed lymphocyte reaction

MLR — (continued)
  mixed lymphocyte response
MLS —
  mean life span
  medial life span
  median life span
  median longitudinal section
  middle lobe syndrome
  mouse leukemia virus
  myelomonocytic leukemia,
    subacute
MLSB — migrating long spike
  burst
MLT —
  mean latency time
  median lethal time
  Medical Laboratory Techni-
    cian
  mentolaeva transversa (Lat.)
    left mentotransverse [fetal
    position]
MLT(AMT) — Medical Laboratory
  Technician (American Medical Technologists)
MLT(ASCP) — Medical Laboratory Technician certified by
  the American Society of Clinical Pathologists
MLTC —
  mixed leukocyte-trophoblast
    culture
  mixed lymphocyte tumor cell
MLTI — mixed lymphocyte target
  interaction
MLU — mean length of utterance
MLV —
  Moloney's leukemogenic virus
  monitored live voice
  mouse leukemia virus
  multilaminar vesicle
  murine leukemia virus
MLVDP — maximum left ventricular developed pressure
MLVSS — mixed liquor–volatile
  suspended solids
mlx — millilux
MM —
  macromolecule

MM — (continued)
  major medical [insurance]
  malignant melanoma
  manubrium of malleus
  Marshall-Marchetti [procedure]
  Master of Management
  medial malleolus
  mediastinal mass
  megamitochondria
  melanoma metastasis
  meningococcal meningitis
  menstrually related migraine
  metastatic melanoma
  methadone maintenance
  middle molecule
  minimal medium
  mismatched
  mixed monitor
  morbidity and mortality
  motor meal
  mucous membrane
  Müller's maneuver
  multiple myeloma
  muscularis mucosae
  myeloid metaplasia
  myelomeningocele
M&M —
  milk and molasses
  morbidity and mortality
Mm — mandible mentum
mM — millimolar
mm —
  methylmalonyl
  millimeter
  mucous membrane
  murmur
mm. —
  muscles
  musculi
mm^2 — square millimeter
mm^3 — cubic millimeter
MMA —
  mastitis-metritis-agalactia [syndrome]
  medical materials account
  methylmalonic acid
  methylmercuric acetate

MMA — (continued)
  methyl methacrylate
  minor morphologic aberration
  monomethyladenosine
MMAC — mini-microaggregated albumin colloid
MMAD — mass median aerodynamic diameter
MMATP — methadone maintenance and aftercare treatment program
MMC —
  migrating motor complex
  migrating myoelectric complex
  minimal medullary concentration
  mitomycin C
  mucosal mast cell
MMD —
  mass median diameter
  mean marrow dose
  minimal morbidostatic dose
  moyamoya disease
  myotonic muscular dystrophy
MMDA — methoxymethylene dioxyamphetamine
MME —
  M-mode echocardiography
  mouse mammary epithelium
MMECT — multiple monitored electroconvulsive therapy
MMed — Master of Medicine
MMEF — maximal midexpiratory flow
MMEFR — maximal midexpiratory flow rate
MMF —
  magnetomotive force
  maximal midexpiratory flow
  mean maximum flow
  Member of the Medical Faculty
MMFG — mouse milk fat globule
MMFR —
  maximal midexpiratory flow rate

MMFR — *(continued)*
  maximal midflow rate
MMFV —
  maximal midexpiratory flow
    volume
  maximum midrespiratory flow
    volume
MMG — mean maternal glucose
MMH — monomethylhydrazine
mmHg — millimeter(s) of mercury
mmH₂O — millimeter(s) of water
MMI —
  macrophage migration index
  macrophage migration inhibi-
    tion
  methimazole
  methylmercaptoimidazole
  mucous membrane irritation
MMIHS — megacystis-microcolon-
  intestinal hypoperistalsis syndrome
MMIS — Medicaid Management
  Information System
MMK — Marshall-Marchetti-
  Krantz [cystourethropexy]
MML —
  Moloney murine leukemia
  monomethyllysine
  myelomonocytic leukemia
MMLV — Moloney murine leukemia virus
MMM —
  microsome-mediated muta-
    genesis
  Minnesota Mining and Manu-
    facturing Company [3M]
  myelofibrosis with myeloid
    metaplasia
  myeloid metaplasia with my-
    elofibrosis
  myelosclerosis with myeloid
    metaplasia
mμm — millimicrometer (nanometer)
μmm — micromillimeter
MMMF — man-made mineral fibers

MMMT —
  malignant mixed müllerian tu-
    mor
  metastatic mixed müllerian tu-
    mor
MMN —
  morbus maculosus neonato-
    rum
  multiple mucosal neuroma
MMNC — marrow mononuclear
  cell
MMO — methane mono-oxy-
  genase
MMOA — maxillary-mandibular
  odontectomy-alveolectomy
MMoL — myelomonoblastic leukemia
mmol — millimole
μmol — micromole
mmol/L — millimoles per liter
MMPI —
  McGill-Melzack Pain Index
  Minnesota Multiphasic Per-
    sonality Inventory
MMPI-D — Minnesota Multiphasic Personality Inventory Depression Scale
MMPNC — Medical Maternal Program for Nuclear Casualties
mmpp — millimeters partial pressure
MMPR — methylmercaptopurine
  riboside
MMPS — Medical Media Production Service
mm-PTH — mid-molecule parathyroid hormone
MMR —
  mass miniature radiography
  mass miniature roentgeno-
    graphy
  maternal mortality rate
  measles-mumps-rubella [vac-
    cine]
  midline malignant reticulosis
  mild mental retardation
  mobile mass x-ray
  monomethylolrutin

MMR — *(continued)*
    myocardial metabolic rate
MMS —
    Master of Medical Science
    methyl methanesulfonate
    Mini-Mental State [examination]
    Moloney's murine sarcoma
MMSA — Master of Midwifery, Society of Apothecaries
MMSc — Master of Medical Science
MMSE — Mini-Mental State Examination
mm/sec — millimeters per second
mm st — muscle strength
MMT —
    alpha-methyl-*m*-tyrosine
    manual muscle test
    Mini-Mental Test
    mouse mammary tumor
MMTA — methylmetatyramine
MMTP — methadone maintenance treatment program
MMTV — mouse mammary tumor virus
MMU —
    Medical Maintenance Unit
    mercaptomethyl uracil
mmu — millimass unit
μμ — micromicron
μM — micromolar
μm — micrometer
μμCi — micromicrocurie
μmg — micromilligram
μμg — micromicrogram
mμCi — millimicrocurie
mμg — millimicrogram
mμm — millimicrometer
MMuLV — Moloney murine leukemia virus
mμs — millimicrosecond
μmμ — meson
MMV —
    mandatory minute ventilation
    mandatory minute volume
MMWR — Morbidity and Mortality Weekly Report

MN —
    a blood group in the MNSs blood group system
    malignant nephrosclerosis
    Master of Nursing
    meganewton
    melanocytic nevus
    melena neonatorum
    membranous nephropathy
    membranous neuropathy
    mesenteric node
    metanephrine
    midnight
    mononuclear
    motor neuron
    mucosal neurolysis
    multinodular
    myoneural
M/N —
    macrocytic/normochromic [anemia]
    microcytic/normochromic [anemia]
M-N — motility nitrate
M&N — morning and night
Mn — manganese
mN —
    micronewton
    millinormal
mn —
    midnight
    modal number
MNA — maximum noise area
MNAP — mixed nerve action potential
MNB — murine neuroblastoma
5-MNBA — 5-mercapto-2-nitrobenzoic acid
MNBCCS — multiple nevoid basal-cell carcinoma syndrome
MNC — mononuclear cell
MNCL — monoclonal
MNCV — motor nerve conduction velocity
MND —
    minimum necrosing dose
    minor neurological dysfunction

MND — (continued)
>   modified neck dissection
>   motor neuron disease

MNG — multinodular goiter

mng — morning

MNGIE — myo-, neuro-, gastrointestinal encephalopathy

MNJ — myoneural junction

MNL —
>   marked neutrophilic leukocytosis
>   maximum number of lamellae
>   mononuclear leukocyte

MN/m^2 — meganewtons per square meter

MNMK — maximal number of microbes killed

MNMS — myonephropathic metabolic syndrome

MNNG — N-methyl N'-nitro-N-nitrosoguanidine

MNO — minocycline

MNP — mononuclear phagocyte

MNPA — methoxy-naphthyl propionic acid

MNR — marrow neutrophil reserve

MNS —
>   medial nuclear stratum
>   Melnick-Needles syndrome

MNSER — mean normalized systolic ejection rate

Mn-SOD — manganese-superoxide dismutase

MNSs — a blood group system consisting of groups M, N, and MN

MnSSEP — median nerve somatosensory evoked potential

MNTB — medial nucleus of trapezoid body

MNU — methylnitrosourea

MNZ — metronidazole

MO —
>   macro-orchidism
>   manually operated
>   Master of Obstetrics
>   Master of Osteopathy

MO — (continued)
>   medial oblique [x-ray view]
>   Medical Officer
>   mesio-occlusal
>   mineral oil
>   minute output
>   mitral orifice
>   molecular orbit
>   mono-oxygenase
>   month
>   months old
>   morbid obesity
>   morbidly obese
>   mother

MO_2 — myocardial oxygen [consumption]

Mo —
>   mode
>   Moloney [strain]
>   molybdenum
>   monoclonal

$M\Omega$ — megohm

$\mu\Omega$ — microhm

mo —
>   mode
>   month
>   months old
>   mother

MOA —
>   mechanism of action
>   medical office assistant

MoAb — monoclonal antibody

MOB — medical office building

mob —
>   mobil
>   mobility
>   mobilization

MOC —
>   maximum oxygen consumption
>   mother of child
>   multiple ocular coloboma
>   myocardial oxygen consumption

MoCM — molybdenum-conditioned medium

MOD —
>   maturity-onset diabetes

MOD — (continued)
  Medical Officer of the Day
  Medical Officer on Duty
  medicine, osteopathy, and
    dentistry
  mesio-occlusodistal
mod —
  modality
  moderate
  moderation
  modification
  modulation
  module
modem — modulator/demodulator
MODM — maturity-onset diabetes
  mellitus
mod. praesc. — modo praescripto
  (Lat.) in the way directed
MODS — medically oriented data
  system
MODY — maturity-onset diabetes
  of youth
MOF —
  marine oxidation/fermenta-
    tion
  methoxyflurane
  multiple organ failure
MOFS — multiple-organ failure
  syndrome
MO&G — Master of Obstetrics
  and Gynaecology
MOH — Medical Officer of
  Health
MOI —
  maximum oxygen intake
  multiplicity of infection
MOIVC — membranous obstruction of the inferior vena cava
MOJAC — mood, orientation,
  judgment, affect, and content
MOL —
  molecular
  molecular layer
mol —
  mole
  molecule
molc — molar concentration
molfr — mole fraction

mol/kg — moles per kilogram
moll. — mollis (Lat.) soft
mol/L —
  molecules per liter
  moles per liter
mol/m³ — moles per cubic meter
mol/s — moles per second
mol. wt. — molecular weight
MOM —
  milk of magnesia
  mucoid otitis media
MoM — multiples of the median
MOMA — methylhydroxymandelic
  acid
MΩ — megohm
mΩ — milliohm
MO-MOM — mineral oil and milk
  of magnesia
MOMS — multiple organ malrota-
  tion syndrome
Mo-MSV — Moloney murine sarcoma virus
MOMX — macro-orchidism-
  marker X chromosome [syn-
  drome]
MON —
  mongolian [gerbil]
  monitor
mon —
  monocyte
  month
MONO — mononucleosis
Mono — Monospot [test]
mono. —
  monocyte
  mononucleosis
monos — monocytes
MOOW — Medical Officer of the
  Watch
MOP —
  major organ profile
  medical outpatient
  medical outpatient program
8-MOP — 8-methoxypsoralen
MOPEG — 3-methoxy-4-hydroxy-
  phenylglycol
MOPV — monovalent oral poliovirus vaccine

MOR — Medical Officer's Report
Mor — morphine
MORA — mandibular orthopedic repositioning appliance
MORC — Medical Officers Reserve Corps
MORD — magnetic optical rotatory dispersion
mor. dict. — *more dicto* (Lat.) in the manner directed
MORE — Management of Radiographic Environments
morph. —
  morphine
  morphological
  morphology
mor. sol. — *more solito* (Lat.) in the usual way
mort. — mortality
MOS —
  medial orbital sulcus
  Medical Outcome Study
  microsomal ethanol-oxidizing system
  mirror optical system
  myelofibrosis osteosclerosis
mOs — milliosmolal
mos — months
MOSF — multiple organ system failure
MOSFET — metal oxide semiconductor field effect transistor
mOsm —
  milliosmol
  milliosmole
μOsm — micro-osmole
mOsm/kg — milliosmoles per kilogram
MOT —
  mini-object test
  motility examination
  mouse ovarian tumor
mot. — motor
MOTT — mycobacteria other than tubercle [bacilli]
MOU — memorandum of understanding
MOUS — multiple occurrences of unexplained symptoms

MOV — multiple oral vitamins
MOVC — membranous obstruction of (inferior) vena cava
MOX — moxalactam
MP —
  macrophage
  matrix protein
  mean pressure
  mechanical percussion
  mechanical percussor
  medial plantar
  medical payment
  melting point
  membrane potential
  menstrual period
  mentoposterior
  mentum posterior [fetal position]
  mercaptopurine
  mesial pit
  mesiopulpal
  metacarpophalangeal
  metaphalangeal
  metatarsophalangeal
  methylprednisolone
  Mibelli's porokeratosis
  middle phalanx
  modo prescripto (Lat.) as directed
  modulator protein
  moist pack
  monophosphate
  mouth piece
  mouth pressure
  mucopolysaccharide
  mucopurulent
  multiparous
  multiprogrammable pacemaker
  muscle potential
  mycoplasmal pneumonia
  myeloma protein
μP — microprocessor
4MP4 — methylpyrazole
6-MP — 6-mercaptopurine
8-MP — 8-methylpsoralen
mp —
  melting point

mp — *(continued)*
  millipond
  myeloma protein
m.p. —
  mane primo (Lat.) early in the
    morning
  modo prescripto (Lat.) in the
    manner prescribed
MPA —
  main pulmonary artery
  medial preoptic area
  Medical Procurement Agency
  medroxyprogesterone acetate
  methylprednisolone acetate
  microscopic polyarteritis
  minor physical anomaly
  mycophenolic acid
MPa — megapascal
μPa — micropascal
MPAG — McGill Pain Assessment
  Questionnaire
MPAP — mean pulmonary arterial
  pressure
MPAS — mild periodic acid–Schiff
  [reaction]
MPB —
  male pattern baldness
  meprobamate
MPC —
  marine protein concentrate
  maximum permissible concen-
    tration
  mean plasma concentration
  meperidine, promethazine,
    and chlorpromazine
  metallophthalocyanine
  minimal protozoacidal con-
    centration
  minimum mycoplasmacidal
    concentration
  mucopurulent cervicitis
  myeloblast-promyelocyte com-
    partment
MPCD — minimal perceptible
  color difference
MPCN — microscopically positive,
  culturally negative

MPCO — micropolycystic ovary
  [syndrome]
MPCUR — maximum permissible
  concentration of unidentified
  radionucleotides
MPCWP — mean pulmonary capillary wedge pressure
MPD —
  main pancreatic duct
  maximum permissible dose
  mean population doubling
  membrane potential differ-
    ence
  minimal perceptible differ-
    ence
  minimal phototoxic dose
  minimal popular dose
  minimal port diameter
  Minnesota Percepto-Diagnos-
    tic [test]
  multiplanar display
  multiple personality disorder
  myeloproliferative disease
  myofascial pain dysfunction
MPDS —
  mandibular pain dysfunction
    syndrome
  myofascial pain dysfunction
    syndrome
MPDT — Minnesota Percepto-
  Diagnostic Test
MPDW — mean percentage of
  desirable weight
MPE —
  maximal permissible exposure
  maximal possible effect
  maximum possible error
MPEC — monopolar electrocoagulation
MPED — minimal phototoxic erythema dose
MPEH — methylphenylethylhydan-
  toin
MPF —
  maturation-promoting factor
  mean power frequency
MPFM — mini-Wright peak flow
  meter

MPG —
  magnetopneumography
  mercaptopropionylglycine
MPGM — monophosphoglycerate
  mutase
MPGN —
  membranoproliferative glo-
    merulonephritis
  mesangioproliferative glomer-
    ulonephritis
MPH —
  male pseudohermaphroditism
  Master of Public Health
  methylphenidate
  milk protein hydrolysate
MPharm — Master in Pharmacy
M phase — phase of mitosis
MPHD — multiple pituitary hormone deficiencies
MPHR — maximum predicted
  heart rate
MPhysA — Member of
  Physiotherapists' Association
  (British)
MPI —
  mannose phosphate isomer-
    ase
  master patient index
  Maudsley Personality Inven-
    tory
  maximum permitted intake
  maximum point of impulse
  Multiphasic Personality In-
    ventory
  Multivariate Personality In-
    ventory
  myocardial perfusion imaging
MPJ —
  metacarpophalangeal joint
  metatarsophalangeal joint
mpk — milligrams per kilogram
MPL —
  maximum permissible level
  melphalan
  mesiopulpolabial
  mesiopulpolingual
MPLa — mesiopulpolabial

MPM —
  malignant papillary mesotheli-
    oma
  medial pterygoid muscle
  minor psychiatric morbidity
  Mortality Prediction Model
  multiple primary malignan-
    cy
  multipurpose meal
MPME — (5R,8R)-8-(4-p-
  methoxy-phenyl)-1-
  piperazynyl-methyl-6-methyl-
  ergolene
MPMP — 10[(1-methyl-3-
  piperidinyl)methyl]-10H-
  phenothiazine
MPMT — Murphy punch maneuver test
MPMV — Mason-Pfizer monkey
  virus
MPN — most probable number
MPO —
  maximum power output
  minimal perceptible odor
  myeloperoxidase
MPOA — medial preoptic area
MPOD — myeloperoxidase deficiency
MPOS — myeloperoxidase system
MPP —
  massive periretinal prolifera-
    tion
  maximal perfusion pressure
  maximal print position
  medial pterygoid plate
  Medical Personnel Pool
  mercaptopyrazidopyrimidine
  metacarpophalangeal profile
  methyl phenylpyridinium
mppcf — millions of particles per
  cubic foot [of air]
MPPEC — mean peak plasma ethanol concentration
MPPG — microphotoelectric plethysmography
MPPN — malignant persistent positional nystagmus

MPPT —
    maximal predicted phonation time
    methylprednisolone pulse therapy
MPQ — McGill Pain Questionnaire
MPR —
    marrow production rate
    massive preretinal retraction
    maximum pulse rate
    mercaptopurine riboside
    myeloproliferative reaction
MPRE — minimal pure radium equivalent
MPS —
    meconium plug syndrome
    Member of the Pharmaceutical Society
    methylprednisolone
    Michigan Picture Stories
    Microbial Profile System
    mononuclear phagocyte system
    Montreal platelet syndrome
    movement-produced stimuli
    mucopolysaccharide
    mucopolysaccharidosis
    multiphasic screening
    myocardiac perfusion scintigraphy
    myofascial pain syndrome
MPSMT — Merrill-Palmer Scale of Mental Tests
MPSRT — matched pairs signed rank test
MPSS — methylprednisolone sodium succinate
MPSV — myeloproliferative sarcomavirus
MPsyMed — Master of Psychological Medicine
MPT —
    Michigan Picture Test
    morphine provocative test
MPTAH — Mallory phosphotungstic acid hematoxylin

MPTP — 1-methyl-4-phenyl-1,2,3,6-tetrahydropyridine
MPTR ↓ — motor, pain, touch, reflex [deficit]
MPT-R — Michigan Picture Test, Revised
MPU — Medical Practitioners Union (British)
MPV —
    mean plasma volume
    mean platelet volume
    metatarsus primus varus
    mitral valve prolapse
mpz — millipièze
MQ —
    memory quotient
    menaquinone
MQC — microbiological quality control
MQL — Medical Query Language [computer]
MR —
    Maddox rods
    magnetic resistance
    magnetic resonance
    mandibular reflex
    mannose-resistant
    maximal right
    may repeat
    measles and rubella [vaccine]
    medial raphe
    medial rectus [muscle]
    median raphe
    medical record(s)
    medical rehabilitation
    medical release
    medication responder
    medium range
    megaroentgen
    mentally retarded
    mental retardation
    menstrual regulation
    mesencephalic raphe
    metabolic rate
    methemoglobin reductase
    methyl red
    milk ring

MR — *(continued)*
    mitral reflux
    mitral regurgitation
    mixed respiratory
    moderate resistance
    modulation rate
    mortality rate
    mortality ratio
    motivation research
    multicentric reticulohistio-
       cytosis
    multiplication rate
    multiplicity reactivation
    muscle receptor
    muscle relaxant
    myotactic reflex
M&R — measure and record
MR × 1 — may repeat one time
M_r —
    molecular weight ratio
    relative molecular mass
Mr — mandible ramus
mr — milliroentgen
μR — microroentgen
MRA —
    magnetic resonance angiogra-
       phy
    magnetic resonance arteriogra-
       phy
    main renal artery
    marrow repopulation activity
    Medical Record Administra-
       tor
    mid-right atrium
    multivariate regression analy-
       sis
MRAA — Mental Retardation As-
    sociation of America
MRACGP — Member of Royal
    Australasian College of Gen-
    eral Practice
MRACO — Member of Royal Aus-
    tralasian College of Ophthal-
    mology
MRACP — Member of Royal Aus-
    tralasian College of Physi-
    cians

MRACR — Member of Royal Aus-
    tralasian College of Radiolo-
    gists
MRad — Master of Radiology
mrad — millirad
MRAN — medical resident admit-
    ting note
MRAP —
    maximal resting anal pressure
    mean right atrial pressure
MRAS — main renal artery steno-
    sis
MRBC —
    monkey red blood cell
    mouse red blood cell
MRBF — mean renal blood flow
MRC —
    maximum recycling capacity
    Medical Registration Council
    Medical Research Council
    Medical Reserve Corps
    methylrosaniline chloride
MRCGP — Member of Royal Col-
    lege of General Practitioners
MRCP — Member of the Royal
    College of Physicians
MRCS — Member of the Royal
    College of Surgeons
MRCVS — Member of the Royal
    College of Veterinary Sur-
    geons
MRD —
    margin reflex distance
    maximum rate of depolariza-
       tion
    measles-rinderpest-distemper
       [virus group]
    medical records department
    method of rapid determina-
       tion
    minimal renal disease
    minimal residual disease
    minimum reacting dose
mrd — millirutherford
MRDM — malnutrition-related
    diabetes mellitus

MRE —
    maximal resistive exercise
    maximal respiratory effective-
      ness
    maximal risk estimate
MR-E — methemoglobin reductase
MREI — mean rate ejection index
mrem —
    millirem
    milliroentgen equivalent, man
mrep — milliroentgen equivalent,
    physical
MRF —
    medical record file
    melanocyte-releasing factor
    melanocyte-stimulating hor-
      mone–releasing factor
    melanophore-stimulating hor-
      mone–releasing factor
    mesencephalic reticular forma-
      tion
    midbrain reticular formation
    mitral regurgitant flow
    moderate renal failure
    monoclonal rheumatoid factor
    müllerian regression factor
mRF — monoclonal rheumatoid
    factor
MRFC — mouse rosette-forming
    cell
MRFIT — Multiple Risk Factor In-
    tervention Trial
MRFT — modified rapid fermenta-
    tion test
MRG — murmurs, rubs, and gal-
    lops
MRH —
    Maddox rod hyperphoria
    melanocyte-stimulating hor-
      mone–releasing hormone
    melanophore-stimulating hor-
      mone–releasing hormone
MRHA — mannose-resistant hem-
    agglutination
MRHD — maximal recommended
    human dose
mrhm — milliroentgen per hour at
    one meter

MRHT — modified rhyme hearing
    test
MRI —
    machine-readable identifier
    magnetic resonance imaging
    medical records information
    Medical Research Institute
    Member of the Royal Institu-
      tion
    Mental Research Institute
    moderate renal insufficiency
MRIF —
    melanocyte(-stimulating
      hormone) release-inhibiting
      factor
    melanophore(-stimulating
      hormone) release-inhibiting
      factor
MRIH — melanocyte(-stimulating
    hormone) release-inhibiting
    hormone
MRIPHH — Member of the Royal
    Institute of Public Health and
    Hygiene
MRK — Mayer-Rokitansky-Küster
    [syndrome]
MRL —
    Medical Record Librarian
    Medical Research Laboratory
    minimal response level
MRM — modified radical mastec-
    tomy
MRN — malignant renal neoplasm
mRNA — messenger ribonucleic
    acid
mRNP — messenger ribonucleo-
    protein
MRO —
    minimal recognizable odor
    muscle receptor organ
MROD — Medical Research and
    Operations Directorate
MRP —
    maximal reimbursement point
    mean resting potential
    medical reimbursement plan
MRPAH — mixed reverse passive
    antiglobulin hemagglutination

MRPN — medical resident progress rate

MRR —
 marrow release rate
 maximal relaxation rate
 maximum relation rate

MRS —
 magnetic resonance spectroscopy
 Mania Rating Scale
 median range score
 Medical Receiving Station
 Melkersson-Rosenthal syndrome
 methicillin-resistant *Staphylococcus aureus*
 multiple representative sections

MRSA — methicillin-resistant *Staphylococcus aureus*

MRSH — Member of the Royal Society of Health

MRSI — magnetic resonance spectroscopic imaging

MRT —
 magnetic resonance tomography
 major role therapy
 maximum relaxation time
 mean residence time
 median range score
 median reaction time
 median recognition threshold
 median relapse time
 Medical Records Technician
 medical records technology
 milk ring test
 modified rhyme test
 muscle response test

MRU —
 Mass Radiography Unit
 measure of resource use
 minimal reproductive unit

MRUS — maximal rate of urea synthesis

MRV —
 minute respiratory volume

MRV — *(continued)*
 mixed respiratory vaccine

MRVI — mixed respiratory virus infection

MRVP —
 mean right ventricular pressure
 methyl red, Voges-Proskauer [medium]

MS —
 Maffuci syndrome
 main scale
 maladjustment score
 mannose-sensitive
 Marfan syndrome
 Marie-Strümpell [syndrome]
 mass spectrometry
 Master of Science
 Master of Surgery
 mean score
 mean square [statistics]
 mechanical stimulation
 Meckel syndrome
 mediastinal shift
 medical science
 Medical Services
 medical student
 medical supplies
 medical-surgical
 medical survey
 Menkes' syndrome
 menopausal syndrome
 mental status
 Meretoja syndrome
 metaproterenol sulfate
 microscope slide
 Mikulicz's syndrome
 milkshake
 minimal support
 mitral sound
 mitral stenosis
 mobile surgical [unit]
 modal sensitivity
 molar solution
 mongolian spot
 morning stiffness
 morphine sulfate

MS — (continued)
    motile sperm
    mucosubstance
    multilaminated structure
    multiple sclerosis
    Münchausen syndrome
    muscle shortening
    muscle strength
    musculoskeletal
M&S — microculture and sensitivity
MS-zzz — tricaine methane sulfonate
MS I, II, III, IV — medical student—first, second, third, and fourth year
Ms —
    murmurs
    musculoskeletal
ms —
    manuscript
    millisecond
    mitral stenosis
    morphine sulfate
μs — microsecond
m/s — meters per second
m/s² — meters per second squared
MSA —
    major serologic antigen
    male-specific antigen
    mannitol salt agar
    Medical Services Administration
    membrane stabilizing action
    metropolitan statistical area
    mouse serum albumin
    multichannel signed averager
    Multidimensional Scalogram Analysis
    multiple system atrophy
    multiplication-stimulating activity
    muscle sympathetic activity
MSAA — multiple sclerosis–associated agent
MSAF — meconium-stained amniotic fluid

MS-AFP — maternal serum alpha-fetoprotein
MSAN — medical student's admission note
MSAP — mean systemic arterial pressure
MSB —
    Martin's scarlet blue
    Master of Science in Bacteriology
    mid-small bowel
    most significant bit
MsB — Master of Science in Bacteriology
MSBC — maximum specific binding capacity
MSBLA — mouse-specific B-lymphocyte antigen
MSBOS — maximal surgical blood order schedule
MSC —
    marrow stromal cell
    Medical Service Corps
    Medical Specialist Corps
    Medical Staff Corps
    multiple sibling case
MSc — Master of Science
MSCA — McCarthy Scales of Children's Abilities
MSCC — midstream clean catch
MScD —
    Doctor of Medical Science
    Master of Dental Science
MSCE — monitored self-care evaluation
MSCLC — mouse stem cell-like cell
MScMed — Master of Science in Medicine
MScN — Master of Science in Nursing
mscp — mean spherical candle power
MSCU — medical special care unit
MSCWP — musculoskeletal chest wall pain

MSD —
    mean square deviation
    metabolic screening disorder
    microsurgical discectomy
    midsleep disturbance
    mild sickle cell disease
    most significant digit
    multiple sulfatase deficiency
MSDC — Mass Spectrometry Data Centre
MSDI — Martin Suicide Depression Inventory
MSDS — material safety data sheet
MSE —
    medical support equipment
    mental status examination
    muscle-specific enolase
mse — mean square error
MSEA — Medical Society Executives Association
msec — millisecond
μsec — microsecond
m/sec — meters per second
MSEL — myasthenic syndrome of Eaton-Lambert
MSER —
    mean systolic ejection rate
    Mental Status Examination Record
MSES — medical school environmental stress
MSET — multistage exercise test
MSF —
    macrophage slowing factor
    macrophage spreading factor
    meconium-stained fluid
    Mediterranean spotted fever
    megakaryocyte-stimulating factor
    melanocyte-stimulating factor
    migration-stimulating factor
    modified sham feeding
MSG —
    massage
    methysergide
    monosodium glutamate

MSGV — mouse salivary gland virus
MSH —
    medical self-help
    melanocyte-stimulating hormone
    melanophore-stimulating hormone
MSHA —
    mannose-sensitive hemagglutination
    Mine Safety and Health Administration
MSHIF —
    melanocyte-stimulating hormone–inhibiting factor
    melanophore-stimulating hormone–inhibiting factor
MSHRF — melanocyte-stimulating hormone–releasing factor
MSHRH — melanocyte-stimulating hormone–releasing hormone
MSHSC — multiple self-healing squamous carcinoma
MSHyg — Master of Science in Hygiene
MSI —
    magnetic source imaging
    medium-scale integration
MSIR — morphine sulfate immediate-release [tablet]
MSIS — multistate information system
MSK —
    medullary sponge kidney
    musculoskeletal
MSKCC — Memorial Sloan-Kettering Cancer Center
MSKP — Medical Sciences Knowledge Profile
MSL —
    midsternal line
    multiple symmetric lipomatosis
MSLA —
    mouse-specific lymphocyte antigen

MSLA — (continued)
  multisample Luer adapter
MSLR — mixed skin cell-leukocyte reaction
MSLT — multiple sleep latency test
MSLVP — mean systolic left ventricular pressure
MSM —
  Master of Medical Science
  medium-size molecule
  mineral salts medium
MSN —
  main sensory nucleus
  Master of Science in Nursing
  medial septal nucleus
  mildly subnormal
MSO — medial superior olive
MSOF — multiple systems organ failure
MSP —
  maximum squeeze pressure
  mouse serum protein
  Münchausen syndrome by proxy
msp — muscle spasm
MSPGN — mesangial proliferative glomerulonephritis
MSPH — Master of Science in Public Health
MSPhar — Master of Science in Pharmacy
MSPN — medical student's progress note
MSPQ — Modified Somatic Perception Questionnaire
MSPS — myocardial stress perfusion scintigraphy
MSPU — medical short procedure unit
MSQ — mental status questionnaire
MSR —
  Member of the Society of Radiographers
  mitral stenoregurgitation
  monosynaptic reflex

MSR — (continued)
  muscle stretch reflex
MS Rad — Master of Science in Radiology
MSRG — Member of Society for Remedial Gymnastics
MSRPP — Multidimensional Scale for Rating Psychiatric Patients
MSRT — Minnesota Spatial Relations Test
MSS —
  Marital Satisfaction Scale
  Marshall-Smith syndrome
  massage
  Medical Service School
  Medical Superintendents' Society
  Medicare Statistical System
  mental status schedule
  Metabolic Support Service
  minor surgery suite
  motion sickness susceptibility
  mucus-stimulating substance
  multiple sclerosis susceptibility
  muscular subaortic stenosis
mss — massage
MSSc — Master of Sanitary Science
MSSE — Master of Science in Sanitary Engineering
MSSG — multiple sclerosis susceptibility gene
MSSR — Medical Society for the Study of Radiesthesia
MSSVD — Medical Society for the Study of Venereal Diseases
MST —
  mean survival time
  mean swell time [botulism test]
  median survival time
MSTA — mumps skin test antigen
MSTh — mesothorium
MSTI — multiple soft tissue injuries

MSU —
  maple sugar urine
  maple syrup urine
  medical studies unit
  midstream urine
  monosodium urate
  myocardial substrate uptake
MSUA — midstream urinalysis
MSUD — maple syrup urine disease
MSUM — monosodium urate monohydrate
MSurg — Master of Surgery
MSV —
  maximum sustained level of ventilation
  mean scale value
  Moloney's sarcoma virus
  murine sarcoma virus
MSVC — maximal sustained ventilatory capacity
MSVL — maximal spatial vector to left
MSW —
  Master of Social Welfare
  Master of Social Work
  Medical Social Worker
  multiple stab wounds
MSWYE — modified sea water yeast extract
MT —
  empty
  malaria therapy
  malignant teratoma
  mammary tumor
  mammillothalamic tract
  manual traction
  Martin-Thayer [plate, medium]
  mastoid tip
  maximal therapy
  medial thalamus
  medial thickening
  medial thickness
  mediastinal tube
  Medical Technologist
  medical therapy

MT — *(continued)*
  Medical Transcriptionist
  medical treatment
  melatonin
  membrana tympani (Lat.) tympanic membrane
  membrane thickness
  mesangial thickening
  metallothioneine
  metatarsal
  methoxytryptamine
  methoxytyramine
  methyltyrosine
  microtome
  microtubule
  middle turbinate
  midtrachea
  minimum threshold
  Monroe tidal drainage
  more than
  movement time
  Muir-Torre [syndrome]
  multiple tics
  multitest [plate]
  muscles and tendons
  muscle test
  music therapy
M/T —
  masses of tenderness
  myringotomy with tubes
M-T — macroglobulin-trypsin [complex]
M&T —
  Monilia and *Trichomonas*
  myringotomy and tubes
3-MT — 3-methoxytyramine
MT6 — mercaptomerin
Mt —
  megatonne
  Mycobacterium tuberculosis
mt — mitochondrial
m.t. — *mitte talis* (Lat.) send of such
MTA —
  malignant teratoma, anaplastic
  mammary tumor agent

MTA — *(continued)*
  Medical Technical Assistant
  metatarsus adductus
  myoclonic twitch activity
mTA — meta-tyramine
MTAC — mass transfer-area coefficient
MTAD — *membrana tympana auris dextrae* (Lat.) tympanic membrane of right ear
MTAL — medullary thick ascending limb
MT(AMT) — Medical Technologist (American Medical Technologists)
MTAS — *membrana tympana auris sinistrae* (Lat.) tympanic membrane of left ear
MT(ASCP) — Medical Technologist certified by the American Society of Clinical Pathologists
MT(ASCP)SBB — Medical Technologist (American Society of Clinical Pathologists) Specialist in Blood Bank (Technology)
MTAU — *membranae tympani aures unitae* (Lat.) tympanic membranes of both ears
MTB —
  methylthymol blue
  Mycobacterium tuberculosis
Mtb — *Mycobacterium tuberculosis*
MTBE —
  meningeal tick-borne encephalitis
  methyl *tert*-butyl ester
MTBF — mean time between (or before) failures
MTC —
  mass transfer coefficient
  maximum tolerated concen-
  .tration
  maximum toxic concentration
  medical test cabinet
  Medical Training Center

MTC — *(continued)*
  medullary thyroid carcinoma
  metoclopramide
MTCS — Madelian Thomas Completion Stories
MTD —
  maximum tolerated dose
  mean total dose
  metastatic trophoblastic disease
  Midwife Teacher's Diploma
  Monroe tidal drainage
  multiple tic disorder
m.t.d. — *mitte tales doses* (Lat.) send such doses
MTDDA — Minnesota Test for Differential Diagnosis of Aphasia
MTDI — maximal tolerable daily intake
MT-DN — multitest, dermatophytes, and *Nocardia* [plate]
mtDNA — mitochondrial deoxyribonucleic acid
MTDT — modified tone decay test
MTE — medical toxic environment
MTET — modified treadmill exercise testing
MTF —
  maximum terminal flow
  medical treatment facility
  modulation transfer factor
  modulation transfer function
MTG — midthigh girth
MTg — mouse thyroglobulin
MTH —
  metharbital
  mithramycin
MTHF — methyl tetrahydrofolic acid
5-MTHF — 5-methyltetrahydrofolate
MTI —
  malignant teratoma, intermediate
  minimum time interval

MTI — *(continued)*
    moving target indicator
MTJ — midtarsal joint
MTLP — metabolic toxemia of
    late pregnancy
MTM — modified Thayer-Martin
    [agar]
MT-M — multitest, mycology
    [plate]
MTO — Medical Transport Officer
MTOC —
    microtubule organizing center
    mitotic organizing center
MTP —
    master treatment plan
    maximum tolerated pressure
    medial tibial plateau
    median time to progression
    medical termination of preg-
    nancy
    metatarsophalangeal
    microtubule protein
MTPJ — metatarsophalangeal joint
MTQ — methaqualone
MTR —
    mass, tenderness, rebound [ab-
    dominal examination]
    Meinicke turbidity reaction
    mental treatment rules
    5-methylthioribose
    metronidazole
MTR-0 — no masses, tenderness,
    or rebound [abdominal exami-
    nation]
MTRX — methotrexate
MTS —
    mesial temporal sclerosis
    moderate tactile stimulus
    monosyllable, trochee, spon-
    dee [test]
    multicellular tumor spheroid
MTSO — medical transcription
    service organization
MTST — maximal treadmill stress
    test
MTT —
    malignant trophoblastic tera-
    toma

MTT — *(continued)*
    maximal treadmill testing
    meal tolerance test
    mean transit time
    methyltetrazolium
    monotetrazolium
MTU —
    malignant teratoma, undiffer-
      entiated
    medical therapy unit
    methylthiouracil
M. tuberc. — Mycobacterium tuber-
    culosis
MTV —
    mammary tumor virus
    metatarsus varus
    mouse (mammary) tumor
    virus
MTX — methotrexate
MT-Y — multitest yeast [plate]
MTZ — mitoxantrone
MU —
    Mache unit
    maternal uncle
    megaunit
    mescaline unit
    methyl-uric [acid]
    million units
    Montevideo unit
    motor unit
4-MU — 4-methylumbelliferone
Mu — Mache unit
mU. — milliunit
μU. — microunit
m.u. — mouse unit
MUA —
    middle uterine artery
    motor unit activity
    multiple unit activity
MUAC — middle upper-arm cir-
    cumference
MUAP — motor unit action poten-
    tial
μb — microbar
μbar — microbar
MUC —
    maximum urinary concentra-
    tion

MUC — (continued)
mucosal ulcerative colitis

muc —
mucous
mucus

muc. — *mucilago* (Lat.) mucilage

μC — microcoulomb

μCi — microcurie

μCi-hr — microcurie-hour

μcoul — microcoulomb

MUD — minimum urticarial dose

MUE — motor unit estimated

μEq — microequivalent

μf — microfarad

μg — microgram

MUGA —
multigated angiogram [scan]
multiple gated acquisition

MU-GAL — methylumbelliferyl-β-galactosidase

μγ — microgamma

MUGEx — multigated blood pool image during exercise

μg/kg — micrograms per kilogram

μg/L — micrograms per liter

MUGR — multigated blood pool image at rest

MUGX — multigated blood pool image during exercise

μGy — microgray

μH — microhenry

μHg — micron of mercury

μin — microinch

μIU — one-millionth of an International Unit

μkat — microkatal

μl — microliter

mult —
multiple
multiplication

multip. —
multipara
multiparous

MuLV — murine leukemia virus

μM — micromolar

μm —
micrometer

μm — (continued)
micromilli-

μmg — micromilligram (nanogram)

μmHg — micrometer of mercury

μmm — micromillimeter (nanometer)

μmμ — meson

μmol/L — micromoles per liter

MUMPS — Massachusetts General Hospital Utility Multi-Programming System

MuMTv — murine mammary tumor virus

μμ — micromicro-

μμC — micromicrocurie (picocurie)

μμF — micromicrofarad (picofarad)

μμg — micromicrogram (picogram)

MUN(WI) — Munich Wistar [rat]

MUO — myocardiopathy of unknown origin

μΩ — microhm

μOsm — micro-osmole

MUP —
major urinary protein
maximal urethral pressure
motor unit potential
mouse urine protein

μP — microprocessor

μPa — micropascal

μR — microroentgen

MURC — measurable undesirable respiratory contaminants

μ/ρ — mass attenuation coefficient

MurNAc — *N*-acetylmuramate

MURP — Master of Urban and Regional Planning

MUS — mouse urologic syndrome

μs — microsecond

musc —
muscle
muscular
musculature

mus-lig — musculoligamentous

μsec — microsecond
MUST — medical unit, self-contained and transportable
MUT — mutagen
μU — microunit
MUU — mouse uterine unit
μV — microvolt
μW — microwatt
MUWU — mouse uterine weight unit
MV —
    malignant (rabbit fibroma) virus
    measles virus
    mechanical ventilation
    Medicus Veterinarius (Lat.) veterinary physician
    megavolt
    microvascular
    microvillus
    minute ventilation
    minute volume
    mitral valve
    mixed venous [blood]
    multivesicular
    multivessel
Mv — mendelevium
mV — millivolt
MVA —
    malignant ventricular arrhythmia
    mechanical ventricular assistance
    mevalonic acid
    mitral valve area
    modified vaccine (virus), Ankara
    motor vehicle accident
MV·A — megavolt-ampere
mV·A — millivolt-ampere
MVB —
    mixed venous blood
    multivesicular body
MVC —
    maximal vital capacity
    maximum voluntary contraction
    myocardial vascular capacity

MVD —
    Doctor of Veterinary Medicine
    Marburg virus disease
    microvascular decompression
    mitral valve disease
    mouse vas deferens
    multivessel (coronary) disease
MVE —
    mitral valve echo
    mitral valve (leaflet) excursion
    Murray Valley encephalitis
MV grad. — mitral valve gradient
MVH —
    massive variceal hemorrhage
    massive vitreous hemorrhage
MVI —
    multiple vitamin infusion
    multiple vitamin injection
    multivalvular involvement
    multivitamin infusion
    multivitamins intravenously
MVL — mitral valve leaflet
MVLS —
    mandibular vestibulolingual sulcoplasty
    Mecham Verbal Language Scale
MVM —
    microvillus membrane
    minute virus of mice
MVMT — movement
MVN — medial ventromedial nucleus
MVO — maximum venous outflow
MVO_2 —
    maximal venous oxygen [consumption]
    myocardial oxygen ventilation rate
    oxygen content of mixed venous blood
mVO_2 —
    minimal venous oxygen [consumption]
    minute venous oxygen [consumption]

MVOA — mitral valve orifice area

MVOS — mixed venous oxygen saturation

MVP —
  mean venous pressure
  microvascular pressure
  mitral valve prolapse

MVPS —
  Medicare Volume Performance Standards
  mitral valve prolapse syndrome

MVP-SC — mitral valve prolapse-systolic click [syndrome]

MVPT — Motor-Free Visual Perception Test

MVR —
  massive vitreous retraction
  massive vitreous retractor [blade]
  maximum ventilation rate
  microvitreoretinal
  minimal vascular resistance
  mitral valve regurgitation
  mitral valve replacement

MVRI —
  mixed vaccine, respiratory infection
  mixed viral respiratory infection

MVS —
  mitral valve stenosis
  motor, vascular, and sensory

mV·s — millivolt-second

MVT — maximal ventilation time

mvt — movement

MVV —
  maximal ventilatory volume
  maximal voluntary ventilation
  maximum voluntary volume
  mixed vespid venom

MVV$_1$ — maximal ventilatory volume in 1 minute

MVV$_x$ — maximal voluntary ventilation in a specified time period

MW —
  Mallory-Weiss [syndrome]
  mean weight
  megawatt
  microwave
  Minot–von Willebrand [syndrome]
  molecular weight
  Munich Wistar [rat]

M-W —
  Mallory-Weiss [syndrome]
  men and women

mW — milliwatt

μW — microwatt

mw — microwave

mWb — milliweber

MWD —
  microwave diathermy
  molecular weight distribution

MWI — Medical Walk-In [clinic]

MWLT — Modified Word Learning Test

MWMT — Monotic Word Memory Test

MWP — mean wedge pressure

MWPC — multiwire proportional chamber

MWS —
  Marden-Walker syndrome
  Mikity-Wilson syndrome
  Moersch-Woltman syndrome

MWT —
  malpositioned wisdom teeth
  myocardial wall thickness

MWt — molecular weight

MX — matrix

Mx —
  mastectomy
  maxillary
  maxwell
  MEDEX: *médecin extension* (Fr.) extension of the physician
  multiple
  myringotomy

mx —
  management
  mixture
M_{xy} — transverse magnetization
My. —
  myopia
  myxedema
  myxedematous
my — mayer [unit of heat capacity]
Myco —
  Mycobacterium
  Mycoplasma
Mycol —
  mycologist
  mycology
MYD — mydriatic
MyD — myotonic dystrophy
MYE — myelotomy
MYEL —
  myelogram
  myeloma
Myel — myelocyte
myel —
  myelin
  myelinated
Myelo —
  myelogram

Myelo — (*continued*)
  myelography
myelo — myelocyte
MyG — myasthenia gravis
Myg — myriagram
Myl — myrialiter
Mym — myriameter
MyMD — myotonic muscular dystrophy
MYO — myoglobin
myo —
  myocardial
  myocardium
myop — myopia
MYS — myasthenia syndrome
MYTGC — Miller-Yoder Test of Grammatical Comprehension
MYX — myxoma
MZ —
  mantle zone
  mezlocillin
  monozygotic
M_z — longitudinal magnetization
m/z — mass-to-charge ratio
MZA — monozygotic twins raised apart
MZL — marginal zone lymphocyte
MZT — monozygotic twins raised together

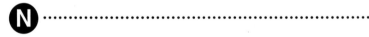

N —
  asparagine
  Avogadro's number
  blood factor in the MNS blood group system
  loudness
  nasal
  nasion
  nausea
  negative
  Negro
  neomycin
  neper
  neural

N — (*continued*)
  neuraminidase
  neurologist
  neurology
  neuropathy
  neutron number
  neutrophil
  newton
  nicotinamide
  nifedipine
  nitrogen
  nodal
  nodule
  non-malignant

N — (*continued*)
  Nonne [test]
  normal [solution]
  normal concentration
  nu (thirteenth letter of the Greek alphabet), uppercase
  nucleoside
  nucleus
  number
  number density
  number in sample
  number of molecules
  number of neutrons in an atomic nucleus
  numerical aptitude
  population size
  radiance
  refractive index
  sample size
  spin density
  unit of neutron dosage

N. —
  Neisseria
  Nocardia

^{15}N — radioactive nitrogen
N/2 — half-normal [solution]
N/10 — tenth-normal [solution]
N/50 — fiftieth-normal [solution]
NI–NXII — first through twelfth cranial nerves
0.02N — fiftieth-normal [solution]
0.1N — tenth-normal [solution]
0.5N — half-normal [solution]
2N — double-normal [solution]

n —
  amount of substance expressed in moles
  haploid chromosome number
  index of refraction
  nano-
  nasal
  neuter
  neutron
  neutron dosage
  neutron number density
  normal
  nostril
  number
  number of density of molecule
  number of observations

n — (*continued*)
  principal quantum number
  refractive index
  rotational frequency
  sample size

ν —
  degrees of freedom
  frequency
  kinematic velocity
  neutrino
  nu (thirteenth letter of the Greek alphabet), lowercase

n. —
  naris (Lat.) nostril
  natus (Lat.) born
  nervus (Lat.) nerve

n_D — refractive index
2n — diploid chromosome number
3n — triploid chromosome number
4n — tetraploidy
5'-N — 5'-nucleotidase
5n — pentaploidy
7n — heptaploidy
8n — octaploidy

NA
  nalidixic acid
  Narcotics Anonymous
  network administrator
  neuraminidase
  neurologic age
  neutralizing antibody
  neutrophil antibody
  nicotinic acid
  nitric acid
  no abnormality
  Nomina Anatomica
  nonadherent
  non-A hepatitis
  nonalcoholic
  nonamnionic
  nonmyelinated axon
  noradrenaline
  not admitted
  not applicable
  not attempted
  not available
  nuclear antibody
  nuclear antigen
  nucleic acid
  nucleus accumbens

NA — *(continued)*
    nucleus ambiguus
    numerical aperture
    nurse's aide
    nurse anesthetist
    nursing assistant
    Nursing Auxiliary (British)
N/A —
    no alternative
    not applicable
N & A — normal and active
Na —
    Avogadro's number
    sodium (Lat., *natrium*)
^{24}Na — radioactive sodium
nA — nanoampere
NAA —
    naphthaleneacetic acid
    neutral amino acid
    neutron activation analysis
    neutrophil aggregation activity
    nicotinic acid amide
    no apparent abnormalities
NAAC — no apparent anesthetic complication
NAACLS — National Accrediting Agency for Clinical Laboratory Sciences
NAACOG — Nurses Association of the American College of Obstetricians and Gynecologists
NAACP — neoplasia, allergy, Addison's disease, collagen vascular disease, and parasites
NAAP — *N*-acetyl-4-aminophenazone
NAB —
    non-A, non-B [hepatitis]
    novarsenobenzene
NABP — National Association of Boards of Pharmacy
NABPLEX — National Association of Boards of Pharmacy Licensing Examination
NaBr — sodium bromide
NABS — normoactive bowel sounds
NAC —
    N-acetyl-L-cysteine

NAC — *(continued)*
    National Asthma Center
    neoadjuvant chemotherapy
    Noise Advisory Council
    nonadherent cell
NACDS — North American Clinical Dermatological Society
NACED — National Advisory Council on the Employment of the Disabled
NAC-EDTA — *N*-acetyl-L-cysteine ethylenediaminetetraacetic acid
nAChR — nicotinic acetylcholine receptor
NACI — National Advisory Committee on Immunization
NaCl — sodium chloride
NaClO — sodium hypochlorite
NaClO$_3$ — sodium chlorate
Na$_2$CO$_3$ — sodium carbonate
Na$_2$C$_2$O$_4$ — sodium oxalate
NACOR — National Advisory Committee on Radiation
NACSAP — National Alliance Concerned with School-Age Parents
NACT — National Alliance of Cardiovascular Technologists
NAD —
    new antigenic determinant
    nicotinamide adenine dinucleotide
    nicotinic acid dehydrogenase
    no abnormal discovery
    no abnormality demonstrable
    no active disease
    no acute distress
    no apparent distress
    no appreciable disease
    normal axis deviation
    nothing abnormal detected
    nothing abnormal discovered
NAD$^-$ — nicotinamide adenine dinucleotide, oxidized form
NaD — sodium dialysate
NADA — New Animal Drug Application

NADABA — N-adenoxyldiamino-
butyric acid

NADG — nicotinamide adenine
dinucleotide glycohydrolase

NADH — nicotinamide adenine
dinucleotide, reduced form

NADL — National Association of
Dental Laboratories

NaDodSO$_4$ — sodium dodecyl sulfate

NADP — nicotinamide adenine dinucleotide phosphate

NADP$^+$ — nicotinamide adenine
dinucleotide phosphate, oxidized form

NADPH — nicotinamide adenine
dinucleotide phosphate, reduced form

NAE — net acid excretion

Na$_e$ — exchangeable body sodium

NAEMT — National Association
of Emergency Medical Technicians

NaERC — sodium efflux rate constant

NAF —
nafcillin
National Amputation Foundation
National Ataxia Foundation
net acid flux

NaF — sodium fluoride

NAG —
N-acetyl-D-glucosaminidase
narrow-angle glaucoma
non-agglutinating

NAGO — neuraminidase and galactose oxidase

NAH — 2-hydroxy-3-naphthoic
acid hydrazide

NAHA — National Association of
Health Authorities

NaHCO$_3$ — sodium bicarbonate

NAHCS — National Association
of Health Career Schools

NAHG — National Association of
Humanistic Gerontology

NAHI — National Athletic
Health Institute

NAHMOR — National Association of Health Maintenance
Organization Regulators

NAHPA — National Association
of Hospital Purchasing
Agents

NaH$_2$PO$_4$ — monosodium acid
phosphate (sodium biphos-
phate)

Na$_2$HPO$_2$ — disodium acid phosphate (sodium phosphate)

NAHSA — National Association
for Hearing and Speech Agencies

NAHSE — National Association
of Health Services Executives

NAHU — National Association of
Health Underwriters

NAHUC — National Association
of Health Unit Clerks-Coordi-
nators

NAI —
net acid input
neural amidase inhibition
non-accidental injury
no acute inflammation
nonadherence index

NaI — sodium iodide

NaI (TI) crystal — thallium-acti-
vated sodium iodide crystal

NAIC — National Association of
Insurance Commissioners

NAIR — nonadrenergic inhibitory
response

Na & K — sodium and potassium

Na & KSP — sodium and potassium spot

NAL — nonadherent leukocyte

NALC — N-acetyl-L-cysteine

NALD — neonatal adrenoleuko-
dystrophy

NALP — neuroadenolysis of pituitary

NAM — natural actomyosin

NAMCS — National Ambulatory
Medical Care Survey

NAME —
National Association of Medical Examiners

NAME — *(continued)*
nevi, atrial myxoma, myxoid neurofibroma, ephelides [syndrome]

NAMH — National Association of Mental Health

NAMN — nicotinic acid mononucleotide

NAMRU — Navy Medical Reserve Unit

NAMS — Nurses and Army Medical Specialists

NAMT — National Association for Music Therapy

NAN — *N*-acetylneuraminic acid

NANBH — non-A, non-B hepatitis

NaOH — sodium hydroxide

NAON — National Association of Orthopedic Nurses

NAOO — National Association of Optometrists and Opticians

NAOP — National Alliance for Optional Parenthood

NAOT — National Association of Orthopaedic Technologists

NAP —
narrative, assessment, and plan
nasion, point A, pogonion [angle of convexity]
nerve action potential
neutrophil alkaline phosphatase
nodular adrenocortical pathology
nucleic acid phosphatase
nucleic acid phosphorus

NAPA —
N-acetyl-*p*-aminophenol
N-acetyl procainamide

NAPCA — National Air Pollution Control Administration

NAPD — no active pulmonary disease

NaPent — sodium pentothal

NaPG — sodium pregnanediol glucuronide

NAPH —
naphthyl
nicotinamide adenine dinucleotide phosphate

NAPHT — National Association of Patients on Hemodialysis and Transplantation

NAPM — National Association of Pharmaceutical Manufacturers

NAPN — National Association of Physicians' Nurses

NAPNAP — National Association of Pediatric Nurse Associates and Practitioners

NAPNES — National Association for Practical Nurse Education and Services

NAPPH — National Association of Private Psychiatric Hospitals

NAPT — National Association for the Prevention of Tuberculosis

NAR —
nasal airway resistance
National Association for Retarded [Children, Citizens]
no action required
not at risk

NARA —
Narcotics Addict Rehabilitation Act
National Association of Recovered Alcoholics

NARAL — National Abortion Rights Action League

NARC — National Association for Retarded Children

NARC — nucleus arcuatus

narc. —
narcotic
narcotism

narco. — narcolepsy

NARD — National Association of Retail Druggists

NARES — nonallergic rhinitis–eosinophilia syndrome

NARF — National Association of Rehabilitation Facilities

NARMC — Naval Aerospace and Regional Medical Center

NARMH — National Association for Rural Mental Health

NARS — National Acupuncture Research Society

NAS —
nasal
National Academy of Sciences
National Association of Sanitarians
neonatal abstinence syndrome
neonatal airleak syndrome
neuroallergic syndrome
no added salt
normalized alignment score

NASA — National Aeronautics and Space Administration

NASCET — North American Symptomatic Carotid Artery Trial

NASE — National Association for the Study of Epilepsy

NASEAN — National Association for State Enrolled Assistant Nurses

NASM — Naval Aviation School of Medicine

NASMV — National Association on Standard Medical Vocabulary

NAS-NRC — National Academy of Science — National Research Council

Na_2SO_4 — sodium sulfate

$Na_2S_2O_3$ — sodium thiosulfate

NASW — National Association of Social Workers

NAT —
N-acetyltransferase
natal
neonatal alloimmune thrombocytopenia
no action taken
nonaccidental trauma

NaT — sodium tartrate

nat —
national

nat — *(continued)*
native
natural

NATB — Nonreading Aptitude Test Battery

NATCO — North American Transplant Coordinator Organization

NATP — neonatal autoimmune thrombocytopenic purpura

natr. — *natrium* (Lat.) sodium

NB —
nail bed
needle biopsy
Negri bodies
nervus buccalis
neuro-Behçet [syndrome]
neuroblastoma
neurometric battery
newborn
nitrogen balance
nitrous oxide–barbiturate
normal bowel
normoblast
nota bene (Lat.) note well
novobiocin
nutrient broth

N/B — neopterin to biopterin

Nb — niobium

^{95}Nb — radioactive niobium

n.b. — *nota bene* (Lat.) note well

NBA —
neuron-binding activity
non–weight-bearing ambulation

NBC —
non-battle casualty
non-bed care

NBCC — nevoid basal cell carcinoma

NBCCS — nevoid basal cell carcinoma syndrome

NBCIE — nonbullous congenital ichthyosiform erythroderma

NBD —
neurogenic bladder dysfunction
neurologic bladder dysfunction

NBD — *(continued)*
    no brain damage
NBEI — non-butanol-extractable iodine [syndrome]
NBF —
    no breast feeding
    not breast fed
NBI —
    neutrophil bactericidal index
    no bone injury
    non-battle injury
NBICU — newborn intensive care unit
NBIL — neonatal bilirubin
nbl — normoblast
NBM —
    no bowel movement
    normal bone marrow
    normal bowel movement
    nothing by mouth
    nucleus basalis of Meynert
nbM — newborn mouse
nbMb — newborn mouse brain
NBME —
    National Board of Medical Examiners
    normal bone marrow extract
NBN — newborn nursery
NBO — non-bed occupancy
NBOT — National Board of Orthopaedic Technologists
NBP —
    needle biopsy of prostate
    neoplastic brachial plexopathy
NBQC — narrow base quad cane
NBRT — National Board for Respiratory Therapy
NBS —
    N-bromosuccinimide
    National Bureau of Standards
    Neri-Barré syndrome
    nevoid basal cell carcinoma syndrome
    newborn screen
    Nijmegen breakage syndrome
    no bacteria seen
    normal blood serum

NBS — *(continued)*
    normal bowel sounds
    normal brainstem
    normal burro serum
    nystagmus blockage syndrome
NBT —
    nitroblue tetrazolium
    non–tumor-bearing
    normal breast tissue
NBTE — nonbacterial thrombotic endocarditis
NBTNF — newborn, term, normal, female
NBTNM — newborn, term, normal, male
NBT PABA — *N*-benzoyl-L-tyrosyl paraaminobenzoic acid
NBTS — National Blood Transfusion Service
n-Bu — *n*-butyl
NBW — normal birth weight
NC —
    nabothian cyst
    nasal cannula
    nasal clearance
    natural cytotoxicity
    neck complaint
    neonatal cholestasis
    nerve conduction
    neural crest
    neurocirculatory
    neurologic check
    neurologic control
    nevus comedonicus
    night call
    nitrocellulose
    nitrosocarbazole
    no casualty
    no change
    no charge
    noise criterion
    noncirrhotic
    noncompliance
    noncompliant
    noncontributory
    noncultured
    normocephalic
    nose clip

NC — (continued)
    nose cone
    not classified
    not completed
    not cultured
    nucleocapsid
    Nurse Corps
    nursing coordinator
N:C — nuclear-cytoplasmic ratio
N/c —
    neurocirculatory
    no complaints
N & C — nerves and circulation
nC — nanocoulomb
nc —
    nanocurie
    no change
    no charge
    not counted
NCA —
    National Certification
      Agency
    National Council on Aging
    National Council on Alcohol-
      ism
    neurocirculatory asthenia
    neutrophil chemotactic activ-
      ity
    no congenital abnormalities
    nodulocystic acne
    noncontractile area
    nonspecific cross-reacting an-
      tigen
    nuclear cerebral angiogram
n-CAD — negative coronoradio-
    graphic documentation
NCADD — National Council on
    Alcoholism and Drug Depen-
    dence
NCAE — National Council for Al-
    cohol Education
N-CAM — nerve cell adhesion
    molecule
NCAMI — National Committee
    Against Mental Illness
NCAMLP — National Certifica-
    tion Agency for Medical Labo-
    ratory Personnel

NcAMP — nephrogenous cyclic
    adenosine monophosphate
NCAT — normocephalic and
    atraumatic
NCB — no code blue
NCBI — National Center for Bio-
    technology Information
NCC —
    neurocysticercosis
    no concentrated carbohy-
      drates
    noncoronary cusp
    nucleus caudalis centralis
    nursing care continuity
NCCDC — National Center for
    Chronic Disease Control
NCCDS — National Cooperative
    Crohn's Disease Study
NCCEA — Neurosensory Center
    Comprehensive Examination
    for Aphasia
NCCIP — National Center for
    Clinical Infant Program
NCCLS — National Committee
    for Clinical Laboratory Stan-
    dards
NCCLVP — National Coordinat-
    ing Committee on Large Vol-
    ume Parenterals
NCCMHC — National Council
    for Community Mental
    Health Centers
NCCPA — National Commission
    on Certification of Physician
    Assistants
NCCU — newborn convalescent
    care unit
NCD —
    National Commission on Dia-
      betes
    National Council on Drugs
    neurocirculatory dystonia
    nitrogen clearance delay
    no congenital deformities
    normal childhood diseases
    not considered disabling
    not considered disqualifying
NCDA — National Council on
    Drug Abuse

NCDC — National Communicable Disease Center

NCDV — Nebraska calf diarrhea virus

NCE —
negative contrast echocardiography
new chemical entity
nonconvulsive epilepsy

NCEP — National Cholesterol Education Program

NCF —
neutrophil chemotactic factor
no cold fluids

NCFA — Narcolepsy and Cataplepsy Foundation of America

NCF (C) — neutrophil chemotactic factor (complement)

NCGS — National Cooperative Gallstone Study

NCHC — National Council of Health Centers

NCHCA — National Commission for Health Certifying Agencies

NCHCT — National Center for Health Care Technology

NCHLS — National Council of Health Laboratory Services

NCHPD — National Council on Health Planning and Development

NCHS — National Center for Health Statistics

NCHSR — National Center for Health Services Research

NCI —
naphthalene creosote iodoform
National Cancer Institute
noncriterion ischemic [animal]
nuclear contour index
nursing care integration

nCi — nanocurie

NCIB — National Collection of Industrial Bacteria

NCIH — National Council for International Health

NCJ — needle catheter jejunostomy

NCL —
National Chemical Laboratory
neuronal ceroid lipofuscinosis
nuclear cardiology laboratory

NCLEX-RN — National Council Licensure Examination for Registered Nurses

NCM — nailfold capillary microscope

N/cm^2 — newtons per square centimeter

NCMC — natural cell-mediated cytotoxicity

NCME — Network for Continuing Medical Education

NCMH —
National Committee for Mental Health
National Committee for Mental Hygiene

NCMHI — National Clearinghouse for Mental Health Information

NCMI — National Committee Against Mental Illness

NCN — National Council of Nurses

NCNCA — normochromic normocytic anemia

NCNR — National Center for Nursing Research

NCP —
no caffeine or pepper
noncollagen protein
nursing care plan

n-CPAP — nasal continuous positive airway pressure

NCPE — noncardiac pulmonary edema

NCPPB — National Collection of Plant Pathogenic Bacteria

NCPR — no cardiopulmonary resuscitation

NCQA — National Committee for Quality Assurance

NCR —
    neutrophil chemotactic response
    nuclear-cytoplasmic ratio
NCRE — National Council on Rehabilitation Education
NCRND — National Committee for Research in Neurological Diseases
NCRP — National Council on Radiation Protection
NCRPM — National Council on Radiation Protection and Measurements
NCRV — National Committee for Radiation Victims
NCS —
    National Collaborative Study
    neocarzinostatin
    nerve conduction study
    newborn calf serum
    no concentrated sweets
    noncircumferential stenosis
    nystagmus compensation syndrome
NCSC — National Council on Senior Citizens
NCSN — National Council for School Nurses
NCT —
    nerve conduction test
    neural crest tumor
    neutron capture therapy
    noncontact tonometry
    number connection test
NCTC —
    National Cancer Tissue Culture
    National Collection of Type Cultures
NCV —
    nerve conduction velocity
    noncholera vibrio
NCVS — nerve conduction velocity study
NCYC — National Collection of Yeast Cultures
ND —
    Doctor of Naturopathy

ND — (continued)
    nasal deformity
    nasolacrimal duct
    natural death
    Naval Dispensary
    neonatal death
    neoplastic disease
    nervous debility
    neuropsychological deficit
    neurotic depression
    neutral density
    Newcastle disease
    new drugs
    no data
    no disease
    nondetectable
    nondetermined
    nondiabetic
    nondisabling
    none detectable
    normal delivery
    normal development
    Norrie disease
    nose drops
    not detectable
    not detected
    not determined
    not diagnosed
    not done
    nothing done
    nucleus of Darkshevich
    nurse's diagnosis
    Nursing Doctorate
    nutritionally deprived
N/D —
    no defects
    not done
N&D — nodular and diffuse
N_D — refractive index
Nd — neodymium
n_D — refractive index
NDA —
    National Dental Association
    new drug application
    no data available
    no demonstrable antibodies
    no detectable activity

NDA — *(continued)*
  no detectable antibody
NDC —
  National Data Communications
  National Drug Code
  Naval Dental Clinic
  nondifferentiated cell
  nuclear dehydrogenating clostridia
NDCD — National Drug Code Directory
NDD — no dialysis days
NDDG — National Diabetes Data Group
NDE —
  near-death experience
  nondiabetic extremity
NDEA — no deviation of electrical axis
NDF —
  neutrophil diffraction factor
  new dosage form
  Nicolas-Durand-Faure [disease]
  no disease found
NDFDA — nonadecafluoro-*n*-decanoic acid
NDGA — nordihydroguaiaretic acid
NDH — Natural Disaster Hospital
NDI —
  naphthalene diisocyanate
  nephrogenic diabetes insipidus
NDIR — nondispersive infrared analyzer
NDMA — nitrosodimethylamine
nDNA — nuclear deoxyribonucleic acid
N/D NHL — nodular/diffuse non-Hodgkin's lymphoma
Nd/Nt — nondistended/nontender
NDP —
  net dietary protein
  nucleoside diphosphate
NDR —
  neonatal death rate

NDR — *(continued)*
  neurotic depressive reaction
  normal detrusor reflex
  nucleus dorsalis raphe
NDS —
  Naval Dental School
  new drug submission
  normal dog serum
NDSB — Narcotic Drugs Supervisory Board
NDSC — National Down's Syndrome Congress
NDT —
  neurodevelopmental treatment
  noise detection threshold
  nondestructive testing
NDTA — National Dental Technicians Association
NDTI — National Disease and Therapeutic Index
NDV — Newcastle disease virus
NDX — nondiagnostic
Nd:YAG — neodymium:yttrium-aluminum-garnet [laser]
NE —
  national emergency
  necrotic enteritis
  neomycin
  nephropathia epidemica
  nerve ending
  nerve excitability
  neural excitation
  neuroendocrinology
  neuroepithelium
  neurologic examination
  neutrophil elastase
  no ectopia
  no effect
  no enlargement
  no exposure
  nocturnal exacerbation
  nonelastic
  nonendogenous
  noninvasine evaluation
  norepinephrine
  not elevated
  not enlarged

NE — *(continued)*
  not equal
  not evaluated
  not examined
  nutcracker esophagus
Ne — neon
NEA —
  neoplasm embryonic antigen
  no evidence of abnormality
NEB — neuroendocrine body
nebul. — *nebula* (Lat.) spray
NEC —
  National Electrical Code
  necrotizing enterocolitis
  neuroendocrine cell
  no essential changes
  nonesterified cholesterol
  not elsewhere classifiable
  not elsewhere classified
NECHI — Northeastern Consortium for Health Information
NECP — New England College of Pharmacy
NECT — non-enhanced computed tomography
NED —
  no evidence of disease
  no expiration date
  normal equivalent deviation
NEE — needle electrode examination
NEEE — Near East equine encephalomyelitis
NEEP — negative end-expiratory pressure
NEF —
  negative expiratory force
  nephritic factor
NEFA — nonesterified fatty acids
NEFG — normal external female genitalia
NEG — nonenzymatic glycosylation
neg. —
  negative
  Negro
NEHA — National Environmental Health Association

NEHE — Nurses for Environmental Health Education
NEI — National Eye Institute
NEISS — National Electronic Injury Surveillance System
NEJ — neuroeffector junction
NEJM — New England Journal of Medicine
NEM —
  N-ethylmaleimide
  no evidence of malignancy
  nonspecific esophageal motility
nem — *Nährungs Einheit Milch* (Ger.) nutritional milk unit
NEMA — National Eclectic Medical Association
nema. — nematode
Nemb — Nembutal
NEMD —
  nonspecific esophageal motility disorder
  nonspecific esophageal motor dysfunction
NEO — neonatology
Neo — neomycin
neo —
  neoarsphenamine
  neonatal
NEP —
  negative expiratory pressure
  nephrology
  neutral endopeptidase
  no evidence of pathology
  noise equivalent power
nep. — nephrectomy
NEPD — no evidence of pulmonary disease
NEPH — nephrology
neph — nephritis
NEPHGE — nonequilibrated pH gradient electrophoresis
NEPHRO — nephrogram
NER —
  no evidence of recurrence
  nonionizing electromagnetic radiation
NERD — no evidence of recurrent disease

NERHL — Northeastern Radiological Health Laboratory

NERO — noninvasive evaluation of radiation output

nerv. —
nervous
nervousness

NES — not elsewhere specified

NESO — Northeastern Society of Orthodontists

NESP — Nurse Education Support Program

NET —
nasoendotracheal tube
nerve excitability test
netilmicin
norethisterone

NETEN — norethisterone enanthate

n. et m. — *nocte et mane* (Lat.) night and morning

Neu — neuraminidase

neu — neurilemma

neur. —
neurologist
neurology

neuro. —
neurologic
neurological

neuropath —
neuropathologist
neuropathology

neurosurg —
neurosurgeon
neurosurgery

neut —
neuter
neutral
neutralize
neutrophil

NEX — nose to ear to xiphoid

NEYA — neomycin egg-yolk agar

NF —
nafcillin
nasopharyngeal fibroma
National Formulary
Negro female
nephritic factor

NF — *(continued)*
neurofibromatosis
neurofilament
neutral fraction
noise factor
none found
nonfiltered
nonfluent
nonfunction
Nonne-Froin [syndrome]
normal flow
not found

nF — nanofarad

NFAR — no further action required

NFAIS — National Federation of Abstracting and Indexing Services

NFB —
National Foundation for the Blind
nonfermenting bacteria

NFC —
National Fertility Center
not favorably considered

NFD —
neurofibrillary degeneration
no family doctor

NFDM — nonfat dry milk

NFDR — neurofaciodigitorenal [syndrome]

NFE — nonferrous extract

NFH — nonfamilial hematuria

NFIC — National Foundation for Ileitis and Colitis

NFID — National Foundation for Infectious Diseases

NFIP — National Foundation for Infantile Paralysis

NFL — nerve fiber layer

NFLD — nerve fiber layer defect

NFLPN — National Federation for Licensed Practical Nurses

NFMD — National Foundation for Muscular Dystrophy

NFME — National Fund for Medical Education

NFND — National Foundation for Neuromuscular Diseases

NFNID — National Foundation for Non-Invasive Diagnostics

NFP — no family physician

NFPA — National Fire Protection Association

NFS — National Fertility Study

NFT — neurofibrillary tangle

NFTD — normal full-term delivery

NFTSD — normal full-term spontaneous delivery

NFTT — nonorganic failure to thrive

NFW — nursed fairly well

NG —
nasogastric
new growth
nitroglycerin
nodose ganglion
no good
no growth
nongenetic
not given

ng — nanogram

NGA — nutrient gelatin agar

NGB — neurogenic bladder

NGC — nucleus reticularis gigantocellularis

NGF — nerve growth factor

NGGR — nonglucogenic/glucogenic ratio

NGI — nuclear globulin inclusions

ngiv — not given

NGL — neutral glycolipid

NGR —
narrow gauze roll
nasogastric replacement

NGS — normal goat serum

NGSA — nerve growth stimulating activity

NGSF — nongenital skin fibroblast

NGT —
nasogastric tube
normal glucose tolerance

NGU — nongonoccal urethritis

NH —
natriuretic hormone
Naval Hospital
neonatal hepatitis

NH — (continued)
neurologically handicapped
nocturnal hypoventilation
nodular histiocytic [lymphoma]
nonhuman
nursing home

N(H) — proton density

NH_3 — ammonia

$(NH_4)_2SO_2$ — ammonium sulfate

NHA —
National Health Association
National Hearing Association
National Hemophilia Association
nonspecific hepatocellular abnormality

NHAIS — Naylor-Harwood Adult Intelligence Scale

NHANES — National Health and Nutrition Examination Survey

NHAS — National Hearing Aid Association

NHBPCC — National High Blood Pressure Coordinating Committee

NH_4Br — ammonium bromide

NHC —
National Health Council
neighborhood health center
neonatal hypocalcemia
nonhistone chromatin
nursing home care

NH_4Cl — ammonium chloride

NH_4CNO — ammonium cyanate

$(NH_2)_2CO$ — urea

$(NH_4)_2CO_3$ — ammonium carbonate

NHCP — nonhistone chromosomal protein

NHD — normal hair distribution

NHDC — National Hansen's Disease Center

NHDF — normal human diploid fibroblast

NHDL — non–high-density lipoprotein

NHDS — National Hospital Discharge Survey

NHEFS — National Health Epidemiologic Follow-up Study

NHF —
National Health Federation
National Hemophilia Foundation
nonimmune hydrops fetalis

NHG — normal human globulin

NHGJ — normal human gastric juice

NHH — neurohypophyseal hormone

(NH₄)HS — ammonium hydrosulfide

NHI —
National Health Institute
National Health Insurance
National Heart Institute

NHIF — National Head Injury Foundation

NHIS — National Health Interview Survey

NHK — normal human kidney

NHL —
nodular histiocytic lymphoma
non-Hodgkin's lymphoma

nHL — normalized hearing level

NHLBI — National Heart, Lung, and Blood Institute

NHLI — National Heart and Lung Institute

NHML — non-Hodgkin's malignant lymphoma

NHMRC — National Health and Medical Research Council

NH₄NO₃ — ammonium nitrate

NH₄O-CO-NH₂ — ammonium carbonate

NHP —
New Health Practitioners
nonhemoglobin protein
nonhistone protein
normal human pooled plasma
nursing home placement

NHPC — National Health Planning Council

NHPF — National Health Policy Forum

NHPIC — National Health Planning Information Center

NHPP — normal human pooled plasma

NHPPN — National Health Professions Placement Network

NHR — net histocompatibility ratio

NHRC — National Health Research Center

NHS —
Nance-Horan syndrome
National Health Service (British)
native human serum (pooled)
normal horse serum
normal human serum

NHSAS — National Health Service Audit Staff

NHSC — National Health Service Corps

NHSM — no hepatosplenomegaly

NHSR — National Hospital Service Reserve

NHT — nonpenetrating head trauma

NHWM — normal human white matter

NI —
neuraminidase inhibition
neurological improvement
neutralization index
no improvement
no information
noise index
not identified
not indicated
not isolated
nucleus intercalatus

Ni — nickel

NIA —
National Institute on Aging
nephelometric inhibition assay

NIA — *(continued)*
    neutrophil-inducing activity
    niacin
    no information available
    Nutritional Institute of
        America
nia — niacin
NIAAA — National Institute of
    Alcohol Abuse and Alcohol-
    ism
NIADDK — National Institute of
    Arthritis, Diabetes, Digestive
    and Kidney Diseases
NIAID — National Institute of Al-
    lergy and Infectious Diseases
NIAL — not in active labor
NIAMD — National Institute of
    Arthritis and Metabolic Dis-
    eases
NIAMDD — National Institute of
    Arthritis, Metabolism, and Di-
    gestive Diseases
NIAMSD — National Institute of
    Arthritis and Musculoskeletal
    and Skin Diseases
NIB —
    National Institute for the
        Blind
    noninvolved bone
NIBP — noninvasive blood pres-
    sure
NIBS — Nippon Institute of Bio-
    logical Sciences
NIBSC — National Institute for
    Biological Standards and Con-
    trol
NIC —
    neonatal intensive care
    neurogenic intermittent clau-
        dication
    newborn intensive care
    Nomarsky interference con-
        trast
    noninvasive carotid [study]
    nursing interim care
Nic. — nicotinyl alcohol
NICC — neonatal intensive care
    center

NICE — noninvasive carotid ex-
    amination
NICHHD — National Institute of
    Child Health and Human De-
    velopment
NICN — National Institute of
    Comparative Medicine
NICU —
    neonatal intensive care unit
    neurological intensive care
        unit
    neurosurgical intensive care
        unit
    newborn intensive care unit
    nonimmunologic contact urti-
        caria
NID —
    nonimmunological disease
    non–insulin-dependent [dia-
    betes]
NIDA — National Institute on
    Drug Abuse
NIDD — non–insulin-dependent
    diabetes
NIDDK — National Institute of
    Diabetes and Digestive and
    Kidney Diseases
NIDDM — non–insulin-dependent
    diabetes mellitus
NIDDY — non–insulin-dependent
    diabetes in the young
NIDM — National Institute for Di-
    saster Mobilization
NIDR — National Institute of
    Dental Research
NIDS — nonionic detergent–
    soluble
NIEHS — National Institutes of
    Environmental Health Sci-
    ences
NIF —
    negative inspiratory force
    neutrophil immobilizing fac-
        tor
    nifedipine
    nonintestinal fibroblast
NIg — non-immunoglobulin
nig. — *niger* (Lat.) black

NIGMS — National Institute of General Medical Sciences

NIH — National Institutes of Health

NIHD — noise-induced hearing damage

NIHL — noise-induced hearing loss

NIHR — National Institute of Handicapped Research

NIHS — National Institute of Hypertension Studies

NIIC — National Injury Information Clearinghouse

NIIP — National Institute of Industrial Psychology

NIIS — National Institute of Infant Services

NIL — noise interference level

nil — not in labor

NIMH — National Institute of Mental Health

NIMP — National Intern Matching Program

NIMR — National Institute for Medical Research

NIMS — National Infant Mortality Surveillance

NINCDS — National Institute of Neurological and Communicative Disorders and Stroke

NINDB — National Institute of Neurological Diseases and Blindness

NINDS — National Institute of Neurological Diseases and Stroke

NINR — National Institute For Nursing Research

NINVS — noninvasive neurovascular studies

NIOSH — National Institute of Occupational Safety and Health

NIP —
National Inpatient Profile
negative inspiratory pressure

NIP — (continued)
nipple
nitroiodophenyl
no infection present
no inflammation present

NIPH — National Institute of Public Health

NIPS —
neuroleptic-induced Parkinson syndrome
noninvolved psoriatic skin

NIPTS — noise-induced permanent threshold shift

NIR — near infrared

nIR — non-insulin resistance

NIRA — nitrite reductase

NIRD — nonimmune renal disease

NIRMP — National Intern and Resident Matching Program

NIRNS — National Institute for Research in Nuclear Science

NIROS — near infrared oxygen sufficiency [scope]

NIRR — non–insulin-requiring remission

NIRS — normal inactivated rabbit serum

NIS —
N-iodosuccinimide
no inflammatory signs

NISM — nucleus of stria medullaris

NIST —
nucleus of stria terminalis
nasointestinal tube

NIT —
National Intelligence Test
neonatal isoimmune thrombocytopenia

NITD — non–insulin-treated disease

nit — nitrous

nitro — nitroglycerin

NITTS — noise-induced temporary threshold shift

NIV — nodule-inducing virus

NJ — nasojejunal

NJPC — National Joint Practice Commission

NK —
    natural killer [cell]
    no ketones
    Nomenklatur Kommission
        (Ger.) Commission on (An-
        atomical) Nomenclature
    not known
NKA —
    neurokinin A
    no known allergies
nkat — nanokatal
NKC —
    natural killer cells
    nonketotic coma
NKCA — natural killer cell activity
NK cells — natural killer cells
NKCF — natural killer cytotoxic
    factor
NKDA — no known drug allergies
NKFA — no known food allergies
NKH —
    nonketogenic hyperglycemia
    nonketotic hyperosmosis
NKHA — nonketotic hyperosmo-
    lar acidosis
NKHS —
    nonketotic hyperosmolar syn-
        drome
    normal Krebs-Henseleit solu-
        tion
NKMA — no known medication
    allergies
NKTS — natural killer target struc-
    ture
NL —
    nasolacrimal
    neural lobe
    neutral lipid
    nodular lymphoma
    normal
    normal libido
    normal limits
    normolipemic
    Nyhan-Lesch [syndrome]
nl — nanoliter
n.l. —
    non licet (Lat.) it is not per-
        mitted

n.l. — *(continued)*
    non liquet (Lat.) it is not clear
NLA —
    National Leukemia Associa-
        tion
    neuroleptanalgesia
    neuroleptanesthesia
    normal lactase activity
NLAL — nodule-like alveolar le-
    sion
NLB — needle liver biopsy
NLD —
    nasolacrimal duct
    necrobiosis lipoidica diabet-
        icorum
NLDL — normal low-density lipo-
    protein
NLE — neonatal lupus erythemato-
    sus
Nle — norleucine
NLEF — National Lupus Erythe-
    matosus Association
NLF —
    nasolabial fold
    neonatal lung fibroblast
    nonlactose fermentation
NLK — neuroleukin
NLM —
    National Library of Medicine
    noise level monitor
NLMC — nocturnal leg muscle
    cramp
NLN —
    National League for Nursing
    no longer needed
NLNE — National League for
    Nursing Education
NLP —
    neurolinguistic programming
    no light perception
    nodular liquefying panicul-
        itis
    normal light perception
    normal luteal phase
NLPD — nodular lymphocytic,
    poorly differentiated
NLS —
    neonatal lupus syndrome

NLS — (continued)
>   nonlinear least squares
>   normal lymphocyte supernatant
NLT —
>   Names Learning Test
>   normal lymphocyte transfer [test]
>   not later than
>   not less than
>   nucleus lateralis tuberis
NLX — naloxone
NM —
>   near-miss
>   neomycin
>   neuromotor
>   neuromuscular
>   nictitating membrane
>   nitrogen mustard
>   nocturnal myoclonus
>   nodular melanoma
>   nodular mixed [lymphoma]
>   nonmalignant
>   nonmotile
>   normetanephrine
>   not measurable
>   not measured
>   not mentioned
>   not motile
>   nuclear medicine
N&M —
>   nerves and muscles
>   night and morning
Nm — newton-meter
N/m^2 — newtons per square meter
nM — nanomolar
nm —
>   nanometer
>   nonmetallic
n.m. —
>   *nocte et mane* (Lat.) night and morning
>   *nux moschata* (Lat.) nutmeg
NMA —
>   National Malaria Association
>   National Medical Association
>   neurogenic muscular atrophy
>   *N*-nitroso-*N*-methylalanine
NMAC — National Medical Audiovisual Center

NM(ASCP) — Technologist in Nuclear Medicine certified by the American Society of Clinical Pathologists
NMC —
>   National Medical Care
>   Naval Medical Center
>   neuromuscular control
>   nodular mixed-cell [lymphoma]
>   nonmotor condition
>   nucleus reticularis magnocellularis
>   nurse-managed center
NMCD — nephrophthisis-medullary cystic disease
NMCES — National Medical Care Expenditure Survey
NMCUES — National Medical Care Utilization and Expenditure Survey
NMD —
>   neuromyodysplasia
>   normal muscle development
NMDA — *N*-methyl-D-aspartate
NMDP — National Marrow Donor Program
NME —
>   National Medical Enterprises
>   neuromyeloencephalopathy
NMF —
>   *N*-methylformamide
>   National Medical Fellowship
>   National Migraine Foundation
>   nonmigrating fraction
NMFI — National Master Facility Inventory
NMI —
>   no mental illness
>   no middle initial
>   normal male infant
NMJ — neuromuscular junction
NML —
>   National Medical Library
>   nodular mixed lymphoma
NMM —
>   nodular malignant melanoma

NMM — (continued)
   Nonne-Milroy-Meige [syndrome]
NMN —
   nicotinamide mononucleotide
   normetanephrine
NMN$^+$ — nicotinamide mononucleotide (reduced form)
NMNA — National Male Nurse Association
NMNRU — National Medical Neuropsychiatric Research Unit
NMO — nitrogen mustard oxide
nmol — nanomole
NMOR — N-nitrosomorpholine
NMOS — N-type metal oxide semiconductor
NMP —
   Naval Medical Publication
   normal menstrual period
   nucleoside 5'-monophosphate
NMPCA — nonmetric principal component analysis
NMPTP — N-methyl-4-phenyl-1,2,3,6-tetrahydropyridine
NMR —
   Neill-Mooser reaction
   neonatal mortality rate
   nictitating membrane response
   nuclear magnetic resonance
NMRDC — Naval Medical Research and Development Command
NMRI —
   National Medical Research Institute
   Naval Medical Research Institute
   nuclear magnetic resonance imaging
NMRL — Naval Medical Research Laboratory
NMRU — Naval Medical Research Unit
NMS —
   Naval Medical School

NMS — (continued)
   neuroleptic malignant syndrome
   neuromuscular spindle
   neuromuscular stimulator
   normal mouse serum
N·m/s — newton meter per second
NMSIDS — near-miss sudden infant death syndrome
NMSS — National Multiple Sclerosis Society
NMT —
   neuromuscular tension
   neuromuscular transmission
   N-methyltransferase
   no more than
   Nuclear Medicine Technologist
NMTB — neuromuscular transmission blockade
NMTCB — Nuclear Medicine Technology Certification Board
NMTD — nonmetastatic trophoblastic disease
NMTS — neuromuscular tension state
NMU —
   neuromuscular unit
   nitrosomethylurea
NN —
   neonatal
   nevocellular nevus
   normally nourished
   normal nutrition
   nurses' notes
n/n — negative/negative
nn. — nervi (Lat.) nerves
n.n. — nomen novum (Lat.) new name
nna — normochromic normocytic anemia
NNAS — neonatal narcotic abstinence syndrome
NNC — National Nutrition Consortium

NND —
    neonatal death
    New and Nonofficial Drugs
    nonspecific nonerosive duode-
      nitis
NNDC — National Naval Dental
    Center
NNE —
    neonatal necrotizing enteroco-
      litis
    non-neuronal enolase
NNEB — National Nursery Exami-
    nation Board
NNG — nonspecific nonerosive
    gastritis
NNHS — National Nursing Home
    Survey
NNI — noise and number index
NNIS — National Nosocomial In-
    fections Study
NNM —
    neonatal mortality
    Nicolle-Novy-Macneal [me-
      dium]
NNMC — National Naval Medi-
    cal Center
NNNMU — *N*-nitroso-*N*-methyl-
    urethane
NNO — no new orders
n. nov. — *nomen novum* (Lat.) new
    name
NNP —
    neonatal nurse practitioner
    nerve net pulse
NNR — New and Nonofficial
    Remedies
NNS —
    neonatal screen
    non-neoplastic syndrome
    non-nutritive sucking
NNT —
    neonatally tolerant
    nuclei nervi trigemini
NNU — net nitrogen utilization
NNWI — Neonatal Narcotic
    Withdrawal Index
NO —
    narcotics officer

NO — *(continued)*
    nasal oxygen
    nitric oxide
    none obtained
    nonobese
    number
    nurse's office
N_2O — dinitrogen monoxide (ni-
    trous oxide)
No — nobelium
no. — *numero* (Lat.) to the num-
    ber of
NOA —
    National Optometric Associa-
      tion
    nurse obstetric assistant
NOAPP — National Organization
    of Adolescent Pregnancy and
    Parenting
NOBT — nonoperative biopsy
    technique
NOC — not otherwise classified
NO-CCE — no clubbing, cyanosis,
    or edema
NOCT — National Occupation
    Competency Testing
noct —
    nocturia
    nocturnal
noct. — *nocte* (Lat.) at night
noct. maneq. — *nocte maneque*
    (Lat.) at night and in the
    morning
NOD —
    nodular melanoma
    nonobese diabetic
    notify of death
NOEL — no observed effect level
NOF — National Osteopathic
    Foundation
NOFT — nonorganic failure-to-
    thrive
NOGM — no gammopathy
NOII — nonocclusive intestinal
    ischemia
NOK — next of kin
NOM —
    nonsuppurative otitis media

NOM — *(continued)*
    normal extraocular movements

nom. dub. — *nomen dubium* (Lat.) a doubtful name

NOMI — nonocclusive mesenteric infarction

nom. nov. — *nomen novum* (Lat.) new name

nom. nud. — *nomen nudum* (Lat.) a name without designation

non D — none detected

non F — nonfasting

non-REM — non-rapid eye movement

non rep., non repetat. — *non repetatur* (Lat.) do not repeat

NONS — nonspecific

NON-VIS —
    non visualization
    non visualized

NOOB — not out of bed

$N_2O:O_2$ — nitrous oxide to oxygen ratio

NOP — not otherwise provided for

NOPHN — National Organization for Public Health Nursing

NOR —
    noradrenaline
    normal
    nortriptyline
    nucleolar organizing region

NORC —
    National Opinion Research Center
    normal curve

NOR-EPI — norepinephrine

norleu — norleucine

norm — normal

NOS —
    network operating system
    non–organ-specific
    no synthase
    not on staff
    not otherwise specified

NOSAC — nonsteroidal anti-inflammatory compound

NOSIE — Nurses' Observation Scale for Inpatient Evaluation

NOSTA — Naval Ophthalmic Support and Training Activity

NOT —
    nocturnal oxygen therapy
    nucleus of optic tract

NOTB — National Ophthalmic Treatment Board (British)

NOTT — nocturnal oxygen therapy trial

Nov — novobiocin

nov. n. — *novum nomen* (Lat.) new name

NOVS — National Office of Vital Statistics

nov. sp. — *novum species* (Lat.) new species

NP —
    nasal prongs
    nasopharyngeal
    nasopharynx
    near point
    neonatal-perinatal
    nerve palsy
    neuritic plaque
    neuropathology
    neuropeptide
    neurophysin
    neuropsychiatric
    neuropsychiatry
    new patient
    newly presented
    Niemann-Pick [disease]
    nitrogen-phosphorus
    nitrophenol
    nitroprusside
    no pain
    no pressure
    nonpalpable
    nonparalytic
    nonpathogenic
    nonphagocytic
    nonpracticing
    normal plasma
    normal pressure
    not perceptible
    not performed
    not practiced

NP — (continued)
    not pregnant
    not present
    nucleoplasmic [index]
    nucleoprotein
    nucleoside phosphorylase
    nucleus pulposus
    Nurse Practitioner
    nursed poorly
    nursing procedure
N-P — need-persistence
Np-59 — iodomethylnorcholesterol
Np —
    neper
    neptunium
    neurophysin
np — nucleotide pair
n.p. — *nomen proprium* (Lat.)
    proper name
NPA —
    nasal pharyngeal airway
    National Perinatal Association
    National Pharmaceutical Association
    National Pituitary Agency
    near point accommodation
    no previous admission
NPA-NIHHDP — National Pituitary Agency — National Institutes of Health Hormone Distribution Program
NPAT — nonparoxysmal atrial tachycardia
NPB —
    nodal premature beat
    nonprotein bound
NPBF — nonplacental blood flow
NPC —
    nasopharyngeal carcinoma
    near point of convergence
    no prenatal care
    no previous complaint
    nodal premature contractions
    nonparenchymal (liver) cell
    nonproductive cough

NPC — (continued)
    non protein calorie
    nucleus of posterior commissure
NPCa — nasopharyngeal carcinoma
NPCC — National Poison Control Center
NPCP —
    National Prostatic Cancer Project
    non-*Pneumocystis* pneumonia
NP cult — nasopharyngeal culture
NPD —
    narcissistic personality disorder
    natriuretic plasma dialysate
    negative pressure device
    Niemann-Pick disease
    nitrogen-phosphorus detector
    nonpathologic diagnosis
    nonprescription drug
    normal protein diet
NPDL — nodular, poorly differentiated lymphocytic lymphoma
NPDR — nonproliferative diabetic retinopathy
NPE —
    neurogenic pulmonary edema
    neuropsychologic examination
    no palpable enlargement
    normal pelvic examination
NPEV — nonpolio enterovirus
NPF —
    nasopharyngeal fiberscope
    National Parkinson Foundation
    National Pharmaceutical Foundation
    National Psoriasis Foundation
    no predisposing factor
NPFT — Neurotic Personality Factor Test
NPG — nonpregnant
NPH —
    neutral protamine Hagedorn [insulin]
    no previous history

NPH — *(continued)*
    normal pressure hydrocephalus
    nucleus pulposus herniation
NPHS — Northwick Park Heart Study
NPhx — nasopharynx
NPI —
    Narcissistic Personality Inventory
    neonatal perception inventory
    Neuropsychiatric Institute
    no present illness
    nucleoplasmic index
NPIC — neurogenic peripheral intermittent claudication
NPII — Neonatal Pulmonary Insufficiency Index
NPJT — nonparoxysmal atrioventricular junctional tachycardia
NPK — neuropeptide K
NPL —
    National Physics Laboratory
    neoproteolipid
    nodular poorly differentiated lymphoma
NPM — nothing per mouth
NPN — nonprotein nitrogen
NPO —
    nothing by mouth
    nucleus preopticus
n.p.o. — *nil per os* (Lat.) nothing by mouth
NPO/HS — *nulla per os hora somni* (Lat.) nothing by mouth at bedtime
NPOS — nitrite positive
NPP —
    normal pool plasma
    normal postpartum
    nucleus [tegmenti] pedunculopontinus
4-NPP — 4-nitrophenylphosphate
NPPase — nucleotide pyrophosphatase
NPPH — nucleotide pyrophosphohydrolase
NPPNG — nonpenicillinase-producing *Neisseria gonorrhoeae*

NP polio — nonparalytic poliomyelitis
NPR —
    net protein ratio
    normal pulse rate
    nothing per rectum
    nucleoside phosphoribosyl
NPRL — Navy Prosthetics Research Laboratory
NPS — nail-patella syndrome
NPSA — normal pilosebaceous apparatus
NPSG — nocturnal polysomnogram
NPSH — nonprotein sulfhydryl [group]
NPT —
    neoprecipitin test
    neopyrithiamine
    nocturnal penile tumescence
    normal pressure and temperature
NPTR — National Pediatric Trauma Registry
NPU — net protein utilization
NPV —
    negative pressure valve
    negative pressure ventilation
    nucleopolyhidrosis virus
    nucleus paraventricularis
NQA — nursing quality assurance
NQMI — non–Q-wave myocardial infarction
4NQO — 4-nitroquinoline 1-oxide
NQR — nuclear quadruple resonance
NR —
    nerve root
    neural retina
    neutral red
    non repetatur (Lat.) do not repeat
    no radiation
    no reaction
    no recurrence
    no refill
    no report
    no respiration

NR — (continued)
  no response
  no result
  nodal rhythm
  noise reduction
  nonreactive
  non-rebreathing
  nonresponder
  nonretarded
  normal range
  normal reaction
  normotensive rat
  not readable
  not recorded
  not resolved
  nurse
  nursing representative
  nutrition ratio
N/R — not remarkable
N_R — Reynolds' number
nr — near
NRA —
  nitrate reductase
  nucleus raphe alatus
  nucleus retroambigualis
NRAF — nonrheumatic atrial fibrillation
NRB — nonrejoining break
NRBC —
  National Rare Blood Club
  normal red blood cell
  nucleated red blood cell
NRBS — non-rebreathing system
NRC —
  National Research Council
  noise reduction coefficient
  normal retinal correspondence
  not routine care
  Nuclear Regulatory Commission
NRCA — National Rehabilitation Counseling Association
NRCC — National Registry in Clinical Chemistry
NRCL — nonrenal clearance
NRD — nonrenal death

NRDC —
  Natural Resources Defense Council
  National Respiratory Disease Conference
NRDL — Naval Radiological Defense Laboratory
NREH — normal renin essential hypertension
NREM — nonrapid eye movements
NREMT — National Registry of Emergency Medical Technicians
NRF —
  Neurosciences Research Foundation
  normal renal function
NRFC — nonrosette-forming cell
NRFD — not ready for data
NRGC — nucleus reticularis gigantocellularis
NRH — nodular regenerative hyperplasia
NRI —
  nerve root involvement
  nerve root irritation
  neutral regular insulin
  nonrespiratory infection
NRK — normal rat kidney
NRL — nucleus reticularis lateralis
NRM —
  National Registry of Microbiologists
  normal range of motion
  normal retinal movement
  nucleus raphe magnus
  nucleus reticularis magnocellularis
NRMP — National Resident Matching Program
nRNA — nuclear ribonucleic acid
nRNP — nuclear ribonucleoprotein
NROM — normal range of motion
NRP — nucleus reticularis parvocellularis
NRPC — nucleus reticularis pontis caudalis

NRPG — nucleus reticularis para-
gigantocellularis
NRR —
net reproduction rate
noise reduction rating
NRRL — Northern Regional Research Laboratory
NRS —
neurobehavioral rating scale
nonimmunized rabbit serum
normal rabbit serum
normal reference serum
numerical rating scale
NRSCC — National Reference
System in Clinical Chemistry
NRSFPS — National Reporting
System for Family Planning
Services
NRT — neuromuscular re-educa-
tion technique
NRV — nucleus reticularis ventralis
NS —
natural science
Neosporin
nephrosclerosis
nephrotic syndrome
nervous system
neurological surgery
neurological survey
neurosecretion
neurosecretory
neurosurgeon
neurosurgery
neurosyphilis
neurotic score
no sample
no sequelae
no specimen
nodular sclerosis
nonsmoker
nonspecific
nonstimulation
nonstructural
nonsymptomatic
Noonan syndrome
normal saline
normal serum

NS — (continued)
normal sodium [diet]
normal study
Norwegian scabies
not seen
not significant
not specified
not stated
not sufficient
not symptomatic
nuclear sclerosis
nursing services
Nursing Sister
nylon suture
N/S — normal saline
Ns —
nasospinale
nerves
ns —
nanosecond
no sequelae
nonspecific
nylon suture
NSA —
Neurological Society of
America
no salt added
no serious abnormality
no significant abnormality
no significant anomaly
normal serum albumin
nutritional status assessment
NSABP — National Surgical
Adjuvant Breast and Bowel
Project
NSAD — no signs of acute disease
NSAE — nonsupported arm exercise
NSAI — nonsteroidal anti-inflammatory [drug]
NSAIA — nonsteroidal anti-inflammatory analgesic
NSAID — nonsteroidal anti-inflammatory drug
NSAM — Naval School of Aviation Medicine
NSC —
neurosecretory cell

NSC — *(continued)*
    nonservice-connected
    nonspecific suppressor cell
    normal child with short stature
    no significant change
NSCC — National Society for Crippled Children
NSCD — nonservice-connected disability
NSCLC — non-small cell lung carcinoma (or cancer)
NSCPT — National Society for Cardiopulmonary Technology
NSD —
    Nairobi sheep disease
    neonatal staphylococcal disease
    neurosecretory dysfunction
    night sleep deprivation
    nitrogen specific detector
    no significant defect
    no significant deficiency
    no significant deviation
    no significant difference
    no significant disease
    nominal single dose
    nominal standard dose
    normal single dose
    normal spontaneous delivery
    normal standard dose
NSDA — nonsteroid-dependent asthmatic
NSDP — National Society of Dental Prosthetists
NSE —
    neuron-specific enolase
    nonspecific esterase
    normal saline enema
N$\bar{s}$E — nausea without (*sine,* Lat.) emesis
nsec — nanosecond
NSF —
    National Sanitation Foundation
    National Science Foundation
    nodular subepidermal fibrosis

NSF — *(continued)*
    no significant findings
NSFTD — normal spontaneous full-term delivery
NSG — neurosecretory granules
nsg. — nursing
NSGCT — nonseminomatous germ cell tumor
NSGCTT — nonseminomatous germ cell testicular tumor
NSG Hx — nursing history
NSGI — nonspecific genital infection
NSH — National Society for Histotechnology
NSHD — nodular sclerosing Hodgkin's disease
NSI —
    negative self-image
    Neurosciences Institute
    no sign of infection
    no sign of inflammation
    non–syncytium-inducing
NSIDS — near sudden infant death syndrome
NSILA — nonsuppressible insulin-like activity
NSILP — nonsuppressible insulin-like protein
NSJ — nevus sebaceus of Jadassohn
NSLF — normal sheep lung fibroblast
NSM —
    neurosecretory material
    neurosecretory motor neuron
    nonantigenic specific mediator
    nutrient sporulation medium
N-s/m^2 — newton-second per square meter
NSMR — National Society for Medical Research
NSN —
    nephrotoxic serum nephritis
    nicotine-stimulated neurophysin
    number of similar negative [matches]

NSNA — National Student Nurse Association

NSND —
    nonsymptomatic and nondisabling
    normal saline nose drops

NSO —
    Neosporin ointment
    nucleus supraopticus

NSOL — nerve to soleus

NSP —
    National Stuttering Project
    neuron specific protein
    not specified
    Nutritional Support Panel
    number of similar positive [matches]

NSPB — National Society for the Prevention of Blindness

NSPE — specimen unobtainable

NSPN — neurosurgery progress note

NSPVT — nonsustained polymorphic ventricular tachycardia

NSQ —
    Neuroticism Scale Questionnaire
    not sufficient quantity

NSR —
    nasal septal reconstruction
    nasoseptal repair
    nonspecific reaction
    nonsystemic reaction
    normal sinus rhythm
    not seen regularly

NSRR — normal sinus rate and rhythm

NSS —
    normal saline solution
    normal size and shape
    not statistically significant
    nutrition support services

NSSC — normal size, shape, and consistency

NSSL — normal size, shape, and location

NSSP — normal size, shape, and position

NSST —
    nonspecific ST [wave]
    Northwestern Syntax Screen Test

NSSTT — nonspecific ST and T [wave]

NST —
    neospinothalamic [tract]
    nonshivering thermogenesis
    nonstress test
    normal sphincter tone
    nutritional status type
    nutritional support team

NSTT — nonseminomatous testicular tumor

NSU —
    neurosurgical unit
    nonspecific urethritis

NSurg —
    neurosurgeon
    neurosurgery

NSV — nonspecific vaginitis

NSVD — normal spontaneous vaginal delivery

NSVT — nonsustained ventricular tachycardia

NSX — neurosurgical examination

nsy — nursery

NT —
    nasotracheal
    neotetrazolium
    nephrostomy tube
    neurotensin
    neutralization test
    nicotine tartrate
    nontender
    nontumoral
    nontypable
    normal temperature
    normal tissue
    normotensive
    nortriptyline
    not tender
    not tested
    nourishment taken
    N-terminal [fragment]
    nucleotidase
    nucleotide

NT — *(continued)*
    nurse technician
N&T — nose and throat
5'NT — 5'-nucleotidase
Nt — amino terminal
nt — nucleotide
NTA —
    National Tuberculosis Association
    natural thymocytotoxic auto-antibody
    nitrilotriacetic acid
    Nurse Training Act
NTAB — nephrotoxic antibody
NTBC — nontuberculous
NTBR — not to be resuscitated
NTC —
    neotetrazolium chloride
    neurotrauma center
NTCC — National Type Culture Collection
NTD —
    neural tube defect
    nitroblue tetrazolium dye
    noise tone difference
    5'-nucleotidase
NTE —
    neuropathy target esterase
    neurotoxic esterase
    not to exceed
    nuclear track emulsion
NTF — normal throat flora
NTG —
    nitroglycerin
    nitrosoguanidine
    nontoxic goiter
    non-treatment group
    normal triglyceridemia
NTGO — nitroglycerin ointment
NTHH — nontumorous, hypergastrinemic hyperchlorhydria
NTI —
    nonthyroid illness
    nonthyroid index
    no treatment indicated
NTIG — nontreated immunoglobulin

NTIS — National Technical Information Service
NTLI — neurotensin-like immunoreactivity
NTM —
    Neuman-Tytell medium
    nocturnal tumescence monitor
    nontuberculous mycobacteria
NTMI — nontransmural myocardial infarction
NTMNG — nontoxic multinodular goiter
NTN — nephrotoxic nephritis
NTND — not tender, not distended
NTOS — neurogenic thoracic outlet syndrome
NTP —
    National Toxicology Program
    nitropaste
    nitroprusside
    normal temperature and pressure
    nucleoside triphosphate
NT&P — normal temperature and pressure
NTR —
    negative therapeutic reaction
    normotensive rat
    nutrition
NTRC — National Toxins Research Center
NTRDA — National Tuberculosis and Respiratory Disease Association
NTRS — National Therapeutic Recreation Society
NTS —
    nasotracheal suction
    nephrotoxic serum
    nucleus tractus solitarius
NTT —
    nasotracheal tube
    nearly total thyroidectomy
NTU — Navy Toxicology Unit
NTV — nerve tissue vaccine

nt wt — net weight
NTX — naltrexone
NTZ — normal transformation
zone
NU — name unknown
Nu —
nucleolus
nucleus
nU — nanounit
nu — nude [mouse]
NUC —
nonspecific ulcerative colitis
sodium urate crystal
Nuc — nucleoside
nuc — nucleated
nucl —
nuclear
nucleus
NUD — nonulcer dyspepsia
NUG — necrotizing ulcerative gingivitis
NUI — number user identification
nullip —
nullipara
nulliparous
num — numerator
numc — number concentration
nun — nonurea nitrogen
NURB — Neville upper reservoir
buffer
Nut — nutrition
NUV — near ultraviolet
NV —
naked vision
near vision
negative variation
neovascularization
next visit
non-vaccinated
non-venereal
nonveteran
non-volatile
normal value
not verified
N&V —
nausea and vomiting

N&V — (continued)
nerve and vein
Nv. — naked vision
NVA —
near visual acuity
normal visual acuity
NVAF — nonvalvular atrial fibrillation
NVB — neurovascular bundle
NVD —
nausea, vomiting, and diarrhea
neck vein distention
neovascularization of disc
neurovesicle dysfunction
Newcastle virus disease
no venereal disease
nonvalvular (heart) disease
number of vessels diseased
NVE —
neovascular edema
neovascularization elsewhere
NVG —
neovascular glaucoma
nonventilated group
NVL — no visible lesion
NVM —
neovascular membrane
nonvolatile matter
NVR — no radiographically visible
recurrence
NVS —
neurological vital signs
nonvaccine serotype
NVSS — normal variant short stature
NVT — nerve, vein, and tendon
NW —
naked weight
nasal wash
NWB — non–weight-bearing
NWD — neuroleptic withdrawal
NWDA — National Wholesale
Druggists Association
NWR — normotensive Wistar rat
NWSN — *Nocardia* water-soluble
nitrogen

NWTS — National Wilms' Tumor
    Study
NX — naloxone
NXG — necrobiotic xanthogranu-
    loma
NY — nystatin
NYAM — New York Academy of
    Medicine
NYAS — New York Academy of
    Science
NYBC — New York Blood Center
NYC — New York City [medi-
    um]
NYD —
    not yet diagnosed

NYD — (continued)
    not yet discovered
NYHAFC — New York Heart As-
    sociation Functional Class
nyst. — nystagmus
NZ — normal zone
NZB — New Zealand black
    [mouse]
NZC — New Zealand chocolate
    [mouse]
NZO — New Zealand obese
    [mouse]
NZR — New Zealand red [rabbit]
NZW — New Zealand white
    [mouse]

O —
    absence of sex chromosome
    blood type in the ABO blood
      group
    nonmotile organism
    objective findings
    observation
    observed frequency in a con-
      tingency table
    obstetrics
    obvious
    occipital electrode placement
      in electroencephalography
    occiput
    occlusal
    octarius (Lat.) pint
    oculus (Lat.) eye
    often
    ohne Hauch (Ger.) nonmotile
      strain of microorganisms
    old
    omicron (fifteenth letter of the
      Greek alphabet), uppercase
    open
    opening
    operator
    operon
    opium

O — (continued)
    oral
    orally
    orange
    orbit
    orderly
    ortho-
    orthopedics
    osteocyte
    other
    output
    ovine
    oxidative
    oxygen
    respirations [anesthesia chart]
    without film
Ω —
    ohm
    omega (twenty-fourth letter
      of the Greek alphabet),
      uppercase
O2 — both eyes
O_2 —
    diatomic oxygen
    molecular oxygen
O_3 — ozone
o —
    opening

o — (continued)
  orally
  ovary transplant
o — omicron (fifteenth letter of the
  Greek alphabet), lowercase
ω —
  ohm
  omega (twenty-fourth letter
    of the Greek alphabet),
    lowercase
o. —
  octarius (Lat.) pint
  oculus (Lat.) eye
ō —
  negative
  nil
  none
  without
OA —
  objective assembly
  obstructive apnea
  occipital artery
  occiput anterior [fetal posi-
    tion]
  octanoic acid
  ocular albinism
  old age
  oleic acid
  opiate analgesia
  opsonic activity
  optic atrophy
  oral airway
  oral alimentation
  orotic acid
  osteoarthritis
  ovalbumin
  overall assessment
  Overeaters Anonymous
  oxalic acid
  oxolinic acid
O&A —
  observation and assessment
  odontectomy and alveo-
    loplasty
O_2a — oxygen availability
OAA —
  Old Age Assistance
  Opticians Association of
    America
  oxaloacetic acid

OAAD — ovarian ascorbic acid
  depletion
OAB —
  ABO blood group
  old age benefits
OABP — organic anion-binding
  protein
OAC —
  oral anticoagulant
  overaction
OAD —
  obstructive airway disease
  occlusive arterial disease
  organic anionic dye
OADC — oleate-albumin-
  dextrose-catalase [medium]
OADMT — Oliphant Auditory
  Discrimination Memory Test
OAE — otoacoustic emission
OAF —
  open air factor
  osteoclast-activating factor
OAG — open-angle glaucoma
OAH — ovarian androgenic hyperfunction
OAISO — overaction of the ipsi-
  lateral superior oblique
OAJ — open apophyseal joint
OALF — organic acid–labile fluid
OALL — ossification of anterior
  longitudinal ligament
o. alt. hor. — *omnibus alternis horis*
  (Lat.) every other hour
OAM —
  Office of Alternative Medi-
    cine
  outer acrosomal membrane
  oxyacetate malonate
OAP —
  occupational ability pattern
  Office of Adolescent Preg-
    nancy
  old age pension
  ophthalmic artery pressure
  osteoarthropathy
  oxygen at atmospheric pres-
    sure
OAPP — Office of Adolescent
  Pregnancy Programs

OAR —
>   orientation-alertness remediation
>   other administrative reasons

OARSA — oxacillin-aminoglycoside–resistant *Staphylococcus aureus*

OAS —
>   Old Age Security
>   oral allergy syndrome
>   osmotically active substance

OASD — ocular albinism–sensorineural deafness [syndrome]

OASDHI — Old-Age, Survivors, Disability, and Health Insurance

OASDI — Old-Age, Survivors, and Disability Insurance

OASI — Old Age and Survivors Insurance

OASO — overactive superior oblique

OASP — organic acid-soluble phosphorus

OASR — overactive superior rectus

OAST — Oliphant Auditory Synthesizing Test

OAT — ornithine aminotransferase

OAV — oculoauriculovertebral [dysplasia]

OAVD — oculoauriculovertebral dysplasia

OAW — oral airway

OAWO — opening abductor wedge osteotomy

OB —
>   obese
>   obesity
>   objective benefit
>   obliterative bronchiolitis
>   obstetrician
>   obstetrics
>   occult bleeding
>   occult blood
>   olfactory bulb
>   oligoclonal band

OB + — occult blood–positive

O&B — opium and belladonna

ob — obese [mouse]

ob. — *obiit* (Lat.) he/she died

OBB — own bed bath

OBD — organic brain disease

OBE —
>   Office of Biological Education
>   out-of-body experience

OBF — organ blood flow

OBG — obstetrician-gynecologist

OBGS — obstetrical and gynecological surgery

OB-GYN — obstetrics and gynecology

obj. —
>   object
>   objective

obl. — oblique

OBN — occult blood–negative

ob/ob — obese [mouse]

OBP —
>   occult blood–positive
>   ova, blood, and parasites

OBRA — Omnibus Reconciliation Act

OBS —
>   obstetrical service
>   obstetrics
>   organic brain syndrome

Obs. —
>   observation
>   observed
>   obsolete

OBSC — field obscured

obst. —
>   obstetrician
>   obstetrics
>   obstructed
>   obstipation
>   obstruction

obt. — obtained

OBUS — obstetrical ultrasound

OC —
>   obstetrical conjugate
>   occlusocervical
>   office call

OC — (continued)
  on call
  only child
  optic chiasma
  oral care
  oral contraceptive
  organ culture
  original claim
  outer canthal [distance]
  ovarian cancer
  oxygen consumed
O&C — onset and course
OCA —
  oculocutaneous albinism
  olivopontocerebellar atrophy
  operant conditioning audiometry
  oral contraceptive agent
OCa — ovarian carcinoma
OCAD — occlusive carotid artery disease
O$_{2cap}$ — oxygen capacity
OCBF — outer cortical blood flow
occ —
  occasional
  occasionally
  occipital
  occiput
  occlusion
  occlusive
  occurrence
OCCC — open chest cardiac compression
OCCM — open chest cardiac massage
OCCPR — open chest cardiopulmonary resuscitation
OccTh —
  occupational therapist
  occupational therapy
occup. —
  occupation
  occupational
occup Rx — occupational therapy
OCD —
  obsessive-compulsive disorder
  Office of Child Development
  Office of Civil Defense

OCD — (continued)
  osteochondritis dissecans
  ovarian cholesterol depletion
OCG —
  omnicardiogram
  oral cholecystogram
OCH — oral contraceptive hormone
OCHAMPUS — Office of the Civilian Health and Medical Program for the Uniformed Services
OCHS — Office of Cooperative Health Statistics
OCIS — Oncology Center Information System
OCL —
  oral colonic lavage
  orthopedic casting laboratory
OCM — oral contraceptive medication
OCN —
  oculomotor nucleus
  Oncology Certified Nurse
OCP —
  octacalcium phosphate
  oral case presentation
  oral contraceptive pill
OCR —
  ocular countertorsion reflex
  oculocardiac reflex
  oculocerebrorenal [syndrome]
  optical character recognition
oCRF — ovine corticotropin-releasing factor
OCRG — oxycardiorespirography
oCRH — ovine corticotropin-releasing hormone
OCRL — oculocerebrorenal (Lowe's) [syndrome]
OCRS — oculocerebrorenal syndrome
OCS —
  occipital condyle syndrome
  Ondine's curse syndrome
  open canalicular system
  oral contraceptive steroid

OCS — *(continued)*
    outpatient clinical substation
    oxycorticosteroid
OCSD — oculocraniosomatic disease
OCT —
    object classification test
    optimal cutting temperature
    oral contraceptive therapy
    ornithine carbamoyltransferase
    orthotopic cardiac transplantation
    oxytocin challenge test
O₂CT — oxygen content

O_2CT — oxygen content
octup. — *octuplus* (Lat.) eight fold
OCU — observation care unit
OCV — ordinary conversational voice
OCVM — occult vascular malformation
OD —
    Doctor of Optometry
    omni die (Lat.) every day
    occipital dysplasia
    occupational dermatitis
    occupational disease
    ocular density
    oculodynamic
    Ollier disease
    on duty
    open drop [anesthesia]
    open duct
    optical density
    optimal dose
    originally derived
    out-of-date
    outside diameter
    overdosage
    overdose
O.D. — *oculus dexter* (Lat.) right eye
O/D — overdose
O-D — obstacle-dominance
o.d. — *omni die* (Lat.) every day

ODA — *occipitodextra anterior* (Lat.) right occipitoanterior [fetal position]
ODB — opiate-directed behavior
ODC —
    ornithine decarboxylase
    ornithine 5′-phosphate decarboxylase
    outpatient diagnostic center
    oxygen dissociation curve
ODD — oculodentodigital dysplasia
OD'd — overdosed
ODM —
    ophthalmodynamometer
    ophthalmodynamometry
ODMC — Office for Dependents' Medical Care
ODOD — oculodento-osseous dysplasia
Odont. —
    odontogenic
    odontology
odoram. — *odoramentum* (Lat.) a perfume
odorat. — *odoratus* (Lat.) odoriferous
ODP —
    occipitodextra posterior (Lat.) right occipitoposterior [fetal position]
    offspring of diabetic parents
ODPHP — Office of Disease Prevention and Health Promotion
ODQ — opponens digiti quinti [muscle]
ODS — osmotic demyelination syndrome
ODSG — ophthalmic Doppler sonogram
ODT —
    occipitodextra transversa (Lat.) right occipitotransverse [fetal position]
    oculodynamic tract
ODTS — organic dust toxic syndrome

ODU — optical density unit

OE —
 on examination
 orthopedic examination
 otitis externa

O/E — observed/expected [ratio]

O&E — observation and examination

Oe — oersted [unit of magnetizing force]

OEC — outer ear canal

OEE —
 osmotic erythrocyte enrichment
 outer enamel epithelium

OEF — oxygen extraction fraction

OEIS — omphalocele, exstrophy, imperforate anus, spinal defects [complex]

OEL — occupational exposure limit

OEM —
 open-end marriage
 opposite ear masked

OER —
 osmotic erythrocyte [enrichment]
 oxygen enhancement ratio

O₂ER — oxygen extraction ratio

OERP — Office of Education and Regional Programming

OES —
 Olympus Endoscopy System
 optical emission spectroscopy
 oral esophageal stethoscope

oesoph — oesophagus (esophagus)

OET —
 oral endotracheal tube
 oral esophageal tube

OF —
 occipitofrontal
 open field [test]
 optical fundus
 orbitofrontal
 osmotic fragility [test]
 osteitis fibrosa
 Ostrum-Furst [syndrome]

OF — (continued)
 Ovenstone factor

O/F — oxidation-fermentation

OFA — oncofetal antigen

OFAGE — orthogonal field alternation gel electrophoresis

OFBM — oxidation-fermentation basal medium

OFC —
 occipitofrontal circumference
 orbitofacial cleft
 osteitis fibrosa cystica

OFCTAD — occipito-facio-cervico-thoraco-abdomino-digital [dysplasia]

OFD —
 object-film distance
 occipitofrontal diameter
 oral-facial-digital [syndrome]

Off. — official

OFHA — occipitofrontal headache

OFM — orofacial malformation

OFPF — optic fundi and peripheral fields

OFTT — organic failure to thrive

OG —
 obstetrics and gynecology
 occlusogingival
 oligodendrocyte
 optic ganglion
 orange green [stain]
 orogastric

O&G — obstetrics and gynecology

OG-A — orogastric gonococcal aspirate

OG-D — old granulomatous disease

OGF —
 orogastric feeding
 ovarian growth factor
 oxygen gain factor

OGH — ovine growth hormone

OGM — outgrowth medium

OGS — oxygenic steroid

OGT — oral glucose tolerance

OGTT — oral glucose tolerance test

OH —
>hydroxycorticosteroid
>obstructive hypopnea
>occipital horn
>occupational health
>occupational history
>on hand
>open heart [surgery]
>oral hygiene
>osteopathic hospital
>out of hospital
>outpatient hospital

17-OH — 17-hydroxycorticosteroid

o.h. — *omni hora* (Lat.) every hour

OHA — oral hypoglycemic agent

OHAHA — ophthalmoplegia-hypotonia-ataxia-hypacusis-athetosis [syndrome]

OHB_{12} — hydroxycobalamin

O_2Hb — oxyhemoglobin

OHC —
>hydroxycholecalciferol
>occupational health center
>outer hair cell

OH-Cbl — hydroxocobalamin

17-OHCS — 17-hydroxycorticosteroid

OHD —
>hydroxyvitamin D
>Office of Human Development
>organic heart disease

25-OH-D — 25-hydroxyvitamin D

OHDA — hydroxydopamine

16-OH-DHAS — 16-alpha-hydroxydehydroepiandrosterone sulfate

OH-DOC — hydroxydeoxycorticosterone

OHDS — Office of Human Development Services

OHF —
>Omsk hemorrhagic fever
>overhead frame

OHFA — hydroxy fatty acid

OHFT — overhead frame trapeze

OHG — oral hypoglycemic

OHI —
>Occupational Health Institute
>ocular hypertension indicator
>oral hygiene index

OHIAA — hydroxyindoleacetic acid

OHI-S — Oral Hygiene Instruction — Simplified

OHL — oral hairy leukoplakia

OHN — Occupational Health Nurse

OHP —
>hydroxyprogesterone
>hydroxyproline
>orthogonal-hold test pattern
>oxygen under high pressure
>oxygen under hyperbaric pressure

17-OHP — 17-hydroxyprogesterone

OHR — Office of Health Research

OHRR — open heart [surgery] recovery room

OHS —
>obesity hypoventilation syndrome
>open heart surgery
>ovarian hyperstimulation syndrome
>Overcontrolled Hostility Scale

OHSD — hydroxysteroid dehydrogenase

OHSS — ovarian hyperstimulation syndrome

OHT —
>Occupational Health Technician
>ocular hypertension

OHTA — Office of Health Technology Assessment

OHU — hydroxyurea

OI —
>obturator internus
>occasional insomnia
>opportunistic infection
>opsonic index

OI — (continued)
    orgasmic impairment
    orientation inventory
    orthoiodohippurate
    osteogenesis imperfecta
    otitis interna
    ouabain insensitivity
    oxygen income
    oxygen index
    oxygen intake
O&I — outer and inner
OIC — osteogenesis imperfecta
    congenita
OID —
    optimal immunomodulating
        dose
    organism identification num-
        ber
OIF —
    observed intrinsic frequency
    oil immersion field
    Osteogenesis Imperfecta Foun-
        dation
OIH —
    Office of International Health
    orthoiodohippurate
    ovulation-inducing hormone
OIHA — orthoiodohippuric acid
OILD — occupational immuno-
    logic lung disease
oint. — ointment
OIP — organizing interstitial pneu-
    monia
OIR — Office of International Re-
    search
OIRD — object-to-image receptor
    distance
OIT — organic integrity test
OJ —
    orange juice
    orthoplast jacket
OKAN — optokinetic after nystag-
    mus
OKN — optokinetic nystagmus
OKT —
    Ollier-Klippel-Trenaunay [syn-
        drome]
    ornithine ketoacid transami-
        nase

O.L. — oculus laevus (Lat.) left eye
ol. — oleum (Lat.) oil
OLA — occipitolaeva anterior (Lat.)
    left occipitoanterior [fetal po-
        sition]
OLB —
    olfactory bulb
    open liver biopsy
OLD —
    obstructive lung disease
    orthochromatic leukodystro-
        phy
OLF — olfactory
OLH — ovine lactogenic hormone
oLH — ovine luteinizing hormone
OLIDS — open-loop insulin deliv-
    ery system
OLMAT — Otis-Lennon Mental
    Ability Test
ol. oliv. — oleum oliva (Lat.) olive oil
OLP — occipitolaeva posterior (Lat.)
    left occipitoposterior [fetal po-
        sition]
OLR — otology, laryngology, and
    rhinology
ol. res. — oleoresin
OLS — ouabain-like substance
OLSIST — Oral Language Sen-
    tence Imitation Screening
    Test
OLT —
    occipitolaeva transversa (Lat.)
        left occipitotransverse [fetal
        position]
    orthotopic liver transplanta-
        tion
OM —
    obtuse marginal
    occipitomental
    occupational medicine
    Ochsner-Mahorner [echocar-
        diogram]
    ocular movement
    oculomotor
    Osborne Mendel [rat]
    osteomalacia
    osteomyelitis
    osteopathic manipulation

OM — (continued)
  otitis media
  outer membrane
  ovulation method
o.m. — *omni mane* (Lat.) every morning
OMA — Ophthalmic Medical Assistant
OMAC — otitis media, acute catarrhal
OMAR — Office of Medical Applications of Research
OMAS —
  occupational maladjustment syndrome
  otitis media, acute, suppurating
OMB — Office of Management and Budget
OMCA — otitis media, catarrhal, acute
OMCC — otitis media, catarrhal, chronic
OMCS — otitis media, chronic, suppurating
OMCT — orientation-memory-concentration test
OMD —
  ocular muscle dystrophy
  oculomandibulodyscephaly
  organic mental disorder
  oromandibular dystonia
OME —
  Office of Medical Examiner
  otitis media with effusions
OMH — Office of Mental Health
OMI — old myocardial infarction
OML — orbitomeatal line
OMM —
  ophthalmomandibulomelic [dysplasia]
  outer mitochondrial membrane

OMN —
  oculomotor nerve
  oculomotor nucleus
omn. bid. — *omni bidendis* (Lat.) every two days
omn. bih. — *omni bihora* (Lat.) every two hours
omn. hor. — *omni hora* (Lat.) every hour
omn. 2 hor. — *omni secunda hora* (Lat.) every second hour
omn. man. — *omni mane* (Lat.) every morning
omn. noct. — *omni nocte* (Lat.) every night
omn. quad. hor. — *omni quadrante hora* (Lat.) every quarter of an hour
omn. sec. hor. — *omni secunda hora* (Lat.) every second hour
OMP —
  olfactory marker protein
  ornithine monophosphate
  outer membrane protein
OMPA —
  octamethyl pyrophosphoramide
  otitis media, purulent, acute
OMPC — otitis media, purulent, chronic
om. quad. hor. — *omni quadrante hora* (Lat.) every quarter of an hour
OMR — operative mortality rate
OMS —
  organic mental syndrome
  otomandibular syndrome
OM&S — osteopathic medicine and surgery
OMSA — otitis media, suppurative, acute
OMSC —
  otitis media, secretory, chronic
  otitis media, suppurative, chronic

OMT —
    O-methyltransferase
    osteopathic manipulative therapy
OMVC — open mitral valve commissurotomy
ON —
    occipitonuchal
    office nurse
    onlay
    optic nerve
    optic neuropathy
    oronasal
    orthopedic nurse
    osteonecrosis
    overnight
o.n. — *omni nocte* (Lat.) every night
ONC —
    oncogene
    oncology
    Orthopaedic Nursing Certificate
    over-the-needle catheter
ONCG-A — oncogenic [virus]—acute
OND —
    Ophthalmic Nursing Diploma
    orbitonasal dislocation
    other neurological disorders
ONDS — Oriental nocturnal death syndrome
ONEG — O-negative [blood]
ONH —
    optic nerve head
    optic nerve hypoplasia
ONP —
    operating nursing procedure
    orthonitrophenyl
ONPG — ortho-nitrophenyl-beta-galactosidase
ONS — Oncology Nursing Society
ONTG — oral nitroglycerin
ONTR — orders not to resuscitate
OO —
    oophorectomized
    oophorectomy
    oral orders
O-O — outer to outer

O&O — on and off
OOA — outer optic anlage
OOB —
    out of bed
    out-of-body [experience]
OOC —
    onset of contractions
    out of control
OOL — onset of labor
OOLR — ophthalmology, otology, laryngology, and rhinology
OOM — oogonial metaphase
OOP —
    out on pass
    out of pelvis
    out of plaster
OORR — orbicularis oculi reflex response
OOW — out of wedlock
OOWS — Objective Opiate Withdrawal Scale
OP —
    oblique presentation
    occipitoparietal
    occipitoposterior
    octapeptide
    olfactory peduncle
    opening pressure
    operation
    operative procedure
    ophthalmology
    opponens pollicis
    organophosphorus
    oropharynx
    orthostatic proteinuria
    oscillatory potential
    osmotic pressure
    osteoporosis
    outpatient
    overproof
    ovine prolactin
O/P — outpatient
O&P — ova and parasites
Op —
    ophthalmology
    opisthocranion
op. —
    operation
    operator

op. — (continued)
   opposite
OPA —
   oral pharyngeal airway
   outpatient anesthesia
OPB — outpatient basis
OPC —
   oculopalatocerebral [syndrome]
   outpatient clinic
   oxypneumocardiogram
OPCA — olivopontocerebellar atrophy
op. cit. — opere citato (Lat.) in the work cited
OPCOS — oligomenorrheic polycystic ovary syndrome
OPD —
   obstetric prediabetic
   optical path difference
   otopalatodigital [syndrome]
   outpatient department
   outpatient dispensary
o,p′-DDD — ortho,para-dichlorodiphenyl-dichlorethane (mitotane)
OpDent — operative dentistry
OPDG — ocular plethysmodynamography
OPE — outpatient evaluation
OPG —
   ocular plethysmography
   ocular pneumoplethysmography
   oculoplethysmograph
   ophthalmoplethysmograph
   oxypolygelatin
opg — opening
OPH —
   obliterative pulmonary hypertension
   ophthalmia
   ophthalmic
   ophthalmologic
   ophthalmologist
   ophthalmology
   ophthalmoscope
   ophthalmoscopy

OphD — Doctor of Ophthalmology
ophth. — ophthalmology
OPI —
   oculoparalytic illusion
   Omnibus Personality Inventory
OPIDN — organophosphorus-induced delayed neuropathy
OPK — optokinetic
OPL —
   outer plexiform layer
   ovine placental lactogen
OPLL — ossification of posterior longitudinal ligament
OPM —
   occult primary malignancy
   ophthalmoplegic migraine
OPN — ophthalmic nurse
OPP —
   occiput posterior [fetal position]
   osmotic pressure of plasma
   ovine pancreatic polypeptide
   oxygen partial pressure
opp. —
   opposed
   opposing
   opposite
OPPES — oil-associated pneumoparalytic eosinophilic syndrome
OPPG — oculopneumoplethysmography
OPRR — Office of Protection from Research Risks
OPRT — orotate phosphoribosyltransferase
OPS —
   osteoporosis-pseudolipoma syndrome
   outpatient service
   outpatient surgery
OPs — operations
OPSA — ovarian papillary serous adenocarcinoma
OpScan — optical scanning
OPSI — overwhelming postsplenectomy infection

OPSR — Office of Professional
    Standards Review
OPT —
    Ohio Pediatric Tent
    outpatient
    outpatient treatment
Opt — optometrist
opt —
    optical
    optician
    optics
    optimal
    optimum
    optional
opt. — *optimus* (Lat.) best
OPTHD — optimal hemodialysis
OPV —
    oral polio vaccine
    oral poliovirus vaccine
OPWL — opiate withdrawal
OQSMAT — Otis Quick Scoring
    Mental Abilities Test
OR —
    oestrogen (estrogen) receptor
    odds ratio
    oil retention [enema]
    open reduction
    operating room
    optic radiation
    oral rehydration
    orienting reflex
    orienting response
    orosomucoid
    orthopedic
    orthopedic research
    own recognizance
O-R — oxidation-reduction
O$_R$ — rate of outflow
Or — orbitale
ORA —
    occiput right anterior [fetal
        position]
    opiate receptor agonist
ORAN — orthopedic resident
    admit note
ORANS — Oak Ridge Analytical
    System
ORBC — ox red blood cell

ORCH — orchiectomy
orch — orchitis
ORD —
    optical rotatory dispersion
Ord —
    orderly
    orotidine
ORDA — Office of Recombinant
    DNA Activities
ORDS — Office of Research, Dem-
    onstration, and Statistics
OREF —
    open reduction and external
        fixation
    Orthopedic Research and Edu-
        cation Foundation
OR enema — oil retention enema
ORF — open reading frame
OR&F — open reduction and fixa-
    tion
Org —
    organ
    organic
    organism
ORIF — open reduction with inter-
    nal fixation
orig. —
    origin
    original
OrJ — orange juice
ORL — otorhinolaryngology
ORM —
    orosomucoid
    other regulated material
ORN —
    operating room nurse
    orthopedic nurse
Orn — ornithine
ORNL — Oak Ridge National Lab-
    oratory
ORO — oil red O
Oro — orotate
OROS — oral osmotic
ORP —
    occiput right posterior [fetal
        position]
    oxidation-reduction potential
ORPM — orthorhythmic pace-
    maker

ORS —
- olfactory reference syndrome
- oral rehydration solution
- oral surgeon
- oral surgery
- Orthopaedic Research Society
- orthopedic surgeon
- orthopedic surgery
- oxygen radical scavengers

ORT —
- object relations technique
- operating room technician
- oral rehydration therapy

orth. — orthopedics

ortho —
- orthodontics
- orthodontist
- orthopedics

orthop — orthopnea

orthopod — orthopedist

OS —
- by mouth
- occipitosacral
- occupational safety
- office surgery
- Omenn syndrome
- opening snap
- operating suite
- oral surgery
- organ-specific
- orthopedic surgeon
- orthopedic surgery
- Osgood-Schlatter [disease]
- osteogenic sarcoma
- osteoid surface
- osteosarcoma
- osteosclerosis
- ouabain sensitivity
- overall survival
- oxygen saturation

O.S. — *oculus sinister* (Lat.) left eye

Os — osmium

OSA —
- obstructive sleep apnea
- Office of Services to the Aging
- Optical Society of America

OSA — (*continued*)
- ovarian sectional area

OSAS — obstructive sleep apnea syndrome

O_2sat — oxygen saturation

osc — oscillation

OSCE — objective structured clinical examination

OSCJ — original squamocolumnar junction

OSD — overside drainage

OSF —
- organ system failure
- outer spiral fibers
- overgrowth stimulating factor

OSH Act — Occupational Safety and Health Act of 1970

OSHA — Occupational Safety and Health Administration

OSL — Osgood-Schlatter lesion

OSM —
- osmolarity
- ovine submaxillary mucin
- oxygen saturation meter

μOsm — microosmole

Osm — osmole

osM — osmolar

osm. —
- osmosis
- osmotic

OSMED — otospondylomegaepiphyseal dystrophy

OSMF — oral submucous fibrosis

Osm/kg — osmoles per kilogram

Osm/l — osmoles per liter

osmo — osmolality

osms — osmolality—serum

osmu — osmolality—urine

OSRD — Office of Scientific Research and Development

OSS —
- object sorting scales
- Office of Space Science
- over-the-shoulder strap

oss — osseous

OS-SPT — osmolality (urine) spot [test]

OST — object sorting test

Ost — osteotomy

osteo. —
>osteoarthritis
>osteomyelitis
>osteopath
>osteopathologist
>osteopathy

OSUK — Ophthalmological Society of the United Kingdom

OT —
>objective test
>oblique talus
>occiput transverse [fetal position]
>occlusion time
>occupational therapist
>occupational therapy
>ocular tension
>Oesterreicher-Turner [syndrome]
>office therapy
>old term [in anatomy]
>old tuberculin
>olfactory threshold
>olfactory tubercule
>optic tract
>orientation test
>original tuberulin
>ornithine transcarbamylase
>orotracheal
>orthopedic treatment
>Otis test
>otolaryngology
>otology
>oxytocin
>oxytryptamine

O/T — oral temperature

Ot —
>otolaryngologist
>otolaryngology

OTA —
>ornithine transaminase
>orthotoluidine arsenite

OTC —
>ornithine transcarbamylase
>oval target cell
>over the counter
>oxytetracycline

OTD —
>oral temperature device
>organ tolerance dose

OTE — optically transparent electrode

OTF — oral transfer factor

OTI — ovomucoid trypsin inhibitor

OTM — orthotoluidine manganese sulfate

oto. —
>otology
>otolaryngology
>otorhinolaryngology

Otol —
>otologist
>otology

OTR —
>Ovarian Tumor Registry
>Occupational Therapist, Registered

OTS —
>occipital temporal sulcus
>orotracheal suction

OTSG — Office of the Surgeon General

OTT — orotracheal tube

OTU —
>olfactory tubercle
>operational taxonomic unit

OU —
>observation unit
>Oppenheimer-Urbach [syndrome]

O.U. —
>*oculus unitas* (Lab.) both eyes
>*oculus uterque* (Lat.) each eye

OULQ — outer upper left quadrant

OURQ — outer upper right quadrant

OUS — overuse syndrome

OV —
>oculovestibular
>office visit
>Osler-Vaquez [disease]
>osteoid volume
>ovalbumin

OV — *(continued)*
   ovary
   overventilation
   ovulating
   ovulation
O_2V — oxygen ventilation equivalent
O_v — outflow volume
Ov. — ovary
ov — ovarian
ov. — *ovum* (Lat.) egg
OVA — ovalbumin
OVAL — ovalocyte
OVALO — ovalocytosis
ovar — ovariectomy
OVC — ovarian cancer
OVD — occlusal vertical dimension
OvDF — ovarian dysfunction
OVDQ — Organizational Value Dimensions Questionnaire
OVIT — Oral Verbal Intelligence Test
OVLT — organum vasculosum of the lamina terminalis
OVR — Office of Vocational Rehabilitation
OVX — ovariectomized
OW —
   off work
   once weekly
   open wedge
   outer wall
   out of wedlock
   oval window
O/W —
   oil in water
   oil-water [ratio]

o/w — otherwise
OWA — organics-in-water analyzer
OWR —
   Osler-Weber-Rendu [syndrome]
   ovarian wedge resection
OWS — outerwear syndrome
OWVI — Ohio Work Value Inventory
OX —
   optic chiasma
   orthopedic examination
   oxacillin
   oxalate
   oxide
   oxytocin
Ox — oxygen
ox — oxymel
ox2, Ox-2 — *Proteus vulgaris* antigen
ox19, Ox-19 — *Proteus vulgaris* antigen
OXA — oxaprotiline
Oxi —
   oximeter
   oximetry
OXP — oxypressin
OXT — oxytocin
oxy — oxygen
OYE — old yellow enzyme
oz. — ounce
oz. ap. — apothecaries' ounce (U.S.)
oz. apoth. — apothecaries' ounce (U.K.)
oz. t. — ounce troy (U.S.)
oz. tr. — ounce troy (U.K.)

P —
an electrocardiographic wave corresponding to a wave of depolarization crossing the atria
form perception [in General Aptitude Test Battery]
gas partial pressure
near point
page
pain
para
parent
parenteral
parietal electrode placement [in electroencephalography]
parity
parous
part
partial pressure
partial tension
passive
pater (Lat.) father
paternal
paternally contributing
patient
pelvis
penicillin
percent
percentile
perceptual speed
percussion
perforation
peripheral
permeability
peta-
peyote
pharmacopeia
phenacetin
phenolphthalein
phenylalanine
phon [unit of loudness]
phosphate [group]
phosphorus

P — (continued)
physiology
pico-
pilocarpine
pint
placebo
plasma
point
poise [unit of dynamic viscosity]
poison
poisoning
polarity
polarization
pole
polymyxin
pondere (Lat.) by weight
pondus (Lat.) weight
pons
poor
popular response
population
porcelain
porcine
porphyrin
position
positive
post (Lat.) after
posterior
postpartum
power
precipitin
precursor
prednisone
premolar
presbyopia
pressure
primary
primipara
primitive [hemoglobin]
private [patient, room]
probability
probable error
product

P — (continued)
    progesterone
    prolactin
    proline
    properdin
    propionate
    propionic
    protein
    proximal
    proximum (Lat.) near
    psoralen
    psychiatrist
    psychiatry
    psychosis
    pugillus (Lat.) a handful
    pulmonary
    pulse
    pupil
    pyroplasty
    radiant flux
    radiant power
    significance probability [value]
    sound power
Π — pi (sixteenth letter of the Greek alphabet), uppercase
Φ — phi (twenty-first letter of the Greek alphabet), uppercase
Ψ — psi (twenty-third letter of the Greek alphabet), uppercase
P. —
    Pasteurella
    Plasmodium
    Pneumocystis
    Proteus
    Pseudomonas
P/ — partial upper denture
/P — partial lower denture
P_0 — opening pressure
P_1 —
    first parental generation
    first pulmonic heart sound
    orthophosphate
P_2 — second pulmonic heart sound
P/3 — proximal third [of bone]
P_3 —
    luminous flux
    proximal third [of bone]
P_4 — progesterone

^{32}P — radioactive phosphorus
P-50 — oxygen half-saturation pressure [of hemoglobin]
P-55 — hydroxypregnanedione
P_{700} — chloroplast pigment bleached by 700 nm
P_{870} — bacterial chromatophore pigment bleached by 870 nm
p —
    after
    atomic orbital with angular momentum quantum number 1
    frequency of the more common allele of a pair
    momentum
    page
    papilla
    para-
    partial pressure
    per
    peripheral
    phosphate
    physiologic
    pico-
    pint
    pond
    post-
    power
    pressure
    probability
    probable error
    proton
    pulse
    pupil
    sample proportion [in statistics]
    short arm of chromosome
    sound pressure
π —
    pi (sixteenth letter of the Greek alphabet), lowercase
    ratio of circumference to diameter (value of 3.1415926536)
ϕ —
    magnetic flux
    osmotic coefficient

φ — *(continued)*
  phi (twenty-first letter of the
    Greek alphabet), lowercase
  phi coefficient
ψ —
  psi (twenty-third letter of the
    Greek alphabet), lowercase
  wave function
p. —
  pater (Lat.) father
  pondere (Lat.) by weight
  pondus (Lat.) weight
  post (Lat.) after
  proximum (Lat.) nearest
  pugillus (Lat.) a handful
p̄ —
  after
  mean pressure [gas]
p — para-
5p− [syndrome] — cri-du-chat
  [syndrome]
PA —
  Paleopathology Association
  panic attack
  pantothenic acid
  paralysis agitans
  paranoia
  parietal (cell) antibody
  passive aggressive
  paternal aunt
  pathology
  per annum (Lat.) yearly
  percentage activity
  periapical
  periarteritis
  peridural artery
  periodic acid
  periodontal abscess
  permeability area
  pernicious anemia
  phakic-aphakic
  phenol alcohol
  phenylalanine
  phenylalkylamine
  phosphatidic acid
  phosphoarginine
  photoallergenic
  photoallergy

PA — *(continued)*
  phthalic anhydride
  physical assistance
  physician assistant
  Picture Arrangement [psychol-
    ogy]
  pineapple [test for butyric
    acid in stomach]
  pituitary-adrenal
  plasma adsorption
  plasma aldosterone
  plasminogen activator
  platelet adhesiveness
  platelet aggregation
  platelet-associated
  polyacrylamide
  polyamine
  polyarteritis
  polyarthritis
  post-aural
  posteroanterior
  prealbumin
  predictive accuracy
  pregnancy-associated
  presents again
  primary aldosteronism
  primary amenorrhea
  primary anemia
  prior to admission
  proactivator
  proanthocyanidin
  procainamide
  professional association
  proinsulin antibody
  prolonged action
  prophylactic antibiotic
  propionic acid
  proprietary association
  prostate antigen
  protective antigen
  proteolytic action
  proteolytic activity
  prothrombin activity
  protrusio acetabuli
  Pseudomonas aeruginosa
  psychiatric aide
  psychoanalysis
  psychoanalyst

PA — (continued)
  psychogenic aspermia
  pulmonary artery
  pulmonary atresia
  pulpoaxial
  puromycin aminonucleoside
  pyrophosphate arthropathy
  pyrrolizidine alkaloid
  pyruvic acid
P_A —
  alveolar pressure
  partial pressure in arterial
    blood
P/A —
  percussion and auscultation
  position and alignment
P-A — posteroanterior
P&A —
  percussion and auscultation
  position and alignment
  present and active [reflex]
$P_2 > A_2$ — pulmonic second heart
  sound greater than aortic second heart sound
$P_2 = A_2$ — pulmonic second heart
  sound equal to aortic second
  heart sound
$P_2 < A_2$ — pulmonic second heart
  sound less than aortic second
  heart sound
Pa —
  arterial pressure
  pascal
  pathologist
  pathology
  protactinium
  Pseudomonas aeruginosa
  pulmonary arterial [pressure]
  pulmonary artery [line]
pA — picoampere
pA_2 — affinity constant [binding
  drug to drug receptor]
p.a. —
  per anum (Lat.) through the
    anus
  per annum (Lat.) yearly
  post applicationem (Lat.) after
    application

p.a. — (continued)
  pro anno (Lat.) for the year
PAA —
  partial agonist activity
  phenylacetic acid
  phosphonoacetic acid
  physical abilities analysis
  plasma angiotensinase activity
  polyacrylamide
  polyamino acid
  pyridine acetic acid
p.a.a. — *parti affectae applicetur*
  (Lat.) let it be applied to the
  affected area
$P(A-a)DO_2$, $P(A-a)O_2$ — alveolar-
  arterial oxygen tension difference
PAAAR — Pioneers Across
  America for Alzheimer's Research
$P(A-awo)$ — pressure gradient from
  alveolus to airway opening
PAB —
  para-aminobenzoate
  performance assessment bat-
    tery
  pharmacologic autonomic
    block
  polyacrylamide bead
  Positive Attention Behavior
  premature atrial beat
  purple agar base
PABA — para-aminobenzoic acid
PABD — predeposit autologous
  blood donation
PABP — pulmonary artery balloon
  pump
PAC —
  papular acrodermatitis of
    childhood
  para-aminoclonidine
  parent-adult-child
  phenacetin, aspirin, and caf-
    feine
  plasma aldosterone concentra-
    tion
  platelet-associated comple-
    ment
  Policy Advisory Committee

PAC — *(continued)*
    preadmission certification
    premature atrial contraction
    premature auricular contraction
    Progress Assessment Chart of Social and Personal Development
pac — pachytene
PACC — protein A (immobilized in) collodion charcoal
PACE —
    Pacing and Clinical Electrophysiology
    performance and cost efficiency
    Personal Assessment for Continuing Education
    personalized aerobics for cardiovascular enhancement
    promoting aphasics' communicative effectiveness
    pulmonary angiotensin I–converting enzyme
PA — mean alveolar gas volume
PA$_{CO2}$ — partial pressure of carbon dioxide in alveolar gas
Pa$_{CO2}$ — partial pressure of carbon dioxide in arterial blood
PACP —
    pulmonary alveolar-capillary permeability
    pulmonary artery counterpulsation
PACS — picture archiving and communications system
PACT —
    papillary carcinoma of thyroid
    precordial acceleration tracing
PACU — postanesthetic care unit
PAD —
    per adjusted discharge
    percutaneous abscess drainage
    percutaneous automated discectomy
    peripheral artery disease
    phenacetin, aspirin, and desoxyephedrine

PAD — *(continued)*
    phonologic acquisition device
    photon absorption densitometry
    pre-aid to the disabled
    primary affective disorder
    psychoaffective disorder
    pulmonary artery diastolic
    pulsatile assist device
PAd — pulmonary artery diastolic
PADDS — photon-activated drug delivery system
PADP — pulmonary artery diastolic pressure
PADUA — progressive augmentation by dilating the urethra anterior
PAE —
    postanoxic encephalopathy
    postantibiotic effect
    progressive assistive exercise
p. ae. — *partes aequales* (Lat.) equal parts
paed. —
    paediatric (pediatric)
    paediatrics (pediatrics)
PAEDP — pulmonary artery end-diastolic pressure
PAES — popliteal artery entrapment syndrome
PAF —
    paroxysmal atrial fibrillation
    paroxysmal auricular fibrillation
    phosphodiesterase-activating factor
    platelet-activating factor
    platelet-aggregating factor
    platelet aggregation factor
    pollen adherence factor
    premenstrual assessment form
    pseudoamniotic fluid
    pulmonary arteriovenous fistula
PA&F — percussion, auscultation, and fremitus
PAF-A — platelet-activating factor of anaphylaxis

PAFD —
  percutaneous abscess and fluid drainage
  pulmonary artery filling defect
PAFG — picric acid formaldehyde-glutaraldehyde
PAFI — platelet-aggregation factor inhibitor
PAFIB — paroxysmal atrial fibrillation
PAFP — pre-Achilles fat pad
PAG —
  periaqueductal gray [matter]
  phenylacetyl-glutamine
  polyacrylamide gel
  pregnancy-associated globulin
pAg — protein A-gold [technique]
PAGE —
  polyacrylamide gel electrophoresis
  Program for Automated Gated Evaluation
PAgF — platelet-aggregating factor
PAGG — penta-acetylgluco-pyranosyl guanine
PAGIF — polyacrylamide gel iso-electric focusing
PAGMK — primary African green monkey kidney
PAH —
  para-aminohippurate
  para-aminohippuric [acid]
  phenylalanine hydroxylase
  polycyclic aromatic hydrocarbon
  pulmonary artery hypertension
  pulmonary artery hypotension
PAHA —
  para-aminohippuric acid
  procainamide-hydroxylamine
PAHO — Pan-American Health Organization
PAHVC — pulmonary alveolar hypoxic vasoconstrictor
PAI —
  Pair Attraction Inventory
  plasminogen activator inhibitor

PAI — (continued)
  platelet accumulation index
PAIC — procedures, alternatives, indications, and complications
PAIDS —
  pediatric-acquired immunodeficiency syndrome
PAIgG — platelet-associated immunoglobulin G
PAIR — Personal Assessment of Intimacy in Relationships
PAIRS — Pain and Impairment Relationship Scale
PAIS —
  partial androgen insensitivity syndrome
  phosphoribosylaminoimidazole synthetase
  Psychosocial Adjustment to Illness Scale
PAIVS — pulmonary atresia with intact ventricular septum
PAJ — paralysis agitans juvenilis
PAL —
  pathology laboratory
  phenylalanine ammonia lyase
  posterior axillary line
  product of activated lymphocytes
  pyogenic abscess of the liver
pal. — palate
PALA — N-phosphonacetyl L-aspartate
PA&Lat — posteroanterior and lateral
PALI — Programmed Accelerated Laboratory Investigation [system]
PALN — para-aortic lymph node
PALP — placental alkaline phosphatase
palp. —
  palpable
  palpate
  palpation
  palpitation
palpi. — palpitation

PALS —
> Paired Associate Learning
> Subtest
> periarteriolar lymphoid sheath
> prison-acquired lymphoprolif-
> erative syndrome

PALST — Picture Articulation
and Language Screening Test

Palv — alveolar pressure

PAM —
> crystalline penicillin G in 2%
> aluminum monostearate
> pancreatic acinar mass
> penicillin aluminum monoste-
> arate
> L-phenylalanine mustard
> *p*-methoxyamphetamine
> postauricular myogenic
> potential acuity meter
> pregnancy-associated α-mac-
> roglobulin
> primary amebic meningoen-
> cephalitis
> pulmonary alveolar macro-
> phage
> pulmonary alveolar microlithi-
> asis
> pulse amplitude modulation
> pyridine aldoxime methylchlo-
> ride

2-PAM — pralidoxime

PAMC — pterygoarthromyodyspla-
sia congenita

PAMD — primary adrenocortical
micronodular dysplasia

PAME — primary amebic meningoencephalitis

PAMP — pulmonary artery mean
pressure

PAN —
> periarteritis nodosa
> periodic alternating nystag-
> mus
> peroxyacetyl nitrate
> polyacrylonitrile
> polyarteritis nodosa
> positional alcohol nystagmus
> puromycin aminonucleoside

pan —
> pancreas
> pancreatectomy
> pancreatic

PAND — primary adrenocortical
nodular dysplasia

PANESS — physical and neurologic examination for soft
signs

PA_{N_2O} — mean alveolar nitrous oxide tension

PANS — puromycin aminonucleoside

PANSS — Positive and Negative
Syndrome Scale

PAO —
> peak acid output
> peripheral airway obstruction
> plasma amine oxidase
> polyamine oxidase
> pustulotic arthro-osteitis

PAo —
> airway pressure
> ascending aortic pressure
> pulmonary artery occlusion
> [pressure]

PA_{O_2} —
> alveolar oxygen pressure
> alveolar oxygen tension

PaO_2 — partial pressure of oxygen
in arterial blood

P_{ao} — airway opening pressure

pAO_2 —
> oxygen pressure in aorta
> oxygen pressure on room air

PAOD —
> peripheral arterial occlusive
> disease
> peripheral arteriosclerotic oc-
> clusive disease

PAOI — peak acid output, insulin-
induced

PAOP — pulmonary artery occlusion pressure

PAO_2–PaO_2 — alveolar-arterial difference in partial pressure of
oxygen

PAOx — phenylacetone oxime

PAP —
　　Papanicolaou (test)
　　papaverine
　　para-aminophenol
　　passive-aggressive personality
　　Patient Assessment Program
　　peak airway pressure
　　peroxidase antibody to peroxidase
　　peroxidase-antiperoxidase [method]
　　phosphoadenosine phosphate
　　placental acid phosphatase
　　placental alkaline phosphatase
　　positive airway pressure
　　primary atypical pneumonia
　　prostatic acid phosphatase
　　pseudoallergic reaction
　　pulmonary alveolar proteinosis
　　pulmonary artery pressure
　　purified alternate pathway
Pap —
　　Papanicolaou [test]
　　papilloma
pap. — papilla
PAPF — platelet adhesiveness plasma factor
pap. in. canthus — papilloma, inner canthus
papova — papilloma-polyoma-vacuolating agent [virus]
PAPP —
　　Pappenheimer bodies
　　para-aminopropiophenone
　　pregnancy-associated plasma protein
PAPPC — pregnancy-associated plasma protein C
PAPS —
　　3'-phosphoadenosine-5'-phosphosulfate
　　phosphoadenosylphosphosulfate
PA/PS — pulmonary atresia/pulmonary stenosis
Pap sm — Papanicolaou smear
PAPUFA — physiologically active polyunsaturated fatty acid

parv. — *parvus* (Lat.) small
Pa-Pv — pulmonary arterial pressure–pulmonary venous pressure
PAPVC — partial anomalous pulmonary venous connection
PAPVR — partial anomalous pulmonary venous return
PAPW — posterior aspect of the pharyngeal wall
PAQ —
　　Personal Attitudes Questionnaire
　　Personal Attributes Questionnaire
　　Position Analysis Questionnaire
PAR —
　　paraffin
　　parallel
　　passive avoidance reaction
　　perennial allergic rhinitis
　　photosynthetically active radiation
　　physiological aging rate
　　platelet aggregate ratio
　　positive attention received
　　postanesthesia recovery
　　postanesthesia room
　　probable allergic rhinitis
　　problem-analysis report
　　Program for Alcohol Recovery
　　proximal alveolar region
　　pulmonary arteriolar resistance
PAr — polyarteritis
Par — paranoid
par. —
　　paraffin
　　parallel
　　paralysis
PARA, Para, para — number of pregnancies producing viable offspring
para. —
　　paracentesis
　　paraparesis

para. — *(continued)*
 paraplegia
 paraplegic
 parathyroid
 parathyroidectomy
Para-A — paratyphoid A
Para-B — paratyphoid B
Para-C — paratyphoid C
para c — paracervical
para 0 — nullipara
para I — primipara
para II — secundipara
para III — tripara
para IV — quadripara
par. aff. — *pars affecta* (Lat.) the part affected
para L — paralumbar
parapsych. — parapsychology
parasit. —
 parasitic
 parasitology
parasym. — parasympathetic
para T — parathoracic
PARD — platelet aggregation as a risk of diabetes
parent. —
 parenteral
 parenterally
PARH — plasminogen activator–releasing hormone
PARIET — parietal cell antibody
parox. —
 paroxysm
 paroxysmal
PARR — postanesthesia recovery room
PARS — Personal Adjustment and Role Skills (Scale)
PaRS — pararectal space
part. —
 partim (Lat.) partly
 partis (Lat.) of a part
 parturition
part. aeq. — *partes aequales* (Lat.) equal parts
part. dolent. — *partes dolentes* (Lat.) painful parts
part. vic. — *partitis vicibus* (Lat.) in divided doses

PARU — postanesthetic recovery unit
parv. — *parvus* (Lat.) small
PAS —
 para-aminosalicylate
 para-aminosalicylic [acid]
 Parent Attitude Scale
 patient appointments and scheduling
 periodic acid–Schiff [stain]
 peripheral anterior synechia
 persistent atrial standstill
 Personality Assessment Scale
 phosphatase acid serum
 photoacoustic spectroscopy
 Physician's Activity Study
 pneumatic antiembolic stocking
 postanesthesia score
 posterior airway space
 preadmission screening
 pregnancy advisory service
 premature atrial stimulus
 premature auricular systole
 Professional Activities Study
 progressive accumulated stress
 pseudoachievement syndrome
 pulmonary artery stenosis
Pa·s — pascal-second
Pa/s — pascals per second
PASA —
 para-aminosalicylic acid
 primary acquired sideroblastic anemia
 proximal articular set angle
PASAT — Paced Auditory Serial Addiction Task
Pa Sat — saturation of oxygen in arterial blood
PAS-C — para-aminosalicylic acid crystallized (with ascorbic acid)
PASD — after diastase digestion
P'ase — alkaline phosphatase
Pas. Ex. — passive exercise
PASG — pneumatic antishock garment
PASH — periodic acid–Schiff hematoxylin

PASI — psoriasis area sensitivity index

PASM — periodic acid–silver methenamine

PAS/MAP — Professional Activities Study/Medical Audit Program

PASP — pulmonary artery systolic pressure

pass. —
passim (Lat.) here and there
passive

PAST — periodic acid–Schiff technique

Past. — *Pasteurella*

PASVR — pulmonary anomalous superior venous return

PAT —
Pain Apperception Test
paroxysmal atrial tachycardia
paroxysmal auricular tachycardia
patella
patient
percentage of acceleration time
phenylaminotetrazole
Photo Articulation Test [psychology]
physical abilities test
picric acid turbidity
platelet aggregation test
polyamine acetyltransferase
preadmission assessment team
preadmission assessment test
preadmission testing
Predictive Ability Test
pregnancy at term
prism adaptation test
psychoacoustic testing
pulmonary artery trunk

pat. —
patella
patent
paternal origin
patient

PATE —
psychodynamic and therapeutic education

PATE — *(continued)*
pulmonary artery thromboembolectomy
pulmonary artery thromboembolism
pulmonary artery thromboendarterectomy

PATH —
Partnership Approach to Health
pathological
pathology
pituitary adrenotropic hormone

path —
pathogen
pathogenesis
pathogenic
pathological
pathologist
pathology

path fx — pathological fracture

PATLC — Progressive Achievement Tests of Listening Comprehension

pat. med. — patent medicine

PA-T-SP — periodic acid–thiocarbohydrazide–silver proteinate

pat. T. — patellar tenderness

PAT/TM — patient's time

p. aur. — *post aurem* (Lat.) behind the ear

PAV —
partial atrioventricular
Pavulon (pancuronium bromide)
percutaneous aortic valvuloplasty
poikiloderma atrophicans vasculare
posterior arch vein

pavaex —
passive vascular exercise
passive venoarterial exercise

PAVF — pulmonary arteriovenous fistula

PAVM — pulmonary arteriovenous malformation

PAVN — paraventricular nucleus
PAVNRT — paroxysmal atrioventricular nodal reciprocal tachycardia
PAW —
    peak airway pressure
    peripheral airways
    pulmonary artery wedge
Paw — mean airway pressure
Pawo — pressure at airway opening
PAWP — pulmonary artery wedge pressure
PAWS — primary withdrawal syndrome
PB —
    Pharmacopoeia Britannica (British Pharmacopoeia)
    pancreaticobiliary
    paraffin bath
    Paul-Bunnell [antibody]
    pentobarbital
    perineal body
    periodic breathing
    peripheral blood
    peroneus brevis
    phenobarbital
    phenoxybenzamine
    phonetically balanced
    piggyback
    pinealoblastoma
    piperonyl butoxide
    polymyxin B
    posterior baffle
    powder bed
    powder board
    power building
    premature beat
    pressure balanced
    pressure breathing
    protein binding
    protein bound
    pudendal block
    punch biopsy
PB% — phonetically balanced percentage [of word lists]
P&B —
    pain and burning
    phenobarbital and belladonna

P_B — barometric pressure
Pb —
    phenobarbital
    lead (Lat., *plumbum*)
    presbyopia
    probenecid
PBA —
    percutaneous bladder aspiration
    phenylboronate agarose
    polyclonal B-cell activity
    pressure breathing assister
    prolactin-binding assay
    prune belly anomaly
    pulpobuccoaxial
P_{BA} — brachial arterial pressure
PBB — polybrominated biphenyl
Pb-B — lead level in blood
PBC —
    peripheral blood cell
    point of basal convergence
    pre-bed care
    pregnancy and birth complications
    primary biliary cirrhosis
    progestin-binding complement
PBD —
    percutaneous biliary drainage
    postburn day
PBE —
    partial breech extraction
    Perlsucht Bacillen-Emulsion (Ger.) tuberculin from *Mycobacterium tuberculosis bovis*
PBF —
    peripheral blood flow
    phosphate-buffered formalin
    placental blood flow
    pulmonary blood flow
PBFe — protein-bound iron
PBG —
    Penassay broth plus glucose
    porphobilinogen
PBGM — Penassay broth plus glucose plus menadione
PBG-Q — porphobilinogen—quantitative

PBG-S — porphobilinogen synthase
PBH — pulling boat hands
PBHB — poly-beta-hydroxybutyrate
PBI —
    parental bonding instrument
    partial bony impaction
    penile-brachial index
    protein-bound iodine
PbI — lead intoxication
PB[131]I — protein-bound radioactive iodine
PBIgG — platelet surface blood immunoglobulin G
PBK —
    phosphorylase b kinase
    pseudophakic bullous keratopathy
PB(K) — phonetically balanced (kindergarten)
PBL —
    peripheral blood leukocyte
    peripheral blood lymphocyte
PBLC — peripheral blood lymphocyte count
PBLI — premature birth, live infant
PBLT — peripheral blood lymphocyte transformation
PBM —
    peripheral basement membrane
    peripheral blood mononuclear [cell]
    placental basement membrane
PBMC — peripheral blood mononuclear cell
PBMV — pulmonary blood mixing volume
PBN —
    paralytic brachial neuritis
    peripheral benign neoplasm
    polymyxin B sulfate, bacitracin, and neomycin
PBNA — partial body neutron activation
PBO —
    penicillin in beeswax and oil

PBO — (continued)
    placebo
PbO — lead monoxide
PBP —
    peak blood pressure
    penicillin-binding protein
    porphyrin biosynthetic pathway
    progressive bulbar palsy
    prostate-binding protein
    pseudobulbar palsy
    pulsatile bypass pump
    purified *Brucella* protein
PBPI — penile-brachial pulse index
PBQ —
    phenylbenzoquinone
    Preschool Behavior Questionnaire
Pb-RBC — lead red blood (cell) count
PBRT — phonetically balanced rhyme test
PBS —
    perfusion-pressure breakthrough syndrome
    peripheral blood smear
    phenobarbital sodium
    phosphate-buffered saline
    phosphate-buffered sodium
    planar bone scan
    polybrominated salicylamide
    primer binding site
    prune belly syndrome
    pulmonary branch stenosis
Pbs — pressure at body surface
PBSP — prognostically bad signs during pregnancy
PBT —
    Paul-Bunnell test
    phenacetin breath test
    profile-based therapy
PBT$_4$ — protein-bound thyroxine
PBV —
    percutaneous balloon valvuloplasty
    predicted blood volume
    pulmonary blood volume

PBW — posterior bite-wing

PBZ —
  personal breathing zone
  phenoxybenzamine
  phenylbutazone
  pyribenzamine (tripelenna-
    mine)

PC —
  packed cells
  palmitoyl carnitine
  paper chromatography
  paracortex
  parent cell
  parent to child
  particulate component
  partition coefficient
  pelvic cramp
  penicillin
  pentose cycle
  percent
  peritoneal cell
  pharmacology
  pheochromocytoma
  phosphate cycle
  phosphatidylcholine (leci-
    thin)
  phosphocreatine
  phosphorylcholine
  photoconduction
  phrase construction
  Physicians' Corporation
  picryl chloride
  picture completion
  pill counter
  piriform cortex
  plasma concentration
  plasma cortisol
  plasmacytoma
  plasmin complex
  platelet concentrate
  platelet concentration
  platelet count
  pneumotaxic center
  polycentric
  polyposis coli
  pondus civile (Lat.) avoirdu-
    pois weight
  poor condition

PC — *(continued)*
  poor coordination
  popliteal cyst
  portacaval [shunt]
  portal cirrhosis
  post cibos (Lat.) after meals
  post cibum (Lat.) after food
  postcoital
  postconception
  posterior cervical
  posterior chamber
  posterior circumflex [artery]
  posterior column
  posterior commissure
  posterior cortex
  precaution category
  precordial
  precordium
  premature contraction
  prenatal care
  prepiriform cortex
  present complaint
  primary cleavage
  primary closure
  printed circuit
  procollagen
  producing cell
  productive cough
  professional corporation
  proliferative capacity
  prostatic carcinoma
  prosthetics center
  protein C
  provisional cortex
  proximal colon
  pseudoconditioning control
  pseudocyst
  Psychodevelopment Checklist
  pubococcygeus [muscle]
  pulmonary capillary
  pulmonary circulation
  pulmonic closure
  Purkinje cell
  pyloric canal
  pyruvate carboxylase

P-C — phlogistic corticoid

P&C — prism and (alternate)
    cover-test [ophthalmology]

Pc — penicillin
pc — percent
p.c. —
  pondus civile (Lat.) avoirdu-
    pois weight
  post cibos (Lat.) after meals
  post cibum (Lat.) after food
pc1 — platelet count pretransfu-
  sion
pc2 — platelet count posttransfu-
  sion
PCA —
  para-chloramphetamine
  parietal cell antibody
  passive cutaneous anaphylaxis
  patient care aide
  patient care assistant
  patient-controlled analgesia
  perchloric acid
  percutaneous carotid angiogra-
    phy
  percutaneous carotid arterio-
    gram
  percutaneous coronary angio-
    plasty
  personal care attendant
  phenylcarboxylic acid
  photocontact, allergic
  polyclonal antibody
  porous-coated anatomic [pros-
    thesis]
  portacaval anastomosis
  postconceptional age
  posterior cerebral artery
  posterior communicating
    aneurysm
  posterior communicating
    artery
  posterior cricoarytenoid
  precoronary care area
  President's Council on Aging
  principal components analysis
  procainamide
  procoagulant activity
  prostatic carcinoma
  pyrrolidine carboxylic acid
PCAS — Psychotherapy Competence Assessment Schedule

PCAVC — persistent complete
  atrioventricular canal
PCB —
  pancuronium bromide
  paracervical block
  polychlorinated biphenyl
  portacaval bypass
  postcoital bleeding
  prepared childbirth
Pc.B. — *punctum convergens basalis*
  (Lat.) near point of convergence to the intercentral base
  line
PC-BMP — phosphorylcholine-
  binding myeloma protein
PCC —
  Pasteur Culture Collection
  percutaneous cecostomy
  personal care clinic
  pheochromocytoma
  phosphate carrier compound
  plasma catecholamine concen-
    tration
  pneumatosis cystoides coli
  Poison Control Center
  precoronary care
  premature chromosome con-
    densation
  primary care clinic
  prothrombin complex concen-
    tration
PCc — periscopic concave
pcc — premature chromosome con-
  densation
PCCC — pediatric critical care
  center
PCCP — percutaneous cord cyst
  puncture
PCCS — parent-child communication schedule
PCCU — post-coronary care unit
PCD —
  papillary collecting duct
  paraneoplastic cerebellar de-
    generation
  paroxysmal cerebral dysrhyth-
    mia
  phosphate-citrate-dextrose

PCD — *(continued)*
    plasma cell dyscrasia
    polycystic disease
    posterior corneal deposits
    postmortem cesarean delivery
    premature centromere division
    primary ciliary dyskinesia
    prolonged contractile duration
    pulmonary clearance delay
PCDC — plasma clot diffusion chamber
PCDF — polychlorinated dibenzofuran
PCDUS — plasma cell dyscrasia of unknown significance
PCE —
    physical capacity evaluation
    polymer-coated erythromycin
    pseudocholinesterase
    pulmocutaneous exchange
PCEN — paracentesis [fluid]
PCF —
    peripheral circulatory failure
    pharyngoconjunctival fever
    platelet complement fixation
    posterior cranial fossa
    prothrombin conversion factor
pcf — pounds per cubic feet
PCFIA — particle concentration fluorescence immunoassay
PCFT — platelet complement fixation test
PCG —
    paracervical ganglion
    phonocardiogram
    Planning Career Goals [psychological test]
    pneumocardiogram
    primate chorionic gonadotropin
    pubococcygeus [muscle]
pcg — picogram
PCGG — percutaneous coagulation of gasserian ganglion

PCH —
    paroxysmal cold hemoglobinuria
    polycyclic hydrocarbon
PCHE — pseudocholinesterase
PC&HS — *post cibos & hora somni* (Lat.) after meals and at bedtime
PCI —
    Pittsburgh Cancer Institute
    pneumatosis cystoides intestinalis
    posterior curve intestinalis [cornea]
    Premarital Communication Inventory
    prophylactic cranial irradiation
    prothrombin consumption index
pCi — picocurie
PCIC — Poison Control Information Center
PCIOL — posterior chamber intraocular lens
PC-IRV — pressure-controlled inverted-ratio ventilation
PCIS —
    Patient-Care Information System
    postcardiac injury syndrome
PCK — polycystic kidney
PCKD — polycystic kidney disease
PCL —
    pacing cycle length
    persistent corpus luteum
    plasma cell leukemia
    posterior chamber lens
    posterior collateral ligament
    posterior cruciate ligament
P closure — plastic closure
PCM —
    primary cutaneous melanoma
    process control monitor
    protein-calorie malnutrition
    protein carboxymethylase
    pulse code modulation
p-CMB — para-chloromercuribenzoate

PCMBSA — para-chloromercuri-benzine sulfonic acid
PCMF — perceptual cognitive motor function
PCMO — Principal Clinical Medical Officer
PCMT — pacemaker circus movement tachycardia
PCMX — para-chloro-*m*-xylenol
PCN —
  penicillin
  percutaneous nephrostomy
  pregnenolone carbonitrile
  primary care network
  primary care nursing
PCNA — proliferating cell nuclear antigen
PCNB — pentachloronitrobenzene
PCNL — percutaneous nephrostolithotomy
PCNV —
  postchemotherapy nausea and vomiting
  Provisional Committee on Nomenclature of Viruses
PCO —
  patient complains of
  polycystic ovary
  predicted cardiac output
P_{CO} — partial pressure of carbon monoxide
P_{CO_2} —
  carbon dioxide pressure
  carbon dioxide tension
  partial pressure of carbon dioxide
pCO_2 — partial pressure of carbon dioxide
PCoA — posterior communicating artery
PCOD — polycystic ovarian disease
PCom — posterior communicating [artery]
PCON — platelet concentration
PCOS — polycystic ovary syndrome
PCP —
  parachlorophenate

PCP — (*continued*)
  parachlorophenol
  patient care plan
  pentachlorophenate
  pentachlorophenol
  peripheral coronary pressure
  persistent cough and phlegm
  phencyclidine palmitate
  1-(1-phenylcyclohexyl)piperidine
  pneumocystic pneumonia
  Pneumocystis carinii pneumonia
  postoperative constrictive pericarditis
  primary care physician
  principal care provider
  prochlorperazine
  procollagen peptide
  pulmonary capillary pressure
  pulse cytophotometry
PCPA — parachlorophenylalanine
PCPL — pulmonary capillary protein leakage
pcpn — precipitation
PCPS — phosphatidylcholine-phosphatidylserine
pCpt —
  perception
  precipitate
  precipitation
PCQ — polychloroquaterphenyl
PCR —
  patient contact record
  personal care residence
  phosphocreatine
  plasma clearance rate
  polymerase chain reaction
  probable causal relationship
  protein catabolism rate
PCr — phosphocreatine
P_{Cr} — plasma creatinine
PCS —
  palliative care service
  Patient Care System
  patterns of care study
  pelvic congestion syndrome
  pharmacogenic confusional syndrome

0

PCS — (continued)
  portacaval shunt
  postcardiac surgery
  postcardiotomy syndrome
  postcholecystectomy syn-
    drome
  postconcussion syndrome
  precordial stethoscope
  premature centromere separa-
    tion
  primary cancer site
  primary cesarean section
  Priority Counseling Survey
  prolonged crush syndrome
  proportional counter spec-
    trometry
  proximal coronary sinus
  pseudotumor cerebri syn-
    drome
P c/s — primary cesarean section
pcs — preconscious
PCSM — percutaneous stone manipulation
PCT —
  peripheral carcinoid tumor
  Physiognomic Cue Test [psy-
    chology]
  plasma clotting time
  plasmacrit test
  plasmacytoma
  polychlorinated triphenyl
  porcine calcitonin
  porphyria cutanea tarda
  portacaval transposition
  positron computed tomogra-
    phy
  postcoital test
  progesterone challenge test
  progestin challenge test
  prothrombin consumption
    time
  proximal convoluted tubule
  pulmonary care team
pct — percent
PCTA — percutaneous coronary
  transluminal angioplasty
PCU —
  pain control unit

PCU — (continued)
  palliative care unit
  patient care unit
  post-coronary (care) unit
  primary care unit
  progressive care unit
  protective care unit
  protein-calorie undernutrition
  pulmonary care unit
p cut — percutaneous
PCV —
  packed cell volume
  parietal cell vagotomy
  polycythemia vera
  postcapillary venule
  premature ventricular contrac-
    tion
PCV-M — polycythemia vera with
  myeloid metaplasia
PCW —
  pericanalicular web
  primary capillary wedge
  pulmonary capillary wedge
  purified cell walls
PCWP — pulmonary capillary
  wedge pressure
PCX — paracervical
PCx — periscopic convex
PCX R —
  portable chest radiograph
  portable chest x-ray [film]
PCZ —
  procarbazine
  prochlorperazine
PD —
  Doctor of Pharmacy
  Dublin Pharmacopoeia
  interpupillary distance
  Paget's disease
  pancreatic duct
  papilla diameter
  paralyzing dose
  Parkinson's disease
  parkinsonian dementia
  paroxysmal discharge
  pars distalis
  patent ductus
  patient day

PD — *(continued)*
    patient demonstration
    pediatric
    pediatrics
    percentage difference
    percutaneous drain
    per diem (Lat.) by the day
    peritoneal dialysis
    personality disorder
    pharmacodynamics
    phenyldichlorarsine
    phosphate dehydrogenase
    phosphate dextrose
    photosensitivity dermatitis
    Pick's disease
    plasma defect
    poorly differentiated
    Porak-Durante [syndrome]
    porphobilinogen deaminase
    posterior division
    postnasal drainage
    postural drainage
    potential difference
    pregnanediol
    present disease
    pressor dose
    preventive dentistry
    primary dendrite
    prism diopter
    problem drinker
    progression of disease
    protein degradation
    protein-deprived
    protein diet
    provocation dose
    psychopathic deviate
    psychotic dementia
    psychotic depression
    psychotic deviate
    pulmonary disease
    pulpodistal
    pulse duration
    pupillary distance
    pyloric dilator
P(D+) — probability of having disease
P(D−) — probability of not having disease

P/D — packs per day [cigarettes]
PD_{50} — median paralyzing dose
2-PD — two-point discrimination
Pd —
    palladium
    pediatrics
pd — period
p.d. —
    papilla diameter
    per diem (Lat.) by the day
    pro die (Lat.) for the day
    prism diopter
PDA —
    parenteral drug abuser
    patent ductus arteriosus
    patient distress alarm
    pediatric allergy
    posterior descending artery
    predialyzed human albumin
    principal diagonal artery
    pulmonary disease anemia
PdA — pediatric allergy
PDAB — para-dimethylamino-benzaldehyde
PD/AR — photosensitivity dermatitis and actinic reticuloid [syndrome]
PDB —
    Paget's disease of bone
    paradichlorobenzene
    phorbol 12,13-dibutyrate
    phosphorus-dissolving bacteria
    preventive dental (health) behavior
PDC —
    parkinsonism-dementia complex
    pediatric cardiology
    penta-decylcatechol
    physical dependence capacity
    plasma dioxin concentration
    plasma disappearance curve
    postdecapitation convulsion
    preliminary diagnostic clinic
    private diagnostic clinic
    Psychodevelopment Checklist
PD&C — postural drainage and clapping

PdC — pediatric cardiology
PDCB — para-dichlorobenzene
PDCD — primary degenerative cerebral disease
PD-CSE — pulsed Doppler cross-sectional echocardiography
PDD —
  pervasive developmental disorder
  platinum diamminedichloride (cisplatin)
  primary degenerative dementia
  pyridoxine-deficient diet
PDDB — phenododecinium bromide
PDDS — Parasitic Disease Drug Service
PDE —
  paroxysmal dyspnea on exertion
  phosphodiesterase
  postoperative diffuse edema
  progressive dialysis encephalopathy
  pulsed Doppler echocardiography
PdE — pediatric endocrinology
PDF —
  Parkinson's Disease Foundation
  peritoneal dialysis fluid
  probability density function
  pyruvate dehydrogenase
PDFC — premature dead female child
PDG —
  parkinsonism-dementia complex of Guam
  phosphate-dependent glutaminase
  phosphogluconate dehydrogenase
PDGA — pteroyldiglutamic acid
PDGF — platelet-derived growth factor
PDGS — partial form of DiGeorge's syndrome

PDGXT — predischarge graded exercise test
PDH —
  packaged disaster hospital
  past dental history
  phosphate dehydrogenase
  progressive disseminated histoplasmosis
  pyruvate dehydrogenase
PDHa — pyruvate dehydrogenase in active form
PDHC — pyruvate dehydrogenase complex
PdHO — pediatric hematology-oncology
PDI —
  periodontal disease index
  plan-do integration
  Psychomotor Development Index
Pdi — transdiaphragmatic pressure
PDIE — phosphodiesterase
P-diol — pregnanediol
PDL —
  pancreatic duct ligation
  periodontal ligament
  poorly differentiated lymphocyte
  population doubling level
  primary dysfunctional labor
  progressive diffuse leukoencephalopathy
pdl —
  poundal [unit of force]
  pudendal
PDLC — poorly differentiated lung cancer
PDL-D — poorly differentiated lymphocytic–diffuse
PDLL — poorly differentiated lymphocytic lymphoma
PDL-N — poorly differentiated lymphocytic–nodular
PDLP — predigested liquid protein
PDM — polymyositis and dermatomyositis
PDMC — premature dead male child

PDMEA — phosphoryldimethyl-
    ethanolamine
PDMS —
    Patient Data Management
        System
    pharmacokinetic drug-moni-
        toring service
PDN —
    prednisone
    private day nurse
    private duty nurse
PdNEO — pediatric neonatology
PdNEP — pediatric nephrology
PDP —
    pattern disruption point
    piperidinopyrimidine
    platelet-depleted plasma
    platelet-derived plasma
    primer-dependent deoxy-
        nucleic acid polymerase
    Product Development Proto-
        col
PD&P — postural drainage and
    percussion
PDPD — prolonged-dwell perito-
    neal dialysis
PDPI — primer-dependent deoxy-
    nucleic acid polymerase index
PDQ —
    parental development ques-
        tionnaire
    Personality Diagnostic Ques-
        tionnaire
    Physician's Data Query
    Premenstrual Distress Ques-
        tionnaire
    Prescreening Development
        Questionnaire
    pretty darn quick
    protocol data query
PDR —
    pandevelopmental retardation
    pediatric radiology
    peripheral diabetic retinopa-
        thy
    Physician's Desk Reference
    pleiotropic drug resistance
    postdelivery room

PDR — (continued)
    primary drug resistance
    proliferative diabetic retinopa-
        thy
PdR — pediatric radiology
pdr — powder
PDRB — Permanent Disability
    Rating Board
PDRc̄VH — proliferative diabetic
    retinopathy with vitreous
    hemorrhage
PDRT — Portland Digit Recogni-
    tion Test
PDS —
    pain-dysfunction syndrome
    paroxysmal depolarizing shift
    patient data system
    pediatric surgery
    peritoneal dialysis system
    plasma-derived serum
    polydioxanone sutures
    predialyzed (human) serum
    primary dependence study
PdS —
    pediatric surgery
    psychiatric deviate, subtle
PDSG — pigment dispersion syn-
    drome glaucoma
PDT —
    phenyldimethyltriazine
    photodynamic therapy
    population doubling time
PDU — pulsed Doppler ultrasonog-
    raphy
PDUF — pulsed Doppler ultrasonic
    flowmeter
PDUR — Predischarge Utilization
    Review
PDV — peak diastolic velocity
PDW — platelet distribution width
PDWHF — platelet-derived wound
    healing factor
PDX — probable diagnosis
PE —
    Edinburgh Pharmacopoeia
    pancreatic extract
    paper electrophoresis
    parallel elastic [muscle compo-
        nent]

PE — (continued)
  partial epilepsy
  Pel-Ebstein [disease]
  pelvic examination
  penile erection
  pericardial effusion
  peritoneal exudate
  phakoemulsification
  pharyngoesophageal
  phenylephrine
  phenylethylamine
  phosphatidylethanolamine
  photoelectric effect
  photographic effect
  phycoerythrin
  physical education
  physical evaluation
  physical examination
  physical exercise
  physiological ecology
  pigmented epithelium
  pilocarpine-epinephrine
  placental extract
  plasma exchange
  plating efficiency
  pleural effusion
  pneumatic equalization
  point of entry
  polyethylene
  polynuclear eosinophil
  potential energy
  powdered extract
  practical exercise
  preeclampsia
  preexcitation
  present evaluation
  pressure equalization
  pressure equalizing
  prior to exposure
  probable error
  probe excision
  professional engineer
  protein electrophoresis
  protein excretion
  pseudoexfoliation
  pulmonary edema
  pulmonary embolism
  pulmonary embolus

PE — (continued)
    pyramidal eminence
    pyroelectric
    pyrogenic exotoxin
PE2 — secondary plating efficiency
PĒ — pressure on expiration
Pe —
    pregnenolone
    pressure on expiration
p.e. — per exemplum (Lat.) for ex-
    ample
PEA —
    pelvic examination under an-
      esthesia
    phenylethyl alcohol
    phenylethyl alcohol [agar]
    phenylethylamine
    polysaccharide egg antigen
PE ↓ A — pelvic examination un-
    der anesthesia
PEACH — Preschool Evaluation
    and Assessment for Children
    with Handicaps
PEAO — phenylethylamine oxi-
    dase
PEAP — positive end-airway pres-
    sure
PEAQ — Personal Experience and
    Attitude Questionnaire
PEARLA — pupils equal and reac-
    tive to light and accommoda-
    tion
PEBG — phenethylbiguanide
PEC —
    parallel elastic component
    patient evaluation center
    peduncle of cerebrum
    peritoneal exudate cell
    pulmonary ejection click
    pyogenic exotoxin C
Pecho — prostatic echogram
PE_{CO_2} — mixed expired carbon di-
    oxide tension
PECT — positron emission com-
    puted tomography
PED —
    pediatrics
    peduncle

PED — (continued)

>pharyngoesophageal diverticulum

>pollution and environmental degradation

>postentry day

>postexertional dyspnea

PEd — physical education

ped —

>pedestrian

>pediatric

ped. ed. — pedal edema

PEDG — phenylethyldiguanide

PED/MVA — pedestrian–motor vehicle accident

PeDS — Pediatric Drug Surveillance

Peds — pediatrics

PEE — parallel elastic element

PEEP —

>peak end-expiratory pressure

>positive end-expiratory pressure

PEEPi — intrinsic peak end-expiratory pressure

PEER — Pediatric Examination of Educational Readiness

PEF —

>peak expiratory flow

>pharyngoepiglottic fold

>Psychiatric Evaluation Form

>pulmonary edema fluid

PEFR — peak expiratory flow rate

PEFSR — partial expiratory flow–static recoil [curve]

PEFT — peak expiratory flow time

PEFV — partial expiratory flow volume

PEG —

>Patient Evaluation Grid

>percutaneous endoscopic gastrostomy

>pneumoencephalogram

>pneumoencephalography

>polyethylene glycol

PEG-ELS — polyethylene glycol (and iso-osmolar) electrolyte solution

PEI —

>phosphate excretion index

>phosphorus excretion index

>physical efficiency index

>polyethyleneimine

PEJ — percutaneous endoscopic jejunostomy

PEL —

>peritoneal exudate lymphocyte

>permissible exposure limit

Pel — elastic recoil pressure of lung

PELG — Pelger-Huët anomaly

PELISA — paper enzyme-linked immunosorbent assay

PEM —

>peritoneal exudate macrophage

>precordial electrocardiographic mapping

>prescription event monitoring

>primary enrichment medium

>probable error of measurement

>protein-energy malnutrition

>pulmonary embolus

>pulmonary endothelial membrane

PEMA — phenylethylmalonamide

PEMF — pulsating electromagnetic field

PEMS — physical, emotional, mental, and safety

PEN —

>parenteral and enteral nutrition

>penicillin

Pen —

>penetrating

>penicillin

PENG — photoelectric nystagmography

pen G — penicillin G

penic. cam. — *penicillum camelinum* (Lat.) camel's hair brush

PEN-O — Penner serotype-O

PENS — percutaneous epidural nerve stimulator

Pent — pentothal

Pen VK — penicillin V potassium

PEO — progressive external ophthalmoplegia

PEP —
    peptidase
    performance evaluation procedure
    phosphoenolpyruvate
    physiologic evaluation of primates
    pigmentation, edema, and plasma cell dyscrasia [syndrome]
    polyestradiol phosphate
    positive expiratory pressure
    postencephalitic parkinsonism
    preejection period
    protein electrophoresis
    Psychiatric Evaluation Profile
    Pulmonary Education Program

Pep — peptidase

PEPA —
    peptidase A
    protected environment (units and) prophylactic antibiotics

PEPB — peptidase B

PEPC — peptidase C

PEPc — corrected preejection period

PEPCK — phosphoenolpyruvate carboxykinase

PEPD — peptidase D

PEPE — peptidase E

PEP/EP — pre-ejection period to ejection period

PEPI — pre-ejection period index

PEP/LVET — pre-injection period/ left ventricular ejection time

PEPP — positive expiratory pressure plateau

PEPR — precision encoder and pattern recognizer

PEPS — peptidase S

PER —
    peak ejection rate

PER — (continued)
    pediatric emergency room
    periodic evaluation record
    protein efficiency ratio
    pudendal evoked response

per. —
    perineal
    periodic
    periodicity
    permission
    person

per an. — per annum (Lat.) by year

per bid. — per biduum (Lat.) for a period of 2 days

PERC —
    perceptual
    percutaneous
    potential erythropoietin-responsive cell

percs — Percodan [tablets]

percus — percussion

PERD — photoelectric registration device

PERF — peak expiratory flow rate

perf —
    perfect
    perforation

PERG — pattern electroretinogram

PERI —
    peritoneal fluid
    Psychiatric Epidemiology Research Interview

peri. — perineal

periap. — periapical

PERI/M — perimortem

perim. — perimeter

Perio
    periodontics
    periodontist

PERK — prospective evaluation of radial keratotomy [protocol]

PERL — pupils equal and reactive to light

PERLA — pupils equal and reactive to light and accommodation

perm. —
    permanent

perm. — (continued)
  permutation
per. op. emet. — *peracta operatione emetici* (Lat.) when the action of emetic is over
PEROX — peroxidase stain
perp. —
  perpendicular
  perpetrator
PERR — pattern-evoked retinal response
PERRLA — pupils equal, round, reactive to light and accommodation
PERRLA(DC) — pupils equal, round, reactive to light and accommodation (directly and consensually)
PERS — Patient Evaluation Rating Scale
pers. — personal
PERT — program evaluation and review technique
pert. — pertussis
PES —
  photoelectron spectroscopy
  physicians' equity services
  polyethylene sulfonate
  postextrasystolic
  pre-epiglottic space
  preexcitation syndrome
  primary empty sella [syndrome]
  programmed electrical stimulation
  pseudoexfoliative syndrome
Pes — esophageal pressure
PESP — postextrasystolic potentiation
peSPL — peak equivalent sound pressure level
Pess. — pessary
PEST — point estimation by sequential testing
PET —
  parent effectiveness training
  peak ejection time
  pear-shaped extension tube

PET — (continued)
  polyethylene tube
  poor exercise tolerance
  positron-emission tomography
  preeclamptic toxemia
  pressure-equalizing tube
  progressive exercise test
  Psychiatric Emergency Team
PETA — pentaerythritol triacrylate
PET_{CO_2} — end-tidal partial pressure of carbon dioxide
PETH — pink-eyed, tan-hooded [rat]
PETINIA — particle-enhanced turbidimetric inhibition immunoassay
PETN —
  pentaerythritol tetraniconitate
  pentaerythritol tetranitrate
petr. — petroleum
PETT —
  pendular eye-tracking test
  positron emission transaxial tomography
  positron emission transverse tomography
PEU —
  plasma equivalent unit
  polyether urethane
PEV —
  peak expiratory velocity
  pulmonary extravascular (fluid) volume
PeV — peripheral vein
peV — peak electron volt
PEVN — periventricular nucleus
PEW — pulmonary extravascular water
PEWV — pulmonary extravascular water volume
PEx — physical examination
PF —
  pair feeding
  parafascicular [nucleus]
  parallel fiber
  parotid fluid
  partially follicular
  patellofemoral [joint]

PF — (continued)
  peak factor
  peak flow
  perfusion fluid
  pericardial fluid
  peripheral field
  peritoneal fluid
  permeability factor
  personality factor
  phenol formaldehyde
  physicians' forum
  picture-frustration [study]
  plantar flexion
  plasma factor
  plasma fibronectin
  platelet factor
  pleural fluid
  posterior fontanelle
  power factor
  precursor fluid
  preservative-free
  primary fibrinolysin
  proflavin
  prostatic fluid
  protection factor
  pterygoid fossa
  pulmonary factor
  pulmonary function
  Purkinje fiber
  purpura fulminans
  push fluids
P-F — picture-frustration [test]
Pf —
  Pfeifferella
  Plasmodium falciparum
P_f — final pressure
PF_{1-4} — platelet factors 1 to 4
pF — picofarad
PFA —
  p-fluorophenylalanine
  phosphofructoaldolase
  phosphonoformic acid
  profunda femoris artery
PF3a — platelet factor 3 availability
PFAGH — penalty, frustration, anxiety, guilt, hostility
PFAS — performic acid–Schiff [reaction]

PFB —
  properdin factor B
  pseudofolliculitis barbae
PFC —
  pair-fed control [mice]
  pelvic flexion contracture
  perfluorocarbon
  pericardial fluid culture
  persistent fetal circulation
  plaque-forming cell(s)
pFc — noncovalently bonded dimer of the C-terminal immunoglobulin of the Fc fragment
PFCPH — persistent fetal circulation with pulmonary hypertension
PFD —
  polyostotic fibrous dysplasia
  primary flash distillate
PFDA — perfluoro-*n*-decanoic acid
PFEAAC — posterior fossa extraaxial arachnoid cyst
PFFD — proximal focal femoral deficiency
PFFFP — Pall-filtered fresh-frozen plasma
PFG — peak-flow gauge
PFGE — pulsed field gel electrophoresis
PFIB — perfluoroisobutylene
PFJS — patellofemoral joint syndrome
PFK — phosphofructokinase
PFKL — phosphofructokinase, liver type
PFKM — phosphofructokinase, muscle type
PFKP — phosphofructokinase, platelet type
PFL — profibrinolysin
PFM —
  peak flow meter
  porcelain fused to metal
PFN — partially functional neutrophil
PFO — patent foramen ovale
PFP —
  pentafluoropropionyl

PFP — *(continued)*
   peripheral facial paralysis
   platelet-free plasma
   preceding foreperiod
PFPS — patellofemoral pain syndrome
PFQ — personality factor questionnaire
PFR —
   parotid flow rate
   peak filling rate
   peak flow rate
   pericardial friction rub
   pulmonary flow rate
PFRC —
   plasma-free red cell
   predicted functional residual capacity
PFS —
   penile flow study
   primary fibromyalgia syndrome
   protein-free supernatant
   pulmonary function score
PFST — positional feedback stimulation trainer
PFT —
   pancreatic function test
   parafascicular thalamotomy
   posterior fossa tumor
   pulmonary function test
PFT$_4$ — proportion-free thyroxine
PFTBE — progressive form of tick-borne encephalitis
PFU —
   plaque-forming unit
   pock-forming unit
PFUO — prolonged fever of unknown origin
PFV — physiological full value
PFW — peak flow whistle
PG —
   paralysie générale (Fr.) general paralysis
   parapsoriasis guttata
   paregoric
   parental guidance
   parotid gland

PG — *(continued)*
   pentagastrin
   pepsinogen
   peptidoglycan
   pergolide
   Pharmacopoeia Germanica
   phosphate glutamate
   phosphatidylglycerol
   phosphatidyl glycine
   6-phosphogluconate
   phosphoglycerate
   pigment granule
   pituitary gonadotropin
   plasma gastrin
   plasma glucose
   plasma triglyceride
   polygalacturonate
   postgraduate
   postgraft
   pregnanediol glucuronide
   pregnant
   progesterone
   propylene glycol
   prostaglandin
   proteoglycan
   pyoderma gangrenosum
P$_G$ — plasma glucose
Pg —
   gastric pressure
   pogonion
   pregnancy
   pregnant
   pregnenolone
pg —
   page
   picogram
   pregnant
PGA —
   pepsinogen A
   phosphoglyceric acid
   polyglandular autoimmune [syndrome]
   polyglycolic acid
   prostaglandin A
   pteroylglutamic acid
PGA$_{1-3}$ — prostaglandins A$_1$ to A$_3$
3PGA — 3-phosphoglycerate
PGAC — phenylglycine acid chloride

PGAM — phosphoglycerate mutase
PGAS —
  persisting galactorrhea-amenorrhea syndrome
  polyglandular autoimmune syndrome
PGB — prostaglandin B
PGC —
  percentage of goblet cells
  primordial germ cell
  prostaglandin C
PGD —
  phosphogluconate dehydrogenase
  phosphogluconic dehydrogenase
  phosphoglyceraldehyde dehydrogenase
  prostaglandin D
PGD_2 — prostaglandin D_2
6-PDG — 6-phosphogluconate dehydrogenase
PGDF — Pilot Guide Dog Foundation
PGDH — phosphogluconate dehydrogenase
PGDR — plasma glucose disappearance rate
PGE —
  platelet granule extract
  posterior gastroenterostomy
  primary generalized epilepsy
  prostaglandin E
PGE_1, PGE_2 — prostaglandins E_1, E_2
PGEM — prostaglandin E metabolite
PGF —
  paternal grandfather
  prostaglandin F
PGF_1, PGF_2 — prostaglandins F_1, F_2
PGFM — prostaglandin F metabolite
PGFT — phosphoribosylglycinamide formyltransferase
PGG —
  polyclonal gamma globulin

PGG — (continued)
  prostaglandin G
PGG_2 — prostaglandin G_2
PGH —
  pituitary growth hormone
  plasma growth hormone
  porcine growth hormone
  prostaglandin H
PGH_2 — prostaglandin H_2
PGI —
  pepsinogen I
  phosphoglucose isomerase
  potassium, glucose, and insulin
  prostaglandin I
PGI_2 — prostaglandin I_2
PGK —
  phosphoglycerate kinase
  phosphoglycerokinase
PGL —
  persistent generalized lymphadenopathy
  phosphoglycolipid
PGlyM — phosphoglyceromutase
PGM —
  paternal grandmother
  phosphoglucomutase
PGMA — polyglycerol methacrylate
PGN — proliferative glomerulonephritis
PGO — ponto-geniculo-occipital [spike]
PGP —
  phosphoglyceryl phosphatase
  postgamma proteinuria
  prepaid group practice
  progressive general paralysis
PGR —
  progesterone receptor
  psychogalvanic response
PgR — progesterone receptor
P-GRN — progranulocyte
PGS —
  persistent gross splenomegaly
  pineal gonadal syndrome
  plant growth substance
  postsurgical gastroparesis syndrome

PGS — (continued)
  prostaglandin synthetase
  proteoglycan subunit
PGSI — prostaglandin synthetase
  inhibitor
PGSR — phosphogalvanic skin response
PGT — playgroup therapy
PGTR — plasma glucose tolerance
  rate
PGTT — prednisolone glucose tolerance test
PGU —
  peripheral glucose uptake
  postgonococcal urethritis
PGUT — phosphogalactose uridyl
  transferase
PGV — proximal gastric vagotomy
PGX — prostaglandin X
PGY — postgraduate year
PGYE — peptone, glucose, and
  yeast extract
PH —
  parathyroid hormone
  partial hepatectomy
  partial hysterectomy
  passive hemagglutination
  past history
  patient's history
  peliosis hepatitis
  perianal herpes
  persistent hepatitis
  personal history
  pharmacopeia
  phenethicillin
  phenyl
  phenylalanine hydroxylase
  physical history
  physically handicapped
  pinhole
  polycythemia hypertonica
  poor health
  porphyria hepatica
  porta hepatis
  posterior hypothalamus
  previous history
  primary hyperparathyroidism
  prolyl hydroxylase

PH — (continued)
  prostatic hypertrophy
  pseudohermaphroditism
  pubic hair
  public health
  pulmonary hypertension
  pulmonary hypoplasia
  punctate hemorrhage
  purpura hyperglobulinemia
Ph —
  Pharmacopeia
  phenanthrene
  phenyl
  Philadelphia [chromosome]
  phosphate
Ph^1 — Philadelphia chromosome
pH — hydrogen ion concentration
pH$_1$ — isoelectric point
ph —
  phase
  phial
  phot [unit of surface illumination]
  pinhole
PHA —
  passive hemagglutination
  passive hemagglutination(-inhibition) assay
  peripheral hyperalimentation
  phenylalanine
  phytohemagglutinin
  phytohemagglutinin activation
  phytohemagglutinin antigen
  pseudohypoaldosteronism
  pulse-height analyzer
pH$_A$ — arterial blood hydrogen
  tension
pHa — arterial pH
phaeo. — phaeochromocytoma
PHAL — phytohemagglutinin-stimulated lymphocyte
phal. —
  phalangeal
  phalanges
  phalanx
PHAlb — polymerized human albumin

PHA-LCM — phytohemaggluti-
    nin-stimulated leukocyte-con-
    ditioned medium
PHA-M — phytohemagglutinin M
PHA-m — phytohemagglutinin-
    mucopolysaccharide [fraction]
PHA-P — phytohemagglutinin-
    protein [fraction]
phar. —
    pharmaceutical
    pharmacology
    pharmacopeia
    pharmacy
    pharynx
Phar B — *Pharmaciae Baccalaureus*
    (Lat.) Bachelor of Pharmacy
Phar C — Pharmaceutical Chem-
    ist
Phar D — *Pharmaciae Doctor* (Lat.)
    Doctor of Pharmacy
Phar G — Graduate in Pharmacy
PHARM —
    pharmacist
    pharmacy
Phar M — *Pharmaciae Magister*
    (Lat.) Master of Pharmacy
pharm. —
    pharmaceutical
    pharmacist
    pharmacology
    pharmacopeia
    pharmacy
Pharm D — *Pharmaciae Doctor*
    (Lat.) Doctor of Pharmacy
PHB —
    polyhydroxybutyrate
    preventive health behavior
PhB — *Pharmacopoeia Britannica*
    (British Pharmacopoeia)
PHBB — propylhydroxybenzyl
    benzimidazole
PHC —
    personal health costs
    posthospital care
    premolar aplasia, hyper-
        hidrosis, and (premature)
        canities

PHC — *(continued)*
    premolar hypodontia, hyper-
        hidrosis, and canities pre-
        matura (Book syndrome)
    primary health care
    primary hepatic carcinoma
    primary hepatocellular carci-
        noma
    proliferative helper cell
PhC — pharmaceutical chemist
Ph¹c — Philadelphia chromosome
PHCC — primary hepatocellular
    carcinoma
PHD —
    pathological habit disorder
    photoelectron diffraction
    postheparin plasma diamine
        oxidase
    potentially harmful drug
    pulmonary heart disease
PhD —
    Pharmaciae Doctor (Lat.) Doc-
        tor of Pharmacy
    Philosophiae Doctor (Lat.) Doc-
        tor of Philosophy
PHDD — personal history of de-
    pressive disorders
PHDPE — porous high-density
    polyethylene
PHE —
    periodic health examination
    postheparin esterase
    proliferative hemorrhagic
        enteropathy
Phe — phenylalanine
PhEEM — photoemission electron
    microscopy
PHEN — phenotype
Phen. — phenformin
Pheno — phenobarbital
PHENOB — phenobarbital
phenobarb. — phenobarbital
PHENTH — phenothiazine
PHENYL — phenylpropranolol
Pheo — pheochromocytoma
PHF —
    paired helical filament
    personal hygiene facility

PHFG — primary human fetal glia

PHG — phosphatidylglycerol

PhG —
 Graduate in Pharmacy
 Pharmacopoeia Germanica
  (German Pharmacopeia)

phgly — phenylglycine

PHH — posthemorrhagic hydrocephalus

PHI —
 passive hemagglutination inhibition
 past history of illness
 peptide, histidine, isoleucine
 phosphohexose isomerase
 physiological hyaluronidase inhibitor
 prehospital index
 Public Health Inspector

PhI —
 Pharmacopoeia Internationalis

PHIM — posthypoxic intention myoclonus

PHIS —
 Physically Handicapped in Science
 posthead injury syndrome

PHK —
 platelet phosphohexokinase
 postmortem human kidney [cells]

PHKC — postmortem human kidney cell

PHLA — postheparin lipolytic activity

PHLS — Public Health Laboratory Service

PHM —
 peptide, histidine, methionine
 posterior hyaloid membrane
 psyllium hydrophilic mucilloid
 pulmonary hyaline membrane

PhM —
 Pharmaciae Magister (Lat.)
 Master of Pharmacy
 pharyngeal musculature

PHMDP — Pharmacist's Mate, Dental Prosthetic (Technician) [navy]

PhmG — Graduate in Pharmacy

PHN —
 paroxysmal nocturnal hemoglobinuria
 passive Heymann's nephritis
 postherpetic neuralgia
 public health nurse
 public health nursing

PHNO — 4-propyl-9-hydroxynaphthoxazine

PhNCS — phenyl isothiocyanate

PHO — public health official

PH_2O — partial pressure of water vapor

Phono — phonocardiogram

phos. —
 phosphatase
 phosphate
 phosphorus

PHOS-S — phosphorus spot

PHP —
 partial hospitalization program
 passive hyperpolarizing potential
 persistent hyperphenylalaninemia
 phosphorus
 postheparin phospholipase
 postheparin plasma
 prehospital program
 prepaid health plan
 primary hyperparathyroidism
 pseudohypoparathyroidism

PHPPA — *p*-hydroxyphenylpyruvic acid

p-HPPO — *p*-hydroxyphenyl pyruvate oxidase

PHPT —
 primary hyperparathyroidism
 pseudohypoparathyroidism

pHPT — primary hyperparathyroidism

PHPV — persistent hyperplastic primary vitreous

PHR —
    peak heart rate
    photoreactivity
PHS —
    patient-heated serum
    phenylalanine hydroxylase
        stimulator
    Physician's Health Study
    pooled human serum
    posthypnotic suggestion
    Public Health Service
PHSC — pluripotent hemopoietic
    stem cell
pH-stat — apparatus for main-
    taining the pH of a solution
PHT —
    peroxide hemolysis test
    phentolamine
    phenytoin
    portal hypertension
    primary hyperthyroidism
    pulmonary hypertension
PhTD — Doctor of Physical Ther-
    apy
PHTN — portal hypertension
PHTS — Psychiatric Home Treat-
    ment Service
PHV —
    peak height velocity
    persistent hypertrophic vitre-
        ous
    Prospect Hill virus
PHX — pulmonary histiocytosis X
PHx — past history
Phx — pharynx
PHY —
    pharyngitis
    physical
    physiology
    phytohemagglutinin
PHYS —
    physiological
    physiology
PhyS — physiologic saline [solu-
    tion]
phys. —
    physical
    physician

phys. — (continued)
    physiology
phys. dis. — physical disability
Phys Ed — physical education
physio. —
    physiologic
    physiology
    physiotherapist
    physiotherapy
Physiol. —
    physiological
    physiology
Phys Med — physical medicine
Phys Ther — physical therapy
PI —
    first meiotic prophase
    international protocol
    isoelectric point
    pacing impulse
    package insert
    pancreatic insufficiency
    parainfluenza
    paranoid ideation
    pars intermedia
    paternity index
    patient's interest
    performance index
    performance intensity
    perinatal injury
    periodontal index
    peripheral iridectomy
    permanent incidence
    permeability index
    personal injury
    personality inventory
    phagocytic index
    Pharmacopoeia Internationalis
    phosphatidylinositol
    physically impaired
    pineal body
    plaque index
    plasmin inhibitor
    pneumatosis intestinalis
    poison ivy
    ponderal index
    Porch Index
    postictal immobility
    postinfection

PI — *(continued)*
postinfluenza
postinjury
postinoculation
povidone-iodine
pregnancy-induced
preinduction [examination]
premature infant
prematurity index
preparatory interval
present illness
pressure on inspiration
primary infarction
primary infection
principal investigator
proactive inhibition
proactive interference
product information
programmed instruction
proinsulin
prolactin inhibitor
proliferation index
protamine insulin
protease inhibitor
Protocol Internationale
proximal intestine
psychiatric institute
pulmonary incompetence
pulmonary infarction
pulmonary insufficiency
pulsatility index

P_I — inspiratory pressure

P_i — inorganic phosphate

Pi —
parental generation
pressure of inspiration
protease inhibitor
pulmonary insufficiency

pI —
isoelectric point
platelet count increment

PIA —
peripheral interface adapter
phenylisopropyladenosine
photoelectronic intravenous
angiography
plasma insulin activity
porcine intestinal adeno-
matosis

PIA — *(continued)*
preinfarction angina
Psychiatric Institute of
America

PIAT — Peabody Individual
Achievement Test

PIAVA — polydactyly–imperforate
anus–vertebral anomalies [syn-
drome]

PIB —
partial ileal bypass
psi-interactive biomolecules

PIBC —
percutaneous intra-aortic balloon counterpulsation
peripherally inserted catheter

PIC —
Personality Inventory for
Children
polymorphism information
content
postinflammatory corticoid
postintercourse

PICA —
posterior inferior cerebellar
artery
posterior inferior communicating artery
posterior internal cerebral
artery

PICC — peripherally inserted central catheter

PICD — primary irritant contact
dermatitis

PICFS — postinfective chronic fatigue syndrome

PICSO — pressure-controlled
intermittent coronary sinus
occlusion

PICU —
pediatric intensive care unit
pulmonary intensive care unit

PID —
pain intensity difference
[score]
pelvic inflammatory disease
photoionization detector
plasma iron disappearance

PID — (continued)
    postinertia dyskinesia
    prolapsed intervertebral disk
    proportional–integral–
        derivative
    protruded intervertebral disk
PIDRA — portable insulin dosage-
    regulating apparatus
PIDS — primary immunodeficiency
    syndrome
PIDT — plasma iron disappearance
    time
PIE —
    postinfectious encephalomy-
        elitis
    preimplantation embryo
    prosthetic infectious endocar-
        ditis
    pulmonary infiltration with
        eosinophilia
    pulmonary interstitial edema
    pulmonary interstitial emphy-
        sema
PIEF — isoelectric focusing in poly-
    acrylamide
PIF —
    parotid isoelectric focusing
    peak inspiratory flow
    peak inspiratory force
    pigment inspiratory factor
    point of identical flow
    premorbid inferiority feeling
    proinsulin-free
    prolactin-inhibiting factor
    proliferation-inhibitory factor
    prostatic interstitial fluid
PIFG — poor intrauterine fetal
    growth
PIFR — peak inspiratory flow rate
PIFT — platelet immunofluores-
    cence test
PIG — pertussis immune globulin
PIGI — pregnancy-induced glucose
    intolerance
PIG-A — phosphatidylinositol gly-
    can class A
pigm. —
    pigment

pigm. — (continued)
    pigmented
PIGPA — pyruvate, inosine, glu-
    cose phosphate, adenine
PIH —
    periventricular-intraven-
        tricular hemorrhage
    phenyl isopropylhydrazine
    pregnancy-induced hyperten-
        sion
    prolactin-inhibiting hormone
PIHH — postinfluenza-like
    hyposmia and hypogeusia
PII —
    plasma inorganic iodine
    primary irritation index
PIIP — portable insulin infusion
    pump
PIIS — posterior inferior iliac
    spine
PIL — patient information leaflet
pil. —
    pilula (Lat.) pill
    pilulae (Lat.) pills
PILBD — paucity of interlobular
    bile ducts
PIM — penicillamine-induced my-
    asthenia
PIMS — programmable implant-
    able medication system
PIN — product identification num-
    ber
ping. — *pinguis* (Lat.) fat, grease
PINN — proposed international
    nonproprietary name
PINS — person in need of supervi-
    sion
PINV — postimperative negative
    variation
PIO — progesterone in oil
PIO_2 —
    inspired oxygen tension
    intra-alveolar oxygen tension
    partial pressure of inspired ox-
        ygen
PION — posterior ischemic optic
    neuropathy
PIP —
    paralytic infantile paralysis

PIP — (continued)
  peak inflation pressure
  peak inspiratory pressure
  personal injury protection
  phosphatidylinositol-4-
    phosphate
  piperacillin
  posterior interphalangeal
    [joint]
  postinflammatory polyposis
  postinfusion phlebitis
  postinspiratory pressure
  pressure inversion point
  probable intrauterine preg-
    nancy
  proximal interphalangeal
    [joint]
  psychosis, intermittent hypo-
    natremia, polydipsia [syn-
    drome]
  Psychotic Inpatient Profile
PIP_2 — phosphatidylinositol 4,5-bi-
    phosphate
PIPA — platelet ^{125}I-labeled (staph-
    ylococcal) protein A
PI-PB — performance versus inten-
    sity function for phonetically
    balanced words
PIPE — persistent interstitial pul-
    monary emphysema
PIPIDA — paraisopropylimino-
    diacetic acid [scan]
PIPJ — proximal interphalangeal
    joint
PIQ — Performance Intelligence
    Quotient
PIR —
  piriform
  postinhibition rebound
PIRI — plasma immunoreactive
    insulin
P-IRI — plasma immunoreactive
    insulin
PIRS — plasma immunoreactive
    secretion
PIS —
  preinfarction syndrome
  primary immunodeficiency
    syndrome

PIS — (continued)
  Provisional International
    Standard
pIs — isoelectric point
PISA — phase-invariant signature
    algorithm
PISCES — percutaneously inserted
    spinal cord electrical stimula-
    tion
PIT —
  pacing-induced tachycardia
  patellar inhibition test
  perceived illness threat
  picture identification test
  Pitocin
  Pitressin
  plasma iron turnover
pit. — pituitary
PITC — phenylisothiocyanate
PITP — pseudoidiopathic throm-
    bocytopenic purpura
PITR — plasma iron turnover rate
PITS — parent-infant traumatic
    stress
PIU — polymerase-inducing unit
PIV —
  parainfluenza virus
  peripheral intravenous [line]
  polydactyly–imperforate anus–
    vertebral anomalies [syn-
    drome]
PIVD — protruded intervertebral
    disk
PIVH —
  peripheral intravenous hyper-
    alimentation
  periventricular-intraventric-
    ular hemorrhage
PIVKA — protein induced by vita-
    min K absence or antagonism
PIWT — partially impacted wis-
    dom tooth
PIXE —
  particle-induced x-ray emis-
    sion
  proton-induced x-ray emission
pixel — picture element
PJ —
  pancreatic juice

PJ — *(continued)*
   Peutz-Jeghers [syndrome]
PJB — premature junctional beat
PJC — premature junctional contractions
PJP — pancreatic juice protein
PJRT — permanent junctional reciprocating tachycardia
PJS —
   peritoneojugular shunt
   Peutz-Jeghers syndrome
PJT — paroxysmal junctional tachycardia
PJVT — paroxysmal junctional-ventricular tachycardia
PK —
   pack [cigarette]
   penetrating keratoplasty
   pericardial knock
   pharmacokinetics
   pig kidney
   Prausnitz-Küstner [reaction]
   protein kinase
   psychokinesis
   pyruvate kinase
P_K — plasma potassium
pK —
   ionization constant of acid
   negative logarithm of the dissociation constant
pK' — negative logarithm of the dissociation constant of an acid
pK_a — negative logarithm of the acid ionization constant
pk — peck
PKA —
   prekallikrein activator
   prokininogenase
pKa — measure of acid strength
PKAR — protein kinase activation ratio
PKase — protein kinase
PKB — prone knee bend
PKC — protein kinase C
PKD —
   polycystic kidney disease

PKD — *(continued)*
   proliferative kidney disease
PKF — phagocytosis and killing function
PKI — potato kallikrein inhibitor
PKK —
   plasma prekallikrein
   prekallikrein
PKN — parkinsonism
PKP — penetrating keratoplasty
PKR —
   phased knee rehabilitation
   Prausnitz-Küstner reaction
PKT — Prausnitz-Küstner test
PKU — phenylketonuria
PKV — killed poliomyelitis vaccine
pkV — peak kilovoltage
PL —
   palm leaf reaction
   palmaris longus
   pancreatic lipase
   perception of light
   peroneus longus
   phospholipase
   phospholipid
   photoluminescence
   place
   placebo
   placental lactogen
   plantar
   plasmalemma
   plastic surgeon
   plastic surgery
   platelet
   platelet lactogen
   plural
   polarized light
   polymer of lactic (acid)
   posterior lip [of acetabulum]
   preleukemia platelet
   premature labor
   problem list
   procaine and lactic (acid)
   prolymphocytic leukemia
   psychosocial-labile
   pulpolingual
   Purkinje's layer

PL/1 — programming language 1
PL/I — programming language I
P$_L$ —
  pulmonary venous pressure
  transpulmonary pressure
Pl —
  plasma
  Plasmodium
  poiseuille
pl —
  picoliter
  place
  placenta
  plasma
  plastic surgery
  plate
  platelet
  pleural
  plural
PLA —
  peripheral laser angioplasty
  peroxidase-labeled antibody
    [test]
  phenyl lactate
  phospholipase A
  phospholipid antibody
  placebo therapy
  plasminogen activator
  platelet antigen
  potentially lethal arrhythmia
  procaine/lactic acid
  pulpolabial
  pulpolinguoaxial
P$_{LA}$ — left atrial pressure
PLA$_2$ — phospholipase A$_2$
PLa — pulpolabial
Pla — left atrial pressure
plant.-flex. — plantar flexion
PLAP — placental alkaline phosphatase
Plat. — platelet
PLAX — parasternal long axis
PLB —
  parietal lobe battery
  phospholipase B
  porous layer bead
PLBO — placebo
PLC —
  personal locus of control

PLC — (*continued*)
  phospholipase C
  primary liver cancer
  primary liver cell
  proinsulin-like component
  proinsulin-like compound
  protein-lipid complex
  pseudolymphocytic chorio-
    meningitis
PLCC — primary liver cell cancer
PLCL — polyclonal
PL-CLP — platelet clumps
PLCO — postoperative low cardiac
  output
PLD —
  peripheral light detection
  phospholipase D
  platelet defect
  polycystic liver disease
  posterior latissimus dorsi [mus-
    cle]
  postlaser day
  potentially lethal damage
  pregnancy, labor, and delivery
PLDD — poorly differentiated
  lymphoma, diffuse
PLDH — plasma lactic (acid) dehydrogenase
PLDR — potentially lethal damage
  repair
PL DYL — Placidyl
PLE —
  panlobular emphysema
  paraneoplastic limbic enceph-
    alopathy
  pleura
  polymorphous light eruption
  protein-losing enteropathy
  pseudolupus erythematosus
    [syndrome]
PLED — periodic lateralized epileptiform discharge
PLES — parallel-line equal spac-
  ing
PLET — polymyxin, lysozyme,
  EDTA, and thallous acetate
  [in heart infusion agar]
PLEU — pleural [fluid]

PLEVA — pityriasis lichenoides et varioliformis acuta

PLF —
    perilymphatic fistula
    posterior lung fiber

PLFC — premature living female child

PLFS — perilymphatic fistula syndrome

PLG —
    plasminogen
    L-propyl-L-leucyl-glucinamide

P-LGV — psittacosis–lymphogranuloma venereum

PLH —
    paroxysmal localized hyperhidrosis
    placental lactogenic hormone

PLI — professional liability insurance

PLIF — posterior lumbar interbody fusion

PLISSIT — permission, limited information, specific suggestions, intensive therapy

PLL —
    peripheral light loss
    poly-L-lysine
    posterior longitudinal ligament
    pressure-length loop
    prolymphocytic leukemia

PLM —
    percentage of labeled mitoses
    periodic leg movement
    plasma level monitoring
    polarized light microscopy

PLMC — premature living male child

PLMT — plasmacytoid lymphocyte

PLMV — posterior-leaf mitral valve

PLN —
    pelvic lymph node
    peripheral lymph node
    popliteal lymph node
    posterior lip nerve

PLND — pelvic lymph node dissection

PLO — polycystic lipomembranous osteodysplasia

PLP —
    paraformaldehyde–lysine–periodate
    phospholipid
    plasma leukapheresis
    polypeptide
    polystyrene latex particles
    pyridoxal phosphate

PLPD — pseudoperiodic lateralized paroxysmal discharge

PLR —
    pronation–lateral rotation [fracture]
    pupillary light reflex

PLS —
    Papillon-Lefèvre syndrome
    plastic surgery
    polydactyly-luxation syndrome
    preleukemic syndrome
    Preschool Language Scale
    primary lateral sclerosis
    prostaglandin-like substance
    pulmonary leukostasis syndrome

PLSO — posterior leafspring orthosis

PLT —
    pancreatic lymphocytic infiltration
    platelet [count]
    primed lymphocyte test
    primed lymphocyte typing
    psittacosis–lymphogranuloma venereum–trachoma [group]

Plt. — platelet

PLT EST — platelet estimate

PLT-G — giant platelet

plumb. — *plumbum* (Lat.) lead

PLUT — Plutchnik [geriatric rating scale]

PLV —
    poliomyelitis live vaccine
    panleukopenia virus
    phenylalanine, lysine, and vasopressin

PLV — (*continued*)
   posterior left ventricle
PLWS — Prader-Labhart-Willi syndrome
plx. — plexus
PLYM — prolymphocyte
PLZ — phenelzine
PM —
   after noon
   mean pressure
   pacemaker
   papilla mammae
   papillary muscle
   papular mucinosis
   paromomycin
   partially muscular
   partial meniscectomy
   perinatal mortality
   peritoneal macrophage
   petit mal (Fr.) little sickness
      (petit mal epilepsy)
   photomultiplier [tube]
   physical medicine
   plasma membrane
   platelet membrane
   platelet microsome
   pneumomediastinum
   poliomyelitis
   polymorph
   polymorphonuclear
   polymyositis
   poor metabolizer
   porokeratosis of Mibelli
   posterior mitral [valve]
   postmenopausal
   postmenstrual
   post meridiem (Lat.) after
      noon
   post mortem (Lat.) after death
   premarketing [approval]
   premenstrual
   premolar
   presents mainly
   presystolic murmur
   pretibial myxedema
   preventive medicine
   primary motivation
   prostatic massage

PM — (*continued*)
   protein methylesterase
   protocol management
   pterygoid muscle
   pubertal macromastia
   pulmonary macrophage
   pulpomesial
P/M — parent/metabolite ratio
Pm — promethium
pM — picomolar
pm — picometer
πm — pi meson
p.m. — *post meridiem* (Lat.) after
   noon
PMA —
   papillary gingiva, marginal
      gingiva, attached gingiva
      [index of prevalence and severity of gingivitis]
   para-methoxyamphetamine
   Pharmaceutical Manufacturers
      Association
   phenylmercuric acetate
   phorbol myristate acetate
   phosphomolybdic acid
   premarket approval
   premenstrual asthma
   Primary Mental Abilities
      [test]
   Prinzmetal's angina
   progressive muscular atrophy
   psychomotor agitation
   pyridylmercuric acetate
PMAC — phenylmercuric acetate
PMax — peak inspiratory pressure
PMB —
   papillomacular bundle
   parahydroxymercuribenzoate
   polychrome methylene blue
   polymorphonuclear basophil
      [leukocytes]
   polymyxin B
   postmenopausal bleeding
PMC —
   phenylmercuric chloride
   physical medicine clinic
   pleural mesothelial cell
   pleural mesothelial click

PMC — *(continued)*
    premature mitral closure
    pseudomembranous colitis
PMCP — para-monochlorophenol
PMD —
    perceptual motor development
    posterior mandibular depth
    primary myocardial disease
    private medical doctor
    programmed multiple development
    progressive muscular dystrophy
PM/DM — polymyositis/dermatomyositis
PMDS —
    persistent müllerian duct syndrome
    primary myelodysplastic syndrome
PME —
    polymorphonuclear eosinophil [leukocytes]
    postmenopausal estrogen
    progressive myoclonic epilepsy
PMEA — 9-(2-phosphomethoxyethyl)adenine
PMEC — pseudomembranous enterocolitis
PMF —
    progressive massive fibrosis
    proton motive force
    pterygomaxillary fossa
pmf — proton motive force
PMGCT — primary mediastinal germ-cell tumor
PMH —
    past medical history
    posteromedial hypothalamus
    programmed medical history
PMHR — predicted maximum heart rate
PMHx — past medical history
PMI —
    past medical illness
    patient medical instructions

PMI — *(continued)*
    patient medication instruction
    perioperative myocardial infarction
    phosphomannose isomerase
    plea of mental incompetence
    point of maximal impulse
    point of maximal intensity
    posterior myocardial infarction
    postmyocardial infarction
    present medical illness
    previous medical illness
PMIS —
    postmyocardial infarction syndrome
    PSRO (Professional Standards Review Organization) Management Information System
PMK —
    pacemaker
    primary monkey kidney
PML —
    polymorphonuclear leukocyte
    posterior mitral (valve) leaflet
    progressive multifocal leukodystrophy
    progressive multifocal leukoencephalopathy
    prolapsing mitral leaflet
    promyelocytic leukemia
    pulmonary microlithiasis
pML — posterior mitral (valve) leaflet
PMLE — polymorphous light eruption
PMM —
    pentamethylmelamine
    protoplast maintenance medium
PMMA — polymethyl-methacrylate
PMMF — pectoralis major myocutaneous flap
PMN —
    polymorphonuclear neutrophil [leukocytes]

PMN — (continued)
  polymorphonucleotide
PMNC —
  percentage of multinucleated
    cells
  peripheral blood mononuclear
    cell
  polymorphonuclear cells
PMNG — polymorphonuclear
  granulocyte
PMNL —
  polymorphonuclear leukocyte
PMNN — polymorphonuclear neutrophil
PMNR — periadenitis mucosa ne-
  crotica recurrens
PMO —
  postmenopausal osteoporosis
  Principal Medical Officer
pmol — picomole
P-MONO — promonocytes
PMP —
  pain management program
  past menstrual period
  patient management problem
  patient management program
  patient medication profile
  persistent mentoposterior [fe-
    tal position]
  previous menstrual period
  prior menstrual period
  psychotropic medication plan
PMPO — postmenopausal palpable
  ovary
PMPS — postmastectomy pain syndrome
PMQ — phytylmenaquinone
PMR —
  perinatal morbidity rate
  perinatal mortality rate
  periodic medical review
  physical medicine and rehabil-
    itation
  polymorphic reticulosis
  polymyalgia rheumatica
  posteromedial release
  prior medical record
  proportionate morbidity ratio

PMR — (continued)
  proportionate mortality ratio
  proton magnetic resonance
  psychomotor retardation
PM&R — physical medicine and
  rehabilitation
PMRAFNS — Princess Mary's
  Royal Air Force Nursing Service
PMRS — physical medicine and rehabilitation service
PMS —
  patient management system
  perimenstrual syndrome
  periodic movements during
    sleep
  phenazine methosulfate
  poor miserable soul
  postmarketing surveillance
  postmenopausal syndrome
  postmenstrual stress
  postmitochondrial superna-
    tant
  pregnant mare serum
  premenstrual symptoms
  premenstrual syndrome
  psychotic motor syndrome
  pureed, mechanical, soft [diet]
PMSC — pluripotent myeloid stem
  cell
PMSF — phenylmethylsulfonyl
  fluoride
PMSG — pregnant mare serum gonadotropin
PMT —
  phenol O-methyltransferase
  photoelectric multiplier tube
  photomultiplier tube
  Porteus maze test
  premenstrual tension
  pyridoxyl-methyltryptophan
PMTS — premenstrual tension
  syndrome
PMTT — pulmonary mean transit
  time
PMV —
  paralyzed and mechanically
    ventilated

PMV — (*continued*)
    paramyxovirus
    percutaneous mitral (balloon) valvotomy
    prolapse of mitral valve
PMVL — posterior mitral valve leaflet
PMW — pacemaker wires
PMZ — pentamethylenetetrazol
PN —
    papillary necrosis
    parenteral nutrition
    pavor nocturnus (Lat.) nightmare
    penicillin
    perceived noise
    percussion note
    percutaneous nephrostogram
    periarteritis nodosa
    peripheral nerve
    peripheral neuropathy
    peripheral node
    phrenic nerve
    plaque neutralization
    pneumonia
    polyarteritis nodosa
    polynephritis
    polyneuritis
    polyneuropathy
    polynuclear
    pontine nucleus
    poorly nourished
    positional nystagmus
    posterior nares
    postnasal
    postnatal
    practical nurse
    predicted normal
    premamillary nucleus
    preemie nipple
    primary nurse
    progress note
    propoxyphene napsylate
    protease nexin
    psychiatry and neurology
    psychoneurologist
    psychoneurotic
    pyelonephritis

PN — (*continued*)
    pyridine nucleotide
    pyrrolinitrin
P/N — positive/negative
P&N — psychiatry and neurology
P_{N2} — partial pressure of nitrogen
Pn —
    pneumatic
    pneumonia
pn — pain
PNA —
    Paris Nomina Anatomica
    peanut agglutinin
    pediatric nurse associate
    pentosenucleic acid
P_{Na} — plasma sodium
PNAB — percutaneous needle aspiration biopsy
PNAH — polynuclear aromatic hydrocarbon
PNAS — prudent no-salt-added [diet]
PNAvQ — positive-negative ambivalent quotient
PNB —
    percutaneous needle biopsy
    perineal needle biopsy
    p-nitrobiphenyl
    polymyxin, neomycin, bacitracin
    premature newborn
    premature nodal beat
    prostatic needle biopsy
PNBT — *p*-nitroblue tetrazolium
PNC —
    paranasal cancer
    penicillin
    peripheral nerve conduction
    peripheral nucleated cell
    pneumotaxic center
    postnecrotic cirrhosis
    premature nodal contracture
    prenatal care
    prenatal clinic
    prenodal contraction
    pseudonurse cells
    purine nucleotide cycle
PND —
    paroxysmal nocturnal dyspnea

PND — (continued)
    partial neck dissection
    pelvic node dissection
    postnasal drainage
    postnasal drip
    postneonatal death
    pregnancy, not delivered
    principal neutralizing determinant
    purulent nasal drainage
pnd. — pound
PNdb — perceived noise decibel
PNE —
    peripheral neuroepithelioma
    plasma norepinephrine
    pneumoencephalography
    practical nurse education
    pseudomembranous necrotizing enterocolitis
PNET —
    permeative neuroectodermal tumor
    primitive neuroectodermal tumor
PNET-MB — permeative neuroectodermal tumor–medulloblastoma
pneu. — pneumonia
PNF —
    prenatal fluoride
    proprioceptive neuromuscular fasciculation
PNG — penicillin G
PNH —
    paroxysmal nocturnal hemoglobinuria
    polynuclear hydrocarbon
PNHA — Physicians National Housestaff Association
PNI —
    peripheral nerve injury
    postnatal infection
    prognostic nutrition index
    pseudoneointimal
    psychoneuroimmunology
PNID — Peer Nomination Inventory for Depression
PNK — polynucleotide kinase

PNL —
    percutaneous nephrostolithotomy
    peripheral nerve lesion
    polymorphonuclear neutrophilic leukocyte
PNLA — percutaneous needle lung aspiration
PNM —
    perinatal mortality
    peripheral dysostosis, nasal hypoplasia, and mental retardation [syndrome]
    peripheral nerve myelin
    pneumonia
    postneonatal mortality
PNMG — persistent neonatal myasthenia gravis
PNMR — postnatal mortality risk
PNMT — phenylethanolamine-N-methyltransferase
PNO — Principal Nursing Officer
PNP —
    pancreatic polypeptide
    para-nitrophenol
    para-nitrophenyl
    peak negative pressure
    Pediatric Nurse Practitioner
    peripheral neuropathy
    platelet neutralization procedure
    pneumoperitoneum
    polyneuropathy
    progressive nuclear palsy
    psychogenic nocturnal polydipsia
    purine nucleoside phosphorylase
P-NP — para-nitrophenol
PNPase — polynucleotide phosphorylase
PNPB — positive-negative–pressure breathing
PNPG — para-nitrophenyl-β-galactoside
pNPP — para-nitrophenylphosphate
PNPR — positive-negative–pressure respiration

PNPS — para-nitrophenylsulfate

PNRS — premature nursery

PNS —
    paraneoplastic syndrome
    parasympathetic nervous system
    partial nonprogressive stroke
    peripheral nerve stimulation
    peripheral nervous system
    posterior nasal spine
    practical nursing student

PNSS — Pediatric Nutrition Surveillance System

PNT —
    partial nodular transformation
    patient
    percutaneous nephrostomy tube

Pnt — patient

PNU — protein nitrogen unit

PNV — prenatal vitamins

Pnx —
    pneumonectomy
    pneumothorax

PNZ — posterior necrotic zone

PO —
    parapineal organ
    parietal operculum
    parieto-occipital
    partial pressure of oxygen
    perceptual organization
    period of onset
    perioperative
    per os (Lat.) by mouth, orally
    phone order
    physician only
    posterior
    postoperative
    predominant organism

P/O —
    oxidative phosphorylation [ratio]
    phone order
    protein to osmolar [ratio]

P-O — postoperative

P&O — parasites and ova

PO_2 — partial pressure of oxygen

Po —
    polonium

Po — (continued)
    porion
    position response
    progesterone

p.o. — per os (Lat.) by mouth

POA —
    pancreatic oncofetal antigen
    phalangeal osteoarthritis
    point of application
    preoptic area
    primary optic atrophy

POAG — primary open-angle glaucoma

POA-HA — preoptic anterior hypothalamic area

POB —
    penicillin, oil, beeswax
    phenoxybenzamine
    place of birth
    prevention of blindness

POBE — Profile of Out-of-Body Experiences

POC —
    particulate organic carbon
    postoperative care
    probability of chance
    products of conception
    purgeable organic carbon

Po/C — ocular pressure

pocill. — pocillum (Lat.) small cup

pocul. — poculum (Lat.) cup

POCY — postoperative chronologic year

POD —
    pacing on demand
    peroxidase
    place of death
    podiatry
    polycystic ovary disease
    postoperative day
    postovulatory day

Pod. — podiatry

Pod D — Doctor of Podiatry

PODx — preoperative diagnosis

POE —
    pediatric orthopedic examination
    point of entry

POE — (continued)
   polyoxyethylene
   position of ease
   postoperative endophthalmitis
   postoperative exercise
   proof of eligibility
POEMS — polyneuropathy, organ-
      omegaly, endocrinopathy, M
      protein, skin changes [syn-
      drome]
POET — pulse oximeter/end tidal
POEx — postoperative exercise
POF —
   position of function
   premature ovarian failure
   primary ovarian failure
   pyruvate oxidation factor
PofE — portal of entry
POG —
   Pediatric Oncology Group
   polymyositis ossificans genera-
      lisata
   products of gestation
Pog — pogonion
pOH — hydroxide ion concentra-
      tion in a solution
POHI — physically or otherwise
      health-impaired
POHS — presumed ocular histo-
      plasmosis syndrome
POI —
   Personal Orientation Inven-
      tory
   poison
poik. —
   poikilocyte
   poikilocytosis
POIS — Parkland On-Line Infor-
      mation Systems
pois. —
   poison
   poisoned
   poisoning
POL — premature onset of labor
pol. —
   polish
   polishing
polio — poliomyelitis

poll. — pollex (Lat.) inch
POLY —
   polymorphonuclear
   polymorphonuclear leukocyte
Poly — polymorphonuclear
poly —
   polydipsia
   polymorphonuclear leukocyte
   polymorphonuclear neutro-
      philic granulocyte
   polyphagia
   polyuria
poly-A, poly(A) — polyadenylic
      acid
POLYC — polychromasia
poly-C, poly(C) — polycytidylic
      acid
POLY-CHR — polychromatophilia
poly-G, poly(G) — polyguanylic
      acid
poly-I, poly(I) — polyinosinic acid
poly-IC, poly-I:C —
   copolymer of polyinosinic and
      polycytidylic acids
   synthetic RNA polymer
% POLYS — percent of polymor-
      phonuclear leukocytes
polys (segs) — polymorphonuclear
      segmented neutrophils
poly-T, poly(T) — polythymidylic
      acid
poly-U, poly(U) — polyuridylic
      acid
POM —
   pain on motion
   polyoximethylene
   prescription only medicine
POMC — pro-opiomelanocortin
POMP — principal outer material
      protein
POMR — problem-oriented medi-
      cal record
POMS — Profile of Mood States
PON —
   paraxonase
   particulate organic nitrogen
pond. —
   pondere (Lat.) by weight

pond. — (continued)
　　ponderosus (Lat.) heavy
PONI — postoperative narcotic infusion
POOH — postoperative open-heart [surgery]
POP —
　　diphosphate group
　　pain on palpation
　　paroxypropione
　　persistent occipitoposterior [fetal position]
　　pituitary opioid peptide
　　plasma oncotic pressure
　　plasma osmotic pressure
　　plaster of Paris
　　polymyositis ossificans progressiva
　　popliteal
　　postoperative
POp — postoperative
Pop. —
　　popliteal
　　population
poplit. — popliteal
POPOP — 1,4-bis(5-phenyl-oxazol-2-yl) benzene
POR —
　　physician of record
　　postocclusive oscillatory response
　　prevalence odds ratio
　　problem-oriented record
PORH —
　　postocclusive reactive hyperemia
　　postoperative reactive hyperemia
PORP — partial ossicular replacement prosthesis
Porph. — porphyrins
PORT —
　　Patient Outcome Research Team
　　perioperative respiratory therapy
　　postoperative respiratory therapy

port. — portable
POS —
　　parosteal osteosarcoma
　　periosteal osteosarcoma
　　polycystic ovary syndrome
　　positive
　　psycho-organic syndrome
pos. —
　　position
　　positive
POSC — problem-oriented system of charting
POSCH — Program on the Surgical Control of the Hyperlipidemias [study]
POSG — after glucose infusion started
POSM — patient-operated selector mechanism
Posmo — osmotic permeability
pos. pr. — positive pressure
POSS —
　　percutaneous on-surface stimulation
　　proximal over-shoulder strap
poss. — possible
POSSUM — Pictures of Standard Syndromes and Undiagnosed Malformations
post. —
　　posterior
　　postmortem
post cib. —
　　post cibos (Lat.) after meals
　　post cibum (Lat.) after food
postgangl. — postganglionic
post-op — postoperative
post prand. — *post prandium* (Lat.) after dinner
POSTS — positive occipital sharp transients of sleep
post. sag. d. — posterior sagittal diameter
post sing. sed. liq. — *post singulas sedes liquidas* (Lat.) after every loose stool
POT —
　　periostitis ossificans toxica

POT — (continued)
  postoperative treatment
  potential
  purulent otitis [media]
pot —
  potash
  potassa
  potassium
  potential
  potion
pot. — potus (Lat.) a drink
PotAGT — potential abnormality
  of glucose tolerance
potass. — potassium
poten. — potential
POU — placenta, ovary, and
  uterus
PoV — portal vein
POVT — puerperal ovarian vein
  thrombophlebitis
POW — Powassan [encephalitis]
powd. — powder
POX — point of exit
POX-AC — pox battery, acute
PP —
  diphosphate group
  pacesetter potential
  palmoplantar
  pancreatic polypeptide
  paradoxical pulse
  parietal pleura
  partial pressure
  pathology point
  pedal pulse
  pellagra preventive
  pentose pathway
  perfusion pressure
  peripheral pulse
  peritoneal pseudomyxoma
  permanent partial [denture]
  persisting proteinuria
  Peyer's patches
  phosphorylase phosphatase
  "pink puffer" [emphysema]
  pinpoint
  pinprick
  placental protein
  placenta previa

PP — (continued)
  plane polarization
  Planned Parenthood
  plasma pepsinogen
  plasmapheresis
  plasma protein
  plaster of Paris
  plethysmograph pressure
  polypeptide
  polypropylene
  polystyrene (agglutination)
    plate
  poor person
  population planning
  porcine pancreatic
  posterior papillary
  posterior pituitary
  postpartum
  postprandial
  precocious puberty
  preferred provider
  presenting part
  primipara
  private patient
  private practice
  proactivator plasminogen
  prothrombin-proconvertin
  protoporphyria
  protoporphyrin
  proximal phalanx
  pseudomyxoma peritonei
  pterygoid process
  pulmonary pressure
  pulse pressure
  pulsus paradoxus
  punctum proximum (Lat.) near
    point [of accommodation]
  purulent pericarditis
  push pills
  pyrophosphate
P-P — prothrombin-proconvertin
P&P —
  pins and plaster
  policy and procedure
  prothrombin and procon-
    vertin [test]
PP_1 — free pyrophosphate
PP5 — placental protein 5

P-5'-P — pyridoxal-5'-phosphate
pp —
    polyphosphate
    postpartum
    postpill [amenorrhea]
    postprandial
    private patient
p̄p̄ — postprandial
p.p. — *punctum proximum* (Lat.)
    near point of accommodation
PPA —
    palpation, percussion, auscultation
    pepsin A
    phenylpropanolamine
    phenylpyruvic acid
    phiala prius agitata (Lat.) the
        vial having first been well
        shaken
    Pittsburgh pneumonia agent
    polyphosphoric acid
    Population Planning Associates
    postpartum amenorrhea
    postpill amenorrhea
    pure pulmonary atresia
PP&A — palpation, percussion,
    and auscultation
PPA — pulmonary arterial pressure
p.p.a. — *phiala prius agitata* (Lat.)
    the vial having first been well
    shaken
PPA pos. — phenylpyruvic acid–
    positive
PPAS — peripheral pulmonary artery stenosis
Ppaw —
    pulmonary artery wedge pressure
PPB —
    platelet-poor blood
    pneumococcal pneumonia
        and bacteremia
    positive-pressure breathing
PPb — postparotid basic protein
ppb — parts per billion
PPBE —
    postpartum breast engorgement

PPBE — *(continued)*
    protease-peptone beef extract
PPBS — postprandial blood sugar
PPC —
    pentose phosphate cycle
    peripheral posterior curve
    plasma prothrombin conversion
    plaster of Paris cast
    pneumopericardium
    pooled platelet concentrate
    progressive patient care
    proximal palmar crease
PPCA —
    plasma prothrombin conversion accelerator
    proserum prothrombin conversion accelerator
PPCD — polymorphous posterior
    corneal dystrophy
PPCE — postproline cleaving enzyme
PPCF —
    peripartum cardiac failure
    plasma prothrombin conversion factor
PPCH — piperazinylmethyl cyclohexanone
PPCM — postpartum cardiomyopathy
P&P/CT — prothrombin and proconvertin control
PPD —
    packs per day [cigarettes]
    paraphenylenediamine
    percussion and postural drainage
    permanent partial disability
    phenyldiphenyloxadiazole
    posterior polymorphous dystrophy
    postpartum day
    primary physical dependence
    progressive perceptive deafness
    purified protein derivative
    (Siebert) purified protein derivative [of tuberculin]

P&PD — percussion and postural drainage

ppd. — prepared

PPD-B — purified protein derivative–Battey

PPDR — preproliferative diabetic retinopathy

PPDS — phonologic programming deficit syndrome

PPD-S — purified protein derivative–standard

PPE —
palmoplantar erythrodysesthesia
partial plasma exchange
permeable pulmonary edema
personal protective equipment
polyphosphoric ester
porcine pancreatic elastase
programmed physical examination

PPES — palmar-plantar erythrodysesthesia syndrome

PPF —
pellagra preventive factor
phagocytosis-promoting factor
phosphonoformate
plasma protein fraction
prostacyclin production-stimulating factor
purified protein fraction

PPFA — Planned Parenthood Federation of America

PPG —
pediatric pneumogram
photoplethysmography
polymorphonuclear (cells) per glomerulus
polyurethane-polyvinyl graphite
postprandial glucose
pretragal parotid gland
protoporphyrinogen

ppg — picopicogram

PPGA — postpill galactorrhea-amenorrhea

PPGF — polypeptide growth factor

PPGI — psychophysiologic gastrointestinal [reaction]

PPGP — prepaid group practice

ppGpp — 3'-pyrophosphoryl-guanosine-5'-diphosphate

PPH —
past pertinent history
persistent pulmonary hypertension
postpartum hemorrhage
primary pulmonary hypertension
protocollagen proline hydroxylase

pphm — parts per hundred million

PPHN — persistent pulmonary hypertension of the neonate

PPHP — pseudopseudohypoparathyroidism

ppht — parts per hundred thousand

PPHx — previous psychiatric history

PPI —
partial permanent impairment
patient package insert
plan-position-indication
preceding preparatory interval
present pain intensity
purified porcine insulin

PPi — inorganic pyrophosphate

PP_i — inorganic pyrophosphate

PPID — peak pain intensity difference [score]

PPIE — prolonged postictal encephalopathy

PPIM — postperinatal infant mortality

PPK —
palmoplantar keratosis
partial penetrating keratoplasty

PPL —
pars plana lensectomy
penicilloyl polylysine
phospholipid
protein polysaccharide

Ppl — intrapleural pressure

PPLF — postperfusion low flow

PPLO — pleuropneumonia-like organism

PPM —
> permanent pacemaker
> phosphopentomutase
> pigmented pupillary membrane
> posterior papillary muscle

ppm —
> parts per million
> pulses per minute

PPMA —
> postpoliomyelitis muscular atrophy
> progressive postmyelitis muscular atrophy

PPMD — posterior polymorphous dystrophy [of cornea]

PPMM — postpolycythemia myeloid metaplasia

PPMS — psychophysiologic musculoskeletal [reaction]

PPN —
> partial parenteral nutrition
> pedunculopontine nucleus
> peripheral parenteral nutrition

PPNA — peak phrenic nerve activity

PPNAD — primary pigmented nodular adrenocortical disease

PPNG — penicillinase-producing *Neisseria gonorrhoeae*

PPO —
> diphenyloxazole
> peak pepsin output
> platelet peroxidase
> pleuropneumonia organism
> Preferred Provider Organization

PPP —
> palatopharyngoplasty
> palmoplantar pustulosis
> passage, power, and passenger [evaluation of labor progress]
> pedal pulse present
> pentose phosphate pathway
> peripheral pulse palpable
> Pickford's projective pictures

PPP — (*continued*)
> plasma protamine precipitating
> platelet-poor plasma
> polyphoretic phosphate
> porcine pancreatic polypeptide
> portal perfusion pressure
> postpartum psychosis
> protamine paracoagulation phenomenon
> purified placental protein
> pustulosis palmaris et plantaris

PPPBL — peripheral pulses palpable, both legs

PPPG — postprandial plasma glucose

PPPH — purified placental protein, human

PPPI —
> primary private practice income
> primary private practice insurance

PPPPP — pain, pallor, pulse loss, paresthesia, paralysis

PPR —
> patient progress record
> photopalpebral reflex
> patient-physician relation
> poor partial response
> posterior primary ramus
> Price precipitation reaction

PPr — paraprosthetic

PPRC — Physician Payment Review Commission

PPRF —
> paramedian pontine reticular formation
> postpartum renal failure

PPROM — prolonged premature rupture of membranes

PPRP — phosphoribosyl pyrophosphate

PPRWP — poor precordial R-wave progression

PPS —
> peripheral pulmonary stenosis

PPS — (continued)
  Personal Preference Scale
  phosphoribosylpyrophosphate
    synthetase
  polyvalent pneumococcal
    polysaccharide
  popliteal pterygium syndrome
  postpartum sterilization
  postperfusion syndrome
  postpericardiotomy syndrome
  postpolio syndrome
  postpump syndrome
  Prausnitz-Küstner sclerosis
  primary acquired preleukemic
    syndrome
  prospective payment sys-
    tem
  prospective pricing system
  protein plasma substitute
  pulse per second
PPSB — prothrombin, procon-
    vertin, Stuart factor, antihe-
    mophilic B factor
PPSH — pseudovaginal perineo-
    scrotal hypospadias
PPT —
  parietal pleural tissue
  partial prothrombin time
  peak-to-peak threshold
  plant protease test
  polypurine tract
  postpartum thyroiditis
  potassium phosphotungstate
  pulmonary platelet trapping
Ppt —
  parts per trillion
  precipitate
  precipitation
  prepared
ppt. — praeparatus (Lat.) prepared
pptd. — precipitated
PPTL — postpartum tubal ligation
pptn. — precipitation
PPTT — postpartum painless thy-
    roiditis (with transient) thyro-
    toxicosis
PPU — perforated peptic ulcer

PPV —
  pneumococcal polysaccharide
    vaccine
  porcine parvovirus
  positive predictive value
  positive-pressure ventilation
  progressive pneumonia virus
  pulmonary plasma volume
PPVr — regional pulmonary
    plasma volume
PPVT — Peabody Picture Vocabu-
    lary Test
PPVT-R — Peabody Picture Vocab-
    ulary Test, Revised
Ppw — pulmonary wedge pressure
PPY — pancreatic polypeptide
PPZ — perphenazine
PPZ SO — perphenazine sulfoxide
PQ —
  paraquat
  permeability quotient
  physician's questionnaire
  plastoquinone
  pronator quadratus
  pyrimethamine-quinine
PQD — protocol data query
PQNS — protein quantity not suf-
    ficient
PR —
  palindromic rheumatism
  Panama red [variety of
    marijuana]
  parallax and refraction
  pars recta
  partial recanalization
  partial reinforcement
  partial remission
  partial response
  patient relations
  peer review
  pelvic rock
  percentile rank
  perfusion rate
  peripheral resistance
  per rectum (Lat.) by way of
    the rectum
  phenol red

PR — (continued)
  photoreaction
  photoreactivation
  physical rehabilitation
  physician reviewer
  pityriasis rosea
  polymyalgia rheumatica
  posterior repair
  posterior root
  postmyalgia rheumatica
  postural reflex
  potency ratio
  potential relation
  predicted rate
  preference record
  pregnancy
  pregnancy rate
  premature
  preretinal
  presbyopia
  pressoreceptor
  pressure
  prevention
  Preyer's reflex
  proctologist
  proctology
  production rate
  professional relations
  profile
  progesterone receptor
  progressive relaxation
  progressive resistance
  progress report
  prolactin
  prolonged remission
  propicillin
  propranolol
  prosthetic group–removing
  prosthion
  protein
  psychotherapy responder
  public relations
  pulmonary regurgitation
  pulmonary rehabilitation
  pulmonic regurgitation
  pulse rate
  pulse repetition

PR — (continued)
  punctum remotum (Lat.) far
    point [of accommodation]
  pyramidal response
P/R — productivity to respiration
    [ratio]
P-R — the time between the P
    wave and the beginning of
    the QRS complex in electro-
    cardiography [interval]
P&R —
  pelvic and rectal [examination]
  pulse and respiration
Pr —
  praseodymium
  prednisolone
  premature
  presbyopia
  presentation
  pressure
  primary
  prism
  proctologist
  production rate [of steroid
    hormones]
  prolactin
  propyl
  protein
pr — pair
p.r. —
  per rectum (Lat.) by way of
    the rectum
  punctum remotum (Lat.) far
    point [of accommodation]
PRA —
  panel-reactive antibody
  phonation, respiration, articu-
    lation-resonance
  phosphoribosylamine
  physician recognition award
  plasma renin activity
  progesterone receptor assay
prac —
  practice
  practitioner
pract —
  practical

pract — *(continued)*
    practice
    practitioner
PrA-HPA — protein A hemolytic
    plaque assay
prand. — *prandium* (Lat.) dinner
PRAS —
    prereduced anaerobically steri-
        lized [medium]
    pseudo-renal artery syndrome
PRAT — platelet radioactive anti-
    globulin test
p. rat. aetat. — *pro ratione aetatis*
    (Lat.) in proportion to age
PRB —
    Personal Reaction Blank [psy-
        chiatry]
    Population Reference Bureau
    Prosthetics Research Board
PRBC —
    packed red blood cells
    placental residual blood cells
PRBV — placental residual blood
    volume
PRC —
    packed red cells
    peer review committee
    phase response curve
    plasma renin concentration
    professional review committee
PRCA —
    pure red cell agenesis
    pure red cell aplasia
PRD —
    partial reaction of degenera-
        tion
    phosphate-restricted diet
    polycystic renal disease
    postradiation dysplasia
PRE —
    passive resistance exercise
    photoreacting enzyme
    photoreactivity
    physical reconditioning exer-
        cise
    pigmented retinal epithelium
    progressive resistive exercise

pre — preliminary
pre-AIDS — pre-acquired immune
    deficiency syndrome
p. rec. — *per rectum* (Lat.) by way
    of the rectum
precip. —
    precipitate
    precipitated
    precipitation
PRED — prednisone
PreD$_3$ — previtamin D$_3$
pred. — predicted
PREE — partial reinforcement of
    extinction effect
prefd. — preferred
PREG — pregnenolone
preg —
    pregnancy
    pregnant
pregang — preganglionic
pregn —
    pregnancy
    pregnant
prelim. — preliminary
prelim. diag. — preliminary diagno-
    sis
prem. —
    premature
    prematurity
PRE MS — preoperative mental
    state
preop —
    preoperative
    preoperatively
pre-op —
    preoperative
    preoperatively
prep —
    preparation
    prepare
    preposition
prepd. — prepared [for surgery]
PRERLA — pupils round, equal,
    reactive to light, accommoda-
    tion
PREs — progressive resistive exer-
    cises

preserv. —
>   preservation
>   preserve
>   preserved

press. — pressure

prev. —
>   prevent
>   prevention
>   preventive
>   previous

PrevAGT — previous abnormality of glucose tolerance

PrevMed — preventive medicine

PREVMEDU — preventive medicine unit

PRF —
>   partial reinforcement
>   patient report form
>   plasma recognition factor
>   pontine reticular formation
>   progressive renal failure
>   prolactin-releasing factor
>   pyrogen-releasing factor

pRF — polyclonal rheumatoid factor

PRFA — plasma recognition factor activity

PRFM —
>   premature rupture of fetal membranes
>   prolonged rupture of fetal membranes

PRFN — percutaneous radiofrequency

PRFR — pressure-retaining, flow-relieving

PRG —
>   phleborheogram
>   phleborheography
>   purge

PRGI — percutaneous retrogasserian glycerol injection

PRGS — phosphoribosylglycineamide synthetase

PRH —
>   past relevant history
>   preretinal hemorrhage

PRH — (continued)
>   prolactin-releasing hormone

PRHBF — peak reactive hyperemia blood flow

PRI —
>   Pain Rating Index
>   phosphate reabsorption index
>   phosphoribose isomerase
>   plexus rectalis inferior
>   P-R interval

PRIAS — Packard's radioimmunoassay system

PRICES — protection, rest, ice, compression, elevation, support [first aid]

PRIH — prolactin release–inhibiting hormone

prim. — primary

PRIME — Prematriculation Program in Medical Education

PRIMEX — primary care extender

primip. — primipara

prim. luc. — *prima luce* (Lat.) at first light (early in the morning)

prim. m. — *primo mane* (Lat.) first thing in the morning

PRIMP — primipara

PRIND — prolonged reversible ischemic neurologic deficit

PRISM — Pediatric Risk of Mortality Score

PRIST —
>   paper radioimmunosorbent technique
>   paper radioimmunosorbent test

priv. — private

PRK —
>   photorefractive keratectomy
>   primary rabbit kidney

PRL — prolactin

Prl — prolactin

PRLA — pupils reactive to light and accommodation

PRM —
>   phosphoribomutase

PRM — *(continued)*
  photoreceptor membrane
  premature rupture of membranes
  preventive medicine
  Primary Reference Material
  primidone
PrM — preventive medicine
PRM-SDX — pyrimethamine sulfadoxine
PRM-SOX — pyrimethamine sulfadoxine
PRN — polyradiculoneuropathy
p.r.n. — *pro re nata* (Lat.) as required
PRNT — plaque reduction neutralization test
PRO —
  Peer Review Organization
  Professional Review Organization
  projection
  prolapse
  prolactin
  pronation
  protein
Pro —
  proline
  pronation
  prophylactic
  protein
  prothrombin
pro. — protein
prob. —
  probable
  probability
  problem
proc. —
  procedure
  proceedings
  process
Procarb. — procarbazine
proct —
  proctologist
  proctology
procto — proctoscopy

prod. —
  product
  production
pro dos. — *pro dose* (Lat.) for a dose
Pro El — protein electrophoresis
PROG —
  progesterone
  prognathism
  program
  progressive
prog. —
  progesterone
  prognathism
  prognosis
  program
  progress
  progressive
progn. — prognosis
progr. — progress
proj. — project
PROLAC — prolactin
prolong. —
  prolongation
  prolonged
PROM —
  passive range of motion
  premature rupture of (fetal) membranes
  programmable read-only memory
  prolonged rupture of (fetal) membranes
PROMIM — programmable multiple ion monitor
PROMIS — Problem-Oriented Medical Information System
PROMISE — Prospective Randomized Milrinone Survival Evaluation
Promy — promyelocyte
pron. —
  pronation
  pronator
PROP — propranolol
prop. —
  prophylactic

prop. — (continued)
   prophylaxis
ProPac — Prospective Payment Assessment Commission
proph. —
   prophylactic
   prophylaxis
prophy. —
   prophylactic
   prophylaxis
PROPLA — prophospholipase A
pro rat. aet. — pro ratione aetatis (Lat.) according to age
pro rect. — pro recto (Lat.) by rectum
pros. —
   prostate
   prostatic
   prosthetic
PROSO — protamine sulfate
prostat. —
   prostate
   prostatic
prosth. —
   prosthesis
   prosthetic
prot. — protein
PROTO — protoporphyrin
pro-UK — prourokinase
pro us. ext. — pro usum externum (Lat.) for external use
prov. — provisional
PROVIMI — proteins, vitamins, and minerals
prox. — proximal
PRO-XAN — protein-xanthophyll
prox. luc. — proxima luce (Lat.) the day before
PRP —
   panretinal photocoagulation
   penicillinase-resistant penicillin
   physiologic rest position
   pityriasis rubra pilaris
   platelet-rich plasma
   polymer of ribose phosphate
   polyribophosphate
   polyribosyl ribitol phosphate

PRP — (continued)
   postreplication repair
   postural rest position
   pressure rate product
   primary Raynaud's phenomenon
   problem-reporting program
   progressive rubella panencephalitis
   proliferative retinopathy photocoagulation
   Psychotic Reaction Profile
   pulse repetition frequency
PRPP — phosphoribosylpyrophosphate
PRR —
   proton relaxation rate
   pulse repetition rate
PrR — progesterone receptor
PRRE — pupils round, regular, and equal
PR-RSV — Prague (strain) Rous sarcoma virus
PRS —
   parent's rating scale
   Personality Rating Scale
   Pierre Robin syndrome
   plasma renin substrate
   positive rolandic spike
   pupil rating scale
PRSA — plasma renin substrate activity
PRSIS — Prospective Rate Setting Information System
PRSM — peripheral smear
PRSP — penicillinase-resistant synthetic penicillin
PRT —
   Penicillium roqueforti toxin
   pharmaceutical research and testing
   phosphoribosyltransferase
   photoradiation therapy
   postoperative respiratory therapy
   postoperative respiratory treatment

PRT — *(continued)*
    prospective randomized trial
PRTase — phosphoribosyltransferase
PRTH — prothrombin time
PRTH-C — prothrombin (time) control
PRU — peripheral resistance unit
PRV —
    polycythemia rubra vera
    pseudorabies virus
PRVEP — pattern reversal visual evoked potential
PRVR — peak-to-resting velocity ratio
PrVS — prevesical space
PRW — polymerized ragweed
PRWP — poor R-wave progression [electrocardiography]
PRX — pseudoexfoliation
Prx — prognosis
PRZ — prazepam
PRZF — pyrazofurin
PS —
    chloropicrin
    pacemaker syndrome
    paired stimulation
    paradoxical sleep
    paralaryngeal space
    paranoid schizophrenia
    paraspinal
    parasternal
    parasympathetic
    parotid sialography
    partial seizure
    partial shoulder
    pathological stage
    patient's serum
    pediatric surgery
    perceptual speed [test]
    performance status
    performing scale [I.Q.]
    periodic syndrome
    peripheral smear
    permeability surface
    pferdestärke
    phosphate saline [buffer]
    phosphatidylserine

PS — *(continued)*
    photosensitivity
    photosensitization
    photosynthesis
    photosystems
    phrenic (nerve) stimulation
    physical status
    physiologic saline
    pigeon serum
    plastic surgery
    point of symmetry
    polysaccharide
    polystyrene
    population sample
    Porter-Silber [chromogen]
    postmaturity syndrome
    power supply
    pregnancy serum
    prescription
    presenting symptom
    pressure support
    prestimulus
    principal sulcus
    programmed symbols
    prostatic secretion
    protamine sulfate
    protective services
    protein S
    protein synthesis
    Proteus syndrome
    psychiatric
    psychiatry
    pulmonary stenosis
    pulse sequence
    pyloric stenosis
P-S —
    pancreozymin-secretin
    Porter-Silber [chromogen]
    pyramid surface
P/S —
    polisher-stimulator
    polyunsaturated/saturated [fatty acid ratio]
P&S —
    pain and suffering
    paracentesis and suction
    permanent and stationary

P&S — *(continued)*
 pharmacy and supply
 physicians and surgeons
PS I–V — physical status patient
 classification [American Society of Anesthesiologists]
Ps —
 prescription
 pseudocyst
 Pseudomonas
 psoriasis
ps —
 per second
 picosecond
PSA —
 picryl sulfonic acid
 polyethylene sulfonic acid
 product selection allowed
 progressive spinal ataxia
 prolonged sleep apnea
 prostate-specific anticoagulation
 prostate-specific antigen
 psoriatic arthritis
PsA — psoriatic arthritis
Psa — systemic arterial blood pressure
PSAC — President's Science Advisory Committee
PSAD — psychoactive substance
 abuse and dependence
PSAGN — poststreptococcal acute
 glomerulonephritis
PSAn —
 psychoanalysis
 psychoanalyst
 psychoanalytic
PSAP —
 prostate-specific acid phosphatase
 pulmonary surfactant apoprotein
PSAX — parasternal short axis
PSB —
 phosphorus-solubilizing bacteria
 protected specimen brush

PSbetaG — pregnancy-specific
 beta-I-glycoprotein
PSBO — partial small bowel obstruction
PSC —
 partial subligamentous calcification
 patient services coordination
 physiologic squamocolumnar
 pluripotential stem cell
 Porter-Silber chromogen
 posterior semicircular canal
 posterior subcapsular cataract
 primary sclerosing cholangitis
 pulse-synchronized contractions
PSCC — posterior subcapsular cataract
PSCE — presurgical coagulation
 evaluation
PsChE — pseudocholinesterase
PSCI — Primary Self-Concept
 Inventory
Psci — pressure at slow component
 intercept
PSCM — pokeweed-activated
 spleen-conditioned medium
PSCP — posterior subcapsular cataractous plaque
PSCT — peripheral stem cell transplant
P/score — pressure score
PSD —
 particle size distribution
 peptone-starch-dextrose
 periodic synchronous discharge
 phosphate supplemental diet
 photon-stimulated desorption
 posterior sagittal diameter
 poststenotic dilation
 postsynaptic density
PSDES — primary symptomatic
 diffuse esophageal spasm
PSE —
 paradoxical systolic expansion
 partial splenic embolization

PSE — *(continued)*
   penicillin-sensitive enzyme
   point of subjective equality
   portal systemic encephalopathy
   postshunt encephalopathy
   Present State Examination
   purified spleen extract
PSEC — poststress ethanol consumption
psec — picosecond
PSF —
   peak scatter factor
   point spread function
   posterior spinal fusion
   pseudosarcomatous fasciitis
psf — pound per square foot
PSG —
   peak systolic gradient
   phosphate, saline, and glucose
   polysomnogram
   presystolic gallop
PSGN — poststreptococcal glomerulonephritis
PSH —
   postsurgical history
   postspinal headache
PsHD — pseudoheart disease
PSI —
   personal security index
   physiologic stability index
   posterior sagittal index
   posterior superior iliac [spine]
   problem-solving information
   prostaglandin synthetic inhibitor
   psychologic screening inventory
   psychosomatic inventory
psi — pounds per square inch
psia — pounds per square inch absolute
pSIDS — partially unexplained sudden infant death syndrome
PSIFT — platelet suspension immunofluorescence test
psig — pounds per square inch gauge

PSIL — preferred frequency speech interference level
PSIS —
   posterior sacroiliac spine
   posterior superior iliac spine
PSL —
   parasternal line
   percent stroke length
   potassium, sodium chloride, and sodium lactate [solution]
   prednisolone
PSLT — Picture-Story Language Test
PSM —
   pansystolic murmur
   presystolic murmur
PSMA —
   progressive spinal muscular atrophy
   proximal spinal muscular atrophy
PSMed — psychosomatic medicine
PSMF — protein-sparing modified fast
PSMT — psychiatric services management team
PSNS — parasympathetic nervous system
PSO —
   physostigmine salicylate ophthalmic
   proximal subungual onychomycosis
P sol — partly soluble
PSOR — psoralen
P/sore — pressure sore
PSP —
   pacesetter potential
   pancreatic spasmolytic peptide
   paralytic shellfish poisoning
   parathyroid secretory protein
   periodic short pulse
   Personal Security Preview
   phenolsulfonphthalein
   phosphoserine phosphatase

PSP — *(continued)*
    positive spike pattern
    posterior spinal process
    posterior subcapsular plaque
    postsynaptic potential
    prednisone sodium phosphate
    professional simulated patient
    progressive supranuclear palsy
    pseudopregnancy
PSPF — prostacyclin synthesis-
    stimulating plasma factor
PSQ —
    Parent Symptom Question-
        naire
    Patient Satisfaction Question-
        naire
PSR —
    pain sensitivity range
    percutaneous stereotactic ra-
        diofrequency rhizotomy
    portal systemic resistance
    problem status report
    proliferative sickle retinopa-
        thy
    pulmonary stretch receptor
PSRBOW — premature spontane-
    ous rupture of bag of waters
PSRC — Plastic Surgery Research
    Council
PSRO — Professional Standards
    Review Organization
PSS —
    painful shoulder syndrome
    physiological saline solution
    porcine stress syndrome
    primary Sjögren syndrome
    progressive systemic sclero-
        derma
    progressive systemic sclero-
        sis
    psoriasis severity scale
    Psychiatric Services Section
        [of American Hospital As-
        sociation]
    Psychiatric Status Schedule
    pure sensory stroke
pSS — primary Sjögren syndrome

PST —
    pancreatic suppression test
    paroxysmal supraventricular
        tachycardia
    Pascal-Suttle test
    penicillin, streptomycin, and
        tetracycline
    perceptual span time
    peristimulus time
    phenolsulfotransferase
    phonemic segmentation test
    platelet survival time
    poststenotic
    poststimulus time
    prefrontal sonic treatment
    protein-sparing therapy
    proximal straight tubule
Pst — static transpulmonary pres-
    sure
PSTH — poststimulus time histo-
    graph
PSTI — pancreatic secretory tryp-
    sin inhibitor
PSTP — pentasodium triphosphate
PstTLC/TLC — coefficient of lung
    retraction expressed per liter
    of total lung capacity
PSTV — potato spindle tuber vi-
    roid
P'STYL — Pronestyl
PSU —
    photosynthetic unit
    postsurgical unit
    primary sampling unit
P-SURG — presurgery coagulation
    profile
PSurg — plastic surgery
PSV —
    pressure-supported ventila-
        tion
    psychological, social, and vo-
        cational [adjustment fac-
        tors]
PSVER — pattern-shift visual
    evoked response
PSVT — paroxysmal supraventric-
    ular tachycardia

PSW —
  past sleepwalker
  primary surgical ward
  psychiatric social worker
PSWT — psychiatric social work
  training
PSX — pseudoexfoliation
Psy —
  psychiatry
  psychology
psych. —
  psychological
  psychology
PSYCHEM — psychiatric chemistry
psychiat. —
  psychiatric
  psychiatry
psycho — psychopath
psychoan. —
  psychoanalysis
  psychoanalytical
psychol. —
  psychological
  psychology
psychopath. —
  psychopathological
  psychopathology
psychophys —
  psychophysics
  psychophysiology
PsychosMed — psychosomatic
  medicine
psychosom. — psychosomatic
psychother. —
  psychotherapeutic
  psychotherapy
psy-path —
  psychopath
  psychopathic
psy-som — psychosomatic
Ps-ZES — pseudo-Zollinger-Ellison
  syndrome
PT —
  parathormone
  parathyroid
  paroxysmal tachycardia

PT — (continued)
  part time
  patient
  pericardial tamponade
  permanent and total
  pharmacy and therapeu-
    tics
  phenytoin
  phonation time
  photophobia
  phototoxicity
  physical therapist
  physical therapy
  physical training
  physiotherapy
  pine tar
  pint
  plasma thromboplastin
  pneumothorax
  polyvalent tolerance
  posterior tibial [artery pulse]
  post-tetanic
  post-transfusion
  post-transplantation
  post-traumatic
  premature termination [of
    pregnancy]
  preterm
  pronator teres
  propylthiouracil
  prothrombin time
  protriptyline
  psychotherapy
  pulmonary thrombosis
  pulmonary toilet
  pulmonary trunk
  pulmonary tuberculosis
  pure tone
  pyramidal tract
  temporal plane
P&T —
  paracentesis and tubing [of
    ears]
  peak and trough
  permanent and total [disabil-
    ity]
  pharmacy and therapeutics

Pt —
    patient
    platinum
    psychoasthenia
pt —
    part
    patient
    pint
    point
pt. — *perstetur* (Lat.) let it be continued
PTA —
    parallel tubular arrays
    parathyroid adenoma
    percutaneous transluminal angioplasty
    peroxidase-labeled antibody
    persistent trigeminal artery
    persistent truncus arteriosus
    phosphotungstic acid
    physical therapy assistant
    plasma thromboplastin antecedent
    platelet thromboplastin antecedent
    posterior tibial
    post-traumatic amnesia
    pretreatment anxiety
    prior to admission
    prior to arrival
    prothrombin activity
PT(A) —
    pure tone [average]
    pure tone acuity
PTAF — policy target adjustment factor
P-TAG — target-attaching globulin precursor
PTAH — phosphotungstic acid hematoxylin
PTAP — purified (diphtheria) toxoid (precipitated by) aluminum phosphate
p'tase — phosphatase
PTAT — pure tone average threshold
PTB —
    patellar tendon-bearing

PTB — *(continued)*
    prior to birth
    pulmonary tuberculosis
PTb — pulmonary tuberculosis
PTBA — percutaneous transluminal balloon angioplasty
PTBD —
    percutaneous transhepatic biliary drainage
    percutaneous transluminal balloon dilatation
PTBD-EF — percutaneous transhepatic biliary drainage–enteric feeding
PTBE — pyretic tick-borne encephalitis
PTBNA — protected transbronchial needle aspirate
PTBP — para-tertiary butylphenol
PTBPD — post-traumatic borderline personality disorder
PTBS — post-traumatic brain syndrome
PTC —
    patient to call
    percutaneous transhepatic cholangiogram
    percutaneous transhepatic cholangiography
    phase transfer catalyst
    phenothiocarbazine
    phenylthiocarbamide
    phenylthiocarbamoyl
    pheochromocytoma, thyroid carcinoma [syndrome]
    plasma thromboplastin component
    posterior trabeculae carneae
    premature tricuspid closure
    prior to conception
    prothrombin complex
    pseudotumor cerebri
PT-C — prothrombin time control
PTCA — percutaneous transluminal coronary angioplasty
PtcCO$_2$ — transcutaneous partial pressure of carbon dioxide
PTCER — pulmonary transcapillary escape rate

PTCL — peripheral T-cell lymphoma

PTcO$_2$ — transcutaneous oxygen tension

PTCP — pseudothrombocytopenia

PTCR — percutaneous transluminal coronary recanalization

PT-CT — prothrombin time control

PTD —
   para-toluenediamine
   percutaneous transluminal dilatation
   period to discharge
   permanent total disability
   personality trait disorder
   prior to delivery
   prior to discharge

Ptd — phosphatidyl

PtdCho — phosphatidylcholine

PtdEtn — phosphatidylethanolamine

PtdIns — phosphatidylinositol

PTDP — permanent transvenous demand pacemaker

PtdSer — phosphatidylserine

PTE —
   parathyroid extract
   peritumoral edema
   post-traumatic endophthalmitis
   post-traumatic epilepsy
   pretibial edema
   proximal tibial epiphysis
   pulmonary thromboembolism

PTED — pulmonary thromboembolic disease

pt. ed. — patient education

PteGlu — pteroylglutamic [acid]

PTEN — pentaerythritol tetranitrate

pter — end of short arm of chromosome

PTF —
   patient treatment file
   plasma thromboplastin factor
   proximal tubule fluid

PTFA — prothrombin time–fixing agent

PTFE — polytetrafluoroethylene

PTFS — post-traumatic fibromyalgia syndrome

PTG — parathyroid gland teniposide

PTGA — pteroyltriglutamic acid

PTH —
   parathormone
   parathyroid
   parathyroid hormone
   percutaneous transhepatic [drainage]
   phenylthiohydantoin
   plasma thromboplastin [component]
   post-transfusion hepatitis
   prior to hospitalization

pTH — primary thrombocythemia

PTHBD — percutaneous transhepatic biliary drainage

PTHC — percutaneous transhepatic cholangiography

PTHLP — parathyroid-hormone–like protein

PTHrP — parathyroid-hormone–related protein

PTHS — parathyroid hormone secretion [rate]

PTI —
   pancreatic trypsin inhibitor
   persistent tolerant infection
   Pictorial Test of Intelligence
   pressure time index
   pulsatility transmission index

PTJV — percutaneous transtracheal jet ventilation

PTL —
   Pentothal
   perinatal telencephalic leukoencephalopathy
   pharyngotracheal lumen
   plasma thyroxine level
   posterior tricuspid (valve) leaflet
   preterm labor
   protriptyline

PTLC — precipitation thin-layer chromatography

PTLD —
> post-transplantation lympho-
> proliferative disorder
> prescribed tumor lethal dose

PTM —
> posterior trabecular meshwork
> post-transfusion mononucleosis
> post-traumatic meningitis
> pressure time per minute
> preterm milk
> pulse time modulation

Ptm —
> pterygomaxillary [fissure]
> transmural pressure [airway, blood vessel]

PTMA — phenyltrimethylammo-
nium

PTMC — percutaneous transvenous mitral commissurotomy

PTMDF — pupils, tension, media, disc, fundus

PTN —
> pain transmission neuron
> posterior tibial nerve

pTNM — postsurgical tumor, nodes, metastases [staging of tumors]

PTO —
> *Perlsucht Tuberculin original*
> (Ger.) Klemperer's tubercu-
> lin
> percutaneous transhepatic
> obliteration
> personal time off
> please turn over

PTP —
> pancreatic thread protein
> percutaneous transhepatic por-
> tography
> posterior tibial pulse
> post-tetanic potential
> post-tetanic potentiation
> post-transfusion purpura
> prior to program
> prothrombin-proconvertin
> proximal tubular pressure

Ptp — transpulmonary pressure

PTPI — post-traumatic pulmonary insufficiency

PTPM — post-traumatic progressive myelopathy

PTPN — peripheral (vein) total parenteral nutrition

PTPS — post-thrombophlebitis syndrome

PTR —
> patellar tendon reflex
> patient termination record
> patient to return
> peripheral total resistance
> *Perlsucht Tuberculin Rest*
> (Ger.) tuberculin from *My-*
> *cobacterium tuberculosis bovis*
> plasma transfusion reaction
> prothrombin time ratio
> psychotic trigger reaction

PTr — porcine trypsin

PTRA — percutaneous transluminal renal angioplasty

PTRIA — polystyrene-tube radioimmunoassay

Ptrx — pelvic traction

PTS —
> painful tonic seizure
> para-toluenesulfonic [acid]
> patellar tendon socket
> patellar tendon suspension
> permanent threshold shift
> phosphotransferase system
> postthrombotic syndrome
> post-traumatic syndrome
> prior to surgery

Pts. — patients

pts. — patients

PTSD — post-traumatic stress disorder

PTSS — post-traumatic stress syndrome

PTT —
> partial thromboplastin time
> particle transport time
> patellar tendon transfer
> platelet transfusion therapy
> posterior tibial (tendon) trans-
> fer
> pulmonary transit time
> pulse transmission time

ptt — partial thromboplastin time
PTT-CT — partial thromboplastin time control
PTTH — prothoracicotropic hormone
PTU —
    pain treatment unit
    propylthiouracil
PTV — posterior tibial vein
PTWTKG — patient's weight in kilograms
PTX —
    parathyroidectomy
    pelvic traction
    pentoxifylline
    phototoxic reaction
    picrotoxinin
    pneumothorax
PTx —
    parathyroidectomy
    pelvic traction
PTXA — parathyroidectomy and autotransplantation
PTZ —
    pentamethylenetetrazole
    pentylenetetrazol
    phenothiazine
PU —
    palindromic unit
    passed urine
    paternal uncle
    pelvic-ureteric
    pepsin unit
    peptic ulcer
    per urethra (Lat.) by way of the urethra
    posterior urethra
    precursor uptake
    pregnancy urine
    6-propylthiouracil
    prostatic urethra
Pu —
    plutonium
    purine
    purple
    putrescine
pub. — public

publ. — public
PUBS —
    percutaneous umbilical blood sampling
    purple urine bag syndrome
PUC — pediatric urine collector
PUD —
    peptic ulcer disease
    pudendal
    pulmonary disease
PuD — pulmonary disease
PUE — pyrexia of unknown etiology
PUF — pure ultrafiltration
PUFA — polyunsaturated fatty acid
PUH — pregnancy urine hormones
PUI — platelet uptake index
PUL —
    percutaneous ultrasonic lithotripsy
    pulmonary
pul — pulmonary
pulm —
    pulmonary
    pulmonic
pulm. — *pulmentum* (Lat.) gruel
PULSES — (general) physical, upper extremities, lower extremities, sensory, excretory, social support [physical profile]
pulv. — *pulvis* (Lat.) powder
pulv. gros. — *pulvis grossus* (Lat.) coarse powder
pulv. subtil. — *pulvis subtilis* (Lat.) smooth powder
pulv. tenu. — *pulvis tenuis* (Lat.) very fine powder
PUM — peanut-reactive urinary mucin
PUMS — permanently unfit for military service
PUN — plasma urea nitrogen
punc. —
    puncture
    punctured
PUNL — percutaneous ultrasonic nephrolithotripsy

PUO —
>   pyrexia of undetermined origin
>
>   pyrexia of unknown origin

PUP — percutaneous ultrasonic pyelolithotomy

PU-PC — polyunsaturated phosphatidylcholine

PUPPP —
>   pruritic urticarial papules and plaques of pregnancy
>
>   pruritic urticarial papillary plaques of pregnancy

PUR — polyurethane

Pur. — purple

pur. — purulent

purg. — purgative

PUT —
>   provocative use test
>
>   putamen
>
>   putrescine

PUU — puumala [virus]

PUVA —
>   psoralen plus ultraviolet A
>
>   pulsed ultraviolet actinotherapy

PUVD — pulsed ultrasonic (blood) velocity detector

PUW — pick-up walker

PV —
>   pancreatic vein
>
>   papillomavirus
>
>   paraventricular
>
>   paravertebral
>
>   paromomycin-vancomycin
>
>   pemphigus vulgaris
>
>   peripheral vascular
>
>   peripheral vein
>
>   peripheral vessel
>
>   *per vaginam* (Lat.) through the vagina
>
>   phonation volume
>
>   photovoltaic
>
>   pinocytotic vesicle
>
>   pityriasis versicolor
>
>   plasma viscosity
>
>   plasma volume
>
>   pneumococcus vaccine

PV — *(continued)*
>   poliomyelitis vaccine
>
>   polio vaccine
>
>   polycythemia vera
>
>   polyoma virus
>
>   polyvinyl
>
>   popliteal vein
>
>   portal vein
>
>   postvasectomy
>
>   postvoiding
>
>   predictive value
>
>   pressure velocity
>
>   pressure-volume
>
>   process variable
>
>   pulmonary vein
>
>   pulmonic valve
>
>   pure vegetarian

P-V —
>   Panton-Valentine [leukocidin]
>
>   pressure-volume [curve]

P/V — pressure to volume [ratio]

P&V —
>   peak and valley
>
>   percuss and vibrate
>
>   pyloroplasty and vagotomy

Pv —
>   *Proteus vulgaris*
>
>   venous pressure

p.v. — *per vaginam* (Lat.) through the vagina

PVA —
>   partial villous atrophy
>
>   polyvinyl acetate
>
>   polyvinyl alcohol
>
>   Prinzmetal variant angina

PVAc — polyvinyl acetate

PVAS — postvasectomy

PVB —
>   paravertebral block
>
>   premature ventricular beat

PVBS — possible vertebral-basilar system

PVC —
>   persistent vaginal cornification
>
>   polyvinyl chloride
>
>   postvoiding cystogram
>
>   predicted vital capacity

PVC — (continued)

    premature ventricular complex

    premature ventricular contraction

    primary visual cortex

    pulmonary venous capillary

    pulmonary venous congestion

PVCM — paradoxical vocal cord motion

PV_{CO_2} — partial pressure of carbon dioxide in mixed venous blood

$PvCO_2$ — venous carbon dioxide pressure

PVD —

    parent very disturbed

    patient very disturbed

    percussion, vibration, and drainage

    peripheral vascular disease

    portal vein dilation

    posterior vitreous detachment

    postural vertical dimension

    postvagotomy diarrhea

    premature ventricular depolarization

    pulmonary vascular disease

PVE —

    perivenous encephalomyelitis

    periventricular echogenicity

    premature ventricular extrasystole

    prosthetic valve endocarditis

PVEP — pattern visual evoked potential

PVF —

    peripheral visual field

    portal venous flow

    posterior vitreous face

    primary ventricular fibrillation

PVFS — postviral fatigue syndrome

PVG —

    posterior ventricular guide

    pulmonary valve gradient

PVH —

    periventricular hemorrhage

PVH — (continued)

    preventricular hemorrhage

    pulmonary vascular hypertension

PVI —

    peripheral vascular insufficiency

    perivascular infiltration

    periventricular inhibitor

    personal values inhibitor

PVK — penicillin V potassium

PVL —

    perivalvular leakage

    periventricular leukomalacia

    permanent vision loss

P-VL — Panton-Valentine leukocidin

PVM —

    pneumonia virus of mice

    proteins, vitamins, and minerals

PvMed — preventive medicine

PVN —

    paraventricular nucleus

    predictive value of a negative [test]

PVNPS — post-Viet Nam psychiatric syndrome

PVNS — pigmented villonodular synovitis

PVO —

    peripheral vascular occlusion

    pulmonary venous obstruction

    pulmonary venous occlusion

Pv_{O_2} — partial oxygen pressure in mixed venous blood

PVOD —

    peripheral vascular obstructive disease

    pulmonary vascular obstructive disease

    pulmonary veno-occlusive disease

    pulmonary venous obstructive disease

PVP —

    penicillin V potassium

    peripheral vein plasma

PVP — (continued)
  peripheral venous pressure
  polyvinylpyrrolidone
  portal venous pressure
  posteroventral pallidotomy
  predictive value of a positive
    [test]
  pulmonary venous pressure
PVP-I — polyvinylpyrrolidone-
  iodine [povidone-iodine]
PVR —
  peripheral vascular resistance
  postvoid residual
  proliferative vitreoretinopathy
  pulmonary vascular resistance
  pulmonary venous redistribu-
    tion
  pulse-volume recording
PVRA — peripheral vein renin activity
PVRI — pulmonary vascular resistance index
PVS —
  paravesical space
  percussion, vibration, suction
  peripheral vascular surgery
  peritoneovenous shunt
  persistent vegetative state
  persistent viral syndrome
  pigmented villonodular syno-
    vitis
  plexus visibility score
  Plummer-Vinson syndrome
  poliovirus sensitivity
  poliovirus susceptibility
  polyvinyl sponge
  premature ventricular systole
  programmed ventricular stim-
    ulation
  pulmonary valvular stenosis
  pulmonary vein stenosis
  pulmonic valve stenosis
PVT —
  paroxysmal ventricular tachy-
    cardia
  physical volume test
  portal vein thrombosis
  pressure, volume, and temper-
    ature

PVT — (continued)
  private [patient]
pvt — private
PVW — posterior vaginal wall
PVY — potato virus Y
pvz — pulverization
PW —
  pacing wire
  patient waiting
  peristaltic wave
  plantar wart
  posterior wall [of the heart]
  Prader-Willi [syndrome]
  pressure wave
  psychological warfare
  pulmonary wedge [pressure]
  pulsed wave
  puncture wound
P-W — Prader-Willi [syndrome]
P&W — pressures and waves
Pw —
  progesterone withdrawal
  trans–thoracic wall pressure
PWA — person(s) with AIDS
PWB —
  partial weight-bearing
  psychologic well-being
PWBC — peripheral white blood
  cell
PWBRT — prophylactic whole
  brain radiation therapy
PWC —
  peak work capacity
  physical work capacity
PWCA — pure white cell aplasia
PWCR — Prader-Willi chromosome region
PWD —
  precipitated withdrawal diar-
    rhea
  pulsed-wave Doppler
pwd — powder
pwdr — powder
PWDS — postweaning diarrhea
  syndrome
PWE — posterior wall excursion
PWI — posterior wall infarct
PWLV — posterior wall of left ventricle

PWM — pokeweed mitogen
PWP — pulmonary wedge pressure
PWS —
    port wine stain
    Prader-Willi syndrome
    pulse-wave speed
pwt — pennyweight
PWV —
    peak weight velocity
    polistes wasp venom
    posterior wall velocity
    pulse wave velocity
PX —
    pancreatectomized
    peroxidase
    physical examination
Px —
    past history
    physical examination
    pneumothorax
    prognosis
PXA — pleomorphic xanthoastro-
    cytoma
PXE — pseudoxanthoma elasticum
PXM —
    projection x-ray microscopy
    pseudoexfoliation material
PXS — pseudoexfoliation syn-
    drome
PY —
    pack-year [cigarettes]
    person-year
Py —
    phosphopyridoxal
    polyoma [virus]
    pyrene
    pyridine
    pyridoxal
PYA — psychoanalysis
PyC — pyogenic culture

PYE — peptone-yeast extract
PYG — peptone-yeast extract–
    glucose [broth]
PYGM — peptone-yeast-glucose-
    maltose [broth]
PYLL — potential years of life lost
PYP — pyrophosphate
PYR — person-year rad
Pyr —
    pyridine
    pyruvate
PYRKIN — pyruvate kinase
PYKN — pyknocytes
Pyro — pyrophosphate
PyrP — pyridoxal phosphate
PYRUV — pyruvate
PYS — piriform sinus
PZ —
    pancreozymin
    peripheral zone
    prazosin
    pregnancy zone
    proliferative zone
Pz —
    parietal midline zero [elec-
    trode placement in electro-
    encephalography]
    4-phenylazobenzylylcarbonyl
    pièze
PZA — pyrazinamide
PzB — parenzyme, buccal
PZ-CCK — pancreozymin-
    cholecystokinin
PZD — piperazinedione
PZE — piezoelectric
PZI — protamine zinc insulin
PZP — pregnancy zone protein
PZQ — praziquantel
PZT — lead zirconate titanate

Q

Q —
   cardiac output
   coenzyme Q
   coulomb [electric quantity]
   electric charge
   enzyme
   1,4-glucan branching
   glutamine
   heat
   Quaalude
   qualitative
   quantitative
   quantity of electric charge
   quantity of heat
   quart
   quarter
   quartile
   Queensland [fever]
   query
   quest
   question
   quinacrine
   quinidine
   quinone
   quotient
   radiant energy
   reaction energy
   reaction quotient
   reactive power
   temperature coefficient
   ubiquinone
   volume of blood
Q — electric charge
   heat
   reaction quotient
$\dot{Q}$ —
   perfusion
   rate of blood flow
Q^0 — every hour
Q^1 — every hour around the clock
Q^2 — every two hours around the clock
Q-6 — ubiquinone-6

Q_6 — ubiquinone-6
Q-9 —
   ubichromanol-9
   ubichromenol-9
Q-10 — ubiquinone
Q_{10} —
   temperature coefficient
   ubiquinone
q —
   electric charge
   long arm of chromosome
   quant
   quantity
   quart
   quarter
   quintal
   ubiquinone
q. — *quaque* (Lat.) each, every
QA —
   quality assessment
   quality assurance
   quinaldic acid
   quinolinic acid
   quisqualic acid
QAC — quaternary ammonium compound
q.a.d. — *quaque altera die* (Lat.) every other day
QAF — quality adjustment factor
q.a.h. — *quaque altera hora* (Lat.) every other hour
QALE — quality-adjusted life expectancy
QALY — quality-adjusted life years
QAM — quality assurance monitor
q.a.m. — *quaque ante meridiem* (Lat.) every morning
q.a.n. — *quaque altera nocte* (Lat.) every other night
Q angle — quadriceps angle
QAP —
   quality assurance program
   quinine, Atabrine, and pamaquine

QAR —
  quality assurance reagent
  quantitative autoradiography
QA/RM — quality assurance/risk
  management
QAS — quality assurance standard
QAT — quality assurance technical
QAUR — quality assurance and
  utilization review
QB —
  quantitative battery
  whole blood
Q_B — total body clearance
QBC —
  qualitative buffy coat
  quantitative buffy coat
QBCA — quantitative buffy coat
  analysis
QBV — whole blood volume
QC —
  quality control
  quick catheter
  quinine-colchicine
Qc — pulmonary capillary blood
  flow
QCA — quantitative coronary angiography
QCD — quantum chromodynamics
Qcsf — rate of bulk flow of cerebrospinal fluid
QCIM — Quarterly Cumulative
  Index Medicus
QCO_2 — carbon dioxide evolution
  by a tissue
QCT — quantitative computed tomography
q.d. — *quaque die* (Lat.) every day
q.2d. — *quaque secunda die* (Lat.)
  every second day
QDPR — quinoid dehydropteri-
  dine reductase
q.d.s. — *quater die sumendum* (Lat.)
  to be taken four times a day
QEA — quick electrolyte analyzer
QED — quantum electrodynamics
q.e.d. — *quod erat demonstrandum*
  (Lat.) that which was to be
  demonstrated

QEE — quadriceps extension exercise
QEEG — quantitative electroencephalography
QEF — quail embryo fibroblasts
QEH — Queen Elizabeth's Hospital
QENF — quantifying examination
  of neurologic function
Q-enzyme — 1,4-alpha-glucan
  branching enzyme
QET — quality extinction test
QEW — quick early warning
QF —
  quality factor
  query fever (Q fever)
  quick freeze
  relative biological effectiveness
Q fever — query fever
Q fract. — quick fraction
$Q\text{-}H_2$ — ubihydroquinone
q.h. — *quaque hora* (Lat.) every
  hour
q.2h. — *quaque secunda hora* (Lat.)
  every two hours
q.3h. — *quaque tertia hora* (Lat.) every three hours
q.4h. — *quaque quarta hora* (Lat.)
  every four hours
q.h.s. — *quaque hora somni* (Lat.)
  every hour of sleep
q.i.d. — *quater in die* (Lat.) four
  times daily
QIG — quantitative immunoglobulin
QJ — quadriceps jerk
q.l. — *quantum libet* (Lat.) as much
  as desired
QLS — Quality of Life Scale
qlty — quality
QM — quinacrine mustard
q.m. — *quaque mane* (Lat.) every
  morning
QMI — Q-wave myocardial infarction
Q-M sign — Quénu-Muret sign
QMT — quantitative muscle test

QMWS — quasi-morphine withdrawal syndrome
q.n. — *quaque nocte* (Lat.) every
night
QNB — quinuclidinyl benzilate
QNCR — quantitative neutron
capture radiography
QNS — Queen's Nursing Sister
q.n.s. — *quantum non sufficiat*
(Lat.) quantity not sufficient
Qo — oxygen consumption
Q_{O_2} —
oxygen quotient
oxygen utilization
QOC — quality of contact
Q of C — quality of care
QP —
quadrant pain
qualified psychiatrist
quanti-Pirquet [reaction]
q.p. — *quantum placeat* (Lat.) as
much as desired
QPC —
quadrigeminal plate cistern
quality of patient care
Qpc — pulmonary capillary blood
flow
QPEEG — quantitative pharmaco-
electroencephalography
q.p.m. — *quaque post meridiem*
(Lat.) each evening
QPT — quick prothrombin time
QPVT — Quick Picture Vocabulary Test
q.q. — *quoque* (Lat.) each, every
q.q.d. — *quoque die* (Lat.) every
day
q.q.h. — *quaque quarta hora* (Lat.)
every four hours
q.q. hor. — *quaque hora* (Lat.) every hour
QR —
quadriradial
quality review
quick recovery
quiet room
quieting reflex
quieting response

QR — *(continued)*
quinaldine red
qr —
quadriradial
quarter
quarterly
q.r. — *quantum rectum* (Lat.) quantity is correct
QRB — Quality Review Bulletin
QRN — quasiresonant nucleus
QRZ — *Quaddel Reaktion Zeit*
(Ger.) wheal reaction time
QS —
quantity sufficient
quiet sleep
QS_2 — electromechanical systole
QS_2l — shortened electromechanical systole
Qs — systemic blood flow
q.s. —
quantum satis (Lat.) sufficient
quantity
quantum sufficit (Lat.) as
much as will suffice
q.s.ad — *quantum sufficiat ad* (Lat.)
sufficient quantity to make
QSAR — quantitative structure-
activity relationship
q. sat. — *quantum satis* (Lat.) to a
sufficient quantity
QSC — quasistatic compliance
Q sign — Quant's sign
QSPV — quasistatic pressure volume
Qsp — physiologic shunt flow
Qsrel — relative shunt flow
QSS — quantitative sacroiliac scintigraphy
QST — quantitative sensory test
Q-S test — Queckenstedt-Stookey
test
q. suff. — *quantum sufficit* (Lat.) as
much as will suffice
QT —
cardiac output
qualification test
Queckenstedt's test

QT — *(continued)*
  Quick's test
qt —
  quantitative
  quantity
  quart
  quiet
QTC — quantitative tip culture
qter — end of long arm of chromosome
qty. — quantity
quad —
  quadrant
  quadriceps
  quadrilateral
  quadriplegia
  quadriplegic
quad. atrophy — quadriceps atrophy
quad. ex. — quadriceps exercise
quadrupl. — *quadruplicato* (Lat.) four times as much
qual —
  qualitative
  quality
qual anal — qualitative analysis
quant —
  quantitative
  quantity
quant anal — quantitative analysis
quant suff — quantity sufficient
quar —
  quarantine
  quarterly
QUART — quadrantectomy, axillary dissection, and radiotherapy
quart — quarterly

quat — quaternary ammonium compound
quat. —
  quater in die (Lat.) four times a day
  quattuor (Lat.) four
quer — querulous
QUEST — Quality, Utilization, Effectiveness, Statistically Tabulated
quest —
  question
  questionable
QuF — Q (Queensland) fever
QUICHA — quantitative inhalation of challenge apparatus
quinq. — *quinque* (Lat.) five
QUINID — quinidine
QUININ — quinine
quint — quintuplet
quint. — *quintus* (Lat.) fifth
quor. — *quorum* (Lat.) of which
quot — quotient
quot. —
  quotidie (Lat.) daily
  quoties (Lat.) as often as necessary
quotid. — *quotidie* (Lat.) daily
quot. op. sit — *quoties opus sit* (Lat.) as often as you please
q.v. —
  quantum vis (Lat.) as much as you please
  quod vide (Lat.) which see
QW — quality of working life
QWL — quality of working life
QYD — Qi and Yin deficiency

R

R —
- arginine
- Behnken's unit
- Broadbent registration point
- gas constant
- organic radical
- race
- racemic
- radical
- radioactive mineral
- radiology
- radius
- ramus
- range
- Rankine [scale]
- rare
- rate
- ratio
- rational
- reaction
- Réaumur [scale]
- recessive
- rectal
- rectified
- rectum
- *rectus* (Lat.) right
- red
- reference
- regimen
- registered [trademark]
- regression coefficient
- regular
- regular insulin
- regulator [gene]
- *Reiz* (Ger.) stimulus
- rejection [factor]
- relapse
- relaxation
- release [factor]
- remission
- remote [point of convergence]
- *remotum* (Lat.) far point
- repressor
- resazurin

R — *(continued)*
- residue
- residuum
- resistance
- respiration
- respiratory exchange ratio
- response
- responder
- rest
- restricted
- reticulocyte
- reverse [banding]
- rhythm
- ribose
- right
- Rinne's [test]
- roentgen
- rough [colony]
- routine
- rub

P — rho (seventeenth letter of the Greek alphabet), uppercase

R. — *Rickettsia*

+R — Rinne's test positive

−R — Rinne's test negative

°R —
- degree on the Rankine scale
- degree on the Réaumur scale

Rx — *recipe* (Lat.) take

r —
- angle of refraction
- correlation coefficient
- distance radius
- drug resistance
- radius
- ratio
- recombinant
- regional
- reproductive potential
- ribose
- ribosomal
- ring chromosome
- sample correlation coefficient

ρ —
   correlation coefficient
   electric charge density
   electrical resistivity
   mass density
   reactivity
   rho (seventeenth letter of the
      Greek alphabet), lowercase
r^2 — coefficient of determination
RA —
   radioactive
   radionuclide angiography
   ragocyte
   ragweed antigen
   rapidly adapting [receptors]
   reciprocal asymmetrical
   refractory anemia
   refractory ascites
   renal artery
   renin activity
   renin-angiotensin
   repeat action
   residual air
   retinoic acid
   rheumatoid agglutinin
   rheumatoid arthritis
   rifampicin
   right angle
   right arm
   right atrial
   right atrium
   right auricle
   Rokintansky-Aschoff [sinus]
   room air
R_A — airway resistance
Ra —
   radical
   radium
   radius
   Rayleigh number
^{226}Ra — radioactive radium
rA — riboadenylate
RAA —
   renin-angiotensin-
      aldosterone [system]
   right atrial abnormality
   right atrial appendage
RAAMC — Royal Australian
   Army Medical Corps

RAAS — renin-angiotensin-
   aldosterone system
RAB —
   remote afterloading brachy-
      therapy
   Research Advisory Board
   rice, applesauce, and banana
      [diet]
Rab — rabbit
RABA — rabbit antibladder antibody
RABBI — Rapid Access Blood
   Bank Information
RABCA — rabbit antibladder cancer
RABG — room air blood gas
RAbody — right atrium body
RABP — retinoic acid–binding
   protein
RAC —
   radial artery catheter
   right atrial contraction
rac —
   racemate
   racemic
RACCO — right anterior caudo-
   cranial oblique
RACT — recalcified-activated
   clotting time
RAD —
   radial artery catheter
   radiation absorbed dose
   radical
   radiology
   reactive airways disease
   right anterior descending
   right atrium diameter
   right axis deviation
   roentgen administered dose
Rad. —
   radiologist
   radiology
   radiotherapist
   radiotherapy
   radium
rad —
   radial
   radian

rad — (continued)
    radiation-absorbed dose
    radiation-absorbed unit
    radical
    radiculitis
    radius
rad. — radix (Lat.) root
RADA —
    right acromiodorsoanterior
      [fetal position]
    rosin amine-D-acetate
RADC — Royal Army Dental
    Corps
RADCA — right anterior descend-
    ing coronary artery
RADIO — radiotherapy
radiol —
    radiologist
    radiology
RADISH — rheumatoid arthritis
    diffuse idiopathic skeletal hy-
    perostosis
RAD ISO VENO BILAT — radio-
    active isotopic venogram, bi-
    lateral
RADIUS — Routine Antenatal
    Diagnostic Imaging with Ul-
    trasound
RadLV — radiation leukemia virus
RADP — right acromiodorsopos-
    terior [fetal position]
RADS —
    reactive airways dysfunction
      syndrome
    retrospective assessment of
      drug safety
rad/s —
    rads per second
    radians per second
rad ther — radiation therapy
RADTS — rabbit anti-dog thymus
    serum
rad ul — radius-ulna
RAE — right atrial enlargement
RaE — rabbit erythrocyte
RAEB —
    refractive anemia, erythroblas-
    tic

RAEB — (continued)
    refractory anemia with excess
      blasts
RAEB-T — refractory anemia with
    excess blasts in transforma-
    tion
RAEM — refractory anemia with
    excess myeloblasts
RAF —
    repetitive atrial firing
    rheumatoid arthritis factor
RAFMS — Royal Air Force Medi-
    cal Services
RAG —
    ragweed
    room air gas
Ragg — rheumatoid agglutinin
RAH —
    regressing atypical histio-
      cytosis
    right anterior hemiblock
    right atrial hypertrophy
RAHO — rabbit antibody to hu-
    man ovary
RAHTG — rabbit antihuman thy-
    mocyte globulin
RAI —
    radioactive iodine
    resting ankle index
    right atrial involvement
RAID — radioimmunodetection
RAIS — reflection-absorption
    infrared spectroscopy
RAIU — radioactive iodine uptake
RAL — resorcylic acid lactone
RALPH — renal-anal-lung-
    polydactyly-hamartoblastoma
    [syndrome]
RALT —
    Riley Articulation and Lan-
      guage Test
    routine admission laboratory
      tests
RAM —
    radioactive material
    random-access memory
    rapid alternating movements
    rectus abdominis muscle

RAM — *(continued)*
    rectus abdominis myocutaneous [flap]
    Research Aviation Medicine
    right anterior measurement
RAMC — Royal Army Medical Corps
RAMI — Risk-adjusted Mortality Index
RAMP —
    radioactive antigen microprecipitin
    right atrial mean pressure
RAMT — rabbit antimouse thymocyte
RAN — resident's admission notes
RANA — rheumatoid arthritis nuclear antigen
rANP — rat atrial natriuretic peptide
RAO —
    right anterior oblique
    right anterior occipital
RaONC — radiation oncology
RAP —
    recurrent abdominal pain
    regression-associated protein
    renal artery pressure
    rheumatoid arthritis precipitin
    right atrial pressure
RAPD — relative afferent pupillary defect
RAPK — reticulate acropigmentation of Kitamura
RAPM — refractory anemia with partial myeloblastosis
RAPO — rabbit antibody to pig ovary
RAQ — right anterior quadrant
RAR —
    rat insulin receptor
    right arm reclining
    right arm recumbent
RARalpha — retinoic acid receptor–alpha
RARLS — rabbit antirat lymphocyte serum
RARS — refractory anemia with ringed sideroblasts

RARTS — rabbit antirat thymocyte serum
RAS —
    rapid atrial stimulation
    recurrent aphthous stomatitis
    reflex activating stimulus
    renal artery stenosis
    renin-angiotensin system
    reticular activating system
    rheumatoid arthritis serum
RA-S — refractory anemia with ringed sideroblasts
ras — retrovirus-associated DNA sequence
ras. — *rasurae* (Lat.) scrapings or filings
RASS — rheumatoid arthritis and Sjögren syndrome
RAST — radioallergosorbent test
RASV — recovered avian sarcoma virus
RAT —
    repeat action tablet
    rheumatoid arthritis test
    right anterior thigh
RATG — rabbit antithymocyte globulin
RATHAS — rat thymus antiserum
rAT-P — recombinant antitrypsin Pittsburgh
RATS — rabbit antithymocyte serum
RATx — radiation therapy
RAU — radioactive uptake
RAV — Rous-associated virus
RAVC —
    retrograde atrioventricular conduction
    Royal Army Veterinary Corps
RAVLT — Rey Auditory Verbal Learning Test
R_{aw} — airway resistance
RAZ — razoxane
RB —
    radiation burn
    Rating Board
    rebreathing
    Renaut body

RB — (continued)
  respiratory bronchiole
  respiratory burst
  reticulate body
  retinoblastoma
  retrobulbar
  right bundle
Rb —
  retinoblastoma
  rubidium
RBA —
  relative binding affinity
  rescue breathing apparatus
  right basilar artery
  right brachial artery
  rose bengal antigen
RBAF — rheumatoid biologically active factor
RBAP — repetitive bursts of action potential
RBAS — rostral basilar artery syndrome
RBB —
  right breast biopsy
  right bundle branch
RBBB — right bundle-branch block
RBBsB — right bundle-branch system block
RBBx — right breast biopsy
RBC —
  red blood cell
  red blood corpuscle
  red blood [cell] count
RBCC — red blood cell cast
RBCD — right border cardiac dullness
RBCFO — right blood cell fall-out
RBC frag — red blood cell fragility
RBC/hpf — red blood cells per high power field
RBC IT — red blood cell iron turnover
RBCM — red blood cell mass
RBCV — red blood cell volume
RBD —
  recurrent brief depression
  relative biological dose

RBD — (continued)
  right border of dullness
RBE — relative biological effectiveness
RBF —
  regional blood flow
  regional bone mass
  renal blood flow
RBG — random blood glucose
Rb Imp — rubber base impression
RBL —
  rat basophilic leukemia
  Reid's baseline
RBM —
  Raji (cell) binding material
  regional bone mass
RBME — regenerating bone marrow extract
RBN — retrobulbar neuritis
RBNA — Royal British Nurses Association
RBOW — rupture of the bag of waters
RBP —
  resting blood pressure
  retinol-binding protein
  riboflavin-binding protein
RBR — radiation bowel reaction
RBRVS — resource-based relative value scale
RBS —
  random blood smear
  random blood sugar
  Rutherford backscattering
RbSA — rabbit serum albumin
RBTC — Rational Behavior Therapy Center
RBU — Raji (cell) binding unit
RBV — right brachial vein
RBW — relative body weight
RBZ — rubidazone
RC —
  radiocarpal
  reaction center
  receptor-chemoeffector
  recrystallization
  red cell
  red cell casts

RC — (continued)
    red corpuscle
    Red Cross
    referred care
    reflection coefficient
    regenerated cellulose
    respiration ceases
    respiratory care
    respiratory center
    rest cure
    retention catheter
    retrograde cystogram
    rib cage
    root canal
    rotator cuff
    Roussy-Cornil [syndrome]
    routine cholecystectomy
R/C — reclining chair
R&C — resistance and capacitance
Rc —
    conditioned response
    receptor
RCA —
    radionuclide cerebral angiogram
    Raji cell assay
    red cell adherence
    red cell agglutination
    relative chemotactic activity
    renal cell carcinoma
    right carotid artery
    right coronary artery
RCAMC — Royal Canadian Army Medical Corps
rCBF — regional cerebral blood flow
RCBV — regional cerebral blood volume
RCC —
    radiochemical center
    radiographic coronary calcification
    radiological control center
    rape crisis center
    ratio of cost to charges
    receptor-chemoeffector complex

RCC — (continued)
    red cell cast
    red cell concentrate
    red cell count
    renal cell carcinoma
    right common carotid
    right coronary cusp
RCCA — right common carotid artery
RCCM — Regional Committee for Community Medicine (British)
RCCT — random controlled clinical trial
RCD — relative cardiac dullness
RCDA — recurrent chronic dissecting aneurysm
RCDP — rhizomelic chondrodysplasia punctata
RCDR — relative corrected death rate
RCE — reasonable compensation equivalent
RCF —
    red cell ferritin
    red cell filterability
    red cell folate
    Reiter complement fixation
    relative centrifugal force
    ristocetin cofactor
RCFR — Red Cross Field Representative
RCFS — reticulocyte cell-free system
RCG — radioelectrocardiography
RCGP — Royal College of General Practitioners
RCH — rectocolic hemorrhage
RCHF — right congestive heart failure
RCHMS — Regional Committee for Hospital Medical Services
RCI — respiratory control index
RCIA — red cell immune adherence
RCIRF — radiologic contrast-induced renal failure
RCIT — red cell iron turnover

RCITR — red cell iron turnover rate

RCL —
    range of comfortable loudness
    renal clearance

RCM —
    radiographic contrast medium
    red cell mass
    reinforced clostridial medium
    replacement culture medium
    retinal capillary microaneurysm
    rheumatoid cervical myelopathy
    right costal margin
    Roux conditioned medium
    Royal College of Midwives

RCMI — red cell morphology index

rCMRGlc — regional cerebral metabolic rate for glucose

rCMRO$_2$ — regional cerebral metabolic rate for oxygen

RCN —
    right caudate nucleus
    Royal College of Nursing

RCoF — ristocetin cofactor

RCOG — Royal College of Obstetricians and Gynaecologists

R colony — rough colony

RCP —
    random chemistry profile
    red cell protoporphyrin
    retrocorneal pigmentation
    riboflavin carrier protein
    Royal College of Physicians
    Royal College of Psychiatrists

rCP — regional cerebral perfusion

rcp — reciprocal [translocation]

RCPath — Royal College of Pathologists

RCPH — red cell peroxide hemolysis

RCPM — Raven Colored Progressive Matrix

RCPSGlas — Royal College of Physicians and Surgeons, Glasgow

RCQG — right caudal quarter ganglion

RCR —
    relative consumption rate
    respiratory control ratio

RCRA — Resource Conservation and Recovery Act

RCRS — Rehabilitation Client Rating Scale

RCS —
    rabbit aorta–contracting substance
    red cell suspension
    repeat cesarean section
    reticulum cell sarcoma
    right coronary sinus
    Royal College of Science
    Royal College of Surgeons

RCSE — Royal College of Surgeons, Edinburgh

RCT —
    random controlled trial
    red colloidal test
    retrograde conduction time
    root canal therapy
    Rorschach content test

RCU —
    red cell utilization
    respiratory care unit

RCV — red cell volume

RCVS — Royal College of Veterinary Surgeons

RD —
    radial deviation
    rate difference
    Raynaud's disease
    reaction of degeneration
    reaction of denervation
    reading-disabled
    Registered Dietitian
    Reiter's disease
    related donor
    renal disease
    Rénon-Delille [syndrome]
    resistance determinant
    respiratory disease
    respiratory distress
    retinal detachment

RD — (continued)
  Reye's disease
  rheumatoid disease
  right deltoid [muscle]
  Riley-Day [syndrome]
  Rolland-Desbuquois [syndrome]
  rubber dam
  ruminal drinking
  ruptured disk
Rd — rate of disappearance
rd — rutherford
R&D — research and development
RDA —
  recommended daily allowance
  recommended dietary allowance
  Registered Dental Assistant
  right dorsoanterior [fetal position]
  rubidium dihydrogen arsenate
RDB — random double-blind [trial]
RDC — Research Diagnostic Criteria
RDDA — recommended daily dietary allowance
RDDP — ribonucleic acid–dependent deoxynucleic acid polymerase
RDE — receptor-destroying enzyme
RDEB — recessive dystrophic epidermolysis bullosa
RDES — remote data entry system
R determinant — resistance determinant
RDFC — recurring digital fibroma of childhood
RDFS — ratio of decayed and filled surfaces
RDG — right dorsogluteal
RDH — Registered Dental Hygienist
RDHBF — regional distribution of hepatic blood flow
RDI —
  recommended daily intake
  recommended dietary intake

RDI — (continued)
  respiratory disturbance index
  rupture-delivery interval
RDIH — right direct inguinal hernia
RDLBBB — rate-dependent left bundle-branch block
RDLS — Reynell Development Language Scale
RDM —
  readmission
  rod disk membrane
RDMS — Registered Diagnostic Medical Sonographer
rDNA —
  recombinant deoxyribonucleic acid
  ribosomal deoxyribonucleic acid
RDOD — retinal detachment oculus dexter [right eye]
RDOS — retinal detachment oculus sinister [left eye]
RDP — right dorsoposterior [fetal position]
RDPE — reticular degeneration of pigment epithelium
RDQ — respiratory disease questionnaire
Rd Q — reading quotient
RDRC — radioactive drug research committee
RDRV — rhesus diploid rabies vaccine
RDS —
  respiratory distress syndrome
  reticuloendothelial depressing substance
  rhodanese
RDT —
  regular dialysis treatment
  retinal damage threshold
  routine dialysis therapy
RDV — rice dwarf virus
RDVT — recurrent deep vein thrombosis
RDW — red-cell distribution width

RE —
    racemic epinephrine
    radium emanation
    readmission
    rectal examination
    reflux esophagitis
    regarding
    regional enteritis
    renal and electrolyte
    renal excretion
    resistive exercise
    resting energy
    restriction endonuclease
    reticuloendothelial
    reticuloendothelium
    retinol equivalent
    right ear
    right eye
    rostral end

R_E — respiratory exchange ratio

R&E —
    research and education
    rest and exercise
    round and equal

R_E — respiratory exchange ratio

Re —
    regarding
    rhenium

R_e — Reynolds' number

REA —
    Radiation Emergency Area
    radioenzymatic assay
    renal anastomosis
    right ear advantage

REAB — refractory anemia with excess of blasts

REACH — Reassurance to Each

readm — readmission

REAS —
    reasonably expected as safe
    retained, excluded antrum syndrome

REAT — Radiological Emergency Assistance Team

REB — roentgen-equivalent biological

R-EBD-HS — recessive-epidermolysis bullosa dystrophica—Hallopeau-Siemens [syndrome]

REC —
    rear end collision
    receptor
    right external carotid

rec —
    recent
    recessive
    recombinant chromosome
    recommendation
    record
    recovery
    recreation
    recurrence
    recurrent

rec. — *recens* (Lat.) fresh

RECA — right external carotid artery

recd — received

RECEL — reticulum cell

RECG — radioelectrocardiography

recip —
    recipient
    reciprocal

recond —
    reconditioned
    reconditioning

reconstr — reconstruction

recryst — recrystallization

rect —
    rectal
    rectally
    rectification
    rectum
    rectus [muscle]

rect. — *rectificatus* (Lat.) rectified

recumb — recumbent

recur —
    recurrence
    recurrent

RED —
    radiation experience data
    rapid erythrocyte degeneration

Re-D — re-evaluation deadline

red —
    reduce
    reduction

redig. in pulv. — *redigatur in pulverem* (Lat.) let it be reduced to powder

red. in pulv. — *reductus in pulverem* (Lat.) reduced to powder

REDNP — Regent's External Degree Nursing Program

redox — oxidation-reduction

REE —
rapid extinction effect
rare earth element
resting energy expenditure

REEDS — retention of tears, ectrodactyly, ectodermal dysplasia, and strange hair, skin and teeth [syndrome]

REEG — radioelectroencephalography

R-EEG — resting electroencephalography

REEGT — Registered Electroencephalographic Technician

REELS — Receptive-expressive Emergent Language Scale

ReEND — reproductive endocrinology

REEP — right end-expiratory pressure

reev — re-evaluate

reex — re-examine

REF —
ejection fraction at rest
referred
refused
renal erythropoietic factor

ref —
refer
reference
reflex

Ref Doc — referring doctor

REFI — regional ejection fraction image

ref ind — refractive index

refl —
reflection
reflex

REFMS — Recreation and Education for Multiple Sclerosis Victims

Ref Phys — referring physician

REFRAD — released from active duty

REG —
Radiation Exposure Guide
radioencephalogram
radioencephalography

Reg — registered

reg. —
region
regular
regulation

regen —
regenerate
regenerating
regeneration

reg. rhy. — regular rhythm

reg. umb. — *regio umbilici* (Lat.) umbilical region

regurg. — regurgitation

REH — renin essential hypertension

rehab. —
rehabilitated
rehabilitation

REL —
rate of energy loss
recommended exposure limit
resting expiratory level

rel —
related
relation
relative
religion

RELE — resistive exercise of lower extremities

reliq. — *reliquus* (Lat.) remainder

REM —
radiation-equivalent man
rapid eye movement
recent-event memory
reticular erythematous mucinosis
return electrode monitor
roentgen-equivalent-man

rem. — removal

REMA — repetitive excess mixed anhydride

REMAB — radiation-equivalent manikin absorption

REMCAL — radiation-equivalent manikin calibration

remit — remittent

REMP — roentgen-equivalent-man period

REMS — rapid eye movement sleep

REN — renal

ren. — *renovetur* (Lat.) renew

ren. sem. — *renovetum semel* (Lat.) renew only once

REO — respiratory and enteric orphan [virus]

REP —
    rest-exercise program
    retrograde pyelogram
    roentgen equivalent-physical

rep —
    repair
    replication
    report
    roentgen equivalent—physical

rep. — *repetatur* (Lat.) let it be repeated

REPC — reticuloendothelial phagocytic capacity

repol — repolarization

REPS — reactive extensor postural synergy

req —
    requested
    required

RER —
    renal excretion rate
    respiratory exchange ratio
    rough endoplasmic reticulum

RERF — Radiation Effects Research Foundation

RES —
    radionuclide esophageal scintigraphy
    reticuloendothelial system

res —
    research
    resection
    reserve

res — *(continued)*
    resident
    residue
    resistance

RESNA — Rehabilitation Engineering Society of North America

resp —
    respectively
    respiration
    respiratory
    response
    responsible

RESP-A — respiratory battery, acute

respir — respiration

REST —
    Raynaud's phenomenon, esophageal motor dysfunction, sclerodactyly, and telangiectasia [syndrome]
    regressive electroshock therapy
    reticulospinal tract

resus — resuscitation

RET —
    rational emotive therapy
    retained
    retention
    reticular
    reticulocyte
    retina
    right esotropia

ret —
    rad equivalent therapeutic
    retired

retard —
    retardation
    retarded

RETC — rat embryo tissue culture

ret cath — retention catheter

retic — reticulocyte

REV — reticuloendotheliosis virus

ReV — regulator of virion

rev —
    reverse
    review
    revolution

rev/min — revolutions per minute
rev of sys — review of systems
re-x — re-examination
Rex — regulator x
RF —
    radial fiber
    radiofrequency
    rate of flow
    receptive field
    recognition factor
    Reitland-Franklin [unit]
    relative flow [rate]
    relative fluorescence
    releasing factor
    renal failure
    replicative form
    resistance factor
    resorcinol formaldehyde
    respiratory failure
    retardation factor
    reticular formation
    retroperitoneal fibromatosis
    rheumatic fever
    rheumatoid factor
    riboflavin
    Riga-Fede [disease]
    risk factor
    root canal filling
    rosette formation
    Rundles-Falls [syndrome]
R&F — radiographic and fluoroscopic
R_f — rate of flow
Rf —
    respiratory frequency
    rutherfordium
rf — radiofrequency
RFA —
    right femoral artery
    right forearm
    right frontoanterior [fetal position]
R factor — resistance factor
RFB —
    retained foreign body
    rheumatoid factor binding
RFC —
    retrograde femoral catheter

RFC — (continued)
    right frontal craniotomy
    rosette-forming cells
RFE — relative fluorescence efficiency
RFFIT — rapid fluorescent focus inhibition test
RFI —
    recurrence-free interval
    renal failure index
RFL — right frontolateral [fetal position]
RFLA — rheumatoid factor–like activity
RFLP — restriction fragment length polymorphism
RFLS — rheumatoid factor–like substance
Rfm — rifampin
RFOL — results to follow
RFP —
    recurrent facial paralysis
    request for proposal
    right frontoposterior [fetal position]
RFPS (Glasgow) — Royal Faculty of Physicians and Surgeons of Glasgow
RFR —
    rapid filling rate
    refraction
RFS —
    rapid frozen section
    renal function study
RFT —
    right frontotransverse [fetal position]
    rod-and-frame test
    routine fever therapy
RFTB — riboflavin tetrabutyrate
RFV — right femoral vein
RFW — rapid-filling wave
RG —
    retrograde
    right gluteal [muscle]
rG — regular gene
RGAS — retained gastric antrum syndrome

RGBMT — renal glomerular basement membrane thickness
RGC —
   radio-gas chromatography
   remnant gastric cancer
   retinal ganglion cell
   right giant cell
RGD — range-gated Doppler
RGE —
   relative gas expansion
   respiratory gas equation
RGH — rat growth hormone
RGM — right gluteus maximus
rGM-CSF — recombinant granulo-cyte-macrophage colony-stim-ulating factor
RGMT — reciprocal geometric mean titer
RGN — Registered General Nurse
RGO — reciprocating gait orthosis
RGP — retrograde pyelography
RGR — relative growth rate
RGT — reversed gastric tube
RGU — regional glucose utilization
RH —
   radial hemolysis
   radiant heat
   radiological health
   reactive hyperemia
   recurrent herpes
   reduced haloperidol
   regional heparinization
   regulatory hormone
   relative humidity
   releasing hormone
   renal hemolysis
   retinal hemorrhage
   rheumatism
   rheumatology
   Richner-Hanhart [syndrome]
   right hand
   right heart
   right hemisphere
   right hyperphoria
   room humidifier
Rh —
   Rhesus [factor]

Rh — (continued)
   rhinion
   rhodium
   rhonchi
Rh + — Rhesus positive
Rh − — Rhesus negative
Rh$_{null}$ — Rhesus factor null
^{106}Rh — radioactive rhodium
rh. —
   rheumatic
   rhonchi
r/h — roentgens per hour
RHA —
   Regional Health Authority
   right hepatic artery
RhA — rheumatoid arthritis
RHB —
   raise head of bed
   right heart bypass
RHBF — reactive hyperemia blood flow
RHBs — Regional Hospital Boards
RHC —
   resin hemoperfusion column
   respiration has ceased
   right heart catheterization
   right hypochondrium
RHCSA — Regional Hospitals Consultants' and Specialists' Association
RHD —
   radial head dislocation
   Radiological Health Data
   relative hepatic dullness
   renal hypertensive disease
   rheumatic heart disease
RhD — Rhesus hemolytic disease
RHE —
   respiratory heat exchange
   retinohepatoendocrinologic [syndrome]
RHEED — reflection high-energy electron diffraction
rheo —
   rheology
   rheostat
rheum —
   rheumatic

rheum — (continued)
    rheumatism
    rheumatoid
RHF — right heart failure
RHG —
    relative hemoglobin
    right hand grip
rhG-CSF — recombinant human granulocyte colony-stimulating factor
rhGM-CSF — recombinant human granulocyte macrophage colony-stimulating factor
RHH — right homonymous hemianopia
RHI — Rural Health Initiative
RhIG — Rhesus immune globulin
Rhin. —
    rhinologist
    rhinology
rhino — rhinoplasty
Rhiz — Rhizobium
RHJSC — Regional Hospital Junior Staff Committee
RHL —
    recurrent herpes labialis
    right hemisphere lesion
    right hepatic lobe
RHLN — right hilar lymph node
rhm — roentgen per hour at one meter
RhMK — Rhesus monkey kidney
RHMV — right heart mixing volume
RHN — Rockwell hardness number
Rh neg. — Rhesus factor negative
Rh_{null} — Rhesus factor null
RHO — right heeloff
rhom. — rhomboid [muscle]
RHP — right hemiparesis
RHPA — reverse hemolytic plaque assay
Rh pos. — Rhesus factor positive
RHR —
    renal hypertensive rat
    resting heart rate
r/hr — roentgens per hour

RHS —
    Ramsay Hunt syndrome
    reciprocal hindlimb-scratching [syndrome]
    right heelstrike
    right-hand side
RHT —
    renal homotransplantation
    right hypertropia
rH-TNF — recombinant human tumor necrosis factor
RHU —
    Registered Health Underwriter
    rheumatology
rHuEPO — recombinant human erythropoietin
rHuTNF — recombinant human tumor-necrosing factor
RI —
    radiation intensity
    radioactive isotope
    radioimmunology
    radioisotope
    recession index
    recombinant inbred [strain]
    refractive index
    regenerative index
    regional ileitis
    regular insulin
    relative intensity
    release-inhibiting
    remission induction
    renal insufficiency
    replicative intermediate
    resistance index
    respiratory illness
    respiratory index
    reticulocyte index
    retroactive inhibition
    retroactive interference
    ribosome
    rooming-in
    rosette inhibition
R/I — rule in
RIA —
    radioimmunoassay
    reversible ischemic attack

RIA-DA — radioimmunoassay double antibody [test]

RIAS — Roter International Analysis Scheme

RIAST — Reitan Indiana Aphasic Screening Test

Rib —
riboflavin
ribose

RIBA — recombinant immunoblot assay

RIBS — Rutherford ion backscattering

RIC —
renomedullary interstitial cell
right iliac crest
right internal carotid [artery]
Royal Institute of Chemistry

RICA — reverse immune cytoadhesion

RICE — rest, ice, compression, and elevation

RICM — right intercostal margin

RiCoF — ristocetin cofactor

RICS — right intercostal space

RICU — respiratory intensive care unit

RID —
radial immunodiffusion
remission-inducing drug
ruptured intervertebral disc

RIDCSF — radial immunodiffusion cerebrospinal fluid

RIF —
release-inhibiting factor
rifampin
right iliac fossa
rosette-inhibiting factor

RIFA — radioiodinated fatty acid

RIFC — rat intrinsic factor concentrate

rIFN — recombinant interferon

RIG — rabies immune globulin

RIGH — rabies immune globulin, human

RIH — right inguinal hernia

RIHSA — radioactive iodinated human serum albumin

rIL — recombinant interleukin

RILT — rabbit ileal loop test

RIM —
radioisotope medicine
recurrent induced malaria
relative-intensity measure

RIMA —
right internal mammary anastomosis
right internal mammary artery

RIMR — Rockefeller Institute for Medical Research

RIMS — resonance ionization mass spectrometry

RIN — rat insulinoma

RINB — Reitan-Indiana Neuropsychological Battery

RIND —
resolving ischemic neurological deficit
reversible ischemic neurological deficit

RINN — recommended international nonproprietary name

RIO — right inferior oblique

RIOJ — recurrent intrahepatic obstructive jaundice

RIP —
radioimmunoprecipitation [test]
rapid infusion pump
reflex inhibiting pattern
respiratory inductance plethysmography

RIPA — radioimmunoprecipitation assay

RIPH — Royal Institute of Public Health

RIPHH — Royal Institute of Public Health and Hygiene

RIPP — resistive-intermittent positive pressure

RIR —
relative incidence rates
right iliac region
right inferior rectus [muscle]

RIRB — radioiodinated rose bengal

RIS —
   rapid immunofluorescence
      staining
   resonance ionization spectros-
      copy
RISA —
   radioactive iodinated serum
      albumin
   radioimmunosorbent assay
RIST — radioimmunosorbent test
RIT —
   radioimmune trypsin
   radioiodinated triolein
   radioiodine treatment
   Rorschach Inkblot Test
   rosette inhibition titer
RITA — Randomized Intervention
   Treatment of Angina
RITC — rhodamine isothiocyanate
RIU — radioactive iodine uptake
RIV —
   ramus interventricularis
   right innominate vein
RIVC — right inferior vena cava
RIVD — ruptured intervertebral
   disc
RIVS — ruptured intervertebral
   septum
RJ —
   radial jerk
   Robert Jones [dressing]
RJI — radionuclide joint imaging
RK —
   rabbit kidney
   radial keratoplasty
   radial keratotomy
   right kidney
RKG — radiocardiogram
RKH — Rokitansky-Küster-Hauser
   [syndrome]
RKM — rokitamycin
RKS —
   renal kidney stone
   retrograde kidney study
RKV — rabbit kidney vacuolating
   [virus]
RKW — renal kalium (potassium)
   wasting

RKY — roentgenkymography
RL —
   radiation laboratory
   Record Librarian
   reduction level
   resistive load
   reticular lamina
   right lateral
   right leg
   right lower
   right lung
   Ringer's lactate [solution]
$R{\rightarrow}L$ — right to left
R/L — Ringer's lactate
R&L — right and left
R_L —
   respiratory resistance
   total pulmonary resistance
RLA — radiographic lung area
RLBCD — right lower border of
   cardiac dullness
RLC —
   rectus and longus capitus
   residual lung capacity
RLD —
   related living donor
   right lateral decubitus
   ruptured lumbar disc
RLE — right lower extremity
RLF —
   retained lung fluid
   retrolental fibroplasia
   right lateral femoral
RLL —
   right lower limb
   right lower lobe
RLM — right lower medial
RLMD — rat liver mitochondria
RLN —
   recurrent laryngeal nerve
   regional lymph node
RLNC — regional lymph node cell
RLND —
   regional lymph node dissec-
      tion
   retroperitoneal lymph node
      dissection
RLO — residual lymphatic output

RLP—
   radiation leukemia protection
   ribosome-like particle
RLQ — right lower quadrant
RLR — right lateral rectus [muscle]
RLS—
   restless leg syndrome
   Ringer's lactate solution
   Roussy-Levy syndrome
RLSB—
   right lower scapular border
   right lower sternal border
R-Lsh — right-left shunt
RLT — right lateral thigh
RLV — Rauscher leukemia virus
RLWD — routine laboratory work done
RM—
   radical mastectomy
   random migration
   range of motion
   range of movement
   red marrow
   reference material
   regional myocardial
   rehabilitation medicine
   reinforced maneuver
   relative mobility
   repetition maximum
   resistive movement
   respiratory metabolism
   respiratory movement
   Riehl's melanosis
   risk management
   Rosenthal-Melkersson [syndrome]
   Rothmann-Makai [syndrome]
   routine management
   ruptured membranes
R&M — routine and microscopic
Rm—
   relative mobility
   remission
rm—
   remission
   room

RMA—
   Registered Medical Assistant
   relative medullary area
   right mentoanterior [fetal position]
RMAC — Regional Medical Advisory Committee (British)
RMB — right mainstem bronchus
RMBF — regional myocardial blood flow
RMC — reticular magnocellular [nucleus]
RMCA—
   right main coronary artery
   right middle cerebral artery
RMCAT — right middle cerebral artery thrombosis
RMCL — right midclavicular line
RMCP — rat mast cell protease
RMCT — rat mast cell technique
RMD—
   rapid movement disorder
   ratio of midsagittal diameters
   retromanubrial dullness
RME—
   rapid maxillary expansion
   resting metabolic expenditure
   right mediolateral episiotomy
RMEE — right middle ear exploration
RMEC — regional medical education center
RMF — right middle finger
RMK — Rhesus monkey kidney
RML—
   radiation myeloid leukemia
   regional medical library
   right mediolateral
   right mentolateral
   right middle lobe
RMLB — right middle lobe bronchus
RMLS — right middle lobe syndrome
RMLV — Rauscher murine leukemia virus
RMM — rapid micromedia method
RMN — Registered Mental Nurse

RMO —
    Regional Medical Officer
    Resident Medical Officer
RMP —
    rapidly miscible pool
    regional medical program
    resting membrane potential
    ribulose monophosphate pathway
    rifampin
    right mentoposterior [fetal position]
RMPA — Royal Medico-Psychological Association
RMR —
    relative maximum response
    resting metabolic rate
    right medial rectus [muscle]
RMS —
    rectal morphine sulfate [suppository]
    red man syndrome
    repetitive motion syndrome
    respiratory muscle strength
    rheumatic mitral stenosis
    rhodomyosarcoma
    rigid man syndrome
    root-mean-square
rms — root-mean-square
RMSD — root-mean-square deviation
RMSE — root-mean-square error
RMSF — Rocky Mountain spotted fever
RMT —
    Registered Music Therapist
    relative medullary thickness
    retromolar trigone
    right mentotransverse [fetal position]
RMUI — relief medication unit index
RMV — respiratory minute volume
RN —
    radionuclide
    red nucleus
    reflex nephropathy

RN — (continued)
    Registered Nurse
    residual nitrogen
    reticular nucleus
Rn — radon
^{222}Rn — radioactive radon
RNA —
    radionuclide angiography
    Registered Nurse Anesthetist
    ribonucleic acid
    rough, noncapsulated, avirulent [bacterial culture]
RNAA — radiochemical neutron activation analysis
RNase — ribonuclease
RND —
    radical neck dissection
    radionuclide dacryography
    reactive neurotic depression
RNEF — resting nuclide ejection fraction
RNFP — Registered Nurse Fellowship Program
RNIB — Royal National Institute for the Blind
RNICU — regional neonatal intensive care unit
RNID — Royal National Institute for the Deaf
RNL — renal laboratory profile
RNM — red nucleus, magnocellular
RNMD — Registered Nurse for Mental Defectives
RNMS — Registered Nurse for the Mentally Subnormal
RNMT — Registered Nuclear Medicine Technologist
RNP —
    Registered Nurse Practitioner
    ribonucleoprotein
RNR — ribonucleotide reductase
RNS —
    reference normal serum
    repetitive nerve stimulation
RNSC — radionuclide superior cavography
RNT — radioassayable neurotensin

Rnt —
    roentgenologist
    roentgenology
RNTC — rat nephroma tissue culture
RNV — radionuclide venography
rNTP — ribonuclease-5'-triphosphate
RNVG — radionuclide ventriculography
RO —
    radiation output
    ratio of
    reality orientation
    relative odds
    reverse osmosis
    Ritter-Oleson [technique]
    routine order
    rule out
R/O — rule out
Ro — resting radium
ROA — right occipitoanterior [fetal position]
ROAC — repeated oral dose of activated charcoal
ROAD — reversible obstructive airways disease
ROAT — repeat open application test
ROATS — rabbit ovarian antitumor serum
rob — robertsonian translocation
ROC —
    receiver operating characteristic
    receptor-operated channels
    relative operating characteristic
    resident on call
    residual organic carbon
roc — reciprocal ohm centimeter
ROCFT — Rey-Ostreich Complex Figure Test
RODAC — replicate organism detection and counting
rOEF — regional oxygen extraction fraction
roent. —
    roentgenologist

roent. — (continued)
    roentgenology
ROH — rat ovarian hyperemia [test]
ROI —
    reactive oxygen intermediate
    region of interest
ROIH — right oblique inguinal hernia
ROL — right occipitolateral [fetal position]
ROM —
    range of motion
    range of movement
    read-only memory
    right otitis media
    rupture of membranes
Rom — Romberg [sign]
rom — reciprocal ohm meter
ROM CP — range of motion complete and painfree
ROMSA — right otitis media, suppurative, acute
ROMSC — right otitis media, suppurative, chronic
ROMI — rule out myocardial infarction
ROP —
    regional occupational program
    retinopathy of prematurity
    right occipitoposterior [fetal position]
ROPA — Regional Organ Procurement Agency
ROPS — rollover protective structure
Ror — Rorschach [test]
RO&R — Rey-Ostreich and Recall [test]
ROS —
    reactive oxygen species
    review of systems
    rod outer segment
RoS — rostral sulcus
ROSC — restoration of spontaneous circulation
ROSS — review of subjective symptoms

ROT —
  real oxygen transport
  Registered Occupational
    Therapist
  remedial occupational therapy
  right occipitotransverse [fetal
    position]
  rule of thumb
rot. —
  rotate
  rotating
  rotation
  rotator
ROU — recurrent oral ulcer
ROUL — rouleaux
ROW —
  rat ovarian weight
  Rendu-Osler-Weber [syn-
    drome]
RP —
  radial pulse
  radiographic planimetry
  radiopharmaceutical
  rapid processing [of film]
  Raynaud's phenomenon
  reactive protein
  readiness potential
  rectal prolapse
  re-entrant pathway
  refractory period
  Registered Pharmacist
  regulatory protein
  relapsing polychondritis
  relative potency
  respiratory rate
  rest pain
  resting potential
  resting pressure
  retinitis pigmentosa
  retinitis proliferans
  retrograde pyelogram
  retroperitoneal
  reverse phase
  rheumatoid polyarthritis
  ribose phosphate
  ristocetin polymyxin
R/P — respiratory pulse [rate]
R_p — pulmonary resistance

R-5′-P — ribose-5′-phosphate
RPA —
  radial photon absorptiometry
  resultant physiologic accelera-
    tion
  reverse passive anaphylaxis
  right pulmonary artery
RPAC — Regional Paramedic Advisory Committee
RPase — ribonucleic acid polymerase
RPAW — right pulmonary artery
  withdrawal
Rpba — periosteal bone apposition
  rate
RPBF — regional pulmonary blood
  flow
RPC —
  relapsing polychondritis
  relative proliferative capacity
  reticularis pontis caudalis
RPCF — Reiter protein complement fixation [test]
RPCGN — rapidly progressive
  crescenting glomerulonephritis
RPCU — retropubic cytourethro-
  pexy
RPD — removable partial denture
RPE —
  rate of perceived exertion
  recurrent pulmonary embo-
    lism
  retinal pigment epithelium
RPF —
  rapid processing film
  relaxed pelvic floor
  renal plasma flow
RPF[a] — arterial renal plasma flow
RPF[v] — venous renal plasma flow
RPG —
  radiation protection guide
  retrograde pyelogram
  rheoplethysmography
RPGG — retroplacental gamma
  globulin
RPGMEC — Regional Postgraduate Medical Education Committee

RPGN — rapidly progressive glomerulonephritis

RPH — retroperitoneal hemorrhage

RPh — Registered Pharmacist

RPHA — reversed passive hemagglutination

RPHAMCFA — reversed passive hemagglutination by miniature centrifugal fast analysis

RP-HPLC — reverse phase high-performance liquid chromatography

RPI —
    relative percentage index
    reticulocytic production index
    ribose-5'-phosphate isomerase

RPICCE — round pupil intracapsular cataract extraction

RPIPP — reverse phase ion-pair partition

RPK — ribosephosphate kinase

RPLAD — retroperitoneal lymphadenectomy

RPLC — reverse phase liquid chromatography

RPLD — repair of potentially lethal damage

RPLND — retroperitoneal lymph node dissection

RPM —
    rapid processing mode
    Raven's Progressive Matrices

rpm — revolutions per minute

RPMD — rheumatic pain modulation disorder

RPN —
    renal papillary necrosis
    resident's progress note

RPND — retroperitoneal lymph node dissection

RPO — right posterior oblique

RPP — retropubic prostatectomy

RPPI — role perception picture inventory

RPPR — red cell precursor production rate

RPR —
    rapid plasma reagin [test]

RPR — *(continued)*
    Reiter protein reagin

RPr — retinitis proliferans

RPRCF — rapid plasma reagin complement fixation

RPRCT — rapid plasma reagin cord test

RPS — renal pressor substance

rps — revolutions per second

RPT —
    rapid pull-through
    refractory period of transmission
    Registered Physical Therapist

RPTA — renal percutaneous transluminal angioplasty

RPTC — regional poisoning treatment center

Rptd — ruptured

RPU — retropubic urethropexy

RPV —
    right portal vein
    right pulmonary vein

RPVP — right posterior ventricular pre-excitation

RQ —
    recovery quotient
    reportable quantity
    respiratory quotient

RR —
    radiation reaction
    radiation response
    rapid radiometric
    rate ratio
    recovery room
    red reflex
    regular respirations
    regular rhythm
    relative response
    relative risk
    renin release
    respiratory rate
    respiratory reserve
    response rate
    retinal reflex
    rheumatoid rosette
    risk ratio
    Riva-Rocci [sphygmomanometer]

RR — *(continued)*
    ruthenium red
R/R — rales/rhonchi
R&R —
    rate and rhythm
    recent and remote
    rest and recuperation
RRA —
    radioreceptor assay
    Registered Record Adminis-
      trator
    renal renin activity
RRAM — repetitive and rapid al-
    ternating movements
RRBC — rabbit red blood cell
RRC —
    residency review committee
    risk reduction component
    routine respiratory care
    Royal Red Cross
RRE —
    radiation-related eosinophilia
    regressive resistive exercise
RR&E — round, regular, and equal
    [pupils]
RREF — resting radionuclide
    ejection fraction
RRF — residual renal function
RR-HPO — rapid recompression–
    high-pressure oxygen
RRI —
    recurrent respiratory infection
    reflex relaxation index
    relative response index
RRIS — recurrent respiratory infec-
    tion syndrome
RRL — Registered Record Librar-
    ian
rRNA — ribosomal ribonucleic
    acid
RRND — right radical neck dissec-
    tion
rRNP — ribosomal ribonucleopro-
    tein
RROM — resistive range of mo-
    tion
RRP — relative refractory period
RRpm — respiratory rate per min-
    ute

RRQG — right rostral quarter gan-
    glion
RRR —
    regular rate and rhythm
    renin release rate
RR&R — regular rate and rhythm
RRRN — round, regular and react
    normally
RRS —
    retrorectal space
    Richards-Rundle syndrome
RRT —
    random response technique
    Registered Respiratory Thera-
      pist
    relative retention time
    resazurin reduction time
RRU — respiratory resistance unit
RS —
    random sample
    rating schedule
    Raynaud's syndrome
    reading of standard
    recipient's serum
    rectal sinus
    rectal suppository
    rectosigmoid
    reducing substance
    Reed-Sternberg [cell]
    reinforcing stimulus
    Reiter's syndrome
    relative stimulus
    remnant stomach
    renal specialist
    resolved sarcoidosis
    resorcinol-sulfur
    respiratory syncytial [virus]
    response to stimulus
    resting subject
    reticulated siderocyte
    Rett syndrome
    review of symptoms
    Reye's syndrome
    rheumatoid spondylitis
    rhythm strip
    right sacrum
    right septum
    right side

RS — *(continued)*
   right stellate [ganglion]
   right subclavian
   Ringer's solution
   Ritchie sedimentation
   Roberts' syndrome
   Rous sarcoma
R&S — restraint and seclusion
Rs —
   Rauwolfia serpentina
   systemic resistance
R/s — roentgens per second
r_s — Spearman's rank correlation
   coefficient
RSA —
   rabbit serum albumin
   rat serum albumin
   regular spiking activity
   relative specific activity
   relative standard accuracy
   respiratory sinus arrhythmia
   reticulum cell sarcoma
   right sacroanterior [fetal position]
   right subclavian artery
Rsa — systemic arterial resistance
RSB —
   reticulocyte standard buffer
   right sternal border
RSBT — rhythmic sensory bombardment therapy
RSC —
   rat spleen cell
   rested state contraction
   reversible sickle-cell
RScA — right scapuloanterior [fetal position]
RSCN — Registered Sick Children's Nurse
RScP — right scapuloposterior [fetal position]
RSCT —
   Rach Sentence Completion Test
   Rotter Sentence Completion Test
RSD —
   reflex sympathetic dystrophy

RSD — *(continued)*
   relative sagittal depth
   relative standard deviation
RSDS — reflex sympathetic dystrophy syndrome
RSE —
   rat synaptic ending
   reverse sutured eye
   right sternal edge
RSEP — right somatosensory evoked potential
RSES — Rosenberg Self-esteem Scale
RSG — Reitan Strength of Grip
RSH — Royal Society of Health
RSI — repetition strain injury
RSIC — Radiation Shielding Information Center
R-SICU — respiratory-surgical intensive care unit
R-SIRS — Revised, Seriousness of Illness Rating Scale
RSIVP — rapid-sequence intravenous pyelogram
RSL — right sacrolateral [fetal position]
RSLD — repair of sublethal damage
RSLT — reduced-size liver transplant
RSM —
   risk screening model
   Royal Society of Medicine
RSMR — relative standard mortality rate
RSN — right substantia nigra
RSNA — Radiological Society of North America
RSO —
   Resident Surgical Officer
   right salpingo-oophorectomy
   right superior oblique [muscle]
RSP —
   recirculating single pass
   removable silicone plug
   rhinoseptoplasty
   right sacroposterior [fetal position]

RSPCA — Royal Society for the Prevention of Cruelty to Animals
RSPH — Royal Society for the Promotion of Health
RSPK — recurrent spontaneous psychokinesis
RSR —
  regular sinus rhythm
  relative survival rate
  response-stimulus ratio
  right superior rectus [muscle]
RSS —
  rat stomach strip
  rectosigmoidoscopy
  Russell-Silver syndrome
RSSE — Russian spring-summer encephalitis
RSSR — relative slow sinus rate
RST —
  radiosensitivity test
  rapid surfactant test
  reagin screen test
  right sacrotransverse [fetal position]
  Rodney Smith tube
  rubrospinal tract
RSTI — Radiological Service Training Institute
RSTL — relaxed skin tension lines
RSTMH — Royal Society of Tropical Medicine and Hygiene
RSTS — retropharyngeal soft tissue space
RSV —
  respiratory syncytial virus
  right subclavian vein
  Rous sarcoma virus
R-S variation — rough-smooth variation
RSVC — right superior vena cava
RSW — right-sided weakness
RT —
  radiation therapy
  Radiologic Technologist
  radiotelemetry
  radiotherapy
  radium therapy

RT — (continued)
  raphe transection
  rapid tranquilization
  reaction time
  reading test
  receptor transforming
  reciprocating tachycardia
  recreational therapy
  rectal temperature
  red tetrazolium
  reduction time
  Registered Technician
  renal transplantation
  repetition time
  resistance transfer
  respiratory therapist
  respiratory therapy
  response time
  rest tremor
  retransformation
  reverse transcriptase
  right thigh
  room temperature
  Rubinstein-Taybi [syndrome]
R_T — total pulmonary resistance
RT_3 — serum resin triiodothyronine [uptake]
RT_4 — resin thyroxine
rT_3 — reverse triiodothyronine
rT — ribothymidine
rt. — right
RTA —
  radiology telephone access
  renal tubular acidosis
  renal tubular antigen
  reverse transcriptase assay
  road traffic accident
RTAD — renal tubular acidification defect
RT(ARRT) — Registered Technologist certified by the American Registry of Radiologic Technologists
RTC —
  random control trial
  rape treatment center
  renal tubular cell
  research and training center

RTC — *(continued)*
    residential treatment center
    return to clinic
    round the clock
RTD — routine test dilution
rtd. — retarded
RTE — rabbit thymus extract
RTECS — Registry of the Toxic Effects of Chemical Substances
RTF —
    replication and transfer
    resistance transfer factor
    respiratory tract fluid
RTG-2 — rainbow trout gonadal tissue cells
RtH — right-handed
rTHF — recombinant tumor necrosis factor
RTI —
    respiratory tract infection
    reverse transcriptase inhibition
RTKP — radiothermokeratoplasty
RTL — reactive to light
rtl — rectal
rt. lat. — right lateral
RTM —
    registered trademark
    routine medical care
R_{tmf} — total matrix formation rate
RTN — renal tubular necrosis
RT(N)(ARRT) — Registered Technologist in Nuclear Medicine certified by the American Registry of Radiologic Technologists
rtn. — return
rTNM — retreatment tumor, nodes, metastasis
RTO — return to office
RTOG — Radiation Therapy Oncology Group
R to R — Reach to Recovery
RTP —
    renal transplant patient
    reverse transcriptase-producing [agent]
rt-PA — recombinant tissue-plasminogen activator

RT-PCR — reverse transcriptase-polymerase-chain reaction
RTPS — radiation therapy planning system
RTR —
    Recreational Therapist, Registered
    red blood cell turnover rate
    retention time ratio
RT(R)(ARRT) — Registered Technologist in Radiography certified by the American Registry of Radiologic Technologists
RTS —
    real time scan
    right toestrike
    Rubinstein-Taybi syndrome
RTRR — return to recovery room
RTS — relative tumor size
RTT(AART) — Registered Technologist in Radiation Therapy Technology certified by the American Registry of Radiologic Technologists
RTU —
    real-time ultrasonography
    relative time unit
RT_3U — resin triiodothyronine uptake
RTV — room temperature vulcanization
RTW — return to work
RTx — radiation therapy
RU —
    radioactive uptake
    radioulnar
    rat unit
    reading unit
    rectourethral
    recurrent ulcer
    residual urine
    resin uptake
    resistance unit
    retrograde urogram
    retroverted uterus
    right upper
    rodent ulcer
    roentgen unit

RU — *(continued)*
  routine urinalysis
Ru — ruthenium
^{106}Ru — radioactive ruthenium
ru — radiation unit
RU-1 — human embryonic lung fibroblast
RUA — routine urinalysis
rub. — *ruber* (Lat.) red
RuBP — ribulose bisphosphate
RUD — recurrent ulcer of the duodenal bulb
RUE — right upper extremity
RUG — retrograde ureterogram
RUL —
  right upper lateral
  right upper lid
  right upper limb
  right upper lobe
  right upper lung
RuMP — ribulose monophosphate pathway
RUO — right ureteral orifice
RUOQ — right upper outer quadrant
RUP —
  rat urine protein
  right upper pole
rupt — ruptured
RUQ — right upper quadrant
RUR — resin-uptake ratio
RURTI — recurrent upper respiratory tract infection
RUS —
  radioulnar synostosis
  recurrent ulcerative stomatitis
RUSB — right upper sternal border
RUSS — recurrent ulcerative scarifying stomatitis
RUV — residual urine volume
RUX — right upper extremity
RV —
  random variable
  rat virus
  Rauscher virus
  rectal vault
  rectovaginal

RV — *(continued)*
  reinforcement value
  renal vein
  reovirus
  residual volume
  respiratory volume
  retinal vasculitis
  retrovaginal
  retroversion
  return visit
  rheumatoid vasculitis
  rhinovirus
  right ventricle
  right ventricular
  rubella vaccine
  rubella virus
  Russell viper
R_v — radius of view
RVA —
  rabies vaccine, adsorbed
  re-entrant ventricular arrhythmia
  renal vascular resistance
  right ventricle activation
  right vertebral artery
RVAD — right ventricular assist device
RVAW — right ventricle anterior wall
RVB — red venous blood
RVC — rectovaginal constriction
RVD —
  relative vertebral density
  right ventricular dimension
  right ventricular dysplasia
RVDO — right ventricular diastolic overload
RVDV — right ventricular diastolic volume
RVE — right ventricular enlargement
RVECP — right ventricular endocardial potential
RVEDD — right ventricular end-diastolic diameter
RVEDP — right ventricular end-diastolic pressure
RVEDVI — right ventricular end-diastolic volume index

RVEF —
> right ventricular ejection fraction
>
> right ventricular end-flow

RVESP — right ventricular end-systolic pressure

RVESVI — right ventricular end-systolic volume index

RVET — right ventricular ejection time

RVF —
> renal vascular failure
> Rift Valley fever
> right ventricular failure
> right visual field

RVFP — right ventricular filling pressure

RVG —
> radionuclide ventriculogram
> right ventrogluteal
> right visceral ganglion

RVH —
> renovascular hypertension
> right ventricular hypertrophy

RVHD — rheumatic valvular heart disease

RVI —
> relative value index
> right ventricle infarction

RVID — right ventricular internal dimension

RVIDP — right ventricular initial diastolic pressure

RVIT — right ventricular inflow tract

RVL — right vastus lateralis

RVLG — right ventrolateral gluteal

RVM — right ventricular mean

RVO —
> Regional Veterinary Officer
> relaxed vaginal outlet
> retinal vein occlusion
> right ventricular outflow
> right ventricular overactivity

RVOT — right ventricular outflow tract

RVP —
> red veterinary petrolatum
> renovascular pressure
> resting venous pressure
> right ventricular pressure

RVPEP — right ventricular pre-ejection period

RVPFR — right ventricular peak filling rate

RVPRA — renal vein plasma renin activity

RVR —
> rapid ventricular response
> reduced vascular response
> reduced vestibular response
> renal vascular resistance
> repetitive ventricular response
> resistance to venous return

RVRA —
> renal vein renin activity
> renal venous renin assay

RVRC — renal vein renin concentration

RV/RF — retroverted/retroflexed

RVS —
> rectovaginal space
> relative value scale
> relative value schedule
> relative value study
> reported visual sensation
> retrovaginal space
> Rokeach Value Survey

RVSO — right ventricular stroke output

RVSW — right ventricular stroke work

RVSWI — right ventricular stroke work index

RVT —
> Registered Vascular Technologist
> renal vein thrombosis
> Russell viper (venom) time

RVTE — recurring venous thromboembolism

RV/TLC — residual volume/total lung capacity [ratio]

RVU — relative valve unit

RVV —
  rubella vaccine–like virus
  Russell viper venom
RVWD — right ventricular wall
  device
RW —
  radiological warfare
  ragweed
  respiratory work
  Romano-Ward [syndrome]
  round window
R-W — Rideal-Walker [coefficient]
RWAGE — ragweed antigen E
RWIS — restraint and water im-
  mersion stress
RWM — regional wall motion
RWP —
  ragweed pollen
  R-wave progression

RWS — ragweed sensitivity
RWT — R-wave threshold
Rx —
  medication
  pharmacy
  prescribe
  prescription
  recipe (Lat.) take
  therapy
  treatment
r(X) — right X chromosome
RXLI — recessive X-linked ichthyosis
RXN — reaction
RXT —
  radiation therapy
  right exotropia
R-Y — Roux-en-Y [anastomo-
  sis]

S —
  apparent power
  in electrocardiography, a nega-
    tive deflection that follows
    an R wave [wave]
  entropy
  exposure time
  mean dose per unit cumulated
    activity
  midpoint of sella turcica
  sacral vertebrae (S1 through
    S5)
  saline
  saturated
  saturation
  schizophrenia
  screen-containing cassette
  section
  sedimentation coefficient
  sella [turcica]
  semilente [insulin]
  senile
  senility

S — *(continued)*
  sensation
  sensitivity
  sensory
  septum
  sequential
  series
  serine
  serum
  siderocyte
  siemens
  sign
  signature [prescription]
  silicate
  single
  singular
  sinus
  sister
  small
  smooth [colony]
  soft [diet]
  solid
  soluble

S — *(continued)*
   solute
   sone [unit]
   space
   spasm
   spatial
   specificity
   spherical lens
   spleen
   sporadic
   standard normal deviation
   stem [cell]
   stimulus
   streptomycin
   subject
   subjective findings
   substrate
   suction
   sulcus
   sulfur
   sum of an arithmetic series
   supine
   supravergence
   surface
   surgery
   suture
   Svedberg unit
   swine
   Swiss [mouse]
   symmetrical
   synthesis
   systole

Σ —
   sigma (eighteenth letter of the Greek alphabet), uppercase
   syphilis
   summation of series

S. —
   Salmonella
   Schistosoma
   Shigella
   Spirillum
   Staphylococcus
   Streptococcus

S_1–S_4 — first to fourth heart sounds
S1–S5 — first to fifth sacral nerves

s —
   atomic orbital with angular momentum quantum number 0
   distance
   esophoria
   length of path
   sample standard deviation
   satellite [chromosome]
   scruple
   second
   section
   sensation
   sedimentation coefficient
   sensation
   series
   signed
   smooth [colony]
   steady state
   suckling
   systolic

σ —
   conductivity
   cross section
   millisecond
   molecular type or bond
   one-thousandth part of a second
   sigma (eighteenth letter of the Greek alphabet), lowercase
   standard deviation
   stress
   surface tension
   type of molecular bond
   wave number

s. —
   semis (Lat.) half
   signa (Lat.) label, mark, sign, write
   signetur (Lat.) let it be written
   sinister (Lat.) left

$\bar{s}$ — *sine* (Lat.) without
s^{-1} — reciprocal second
s^2 — sample variance

SA —
   sacrum anterior

SA — (continued)
  salicylamide
  salicylic acid
  saline [solution]
  salt added
  sarcoidosis
  sarcoma
  scalenus anticus
  Schizophrenics Anonymous
  secondary amenorrhea
  secondary anemia
  secondary arrest
  self-agglutinating
  self-analysis
  semen analysis
  sensitizing antibody
  serum albumin
  serum aldolase
  sex appeal
  sexual addict
  short-acting
  sialic acid
  sialoadenectomy
  simian adenovirus
  sinoatrial
  sinus arrest
  sinus arrhythmia
  skeletal age
  skin-adipose [unit]
  sleep apnea
  slightly active
  slowly adapting [receptors]
  soluble in alkaline solution
  spatial average
  specific activity
  spectrum analysis
  sperm abnormality
  spermagglutinin
  spiking activity
  splenic artery
  standard accuracy
  Staphylococcus aureus
  sternal angle
  stimulus artifact
  Stokes-Adams [syndrome]
  subarachnoid
  succinylacetone
  suicide alert

SA — (continued)
  suicide attempt
  surface antigen
  surface area
  Surgeon's Assistant
  sustained action
  sympathetic activity
  systemic aspergillosis
S.A. — secundum artem (Lat.) according to art
S/A — sugar/acetone [urine]
S-A —
  sinoatrial
  sinoauricular
S&A —
  Sickness and Accident [insurance]
  sugar and acetone
Sa —
  most anterior point of anterior contour of sella turcica
  saline
  samarium
  Staphylococcus aureus
sA — statampere
s.a. — secundum artem (Lat.) according to art
SAA —
  serum amyloid A
  severe aplastic anemia
  Stokes-Adams attack
SAAABB — Subcommittee on Accreditation of the American Association of Blood Banks
SAARD — slow-acting antirheumatic drug
SAAST — self-administered alcohol screening test
SAB —
  Sabouraud's [dextrose agar]
  serum albumin
  significant asymptomatic bacteriuria
  sinoatrial block
  Society of American Bacteriologists
  spontaneous abortion

SAB — (continued)
    subarachnoid bleed
    subarachnoid block
SABHI — Sabouraud dextrose agar and brain-heart infusion
SABP — spontaneous acute bacterial peritonitis
SAC —
    saccharin
    sacrum
    screening and acute care
    Self-Assessment of Communication [scale]
    short-arm cast
    splenic adherent cell
    subarea advisory council
    substance abuse counselor
SACC — short-arm cylinder cast
SACD — subacute combined degeneration
SACE — serum angiotensin-converting enzyme
SACH —
    small animal care hospital
    solid ankle cushion heel
SACS — secondary anticoagulation system
SACSF — subarachnoid cerebrospinal fluid
SACT — sinoatrial conduction time
SAD —
    Scale of Anxiety and Depression
    seasonal affective disorder
    Self-Assessment Depression [scale]
    separation anxiety disorder
    small airway disease
    source-to-axis distance
    subacute dialysis
    sugar, acetone, and diacetic acid [test]
    sugar and acetone determination
    suppressor-activating determinant

SADD —
    Short-Alcohol Dependence Data [questionnaire]
    Standardized Assessment of Depressive Disorders
    Students Against Drunk Driving
SADL — simulated activities of daily living
SADQ — Self-Administered Dependency Questionnaire
SADR — suspected adverse drug reaction
SADS —
    Schedule for Affective Disorders and Schizophrenia
    Shipman Anxiety Depression Scale
SADS-C — Schedule for Affective Disorders and Schizophrenia—Change
SADS-L — Schedule for Affective Disorders and Schizophrenia—Lifetime
SADT — Stetson Auditory Discrimination Test
SAE —
    short above-elbow [cast]
    specific action exercise
    subcortical arteriosclerotic encephalopathy
    supported arm exercise
SAEB — sinoatrial entrance block
SAECG — signal-averaged electrocardiogram
SAEM — Society for Academic Emergency Medicine
SAEP — *Salmonella abortus equi* pyrogen
SAF —
    scrapie-associated fibrils
    self-articulating femoral [hip replacement]
    serum accelerator factor
    simultaneous auditory feedback
SAFA — soluble antigen fluorescence antibody [test]

SAG —
    salicylacyl glucuronide
    Swiss-type agammaglobuli-
        nemia
sag — sagittal
SAGM — sodium chloride, ade-
    nine glucouse, mannitol
SAH —
    S-adenosyl-L-homocysteine
    subarachnoid hemorrhage
    systemic arterial hypertension
SAHA — seborrhea-hypertrichosis/
    hirsutism-alopecia [syndrome]
SAHH — S-adenosylhomocys-
    teine hydrolase
SAHIGES — Staphylococcus aureus
    hyperimmunoglobulinemia E
    syndrome
SAHS — sleep apnea–hypersom-
    nolence [syndrome]
SAI —
    Self-Analysis Inventory
    Sexual Arousability Inventory
    Social Adequacy Index
    Sodium Amytal interview
    systemic active immunother-
        apy
    succinoaminoimidazole
s.a.i. — sine altera indicatione (Lat.)
    without other qualification
SAICAR — succinoaminoimidazole
    carboxamide
SAID — specific adaptation to im-
    posed demand [principle]
SAIDS —
    sexually acquired immunode-
        ficiency syndrome
    simian acquired immune defi-
        ciency syndrome
SAL —
    sensorineural activity level
    specified antilymphocytic
    suction-assisted lipectomy
SAL 12 — sequential analysis of
    twelve chemistry constituents
Sal. — Salmonella
sAl — serum aluminum
sal —
    salicylate

sal — (continued)
    salicylic
    saline
    saliva
    salt
s.a.l. — secundum artis leges (Lat.)
    according to the rules of art
SAM —
    S-adenosyl-L-methionine
    scanning acoustic microscope
    self-administered medication
    sex arousal mechanism
    staphylococcal absorption
        method
    sulfated acid mucopolysaccha-
        ride
    surface active material
    systolic anterior motion
SAMA — Student American Med-
    ical Association
SAMD — S-adenosyl-L-methio-
    nine decarboxylase
SAMe — S-adenosyl-L-methionine
SAMF — single-antibody millipore
    filtration
SAMO — Senior Administrative
    Medical Officer
S-AMY — serum amylase
SAN —
    sinoatrial node
    sinoauricular node
    slept all night
    solitary autonomous nodule
Sanat — sanatorium
SANC — short-arm navicular cast
SANDR — sinoatrial nodal re-en-
    try
sang. — sanguineous
sanit —
    sanitary
    sanitation
    sanitarium
SANS — Scale for the Assessment
    of Negative Symptoms
SANWS — sinoatrial node weak-
    ness syndrome
SAO —
    small airway obstruction

SAO — *(continued)*
  splanchnic artery occlusion
SaO$_2$ — oxygen saturation in arterial blood
SAP —
  sensory action potential
  serum acid phosphatase
  serum alkaline phosphatase
  serum amyloid P
  situs ambiguus with polysplenia
  Staphylococcus aureus protease
  surfactant-associated protein
  systemic arterial pressure
sap. —
  saponification
  saponify
SAPD — self-administration of psychotropic drug
saph — saphenous
SAPHO — synovitis-acne-pustulosis-hyperostosis-osteomyelitis [syndrome]
SAPP — sodium acid pyrophosphate
SAPS —
  short-arm plaster splint
  Simplified Acute Physiology Score
SAPX — salivary peroxidase
SAQ — short-arc quadriceps
SAQC — statistical analysis of quality control
SAR —
  seasonal allergic rhinitis
  sexual attitude reassessment
  sexual attitude restructuring
  structure-activity relationship
Sar — sulfarsphenamine
SARA —
  sexually acquired reactive arthritis
  Superfund Amendments and Reauthorization
  System for Anesthetic and Respiratory Analysis
sarc. — sarcoma
SART — sinoatrial recovery time

SAS —
  self-rating anxiety scale
  short-arm splint
  Sklar Aphasia Scale
  sleep apnea syndrome
  small animal surgery
  small aorta syndrome
  sodium amylosulfate
  space-adaptation syndrome
  statistical analysis system
  sterile aqueous solution
  sterile aqueous suspension
  subaortic stensois
  subarachnoid space
  sulfasalazine
  supravalvular aortic stenosis
  surface-active substance
  synchronous atrial stimulation
SASE — self-addressed stamped envelope
SASMAS — skin-adipose superficial musculoaponeurotic system
SASP — salicylazosulfapyridine
SASPP — syndrome of absence of septum pellucidum with preencephaly
SAST —
  Self-Administered Alcoholism Screening Test
  selective arterial secretin injection test
  serum aspartate aminotransferase
SAT —
  satellite
  serum antitrypsin
  single-agent chemotherapy
  slide agglutination test
  sodium ammonium thiosulfate
  specific antithymocytic
  speech awareness threshold
  spermatogenic activity test
  spontaneous activity test
  spontaneous autoimmune thyroiditis
  Standard Achievement Test
  subacute thyroiditis

SAT — (continued)
  symptomless autoimmune thyroiditis
  systematic assertive therapy
sat. —
  saturated
  saturation
SATA — spatial average, temporal average
SATB — Special Aptitude Test Battery
SATL — surgical Achilles tendon lengthening
SATM — sodium aurothiomalate
SATP — spatial-averaged temporal peak
SAU — statistical analysis unit
SAV — sequential arterioventricular [pacing]
SAVD — spontaneous assisted vaginal delivery
SAVE — Survival and Ventricular Enlargement [trial]
SAZ — sulfasalazine
SB —
  Scientiae Baccalaureus (Lat.) Bachelor of Science
  safety belt
  Schwartz-Bartter [syndrome]
  scleral buckle
  Sengstaken-Blakemore [tube]
  serum bilirubin
  shortness of breath
  sick bay
  sideroblast
  Silvestroni-Corda [syndrome]
  single blind [study]
  single breath
  sinus bradycardia
  small bowel
  sodium balance
  soybean
  spina bifida
  spontaneous blastogenesis
  spontaneous breathing
  stereotyped behavior
  sternal border
  stillbirth

SB — (continued)
  stillborn
  suction biopsy
  surface binding
Sb —
  antimony (Lat., stibium)
  strabismus
SBA —
  serum bactericidal activity
  serum bile acid
  soybean agglutinin
  spina bifida aperta
  stand-by assistance
SBB —
  small bowel biopsy
  stimulation-bound behavior
SBC —
  serum bactericidal concentration
  standard bicarbonate
  strict bed confinement
SbCl$_3$ — antimony trichloride
SBD —
  senile brain disease
  straight bag drainage
S-BD — seizure-brain damage
SbDH — sorbitol dehydrogenase
SBE —
  breast self-examination
  short below-elbow [cast]
  shortness of breath on exertion
  subacute bacterial endocarditis
SBEP — somatosensory brainstem evoked potential
SBF —
  serologic blocking factor
  specific blocking factor
  splanchnic blood flow
SBFT — small bowel follow-through
SBG — selenite brilliant green
SBGM — self-blood glucose monitoring
SBH —
  sea-blue histiocyte
  State Board of Health

SBI —
  soybean trypsin inhibitor
  systemic bacterial infection
SBIS — Stanford-Binet Intelligence Scale
SBL —
  serum bactericidal level
  soybean lecithin
sBL — sporadic Burkitt's lymphoma
SBLLA — sarcoma, breast and brain tumors, leukemia, laryngeal and lung cancer, and adrenal cortical carcinoma
SBMPL — simultaneous binaural midplace localization
SBN_2 — single-breath nitrogen [test]
SBNS — Society of British Neurological Surgeons
SBNT — single-breath nitrogen test
SBNW — single-breath nitrogen washout
SBO —
  small bowel obstruction
  spina bifida occulta
Sb_2O_3 — antimony trioxide
Sb_2O_5 — antimony pentoxide
SBOD — scleral buckle, right eye (O.D.)
SBOM — soybean oil meal
SBOS — scleral buckle, left eye (O.S.)
SBP —
  schizobipolar
  scleral buckling procedure
  serotonin-binding protein
  spontaneous bacterial peritonitis
  steroid-binding plasma [protein]
  subacute bacterial peritonitis
  sulfobromophthalein
  systemic blood pressure
  systolic blood pressure
SBQ — Smoking Behavior Questionnaire

SBQC — small-based quad cane
SBR —
  small bowel resection
  spleen-to-body (weight) ratio
  stillbirth rate
  strict bed rest
  styrene-butadiene rubber
Sbr — short branches
SBRN — sensory branch of radial nerve
SBS —
  shaken baby syndrome
  short bowel syndrome
  sick building syndrome
  sinobronchial syndrome
  small bowel series
  social breakdown syndrome
  straight back syndrome
SBSM — self-blood sugar monitoring
SBSRT — Spreen-Benton Sentence Repetition Test
SBSS — Seligmann's buffered salt solution
SBT —
  serum bactericidal titer
  single-breath test
  sulbactam
SBTI — soybean trypsin inhibitor
SBTPE — State Boards Test Pool Examination
SBTT — small bowel transit time
SBV — singular binocular vision
SC —
  conditioned stimulus
  sacrococcygeal
  Sanitary Corps
  scalenus [muscle]
  scapula
  schedule change
  Schwann cell
  Scianna [blood group]
  sciatica
  science
  sclerocorneal
  secondary cleavage
  secretory component
  self care

SC — *(continued)*
 semicircular
 semiclosed
 semilunar valve closure
 serum complement
 serum creatinine
 service connected
 sex chromatin
 Sézary cell
 short circuit
 sick call
 sickle cell
 sieving coefficient
 silicone-coated
 single chemical
 skin conduction
 slow component
 Snellen's chart
 sodium citrate
 soluble complex
 special care
 specific characteristic
 spinal canal
 spinal cord
 splenic collateral
 squamous carcinoma
 statistical control
 stellate cell
 sternoclavicular
 stratum corneum
 stroke count
 subcellular
 subclavian
 subcorneal
 subcortical
 subcutaneous
 succinylcholine
 sugar-coated
 sulfur colloid
 superior colliculus
 superior constrictor
 superior cornu
 supportive care
 suppressor cell
 surface colony
 surgical cone
 systemic candidiasis
 systolic click

S-C — sickle cell
S&C — sclerae and conjunctivae
Sc —
 scandium
 scapula
 science
 scientific
 screening
sc —
 scant
 sclera
 subcutaneous
sc. — *scilicet* (Lat.) one may know
SCA —
 selective coronary angiogram
 self-care agency
 severe congenital anomaly
 sickle cell anemia
 single-channel analyzer
 sperm-coating antigen
 spleen colony assay
 steroidal-cell antibody
 subclavian artery
 subcutaneous abdominal
  [block]
 superior cerebellar artery
 suppressor cell activity
S_{Ca} — serum calcium
SCAA —
 Skin Care Association of
  America
 sporadic cerebral amyloid
  angiopathy
SCABG — single coronary artery
 bypass graft
SCAG —
 Sandoz Clinical Assessment—
  Geriatric [Rating]
 single coronary artery graft
SCAMC — Symposium on Com-
 puter Applications in Medical
 Care
SCAMIN — Self-Concept and
 Motivation Inventory
SCAN —
 scintiscan
 suspected child abuse and neglect

SCAN — *(continued)*
    systolic coronary artery narrowing
SCAP — scapula
SCARF — skeletal abnormalities, cutis laxa, craniostenosis, psychomotor retardation, facial abnormalities [syndrome]
SCAT —
    sheep cell agglutination test
    sickle cell anemia test
    Sports Competition Anxiety Test
scat. — *scatula* (Lat.) box
scat. orig. — *scatula originalis* (Lat.) original package, manufacturer's package
SCB — strictly confined to bed
SCBA — self-contained breathing apparatus
SCBC — small-cell bronchogenic carcinoma
SCBE — single-contrast barium enema
SCBF — spinal cord blood flow
SCBG — symmetric calcification of the basal cerebral ganglia
SCBH — systemic cutaneous basophil hypersensitivity
SCBP — stratum corneum basic protein
SCBU — screening bacteriuria
SCC —
    sequential combination chemotherapy
    Services for Crippled Children
    short-course chemotherapy
    sickle cell crisis
    small-cell carcinoma
    small cleaved cell
    spinal cord compression
    squamous cell carcinoma
SCCA — single-cell cytotoxicity assay
SCCB — small-cell carcinoma of the bronchus
SCCC — squamous cell cervical carcinoma

SCCH — sternocostoclavicular hyperostosis
SCCHN — squamous cell carcinoma of the head and neck
SCCHO — sternocostoclavicular hyperostosis
SCCL — small cell carcinoma of the lung
SCCM — Sertoli cell culture medium
SCCT — severe cerebrocranial trauma
SCD —
    sequential compression device
    service-connected disability
    sickle-cell disease
    spinal cord disease
    spinocerebellar degeneration
    subacute combined degeneration
    subacute coronary disease
    sudden cardiac death
    sudden coronary death
    systemic carnitine deficiency
Sc.D. — Doctor of Science
ScDA — *scapulodextra anterior* (Lat.) right scapuloanterior [fetal position]
SCDH — spinal cord dorsal horn
ScDP — *scapulodextra posterior* (Lat.) right scapuloposterior [fetal position]
SCE —
    saturated calomel electrode
    secretory carcinoma of the endometrium
    sister chromatid exchange
    split hand–cleft lip/palate–ectodermal [dysplasia]
    subcutaneous emphysema
SCe — somatic cell
SCEP —
    sandwich counterelectrophoresis
    somatosensory cortical evoked potential
SCER — sister chromatid exchange rate

SCF — Skin Cancer Foundation
SCFA — short-chain fatty acid
SCFE — slipped capital femoral epiphysis
SCFI — specific clotting factor and inhibitor
SCG —
    serum chemistry graft
    serum chemogram
    sodium cromoglycate
    superior cervical ganglion
SCH — Schirmer [test]
SCh —
    succinylchloride
    succinylcholine
SChE — serum cholinesterase
sched. — schedule
schis. — schistocyte
schiz. — schizophrenia
SCHL — subcapsular hematoma of the liver
SCI —
    Science Citation Index
    short crus of incus
    spinal cord injury
    structured clinical interview
Sci —
    science
    scientific
SCID — severe combined immunodeficiency disease
SCII — Strong-Campbell Interest Inventory
SCIPP — sacrococcygeal to inferior pubic point
SCIS —
    severe combined immunodeficiency syndrome
    spinal cord injury service
scint — scintigram
SCIU — spinal cord injury unit
SCIV —
    subclavian intravenous
    subcutaneous intravenous
SCIWORA — spinal cord injury without radiographic abnormality
SCJ —
    sclerocorneal junction

SCJ — (continued)
    squamocolumnar junction
    sternoclavicular joint
    sternocostal joint
SCK — serum creatine kinase
SCL —
    scleroderma
    serum copper level
    sinus cycle length
    skin conductance level
    soft contact lens
    symptom checklist
    syndrome checklist
scl —
    sclerosed
    sclerosis
    sclerotic
ScLA — *scapulolaeva anterior* (Lat.) left scapuloanterior [fetal position]
SCLC — small cell lung carcinoma
SCLD — sickle-cell chronic lung disease
SCLE —
    subacute cutaneous lupus erythematosus
    subcutaneous lupus erythematosus
scler —
    scleroderma
    sclerosis
ScLP — *scapulolaeva posterior* (Lat.) left scapuloposterior [fetal position]
SCLS — systemic capillary leak syndrome
SCM —
    Schwann cell membrane
    sensation, circulation, and motion
    Society of Computer Medicine
    soluble cytotoxic medium
    spleen cell-conditioned medium
    spondylitic caudal myelopathy
    State Certified Midwife

SCM — (continued)
   steatocystoma multiplex
   sternocleidomastoid [muscle]
   streptococcal cell membrane
   surface-connecting membrane
ScM — scalene muscle
SCMC — spontaneous cell-mediated cytotoxicity
SCMD — senile choroidal macular degeneration
SCMO — Senior Clerical Medical Officer
SCN —
   solid cell nests
   special care nursery
   suprachiasmatic nucleus
SC$_{Na}$ — sieving coefficient for sodium
SCNS — subcutaneous nerve stimulation
SCO —
   sclerocystic ovary
   somatic crossing-over
   subcommissural organ
scop. — scopolamine
SCP
   single-celled protein
   sodium cellulose phosphate
   soluble cytoplasmic protein
   standard care plan
   submucous cleft palate
   superior cerebral peduncle
s.c.p. — spherical candle power
SCPK — serum creatine phosphokinase
SCPN — serum carboxypeptidase N
SCPNT — Southern California Postrotary Nystagmus Test
SCR —
   Schick conversion rate
   silicon-controlled rectifier
   skin conductance response
   slow-cycling rhodopsin
   spondylitic caudal radiculopathy
SCr — serum creatinine
scr. — scrupulus (Lat.) scruple

SCRAM — speech-controlled respirometer for ambulation measurement
scRNA — small cytoplasmic ribonucleic acid
SCS —
   Saethre-Chotzen syndrome
   shared computer system
   silicon-controlled switch
   Society of Clinical Surgery
   spinal cord stimulation
   systolic click syndrome
SCSB — static charge–sensitive bed
SCSIT — Southern California Sensory Integration Test
SCT —
   salmon calcitonin
   Sentence Completion Test
   sex chromatin test
   sexual compatibility test
   sickle-cell trait
   sperm cytotoxicity
   spinal computed tomography
   spinocervicothalamic
   staphylococcal clumping test
   sugar-coated tablet
SCTAT — sex cord tumor with annular tubules
SCTx — spinal cervical traction
SCU —
   self-care unit
   special care unit
SCUBA — self-contained underwater breathing apparatus
SCUD — septicemic cutaneous ulcerative disease
SCUF — slow continuous ultrafiltration
SCUM — secondary carcinoma of upper mediastinum
scu-PA — single chain urokinase-type plasminogen activator
SCUT — schizophrenia, chronic undifferentiated type
SCV —
   sensory nerve conduction velocity

SCV — (continued)
  smooth, capsulated, virulent
  squamous-cell carcinoma of
    the vulva
  subclavian vein
SCV-CPR — simultaneous compression ventilation–cardiopulmonary resuscitation
SD —
  sagittal depth
  Sandhoff disease
  scleroderma
  secretion droplet
  senile dementia
  septal defect
  serologically defined
  serologically detectable
  serologically determined
  serum defect
  severe disability
  Shine-Dalgarno [sequence]
  short dialysis
  shoulder disarticulation
  Shy-Draper [syndrome]
  skin destruction
  skin dose
  somatization disorder
  sphincter dilatation
  spontaneous delivery
  sporadic depression
  Sprague-Dawley [rat]
  spreading depression
  stable disease
  standard deviation
  standard diet
  statistical documentation
  Stensen duct
  sterile dressing
  Still's disease
  stone disintegration
  strength duration
  streptodornase
  sudden death
  sulfadiazine
  superoxide dismutase
  surgical drain
  systolic discharge
S/D —
  sharp/dull

S/D — (continued)
  sit and dangle
  systolic/diastolic
S-D —
  sickle-cell (hemoglobin D)
    disease
  strength-duration [curve]
  suicide-depression
S&D — stomach and duodenum
Sd — stimulus drive
S^d — discriminative stimulus
SDA —
  Sabouraud dextrose agar
  sacrodextra anterior (Lat.)
    right sacroanterior [fetal po-
      sition]
  salt-dependent agglutinin
  sialodacryoadenitis
  specific dynamic action
  steroid-dependent asthmatic
  succinic dehydrogenase activ-
    ity
SDAT — senile dementia of Alzheimer type
SDB — sleep-disordered breathing
SDBP — seated (or standing, or supine) diastolic blood pressure
SDC —
  serum digoxin concentration
  sodium deoxycholate
  subacute combined degenera-
    tion
  subclavian hemodialysis cathe-
    ter
  succinyldicholine
SD&C — suction, dilation and curettage
SDCL — symptom distress checklist
SDD —
  sporadic depressive disease
  sterile dry dressing
SDDS — 2-sulfamoyl-4,4'-diami-
  nodiphenylsulfone
SDE — specific dynamic effect
SDEEG — stereotactic depth electroencephalography
SDES — symptomatic diffuse
  esophageal spasm

SDF —
  slow death factor
  stress distribution factor
SDFP — single donor frozen
  plasma
SDG —
  succinate dehydrogenase
  sucrose density gradient
SDH —
  serine dehydrase
  sorbitol dehydrogenase
  spinal dorsal horn
  subdural hematoma
  succinate dehydrogenase
SDHD — sudden death heart disease
SDI —
  standard deviation interval
  survey diagnostic instrument
SDIHD — sudden death ischemic
  heart disease
SDILINE — Selective Dissemina-
  tion of Information On-Line
  [data bank]
SDL —
  serum digoxin level
  speech discrimination level
sdl —
  sideline
  subline
SDM —
  sensory detection method
  standard deviation of the
    mean
SDMS — Society of Diagnostic
  Medical Sonographers
SDN — sexually dimorphic nucleus
SDO — sudden dosage onset
SDP —
  single-donor platelets
  stomach, duodenum, and pan-
    creas
  sacrodextra posterior (Lat.)
    right sacroposterior [fetal
    position]
SDR —
  spontaneously diabetic rat

SDR — (*continued*)
  surgical dressing room
SDRT — Stanford Diagnostic
  Reading Test
SDS —
  same-day surgery
  school dental services
  Self-Rating Depression Scale
  sensory deprivation syndrome
  sexual differentiation scale
  Shy-Drager syndrome
  single-dose suppression
  sodium dodecyl sulfate
  specific diagnosis service
  speech discrimination score
  standard deviation score
  sudden death syndrome
  sulfadiazine silver
  sustained depolarizing shift
SD-SK — streptodornase-streptoki-
  nase
SDS-PAGE — sodium dodecyl sulfate–polyacrylamide gel electrophoresis
SDT —
  sacrodextra transversa (Lat.)
    right sacrotransverse [fetal
    position]
  single-donor transfusion
  speech detection threshold
SD_t — standard deviation of total
  scores
SDU —
  Standard Deviation Unit
  step-down unit
SDUB — short double upright
  brace
SE —
  saline enema
  sanitary engineering
  sheep erythrocyte
  side effect
  smoke exposure
  solid extract
  sphenoethmoidal [suture]
  spherical equivalent
  spin-echo
  spongiform encephalopathy

SE — *(continued)*
    Spurway-Eddowes [syndrome]
    squamous epithelium
    standard error
    staphylococcal endotoxin
    staphylococcal enterotoxin
    starch equivalent
    Starr-Edwards [prosthesis]
    status epilepticus
    subendocardial
    subendothelial
S&E — safety and efficacy
Se —
    secretion
    selenium
SEA —
    sheep erythrocyte agglutina-
       tion
    sheep erythrocyte antibody
    sheep erythrocyte antigen
    shock-elicited aggression
    soluble egg antigen
    spontaneous electrical activity
    staphylococcal enterotoxin A
SEAT — sheep erythrocyte aggluti-
    nation test
SEB —
    seborrhea
    staphylococcal enterotoxin B
SEBA — staphylococcal entero-
    toxin B antiserum
SEBL — self-emptying blind loop
SEBM — Society for Experimental
    Biology and Medicine
SEC —
    secretin
    secretion
    Singapore epidemic
       conjunctivitis
    size exclusion chromatography
    soft elastic capsule
    squamous epithelial cell
Sec — Seconal
sec. —
    second
    secondary
    section
    secundum (Lat.) according to

sec. a. — *secundum artem* (Lat.) ac-
    cording to art
sec-Bu — sec-butyl
SECG — stress electrocardiography
SECPR — standard external car-
    diopulmonary resuscitation
SECSY — spin-echo correlated
    spectroscopy
sect — section
SED —
    sedimentation rate
    skin erythema dose
    spondyloepiphyseal dysplasia
    standard error of deviation
    staphylococcal enterotoxin D
sed. —
    sedative
    sedes (Lat.) stool
    sedimentation
sed rate — sedimentation rate
SEE — standard error of estimate
SEEG — stereotactic electroen-
    cephalography
SEEP — small end-expiratory pres-
    sure
SEER — Surveillance, Epidemiol-
    ogy, and End Results [Pro-
    gram]
SEF —
    somatically evoked field
    staphylococcal enterotoxin F
SEG —
    segment
    segmented
    soft elastic gelatin [capsule]
    sonoencephalogram
seg — segment
segs — segmented neutrophils
SEGNE — secretory granules of
    neural and endocrine [cells]
SEH — subependymal hemorrhage
SEI —
    Self-Esteem Inventory
    subepithelial infiltrate
    superficial epithelial infiltrates
SELF — Self-Evaluation of Life
    Function [scale]

SELFVD — sterile elective low-forceps vaginal delivery

SEM —
sample evaluation method
scanning electron microscopy
secondary enrichment medium
soft ejection murmur
somatosensory evoked potential
standard error of the mean
systolic ejection murmur

sem. —
semen
seminal

SEMDJL — spondyloepimetaphyseal dysplasia with joint laxity

SEMI —
subendocardial myocardial infarction
subendocardial myocardial injury

semi- — one-half

semid. — *semidrachma* (Lat.) half a drachm (dram)

semih. — *semihora* (Lat.) half an hour

sem. in d. — *semel in die* (Lat.) once a day

SEN —
scalp-ear-nipple [syndrome]
State Enrolled Nurse

sen —
sensitive
sensitivity

SENA — sympathetic efferent nerve activity

SENSOR — Sentinel Event Notification System for Occupational Risks

sens —
sensation
sensorium
sensory

SEO — Surgical Emergency Officer

SEP —
sensory evoked potential
septum

SEP — *(continued)*
sepultus (Lat.) buried
serum electrophoresis
somatosensory evoked potential
sperm entry point
spinal evoked potential
surface epithelium
systolic ejection period

sep. — *sepultus* (Lat.) buried

separ. — *separatum* (Lat.) separately

sept. — *septem* (Lat.) seven

SEQ — side-effects questionnaire

seq —
sequel
sequela
sequence
sequestrum

seq. luce — *sequenti luce* (Lat.) the following day

SER —
scanning equalization radiography
sebum excretion rate
sensory evoked response
service
smooth endoplasmic reticulum
smooth-surface endoplasmic reticulum
somatosensory evoked response
supination, external rotation [fracture]
systolic ejection rate

Ser —
serine
serology
serous
service

sER — smooth endoplasmic reticulum

ser —
serial
series

SER–IV — supination–external rotation, type IV fracture

SerCl — serum chloride
SERHOLD — National Biomedical Serials Holding Database
SERLINE — Serials on Line
serol. —
    serological
    serology
SERS — Stimulus Evaluation/Response Selection [test]
SERT — sustained ethanol release tube
Serv. — service
serv. — *serva* (Lat.) keep, preserve
SERVHEL — Service and Health Records
SES —
    seasonal energy syndrome
    Society of Eye Surgeons
    socioeconomic status
    spatial emotional stimulus
    subendothelial space
SESAP — Surgical Educational and Self-Assessment Program
sesquih. — *sesquihora* (Lat.) an hour and a half
sesunc. — *sesuncia* (Lat.) an ounce and a half
SET —
    skin endpoint titration
    systolic ejection time
sev. —
    severe
    severed
SEWHO — shoulder-elbow-wrist-hand orthosis
s. expr. — *sine expressione* (Lat.) without expressing or pressing
SF —
    Sabin-Feldman [test]
    safety factor
    salt-free
    saturated fat
    scarlet fever
    Schilder-Foix disease
    seizure frequency
    seminal fluid
    serosal fluid
    serum factor

SF — (*continued*)
    serum ferritin
    serum fibrinogen
    sham feeding
    shell fragment
    shrapnel fragment
    shunt flow
    sickle cell-hemoglobin F [disease]
    simian foam-virus
    skin fibroblast
    skin fluorescence
    soft feces
    soluble factor
    sound field
    spinal fluid
    spontaneous fibrillation
    spontaneous fission
    spontaneous fracture
    stable factor
    sterile female
    stress formula
    sugar-free
    superior facet
    suprasternal fossa
    supressor factor
    survival fraction
    swine fever
    symptom-free
    synovial fluid
Sf — *Streptococcus faecalis*
S_f — Svedberg's flotation unit
SFA —
    saturated folic acid
    seminal fluid assay
    serum folic acid
    stimulated fibrinolytic activity
    superficial femoral angioplasty
    superior femoral artery
SFB —
    Sanfilippo syndrome type B
    saphenofemoral bypass
    surgical foreign body
SFBL — self-filling blind loop
SFC —
    serum fungicidal
    soluble fibrin–fibrinogen complex

SFC — *(continued)*
  spinal fluid count
SFD —
  sheep factor delta
  silo filler's disease
  skin-film distance
  soy-free diet
  spectral frequency distribution
SFEMG — single fiber electromyography
SFFA — serum free fatty acid
SFFF — sedimentation field flow fractionation
SFFV — spleen focus-forming virus
SFG —
  spotted fever group
  subglottic foreign body
SFH —
  schizophrenia family history
  serum-free hemoglobin
  stroma-free hemoglobin
SFI —
  Sexual Function Index
  Social Function Index
SFL — synovial fluid lymphocyte
SFLE — Stress From Life Experience
SFM — serum-free medium
SFMC — soluble fibrin monomer complex
SFO — subfornical organ
SFP —
  screen filtration pressure
  simultaneous foveal perception
  spinal fluid pressure
  stopped flow pressure
SFPT — standard fixation preference test
SFR —
  screen filtration resistance
  stroke with full recovery
SFS —
  serial focal seizures
  skin and fascia stapler
  split function study
SFT —
  Sabin-Feldman test

SFT — *(continued)*
  sensory feedback therapy
  serum-free thyroxine
  skinfold thickness
SFTR — sagittal, frontal, transverse, rotation
SFU — surgical follow-up
SFV —
  Semliki Forest virus
  shipping fever virus
  Shope fibroma virus
  squirrel fibroma virus
  superficial femoral vein
SFW —
  sexual function of women
  shell fragment wound
  shrapnel fragment wound
  slow-filling wave
SG —
  Sachs-Georgi [test]
  salivary gland
  secretory granule
  serous granule
  serum globulin
  serum glucose
  skin graft
  soluble gelatin
  specific gravity
  subgluteal
  substantia gelatinosa
  Surgeon General
  Swan-Ganz [catheter]
SGA — small for gestational age
SG_{AW} — specific airway conductance
SGB — sparsely granulated basophil
SGC —
  serum gentamicin concentration
  spermicide-germicide compound
SGD —
  specific granule deficiency
  straight gravity drainage
SGE —
  secondary generalized epilepsy
  significant glandular enlargement

SGF —
    sarcoma growth factor
    skeletal growth factor
SGFR — single-nephron glomerular filtration rate
SGH — subgaleal hematoma
SGL — salivary gland lymphocyte
SGM — Society for General Microbiology
SGO —
    Surgeon General's Office
    surgery, gynecology, and obstetrics
SGOT — serum glutamic-oxaloacetic transaminase (aspartate transaminase)
SGP —
    serine glycerophosphatide
    sialoglycoprotein
    Society of General Physiologists
    soluble glycoprotein
SGPT — serum glutamate pyruvate transaminase (alanine transaminase)
SGR —
    Sachs-Georgi reaction
    Shwartzman generalized reaction
    skin galvanic reflex
    submandibular gland renin
    substantia gelatinosa Rolandi
SGS —
    second-generation sulfonylurea
    subglottic stenosis
S-Gt — Sachs-Georgi test
SGTT — standard glucose tolerance test
SGV —
    salivary gland virus
    selective gastric vagotomy
    small granular vesicle
SGVHD — syngeneic graft-versus-host disease
SH —
    Salter-Harris [fracture]
    Schönlein-Henoch [purpura]

SH — (continued)
    self-help
    serum hepatitis
    sex hormone
    sexual harassment
    Sherman [rat]
    sick in hospital
    sinus histiocytosis
    social history
    somatotropic hormone
    spontaneously hypertensive
    state hospital
    sulfhydryl
    surgical history
    symptomatic hypoglycemia
    syndrome of hyporeninemic hypoaldosteronism
    systemic hyperthermia
S/H —
    sample and hold
    suicidal/homicidal ideation
S&H — speech and hearing
Sh —
    sheep
    Sherwood number
    Shigella
sh. —
    short
    shoulder
SHA —
    staphylococcal hemagglutinating antibody
    superheated aerosol
sHa — suckling hamster
SHAA —
    serum hepatitis–associated antigen
    Society of Hearing Aid Audiologists
SHAA-Ab — serum hepatitis–associated antigen-antibody
SHAFT — sad, hostile, anxious, frustrated, tenacious (patient) [syndrome]
SHARP — School Health Additional Referral Program
SHAV — superior hemiazygos vein

SHB —
   sequential hemibody [irradiation]
   subacute hepatitis with bridging

SHb —
   sickle hemoglobin
   sulfhemoglobin

SHBD — serum hydroxybutyrate dehydrogenase

SHBG — sex hormone–binding globulin

SHCC — State Health Coordinating Council

SHCO — sulfated hydrogenated castor oil

SHE — Syrian hamster embryo

SHEENT — skin, head, eyes, ears, nose, and throat

SHF — simian hemorrhagic fever

shf — super-high frequency

SHG — synthetic human gastrin

SHH — syndrome of hyporeninemic hypoaldosteronism

SHHD — Scottish Home and Health Department

SHHP — semihorizontal heart position

SHHV — Society for Health and Human Values

Shig — *Shigella*

SHL —
   sensorineural hearing loss
   supraglottic horizontal laryngectomy

SHLA — soluble human lymphocyte antigen

shld — shoulder

SHML — sinus histiocytosis with massive lymphadenopathy

SHMO — Senior Hospital Medical Officer

SHMT — serine-hydroxymethyl transferase

SHN —
   spontaneous hemorrhagic necrosis
   subacute hepatic necrosis

SHO —
   secondary hypertrophic osteoarthropathy
   Senior House Officer
   Student Health Organization

SHORT — short stature, hyperextensibility of joints or hernia or both, ocular depression, Rieger anomaly, teething delayed

SHP —
   Schönlein-Henoch purpura
   secondary hyperparathyroidism
   state health plan
   surgical hypoparathyroidism

SHPDA — State Health Planning and Development Agency

SHPT — secondary hyperparathyroidism

SHR — spontaneously hypertensive rat

SHS —
   Sayre head sling
   sheep hemolysate supernatant
   Shipley-Hartford Scale

SHSP — spontaneously hypertensive stroke-prone [rat]

SHSS — Stanford Hypnotic Susceptibility Scale

SHT —
   simple hypocalcemic tetany
   subcutaneous histamine test

SHUR — System for Hospital Uniform Reporting

SHV — simian herpes virus

SHx — social history

SI —
   sacroiliac
   saline infusion
   saline injection
   saturation index
   self-inflicted
   sensitive index
   sensory integration
   septic inflammation
   serious illness
   seriously ill

SI — (continued)
>   serum insulin
>   serum iron
>   severity index
>   sex inventory
>   Singh Index
>   single injection
>   small intestine
>   soluble insulin
>   special intervention
>   spirochetosis icterohaemor-
>   rhagica
>   stimulation index
>   stress incontinence
>   strict isolation
>   stroke index
>   suicidal ideation
>   sulfated insulin
>   suppression index
>   systolic index
>   Système International
>   d'Unités (Fr.) International
>   System of Units

Si —
>   the most anterior point on
>   the lower contour of the
>   sella turcica [point]
>   silicon

S/I — sucrose to isomaltase [ratio]

S&I — suction and irrigation

SIA —
>   serum inhibitory activity
>   single intracranial aneurysm
>   stimulation-induced analgesia
>   stress-induced analgesia
>   stress-induced anesthesia
>   subacute infectious arthritis
>   synalbumin-insulin antago-
>   nism
>   syncytia induction assay

SIADH — syndrome of inappropri-
>   ate antidiuretic hormone

SIB — self-injurious behavior

sib — sibling

SIC —
>   serum inhibitory concentra-
>   tion
>   serum insulin concentration

SIC — (continued)
>   Standard Industrial Classifica-
>   tion

sic. — siccus (Lat.) dry

SICD —
>   Sequenced Inventory of Com-
>   municative Development
>   serum isocitric dehydrogenase

SICSVA — sequential impaction
>   cascade sieve volumetric air

SICT — selective intracoronary
>   thrombolysis

SICU —
>   spinal intensive care unit
>   surgical intensive care unit

SID —
>   single intradermal [test]
>   Society for Investigative Der-
>   matology
>   sucrase-isomaltase deficiency
>   sudden inexplicable death
>   sudden infant death
>   suggested indication of diag-
>   nosis
>   systemic inflammatory disease

s.i.d. — semel in die (Lat.) once a
>   day

SIDER — siderocytes

SIDS — sudden infant death syn-
>   drome

SIE — stroke in evolution

SIECUS — Sex Information and
>   Education Council of the
>   United States

SIF — serum-inhibition factor

SI and F — spinal instrumentation
>   and fusion

SIFT — selector ion flow tube

SIg —
>   serum immune globulin
>   surface immunoglobulin

sig —
>   sigmoidoscope
>   sigmoidoscopy
>   signal
>   signature
>   significant

sig. — signetur (Lat.) let it be la-
>   beled

S-IgA — secretory immunoglobulin A

sig. n. pro. — *signa nomine proprio*
(Lat.) label with the proper
name

SIH —
stimulation-induced hypalge-
sia
stress-induced hyperthermia

SIHE — spontaneous intramural
hematoma of the esophagus

SihPTH — serum immunoreactive
human parathyroid hormone

SIJ — sacroiliac joint

SIL —
seriously ill
soluble interleukin
speech interference level

SILD — Sequenced Inventory of
Language Development

SILFVD — sterile indicated low
forceps vaginal delivery

SILS — Shipley Institute of Living
Scale

SIM —
selected ion monitoring
Society of Industrial Microbiology
sucrase-isomaltase
sulfide, indole, motility [me-
dium]

SIMA — single internal mammary
artery

simp. — *simplex* (Lat.) simple

SIMS — secondary ion mass spectroscopy

simul. — simultaneously

SIMV — synchronized intermittent mandatory ventilation

sin. — *sine* (Lat.) without

s.i.n. — *sex in nocte* (Lat.) six
times a night

sine conf. — *sine confectione* (Lat.)
without sweetness

sing. —
singular
singulorum (Lat.) of each

sing. aur. — *singulis auroris* (Lat.)
every morning

sing. hor. quad. — *singulis horae
quadrantibus* (Lat.) every quarter of an hour

si non val. — *si non valeat* (Lat.) if
it is not enough

SIO — sacroiliac orthosis

SiO_2 — silicon dioxide (silica)

si op. sit — *si opus sit* (Lat.) if it is
necessary

SIP —
Sickness Impact Profile
slow inhibitory potential
student intern program
surface inductive plethysmography

sIPTH — serum immunoreactive
parathyroid hormone

SIQ — Symptom Interpretation
Questionnaire

SIR —
single isomorphous replacement
specific immune release
standardized incidence ratio
syndrome of immediate reac-
tivities

SIRA — Scientific Instrument Research Association

SIREF — specific immune response–enhancing factor

SIRF — severely impaired renal
function

SIRS —
soluble immune response suppressor
Structured Interview of Reported Symptoms

SIS —
serotonin irritation syndrome
simian sarcoma
simulator-induced syndrome
social information system
spontaneous interictal spike
sterile injectable solution
sterile injectable suspension

SISI — short increment sensitivity
index

SISS —
    serum inhibitor of streptolysin
        S
    small inducible secreted sub-
        stances
SISV — simian sarcoma virus
SIT —
    serum inhibiting titer
    sperm immobilization test
SIV —
    simian immunodeficiency
        virus
    Sprague-Dawley-Ivanovas [rat]
SIVagm — simian immunodefi-
    ciency virus from African
    green monkeys
si vir. perm. — *si vires permitant*
    (Lat.) if the strength will per-
    mit
SIVMAC — simian immunodefi-
    ciency virus of macaques
SIVP — slow intravenous push
SIW — self-inflicted wound
SIWIP — self-induced water intox-
    ication and psychosis
SIWIS — self-induced water intox-
    ication and schizophrenic dis-
    orders
S_J — Jaccard coefficient
SJR — Shinowara-Jones-Reinhart
    [unit]
SJS —
    Stevens-Johnson syndrome
    stiff joint syndrome
    Swyer-James syndrome
SjS — Sjögren syndrome
SK —
    seborrheic keratosis
    senile keratosis
    solar keratosis
    spontaneous killer [cell]
    streptokinase
    striate keratopathy
    swine kidney
Sk — skin
SKA — supracondylar knee-ankle
    [orthosis]
SKAB — skeletal antibody

SKAO — supracondylar knee-
    ankle orthosis
SKAT — Sex Knowledge and Atti-
    tude Test
skel —
    skeletal
    skeleton
SKI — Sloan-Kettering Institute
SKL — serum killing level
SKSD — streptokinase-streptodor-
    nase
sk trx — skeletal traction
SKW — Sturge-Kalischer-Weber
    [syndrome]
SL —
    sarcolemma
    satellite-like
    sclerosing leukoencephalopa-
    thy
    secondary leukemia
    sensation level
    sensory latency
    short-leg [brace]
    Sibley-Lehninger [unit]
    signal level
    Sinding-Larsen [disease]
    small lymphocyte
    sodium lactate
    solidified liquid
    sound level
    streptolysin
    Strümpell-Lorrain [disease]
    sublingual
S/L —
    slit lamp
    sucrase to lactase [ratio]
S→L — serosa to lumen
Sl — Steel [mouse]
sl —
    slight
    slyke
    stemline
    sublingual
s.l. —
    secundum legum (Lat.) ac-
    cording to law
    sensu lato (Lat.) in a broad
    sense

SLA —
  sacrolaeva anterior (Lat.) left sacroanterior [fetal position]
  single-cell liquid cytotoxic assay
  slide latex agglutination
  soluble liver antigen
  surfactant-like activity
SLAC — scapholunate advanced collapse [wrist]
SLAM — scanning laser acoustic microscope
SLAP — serum leucine aminopeptidase
s. lat. — *sensu lato* (Lat.) in a broad sense
SLB — short-leg brace
SLC —
  short-leg cast
  sodium-lithium countertransport
SLCC — short-leg cylinder cast
SLDH — serum lactate dehydrogenase
SLDS — single-level dynamic scan
SLE —
  St. Louis encephalitis
  slit lamp examination
  systemic lupus erythematosus
SLEP — short latent evoked potential
SLEV — St. Louis encephalitis virus
SLFIA — substrate-labeled fluorescence immunoassay
SLFVD — sterile low forceps vaginal delivery
SLHR — sex-linked hypophosphatemic rickets
SLI —
  secretin-like immunoreactivity
  selective lymphoid irradiation
  somatostatin-like immunoreactivity
  splenic localization index
SLIP — Singer-Loomis Inventory of Personality

SLIR — somatostatin-like immunoreactivity
SLKC — superior limbic keratoconjunctivitis
SLM — sound level meter
SLMC — spontaneous lymphocyte-mediated cytotoxicity
SLMFD — sterile low midforceps delivery
SLN —
  sublentiform nucleus
  superior laryngeal nerve
SLNWBC — short-leg nonweightbearing cast
SLNWC — short-leg nonwalking cast
SLO — streptolysin O
SLOS — Smith-Lemli-Opitz syndrome
SLP —
  sacrolaeva posterior (Lat.) left sacroposterior [fetal position]
  segmental limb (systolic) pressure
  sex-limited protein
  short luteal phase
  speech-language pathologist
  subluxation of the patella
SLPMS — short leg posterior molded splint
SLPP — serum lipophosphoprotein
SLR —
  Shwartzman local reaction
  single lens reflex
  straight leg raising
  Streptococcus lactis–resistant
SLRT —
  straight leg–raising tenderness
  straight leg–raising test
SLS —
  segment long-spacing [collagen]
  short-leg splint
  single limb support
  Sjögren-Larsson syndrome
  stagnant loop syndrome
  Stein-Leventhal syndrome

SLSQ — Speech and Language Screening Questionnaire

SLT —
  sacrolaeva transversa (Lat.) left sacrotransverse [fetal position]
  solid logic technology
  swing light test

SLUD — salivation, lacrimation, urination, defecation

SLWC — short-leg walking cast

SLZ — serum lysozyme

SM —
  Master of Science
  sadomasochism
  self-monitoring
  semimembranous
  Serratia marcescens
  Shigella mutant
  simple mastectomy
  skim milk
  smooth muscle
  somatomedin
  Space Medicine
  sphingomyelin
  splenic macrophage
  Sports Medicine
  stapedius muscle
  Staphylococcus medium
  Strümpell-Marie [syndrome]
  submandibular
  submaxillary
  submucosal
  submucous [gland]
  suckling mouse
  sucrose medium
  suction method
  superior mesenteric
  supramamillary
  sustained medication
  symptoms
  synaptic membrane
  synovial membrane
  systolic mean
  systolic motion
  systolic murmur

S/M — sadism/masochism

Sm —
  samarium

Sm — (*continued*)
  Serratia marcescens
  Smith [antigen]

sM — suckling mouse

sm. —
  small
  smear

SMA —
  schedule of maximal allowance
  sequential multiple analysis
  serum muramidase activity
  sequential multichannel autoanalyzer
  smooth muscle antibody
  Society for Medical Anthropology
  somatomedin A
  spinal muscular atrophy
  spontaneous motor activity
  standard method agar
  superior mesenteric artery
  supplementary motor area

SM-A — somatomedin A

SMA-6 — Sequential Multiple Analyzer [six different serum tests]

SMA-6/60 — Sequential Multiple Analyzer [six tests in 60 minutes]

SMA 12/60 — Sequential Multiple Analyzer [twelve tests in 60 minutes]

SMABF — superior mesenteric artery blood flow

SMABV — superior mesenteric artery blood velocity

SMAC — Sequential Multiple Analyzer Computer

SMAE — superior mesenteric artery embolism

SMAF —
  smooth muscle–activating factor
  specific macrophage–arming factor
  superior mesenteric artery (blood) flow

SMAG — Special Medical Advisory Group

SMAL — serum methyl alcohol level

sm an — small animal

SMAO — superior mesenteric artery occlusion

SMART — simultaneous multiple angle reconstruction technique

SMAS —
    submuscular aponeurotic system
    superficial musculoaponeurotic system
    superior mesenteric artery syndrome

SMAST — Short Michigan Alcoholism Screening Test

SMB —
    selected mucosal biopsy
    standard mineral base

sMb — suckling mouse brain

SMBG — self-monitored blood glucose

SMBP — serum myelin basic protein

SMC —
    Scientific Manpower Commission
    selenomethylnorcholesterol
    smooth muscle cell
    somatomedin C
    succinylmonocholine

SM-C — somatomedin C

SMCA —
    smooth muscle–contracting agent
    suckling mouse cataract agent

SMCD —
    senile macular choroidal degeneration
    systemic mast cell disease
    systemic meningococcal disease

SM-C/IGF — somatomedin C/insulin-like growth factor

SMCPA — System of Multi-Cultural Pluralistic Assessment

SMD —
    senile macular degeneration
    sternocleidomastoid diameter
    submanubrial dullness

SMDA —
    Safe Medical Devices Act [of 1990]
    starch methylenedianiline

SMDC — sodium-N-methyl dithiocarbamate

SMDS — secondary myelodysplastic syndrome

SME — severe myoclonic epilepsy

SMEDI — stillbirth-mummification, embryonic death, infertility [syndrome]

SMEI — severe myoclonic epilepsy of infancy

smf — sodium motive force

SMFP — state medical facilities plan

SMFVD — sterile midforceps vaginal delivery

SMG — submandibular gland

SMH —
    state mental hospital
    strongyloidiasis with massive hyperinfection

SMI —
    Self-Motivation Inventory
    Senior Medical Investigator
    sensory motor integration
    severe mental impairment
    small volume infusion
    stress myocardial image
    Style of Mind Inventory
    supplementary medical insurance
    sustained maximum inspiration

SmIg — surface membrane immunoglobulin

SMILE — sustained maximal inspiratory lung exercises

SML —
    single major locus
    smouldering leukemia

SMM — supplemental minimal medium

SMMD — specimen mass measurement device
SMN — second malignant neoplasm
SMNB — submaximal neuromuscular block
SMO —
    Senior Medical Officer
    serum monoamine oxidase
SMOH —
    Senior Medical Officer of Health
    Society of Medical Officers of Health
SMON — subacute myelo-optico-neuropathy
SMP —
    slow-moving protease
    standard medical practice
    standard medical procedure
    submitochondrial particle
    sulfamethoxypyrazine
SMR —
    senior medical resident
    sensorimotor rhythm
    severe mental retardation
    skeletal muscle relaxant
    somnolent metabolic rate
    standard morbidity ratio
    standard mortality residuum
    submucous resection
SMRR — submucous resection and rhinoplasty
SMRV — squirrel monkey retrovirus
SMS —
    senior medical student
    serial motor seizures
    Shared Medical Systems
    somatostatin
    State Medical Society
    stiff-man syndrome
    supplemental minimum sodium
SMSA — Standard Metropolitan Statistical Area
SMSV — San Miguel sea lion virus

SMT —
    Sertoli cell/mesenchyme tumor
    spontaneous mammary tumor
    stereotactic mesencephalic tractotomy
SMuLV — Scripps murine leukemia virus
SMV —
    submental vertex
    superior mesenteric vein
SMVT — sustained monomorphic ventricular tachycardia
SMX — sulfamethoxazole
SMZ — sulfamethazine
SN —
    sciatic notch
    sclerema neonatorum
    scrub nurse
    sensorineural
    sensory neuron
    seronegative
    serum neutralizing
    single nephron
    sinus node
    spinal needle
    spontaneous nystagmus
    staff nurse
    Standard Nomenclature
    sternal notch
    student nurse
    subnormal
    substantia nigra
    supernatant
    suprasternal notch
S/N — signal-to-noise [ratio]
Sn —
    subnasale
    tin (Lat., *stannum*)
s.n. — *secundum naturam* (Lat.) according to nature
SNA —
    specimen not available
    Student Nurses Association
    superior nasal artery
S_{Na} — serum sodium [concentration]
SNagg — serum normal agglutinator

SNAI — Standard Nomenclature of Athletic Injuries

SNAP — sensory nerve action potential

SNAT — suspected nonaccidental trauma

SNB —
scalene node biopsy
Silverman needle biopsy

SNC —
sistema nervosum centrale (Lat.) central nervous system
spontaneous neonatal chylothorax

SNCL — sinus node cycle length

SNCS — sensory nerve conduction studies

SNCV — sensory nerve conduction velocity

SND —
sinus node dysfunction
striatonigral degeneration

SNDA — Student National Dental Association

SNDO — Standard Nomenclature of Diseases and Operations

SNE —
sinus node electrogram
subacute necrotizing encephalomyelopathy

SNES — supracapsular nerve entrapment syndrome

SNF —
sinus node formation
skilled nursing facility

SNGBF — single nephron glomerular blood flow

SNGFR — single nephron glomerular filtration rate

SNGPF — single nephron glomerular plasma flow

SNHL — sensorineural hearing loss

SNIVT — Society of NonInvasive Vascular Technology

SNM —
Society of Nuclear Medicine

SNM — *(continued)*
sulfanilamide

SNMA — Student National Medical Association

SNMT — Society of Nuclear Medical Technologists

SNOBOL — String-Oriented Symbolic Language

SNODO — Standard Nomenclature of Diseases and Operations

SNOMED — Symmetrical Nomenclature of Medicine

SNOOP — Systematic Nursing Observation of Psychopathology

SNOP —
Standard Nomenclature of Pathology
Systematized Nomenclature of Pathology

SNP —
School Nurse Practitioner
sinus node potential
sodium nitroprusside

SNQ — superior nasal quadrant

SNR —
signal-to-noise ratio
substantia nigra zona reticulata
supernumerary rib

SNRB — selective nerve root block

snRNA — small nuclear ribonucleic acid

snRNP — small nuclear ribonucleoprotein

SNRT — sinus node recovery time

SNRTd — sinus node recovery time, direct measuring

SNRTi — sinus node recovery time, indirect measuring

SNS —
Senior Nursing Sister (British)
Society of Neurological Surgeons
sterile normal saline

SNS — (continued)
    sympathetic nervous system
SNSA — seronegative spondy-
    loarthropathy
SNST — sciatic nerve stretch test
SNT — sinuses, nose, and throat
SNV —
    spleen necrosis virus
    superior nasal vein
SNW — slow negative wave
SO —
    salpingo-oophorectomy
    Schlatter-Osgood [disease]
    second opinion
    sex offender
    shoulder orthosis
    spheno-occipital [syn-
      chondrosis]
    sphincter of Oddi
    standing orders
    suboccipital
    superior oblique [muscle]
    supraoptic
    supraorbital
S&O — salpingectomy and oopho-
    rectomy
SO_2 —
    oxygen saturation
    sulfur dioxide
SOA —
    serum opsonic activity
    supraorbital artery
    swelling of ankles
SoA — symptoms of asthma
SOAA — signed out against ad-
    vice
SOAMA — signed out against
    medical advice
SOA-MCA — superficial occipital
    artery to middle cerebral ar-
    tery
SOAP — subjective data, objective
    data, assessment, and plan
    [problem-oriented record]
SOAPIE — subjective, objective,
    assessment, plan, implementa-
    tion, and evaluation [prob-
    lem-oriented record]

SOB —
    see order blank
    shortness of breath
    suboccipitobregmatic
SOBOE — shortness of breath on
    exertion
SOC —
    sequential-type oral contra-
      ceptive
    Standard Occupational Classi-
      fication
    standard of care
    state of consciousness
    syphilitic osteochondritis
SoC — state of consciousness
SocSec — Social Security
SocServ — social services
S-OCT — serum ornithine carba-
    moxyltransferase
SOD —
    septo-optic dysplasia
    sinovenous occlusive disease
    superoxide dismutase
    surgical officer of the day
sod — sodium
SODAS — spheroidal oral drug ab-
    sorption system
sod. bicarb. — sodium bicarbonate
SODH — sorbitol dehydrogenase
SOF — superior orbital fissure
SOFS — spontaneous osteoporotic
    fracture of sacrum
SOH — sympathetic orthostatic
    hypotension
SOHN — supraoptic hypothalamic
    nucleus
SOL — space-occupying lesion
Sol. — soluble
sol. — solutio (Lat.) solution
SOLEC — stand on one leg, eyes
    closed
SOLST — Stephens Oral Lan-
    guage Screening Test
solv. — solve (Lat.) dissolve
SOLVD — Studies of Left Ventric-
    ular Dysfunction [trial]
SOM —
    secretory otitis media

SOM — (continued)
    sensitivity of method
    serous otitis media
    somatotropin
    somnolent
    sulformethoxine
    superior oblique muscle
    suppurative otitis media
SOMA — Student Osteopathic
    Medical Association
somat — somatic
SOMI — sternal-occipital-mandibular immobilization
SOMOS — Society of Military
    Orthopedic Surgeons
SON —
    superior olivary nucleus
    supraoptic nucleus
SONK — spontaneous osteonecrosis of the knee
sono —
    sonogram
    sonography
SOP — standard operating procedure
SoP — standard of performance
SOPA — syndrome of primary aldosteronism
SOPCA — sporadic olivopontocerebellar ataxia
SOPP — splanchnic occluded portal pressure
s. op. s. — si opus sit (Lat.) if it is
    necessary
SOQ — Suicide Opinion Questionnaire
SOR —
    stimulus-organism response
    superoxide release
SOr — supraorbitale
Sorb — sorbitol
SORD — sorbitol dehydrogenase
SOREMP — sleep-onset rapid eye
    movement period
SORT — Slosson Oral Reading
    Test
SOS —
    self-obtained smear

SOS — (continued)
    stimulation of senses
    supplemental oxygen system
s.o.s. — si opus sit (Lat.) if it is necessary
SOSF — single organ system failure
SOT —
    sensory organization test
    stream of thought
    systemic oxygen transport
SOTT — synthetic old tuberculin
    trichloroacetic acid
SOWS — subjective opiate withdrawal scale
SP —
    sacroposterior
    sacrum to pubis
    salivary progesterone
    schizotypal personality
    semi-private [room]
    senile plaque
    septum pellucidum
    sequential pulse
    seropositive
    serum protein
    shunt pressure
    shunt procedure
    silent period
    skin potential
    sleep deprivation
    soft palate
    solid phase
    spatial peak
    species
    speech pathology
    sphingomyelin
    spine
    spiramycin
    spirometry
    spleen
    spontaneous proliferation
    standard practice
    standard procedure
    staphylococcal protease
    status post
    steady potential
    stool preservative

SP — *(continued)*
    subliminal perception
    substance P
    suicide precautions
    summating potential
    suprapatellar
    suprapubic
    surfactant protein
    symphysis pubis
    synthase phosphatase
    systolic pressure

Sp —
    most posterior point on the posterior contour of the sella turcica
    sacropubic
    species
    sphenoid
    spine
    Spirillum
    summation potential

sP — senile parkinsonism

sp —
    space
    species
    specific
    spinal
    spine

sp. — *spiritus* (Lat.) spirit

s/p — status post

SPA —
    salt-poor albumin [albumin human]
    serum prothrombin activity
    sheep pulmonary adenomatosis
    sperm penetration assay
    spinal progressive amyotrophy
    spondyloarthropathy
    spontaneous platelet aggregation
    staphylococcal protein A
    stimulation-produced analgesia
    suprapubic aspiration

SP-A — surfactant protein A

sp act — specific activity

SPAD —
    stenosing peripheral arterial disease
    subcutaneous peritoneal access device

SPAF — Stroke Prevention in Atrial Fibrillation [study]

SPAG — small-particle aerosol generator

SPAI — steroid protein activity index

SPAM — scanning photoacoustic microscopy

span. — spansule

sp an — spinal anesthesia

SPAR — sensitivity prediction by acoustic reflex

SPAT — slow paroxysmal atrial tachycardia

SP-B — surfactant protein B

SPBI — serum protein-bound iodine

SPBT — suprapubic bladder tap

SPC —
    salicylamide, phenacetin, and caffeine
    seropositive carrier
    serum phenylalanine concentration
    single palmar crease
    single photoelectron count
    small pyramidal cell
    spleen cell
    standard platelet count
    statistical process control
    synthesizing protein complex

SPCA —
    serum prothrombin conversion accelerator (factor VII)
    Society for Prevention of Cruelty to Animals

SPCC — Spill Prevention, Control, and Countermeasure [plan]

SPCD — syndrome of primary ciliary dyskinesia

sp. cd. — spinal cord

SPD —
- schizotypal personality disorder
- sociopathic personality disorder
- specific paroxysmal discharge
- standard peak dilution
- storage pool deficiency

SPDC — striopallidodentate calcinosis

SPE —
- septic pulmonary edema
- serum protein electrolyte
- serum protein electrophoresis
- streptococcal pyrogenic exotoxin
- sucrose polyester
- superficial punctate erosions
- sustained physical exercise

SPEAR — selective parenteral and enteral anti-sepsis regimen

SPE-C — streptococcal pyrogenic exotoxin type C

Spec —
- specialist
- specialty

spec. —
- special
- specific
- specification
- specimen
- speculum

SPECT — single photon emission computed tomography

SPEG — serum protein electrophoretogram

SPEM — smooth pursuit eye movement

SPEP — serum protein electrophoresis

SPET — single photon emission tomography

SPF —
- skin protection factor
- specific-pathogen free
- spectrophotofluorometer
- S-phase fraction
- split products of fibrin

SPF — (continued)
- standard perfusion fluid
- streptococcal proliferative factor
- Stuart-Prower factor
- sun protection factor
- systemic pulmonary fistula

SPFI — solid phase fluorescence immunoassay

sp. fl. — spinal fluid

SPFT — Sixteen Personality Factors Test

SPG —
- serine phosphoglyceride
- sphenopalatine ganglion
- sucrose, phosphate, and glutamate
- symmetrical peripheral gangrene

spg — sponge

sp gr — specific gravity

SPH —
- secondary pulmonary hemosiderosis
- severely and profoundly handicapped
- spherocyte
- spherocytosis
- sphingomyelin

Sph —
- sphenoidal
- sphingomyelin

sph —
- spherical
- spherical lens
- spheroid

SPHE — Society of Public Health Educators

sp ht — specific heat

SPI —
- selective protein index
- Self-Perception Inventory
- serum precipitable iodine
- serum protein index
- Shipley Personal Inventory
- subclinical papillomavirus infection

SPIA —
- solid-phase immunoabsorption

SPIA — *(continued)*
   solid-phase immunoassay
SPICU — surgical pulmonary intensive care unit
SPID — summed pain intensity difference
SPIF —
   solid-phase immunoassay fluorescence
   spontaneous peak inspiratory force
SPIH — superimposed pregnancy-induced hypertension
spin —
   spinal
   spine
sp. indet. — *species indeterminata* (Lat.) indeterminate species
sp. inquir. — *species inquirenda* (Lat.) species of doubtful status
spir. —
   spiral
   spiritus (Lat.) spirit
spiss. —
   spissatus (Lat.) inspissated, thickened by evaporation
   spissus (Lat.) dried
SPK —
   serum pyruvate kinase
   spinnbarkeit
   superficial punctate keratitis
SPL —
   skin potential level
   sound pressure level
   splanchnic
   spontaneous lesion
   staphylococcal phage lysate
   superior parietal lobule
   syringopleural [shunt]
SPLATT — split anterior tibial tendon [transfer]
sPLM — sleep-related periodic leg movements
SPLV — serum parvovirus-like virus
SPM —
   shocks per minute

SPM — *(continued)*
   significance probability mapping
   subhuman primate model
   suspended particulate matter
   synaptic plasma membrane
SpM — spiriformis medialis [nucleus]
SPMA — spinal progressive muscular atrophy
SPMB — strong partial maternal behavior
SPMI — status post myocardial infarction
SPMR — standard proportionate mortality ratio (or rate)
SPMSQ — Short Portable Mental Status Questionnaire
SPN —
   solitary pulmonary nodule
   Student Practical Nurse
   supplemental parenteral nutrition
   sympathetic preganglionic neuron
sp. nov. — *species novum* (Lat.) new species
SPO — status postoperative
SpO_2 — pulse oximetry
SPOD — spouse's perception of disease
spont. — spontaneous
spont. ab. — spontaneous abortion
SPOOL — simultaneous peripheral operation on-line
SPORO — sporotrichosis
SPP —
   Sexuality Preference Profile
   skin perfusion pressure
   suprapubic prostatectomy
spp — species [plural form]
SPPS —
   solid phase peptide synthesis
   stable plasma protein solution
SPPT — superprecipitation response
SPR —
   scan projection radiography

SPR — (continued)
  serial probe recognition
  skin potential reflex
  Society for Pediatric Radiology
  Society for Pediatric Research
  solid phase radioimmunoassay
  solid phase receptacle
Spr — scan projection radiography
spr — sprain
SPRIA — solid phase radioimmunoassay
SPROM — spontaneous premature rupture of membrane
SPRT — sequential probability ratio test
SPS —
  scapuloperoneal syndrome
  shoulder pain and stiffness
  simple partial seizure
  slow-progressive schizophrenia
  Society of Pelvic Surgeons
  sodium polyethylene sulfonate
  sound production sample
  stimulated protein synthesis
  Suicide Probability Scale
  sulfite polymyxin sulfadiazine [agar]
  systemic progressive sclerosis
SpS — sphenoid sinus
spSHR — stroke-prone spontaneously hypertensive rat
SPST — Symonds Picture-Story Test
SPT —
  secretin-pancreozymin [test]
  single patch technique
  skin prick test
  sleep period time
  slow pull-through
  station pull-through [technique]
SpT — spinal tap
spt. — spiritus (Lat.) spirit
Sp. tap. — spinal tap
SPTI — systolic pressure time index
SPTS — subjective post-traumatic syndrome

S-P tube — suprapubic tube
SPTURP — status post transurethral resection of the prostate
SPTx — static pelvic traction
SPU —
  short procedure unit
  Society of Pediatric Urology
sput — sputum
SPV —
  selective proximal vagotomy
  Shope papillomavirus
  slow-phase velocity
  sulfophosphovanillin
SPVR — systemic peripheral vascular resistance
SPZ —
  secretin-pancreozymin
  sulfinpyrazone
SQ —
  social quotient
  status quo
  subcutaneous
  survey question
  symptom questionnaire
Sq — subcutaneous
sq. —
  square
  squamous
SQC —
  semiquantitative culture
  statistical quality control
SqCCa — squamous cell carcinoma
sq cm — square centimeter
sq m — square meter
sq mm — square millimeter
sqq. — sequentia (Lat.) and following
SQUID — superconducting quantum interference device
SR —
  sarcoplasmic reticulum
  scanning radiometer
  screen
  secretion rate
  sedimentation rate
  seizure resistant
  senior

SR — *(continued)*
  sensitivity response
  sensitization response
  sentence repetition
  service record
  sex ratio
  shorthair [guinea pig]
  short range
  side rails
  sigma reaction
  sinus rhythm
  skin resistance
  slow release
  smooth-rough [colony]
  soluble repository
  specific release
  specific response
  spontaneous discharge rate
  spontaneous respiration
  stage of resistance
  steroid resistance
  stimulation ratio
  stimulus response
  stomach rumble
  stress-related
  stress relaxation
  stretch reflex
  sulfonamide-resistant
  superficial reflex
  superior rectus
  surgical removal
  sustained release
  suture removal
  systemic reaction
  systemic resistance
  systems research
  systems review
S-R — smooth-rough
S&R — seclusion and restraint
Sr — strontium
^{85}Sr — radioactive strontium
sr — steradian
SRA —
  segmented renal artery
  serum renin activity
  spleen repopulating activity
SRAM — static random access
  memory

SR$_{aw}$ — specific airway resistance
SRBC —
  sheep red blood cell
  sickle red blood cell
SRBD — sleep-related breathing
  disorder
SRBOW — spontaneous rupture of
  bag of waters
SRC —
  sedimented red cells
  sheep red cells
src — Rous sarcoma oncogene
SRCA — specific red cell adherence
SRCBC — serum reserve choles-
  terol-binding capacity
SR/CP — schizophrenic reaction,
  chronic paranoid
SRD —
  service-related disability
  Society for the Relief of Distress
  Society for the Right to Die
  sodium-restricted diet
  specific reading disability
SRDS — severe respiratory distress
  syndrome
SRDT — single radial diffusion
  test
SRE — Schedule of Recent Experiences
sREM — stage rapid eye movement
SRF —
  severe renal failure
  skin reactive factor
  slow-reacting factor
  somatotropin-releasing factor
  split renal function
  subretinal fluid
SRF-A — slow-reacting factor of
  anaphylaxis
SRFC — sheep rosette-forming
  (red blood) cell
SRFS — split renal function study
SRH —
  single radial hemolysis
  somatotropin-releasing hormone

SRH — *(continued)*
>> spontaneously responding hyperthyroidism
>> stigmata of recent hemorrhage

SRHL — Southwestern Radiological Health Laboratory

SRI —
>> severe renal insufficiency
>> Stanford Research Institute

SRID — single radial immunodiffusion

SRIF — somatotropin-release inhibiting factor

SRM —
>> spontaneous rupture of membranes
>> Standard Reference Material
>> superior rectus muscle

SRMD — stress-related mucosal damage

SRN —
>> State Registered Nurse (England and Wales)
>> Student Registered Nurse
>> subretinal neovascularization

sRNA — soluble ribonucleic acid

SRNE — sinus rhythm, no ectopy

SRNG — sustained-release nitroglycerin

SRNP — soluble ribonuclear protein

SRNS — steroid-responsive nephrotic syndrome

SRNVM — senile retinal neovascular membrane

SRO —
>> single room occupancy
>> smallest region of overlap
>> Steele-Richardson-Olszewski [syndrome]

SROM — spontaneous rupture of membrane

SRP —
>> short rib–polydactyly [syndrome]
>> signal recognition particle
>> Society for Radiological Protection

SRP — *(continued)*
>> stapes replacement prosthesis
>> State Registered Physiotherapist
>> synchronized retroperfusion

SRPS — short rib–polydactyly syndrome

SRQ — Self-Reporting Questionnaire

SRR —
>> slow rotation room
>> standardized rate ratio
>> surgery recovery room

SRRS — Social Readjustment Rating Scale

SRS —
>> schizophrenic residual state
>> selective rootless section
>> sex reassignment surgery
>> Silver-Russell syndrome
>> slow-reacting substance
>> Social and Rehabilitation Service
>> stereotactic radiosurgery
>> Symptom Rating Scale

SRS-A — slow-reacting substance of anaphylaxis

SRS-RSV — Schmidt-Ruppin strain–Rous sarcoma virus

SRT —
>> sedimentation rate test
>> simple reaction time
>> sinus node recovery time
>> smoke removal tube
>> speech reception test
>> speech reception threshold
>> spontaneously resolving thyrotoxicosis
>> Stroke Rehabilitation Technician
>> surfactant replacement therapy
>> sustained-release theophylline
>> symptom rating test

SRU —
>> sample ratio units
>> side rails up
>> solitary rectal ulcer

SRU — (*continued*)
    structural repeating unit
SRUS — solitary rectal ulcer syndrome
SRV —
    Schmidt-Ruppin virus
    simian retrovirus
    superior radicular vein
SRVT — sustained re-entrant ventricular tachyarrhythmia
SRW — short ragweed [test]
SS —
    sacrosciatic
    saline soak
    saline solution
    saliva sample
    saliva substitute
    Salmonella-Shigella [agar]
    salt substitute
    Sanarelli-Shwartzman [reaction]
    saturated solution
    schizophrenia spectrum
    Schizophrenia Subscale
    seizure-sensitive
    selective shunt
    serum sickness
    Sézary syndrome
    Shigella sonnei
    short sleep
    short stay
    siblings
    sickle cell
    side-to-side
    signs and symptoms
    single-stranded [DNA]
    Sjögren's syndrome
    skull series [radiographs]
    slow wave sleep
    soap solution
    soapsuds
    Social Security
    social services
    sodium salicylate
    somatostatin
    sparingly soluble
    stable sarcoidosis
    stainless steel

SS — (*continued*)
    standard score
    statistically significant
    steady state
    sterile solution
    steroid sensitivity
    Stickler syndrome
    Strachan-Scott [syndrome]
    subaortic stenosis
    subscapular
    subsegmental
    substernal
    suction socket
    sum of squares
    supersaturated
    support and stimulation
    Sweet syndrome
    symmetrical strength
    systemic sclerosis
S/S —
    Salmonella and *Shigella*
    salt substitute
S&S — signs and symptoms
Ss —
    serum soluble [antigen]
    Shigella sonnei
    subjects
ss —
    semis (Lat.) one half
    sensu stricto (Lat.) in the strict sense
    single-stranded
    soapsuds
    subspinale
$\overline{ss}$ — *sans* (Fr.) without
SSA —
    sagittal split advancement
    salicylsalicylic acid
    Salmonella-Shigella agar
    sickle cell anemia
    skin-sensitizing antibody
    skin sympathetic activity
    Smith surface antigen
    Social Security Administration
    sperm-specific antigen
    sperm-specific antiserum
    subsegmental airway

SSA — *(continued)*
   subsegmental atelectasis
   sulfosalicylic acid [test]
   syringosubarachnoid
SS-A — Sjögren's syndrome antigen A
SSAI — Smallest Space Analysis
SSAV — simian sarcoma–associated virus
SSB —
   short spike burst
   single-stranded binding [protein]
   stereospecific binding
SS-B — Sjögren's syndrome antigen B
SSBG — sex steroid–binding globulin
SSC —
   sister strand crossover
   somatosensory cortex
   standard saline citrate
   standard sodium citrate
   Stein Sentence Completion [test]
   superior semicircular canal
   syngeneic spleen cell
SSc —
   systemic scleroderma
   systemic sclerosis
SSCA —
   sensitized sheep cell agglutination
   single shoulder contrast arthrography
   spontaneous suppressor cell activity
SSCCS — slow spinal cord compression syndrome
ss(c)DNA — single-stranded circular deoxyribonucleic acid
SSCF — sleep stage change frequency
SSCP — substernal chest pain
SSCr — stainless steel crown
SSCT — Sacks Sentence Completion Test
SSCVD — sterile spontaneous controlled vaginal delivery

SSD —
   silver sulfadiazine
   single saturating dose
   source-skin distance
   source-surface distance
   speech-sound discrimination
   succinate semialdehyde dehydrogenase
   sudden sniffing death
   sum of square deviations
   syndrome of sudden death
SSDBS — symptom schedule for the diagnosis of borderline schizophrenia
ssDNA — single-stranded deoxyribonucleic acid
SSE —
   saline solution enema
   skin self-examination
   soapsuds enema
   steady state exercise
   subacute spongiform encephalopathy
   systemic side effects
SSEA — stage-specific embryonic antigen
SSEP — somatosensory evoked potential
s. seq. — *sine sequela* (Lat.) without sequel
SSER — somatosensory evoked response
SSES — Sexual Self-Efficacy Scale
SSF —
   soluble suppressor factor
   subscapular skinfold
   supplemental sensory feedback
SSFP — steady state free precession
SSG — sublabial salivary gland
SSHL — severe sensorineural hearing
SSI —
   segmental sequential irradiation
   shoulder subluxation inhibition

SSI — *(continued)*
    small-scale integration
    Social Security Income
    Somatic Symptom Inventory
    Stuttering Severity Index
    subshock insulin
    Supplemental Security Income
    Synthetic Sentence Identification
    System Sign Inventory

SSIDS — sibling of sudden infant death syndrome [victim]

SSIE — Smithsonian Science Information Exchange

SSKI — saturated solution of potassium iodide

SSL —
    skin surface lipid
    sufficient sleep

SSLI — serum sickness–like illness

SSM —
    subsynaptic membrane
    superficial spreading melanoma

SSMS — saturated solution of magnesium iodide

SSN —
    severely subnormal
    Social Security number
    subacute sensory neuropathy
    suprasternal notch

SSNS — steroid-sensitive nephrotic syndrome

SSO —
    Society of Surgical Oncology
    Spanish-speaking only
    special sense organ

SSOP — Second Surgical Opinion Program

SSP —
    Sanarelli-Shwartzman phenomenon
    small spherical particle
    subacute sclerosing panencephalitis
    subspecies
    supersensitivity perception

ssp — subspecies

SSPG — steady state plasma glucose

SSPI — steady state plasma insulin

SSPL — saturation sound pressure level

SSPP — subsynaptic plate perforation

SSPS — side-to-side portacaval shunt

SS-PSE — Schizophrenic Subscale of the Present State Examination

SSPU — surgical short procedure unit

SSQ — Social Support Questionnaire

SSR —
    site-specific recombination
    somatosensory response
    surgical supply room

ssRNA — single-stranded ribonucleic acid

SSS —
    scalded skin syndrome
    secondary Sjögren syndrome
    skin sinus syndrome
    specific soluble substance
    Stanford Sleepiness Scale
    sterile saline soak
    structured sensory stimulation
    systemic sicca syndrome

s.s.s. — *stratum super stratum* (Lat.) layer upon layer

SSSB — sagittal split setback

SSSS — staphylococcal scalded skin syndrome

SSST — superior sagittal sinus thrombosis

SSSV — superior sagittal sinus velocity

SST —
    sagittal sinus thrombosis
    sodium sulfite titration
    somatosensory thalamus
    somatostatin

s. str. — *sensu stricto* (Lat.) in the strict sense

SSU —
    self-service unit
    sterile supply unit
SSV —
    Schoolman-Schwartz virus
    sheep seminal vesicle
    simian sarcoma virus
s.s.v. — *sub signo veneni* (Lat.) under a poison label
SSW — staggered spondaic word [test]
SSX — sulfisoxazole
ST —
    esotropia
    scala tympani
    sclerotherapy
    sedimentation time
    semitendinosus
    septal thickness
    serum transferrin
    shock therapy
    sickle (cell) thalassemia
    sinus tachycardia
    sinus tympani
    skin temperature
    skin test
    skin thickness
    slight trace
    slow twitch
    spastic torticollis
    speech therapist
    speech therapy
    speech threshold
    sphincter tone
    split thickness
    stable toxin
    standardized test
    starting time
    sternothyroid
    stimulus
    stomach
    store
    straight
    stress test
    stretcher
    stria terminalis
    striation
    sublingual tablet

ST — (*continued*)
    subtalar
    sutotal
    superior turbinate
    surface tension
    Surgical Technologist
    survival time
    syndrome of the trephined
    systolic time
S-T —
    in electrocardiography, the interval between the end of the S wave and the beginning of the T wave [segment]
    sickle-cell thalassemia
St. — saint [as in St. Anthony's fire, St. Jude's staging system, St. Louis encephalitis virus]
St — stoke
st —
    stage [of disease]
    state [of disease]
    status
    stere
    sterile
    stimulation
    stone [unit]
    stool
    straight
    stroke
    stomach
    stomion
    subtype
st. —
    stent (Lat.) let them stand
    stet (Lat.) let it stand
STA —
    second trimester abortion
    serum thrombotic accelerator
    serum tobramycin assay
    superficial temporal artery
    superior temporal artery
Sta — staphylion
stab —
    stab cell
    stabilization
    stab neutrophil

STACL — Screening Test for Auditory Comprehension of Language

STAG —
slow target-attaching globulin
split-thickness autogenous graft

STAI — State Trait Anxiety Inventory

STA-MCA — superior temporal artery to middle cerebral artery

StanPsych — standard psychiatric [nomenclature]

Staph. — *Staphylococcus*

stat — German unit of radiation emanation

stat. — *statim* (Lat.) immediately

Stb — stillborn

STC —
serum theophylline concentration
soft tissue calcification
stimulate to cry
Stroke Treatment Center
subtotal colectomy

STD —
sexually transmitted disease
skin test dose
skin-to-tumor distance
sodium tetradecyl sulfate
standard density
standard test dose

std. —
saturated
standard
standardized

STDH — skin test for delayed hypersensitivity

STEL — short-term exposure limit

STEM — scanning transmission electron microscope

sten —
stenosed
stenosis

stereo. —
stereogram
stereophonic

STESS — subject's treatment emergent symptom scale

STET — submaximal treadmill exercise test

STEV — short-term exposure value

STF —
serum thymus factor
slow-twitch fiber
small third trimester fetus
specialized treatment facility
special tube feeding
standard tube feeding
sudden transient freezing

STFM — Society of Teachers of Family Medicine

STG —
short-term goal
split-thickness graft

STGC — syncytiotrophoblastic giant cell

STH —
soft tissue hematoma
soft tissue hemorrhage
somatotropic hormone
subtotal hysterectomy
supplemental thyroid hormone

STh — sickle cell thalassemia

ST/HR — S-T segment heart rate

STHRF — somatotropic hormone–releasing factor

STI —
scientific and technical information
serum trypsin inhibitor
soft tissue injury
soybean trypsin inhibitor
systolic time interval

STIC —
serum trypsin inhibition capacity
solid-state transducer intracompartment

stillat. — *stillatim* (Lat.) drop by drop

still b. — stillborn

stim. —
stimulated
stimulation

stim. — (continued)
    stimulus
stip — stippling [basophilic]
STJ — subtalar joint
STK — streptokinase
STL —
    serum theophylline level
    status thymicolymphaticus
    swelling, tenderness and limitation
STLOM — swelling, tenderness, and limitation of motion
STLS — subacute thyroiditis-like syndrome
STLV — simian T-cell lymphotropic virus
STM —
    scanning tunneling microscope
    short-term memory
    streptomycin
STN —
    subthalamic nucleus
    supratrochlear nucleus
STNR — symmetric tonic neck reflex
STNS — sham transcutaneous nerve stimulation
STNV — satellite tobacco necrosis virus
STO — store
STOM — stomatocytes
stom — stomach
STORCH — syphilis, toxoplasmosis, other agents, rubella, cytomegalovirus, and herpesvirus
STP —
    scientifically treated petroleum
    Sibling Training Program
    sodium thiopental
    standard temperature and pressure
    standard temperature and pulse
STPD — standard temperature and pressure, dry [0°C, 760 mm Hg]

STPI — State-Trait Personality Inventory
STPS — specific thalamic projection system
STQ — superior temporal quadrant
STR —
    special treatment room
    stirred tank reactor
strab — strabismus
STRCT — selective tractotomy
Strep —
    Streptococcus
    streptomycin
STRT — skin temperature recovery time
struct —
    structural
    structure
STS —
    serologic test for syphilis
    Society of Thoracic Surgeons
    sodium tetradecyl sulfate
    sodium thiosulfate
    soft tissue swelling
    standard test for syphilis
    steroid sulfatase
    subtrapezial space
STSA — Southern Thoracic Surgical Association
STSE — split-thickness skin excision
STSG — split-thickness skin graft
STSS — staphylococcal toxic shock syndrome
STT —
    scaphotrapeziotrapezoid [joint]
    serial thrombin time
    skin temperature test
    standard triple therapy
STU —
    shock trauma unit
    skin test unit
STV —
    soft tissue view
    superior temporal vein
STVA — subtotal villous atrophy
STVS — short-term visual storage

STX — saxitoxin
STYCAR — Screening Tests for Young Children and Retardates
STZ —
  streptozocin
  streptozyme
SU —
  salicyluric acid
  secretory unit
  sensation unit
  sensory urgency
  solar urticaria
  Somogyi unit
  sorbent unit
  spectrophotometric unit
  status uncertain
  strontium unit
  subunit
  sulfonamide
  sulfonylurea
  supine
su. — *sumat* (Lat.) let [the patient] take
s&u — supine and upright
SUA —
  sedative urinary antibiotic
  serum uric acid
  single umbilical artery
  single unit activity
SUB — Skene, urethral and Bartholin [glands]
subac — subacute
subclav. —
  subclavian
  subclavicular
subconj — subconjunctival
subcr — subcrepitant
subcut. —
  subcutaneous
  subcuticular
sub fin. coct. — *sub finem coctionis* (Lat.) toward the end of boiling
subling. — sublingual
submand. — submandibular
SubN — subthalamic nucleus
subq. — subcutaneous

subsp — subspecies
substd — substandard
suc. — *succus* (Lat.) juice
Succ —
  succinate
  succinic
SUD —
  skin unit dose
  sudden unexpected death
  sudden unexplained death
SUDH — succinyldehydrogenase
SUDS —
  sudden explained death syndrome
  single unit diagnostic system
  Subjective Unit of Distress Scale
SUF — sequential ultrafiltration
SUI — stress urinary incontinence
SUID — sudden unexplained infant death
sulf —
  sulfate
  sulfur
sulfa — sulfonamide
SULF-PRIM — sulfamethoxazole and trimethoprim
sum. —
  sumantur (Lat.) let them be taken
  sumat (Lat.) let [the patient] take
  sume (Lat.) take
  sumendum (Lat.) to be taken
SUMA — sporadic ulcerating and mutilating acropathy
SUMIT — streptokinase-urokinase myocardial infarct test
sum. tal. — *sumat talem* (Lat.) let [the patient] take one like this
SUN —
  Standard Units and Nomenclature
  serum urea nitrogen
SUO — syncope of unknown origin
SUP —
  schizo-unipolar

SUP — (continued)
    symptomatic uterine prolapse
sup. —
    superficial
    superior
    supervised
    supination
    supinator
    supine
    supra (Lat.) above, superior
supp. —
    support
    suppository
suppl —
    supplement
    supplementary
surg. —
    surgeon
    surgery
    surgical
SURS — solitary ulcer of rectum
    syndrome
SUS —
    Saybolt Universal Seconds
    solitary ulcer syndrome
    stained urinary sediment
    suppressor-sensitive
susp —
    suspended
    suspension
SUTI — symptomatic urinary tract
    infection
SUUD — sudden unexpected, un-
    explained death
SUV — small unilamellar vessel
SUX — succinylcholine
SV —
    saphenous vein
    sarcoma virus
    satellite virus
    scalp vein
    selective vagotomy
    semilunar valve
    seminal vesicle
    Sendai virus
    severe
    sigmoid volvulus
    simian virus

SV — (continued)
    single ventricle
    sinus venosus
    snake venom
    splenic vein
    spoken voice
    spontaneous ventilation
    stimulus valve
    stroke volume
    subclavian vein
    subventricular
    supraventricular
    supravital
S/V — surface/volume [ratio]
SV40 — simian virus 40 [vacuolat-
    ing]
Sv — sievert [unit]
sv — single vibration
s.v. — *spiritus vini* (Lat.) spirit of
    wine
SVA —
    selective vagotomy and an-
        trectomy
    selective visceral angiography
    sequential ventriculoatrial
        [pacing]
    spatial voltage, anterior
    subtotal villous atrophy
SVAS —
    supravalvular aortic stenosis
    supraventricular aortic steno-
        sis
SVB — saphenous vein bypass
SVBG — saphenous vein bypass
    grafting
SVC —
    segmental venous capacitance
    selective venous catheteriza-
        tion
    slow vital capacity
    subclavian vein catheteriza-
        tion
    superior vena cava
    suprahepatic vena cava
SVCCS — superior vena cava com-
    pression syndrome
SVCG — spatial vectorcardiogram
SVCO — superior vena cava ob-
    struction

SVCP — Special Virus Cancer Program

SVCR — segmental venous capacitance ratio

SVC-RPA shunt — superior vena cava–right pulmonary artery shunt

SVCS — superior vena cava syndrome

SVD —
single vessel disease
singular value decomposition
small vessel disease
spontaneous vaginal delivery
spontaneous vertex delivery
swine vesicular disease

SVE —
slow volume encephalography
soluble viral extract
special visceral efferent
sterile vaginal examination
Streptococcus viridans endocarditis

SVG — saphenous vein graft

SVI —
stroke volume index
systolic velocity integral

SVL —
severe visual loss
superficial vastus lateralis

SVM —
seminal vesicle microsome
spatial voltage, maximal
syncytiovascular membrane

SVN —
sinuvertebral nerve
small volume nebulizer

SvO_2 — venous oxygen saturation

SVOM — sequential volitional oral movement

SVP —
selective vagotomy and pyloroplasty
small volume parenteral [infusion]
spontaneous venous pulse
standing venous pressure
static volume pressure

SVP — (*continued*)
superior vascular plexus

SVPB — supraventricular premature beat

SVPC — supraventricular premature contraction

SVPT — supraventricular paroxysmal tachycardia

SVR —
sequential vascular response
supraventricular rhythm
systemic vascular resistance

s.v.r. — *spiritus vini rectificatus* (Lat.) rectified spirit of wine

SVRI — systemic vascular resistance index

SVS —
slit ventricle syndrome
Society for Vascular Surgery

SVSe — supravaginal septum

SVT —
sinoventricular tachyarrhythmia
sinoventricular tachycardia
subclavian vein thrombosis
supraventricular tachyarrhythmia
supraventricular tachycardia

s.v.t. — *spiritus vini tenuis* (Lat.) proof spirit

SW —
Schwartz-Watson [test]
seriously wounded
short wave
sinewave
slow wave
soap and water
Social Worker
spike wave
spiral wound
stab wound
sterile water
stroke work
Swiss Webster [mouse]

Sw — swine

SWA — seriously wounded in action

SWAMP — swine-associated mucoprotein

SWC — submaximal working capacity
SWD — short-wave diathermy
SWE — slow wave encephalography
SWG —
   silkworm gut
   standard wire gauge
SWI —
   skin and wound isolation
   sterile water for injection
   stroke work index
   surgical wound infection
SWIM — sperm-washing insemination method
SWIORA — spinal cord injury without radiologic abnormality
SWM — segmental wall motion
SWO — superficial white onychomycosis
SWOG — Southwest Oncology Group
SWP — small whirlpool
SWR — serum Wassermann reaction
SWS —
   slow-wave sleep
   spike-wave stupor
   steroid-wasting syndrome
   Sturge-Weber syndrome
SWT —
   sinewave threshold
   stab wound of throat
SWU — septic work-up
Sx. —
   signs
   surgery
   symptoms
SXR — skull x-ray
Sxs — serological sex-specific [antigen]
SXT — sulfamethoxazole-trimethoprim
SY —
   syphilis

SY — (continued)
   syphilitic
SYA — subacute yellow atrophy
SYC — small, yellow, constipated [stool]
SYDS — stomach yin deficiency syndrome
sym. — symmetrical
symb. —
   symbol
   symbolic
symp. — symptom
sympath — sympathetic
symph — symphysis
SYN — synovitis
syn. —
   synergistic
   synonym
   synovial
sync — synchronous
synd — syndrome
syn fl — synovial fluid
synth — synthetic
syph. —
   syphilis
   syphilitic
   syphilologist
SYR — Syrian [hamster]
Syr — syringe
syr. — *syrupus* (Lat.) syrup
SYS — stretching-yawning syndrome
sys —
   system
   systemic
SYS-BP — systolic blood pressure
syst —
   system
   systemic
   systole
   systolic
SZ —
   schizophrenia
   schizophrenic
   seizure
   streptozocin
SZN — streptozocin

T

T —
  absolute temperature
  electrocardiographic wave corresponding to repolarization of the ventricles [wave]
  life [time]
  period [time]
  tablespoonful
  tamoxifen
  telomere or terminal banding
  temperature
  temporal electrode placement in electroencephalography
  temporary
  tenderness
  tension [intraocular]
  tera-
  tesla
  testosterone
  tetra-
  tetracycline
  theophylline
  therapy
  thoracic vertebrae [T1 through T12]
  thorax
  threatened [animal]
  threonine
  thrombosis
  thrombus
  thymidine
  thymine
  thymus [cell]
  thymus-derived
  thyroid
  tidal gas
  tidal volume
  time
  timolol
  tincture
  tocopherol
  tonometer
  topical
  torque

T — (continued)
  total
  toxicity
  training [group]
  transition
  transmittance
  transverse
  treatment
  triangulation number
  triggered
  tritium
  tryptamine
  tuberculin
  tuberculosis
  tuberculum
  tuberosity .
  tumor
  turnkey system
  type
T — tesla
T — tau (nineteenth letter of the Greek alphabet), uppercase
Θ — theta (eighth letter of the Greek alphabet), uppercase
T. —
  Taenia
  Treponema
  Trichophyton
  Trypanosoma
T_0 — no evidence of primary tumor
$T_{1/2}$ —
  half-life
  half-time
T + — increased intraocular tension
T − — decreased intraocular tension
T_1 —
  spin-lattice or longitudinal relaxation time
  tricuspid valve closure
T_2 —
  diiodothyronine

T$_2$ — (continued)
    spin-spin or transverse relaxation time
T$_3$ — triiodothyronine
T$_4$ — thyroxine
T-7 — free thyroxine factor
T$_{90}$ — time required for 90% mortality in a population of microorganisms exposed to a toxic agent
2,4,5-T — 2,4,5-trichlorophenoxyacetic acid
T-1824 — Evans Blue [dye]
t —
    duration
    teaspoonful
    temperature
    temporal
τ —
    life [of radioisotope]
    relaxation time
    shear stress
    spectral transmittance
    tau (nineteenth letter of the Greek alphabet), lowercase
    transmission coefficient
θ —
    angular coordinate variable
    customary temperature
    temperature interval
    thermodynamic temperature
    theta (eighth letter of the Greek alphabet), lowercase
t. —
    terminal
    tertiary
    test of significance
    tissue
    tonne
    translocation
    ter (Lat.) three times
TA —
    alkaline tuberculin
    arterial tension
    axillary temperature
    tactile afferent
    Takayasu arteritis
    tannic acid

TA — (continued)
    technical assistance
    teichoic acid
    temporal arteritis
    tendon of Achilles
    tension applanation
    terminal antrum
    therapeutic abortion
    thermophilic *Actinomyces*
    thoracoabdominal [stapler]
    thymocytotoxic autoantibody
    thyroglobulin autoprecipitation
    thyroid antibody
    thyroid autoimmunity
    tibialis anterior
    titratable acid
    total alkaloids
    total antibody
    toxic adenoma
    toxin-antitoxin
    tracheal aspirate
    traffic accident
    Transactional Analysis
    transaldolase
    transantral
    transplantation antigen
    transposition of aorta
    trapped air
    triamcinolone acetonide
    tricuspid annuloplasty
    tricuspid atresia
    trophoblast antigen
    true anomaly
    truncus arteriosus
    tryptamine
    tryptophan acid
    tryptose agar
    tube agglutination
    tumor-associated
T/A — time and amount
T-A — toxin-antitoxin
T&A —
    tonsillectomy and adenoidectomy
    tonsillitis and adenoiditis
    tonsils and adenoids
Ta —
    tantalum

Ta — *(continued)*
    tarsal
    tonometry applanation
TA-4 —
    squamous cell carcinoma anti-
        gen
    tetraiodothyroacetic acid
TAA —
    thioacetamide
    thoracic aortic aneurysm
    total ankle arthroplasty
    transverse aortic arch
    triamcinolone acetonide
    tumor-associated antigen
TAAF — thromboplastic activity
    of the amniotic fluid
TA-AIDS — transfusion-associated
    acquired immunodeficiency
    syndrome
TAB —
    total autoimmune blockage
    typhoid, paratyphoid A, and
        paratyphoid B [vaccine]
TAb — therapeutic abortion
tab. — *tabella* (Lat.) tablet
TABC —
    total aerobic bacteria count
    typhoid, paratyphoid A, para-
        typhoid B, and paratyphoid
        C [vaccine]
TABP — type A behavior pattern
Tabs — tablets
TABT — typhoid, paratyphoid A,
    paratyphoid B, and tetanus
    toxoid [vaccine]
TABTD — typhoid, paratyphoid
    A, paratyphoid B, tetanus tox-
    oid, and diphtheria toxoid
    [vaccine]
TAC —
    terminal atrial contraction
    tetracaine and cocaine
    time activity curve
    total abdominal colectomy
    total aganglionosis coli
    Toxicant Analysis Center
    triamcinolone acetonide
        cream

TACE —
    chlorotrianisene
    teichoic acid crude extract
    tripara-anisylchloroethylene
tachy. — tachycardia
TACL — Test for Auditory Com-
    prehension of Language
TAD —
    test of auditory discrimination
    thoracic asphyxiant dystrophy
    time of analog to digital con-
        version
    total administered dose
    transient acantholytic derma-
        tosis
    transverse abdominal diame-
        ter
    tricyclic antidepressant drug
TADAC — therapeutic abortion,
    dilation, aspiration, curettage
TAE — transcatheter arterial em-
    bolization
TAF —
    tissue angiogenesis factor
    toxin-antitoxin floccules
    toxoid-antitoxin floccules
    transabdominal hysterectomy
    trypsin-aldehyde-fuchsin
    Tuberculin Albumose frei
        (Ger.) albumose-free tuber-
        culin
    tumor angiogenesis factor
TAG —
    target-attaching globulin
    technical advisory group
    thymine, adenine, and gua-
        nine
    triacylglycerol
TAGH — triiodothyronine, amino
    acids, glucagon, and heparin
TAGVHD — transfusion-associ-
    ated graft-versus-host disease
TAH —
    total abdominal hysterectomy
    total artificial heart
    transabdominal hysterectomy
TAH BSO — total abdominal hys-
    terectomy and bilateral sal-
    pingo-oophorectomy

TAI —
    Test Anxiety Inventory
    tissue antagonist of interferon
TAL —
    tendon of Achilles lengthening
    thymic alymphoplasia
    total arm length
tal. — *talis* (Lat.) such a one
talc. — talcum
TALH — thick ascending limb of Henle's loop
T-ALL — T-cell acute lymphoblastic leukemia
TALLA — T-cell acute lymphoblastic leukemia antigen
TALTFR — tendo Achillis lengthening and toe flexor release
TAM —
    tamoxifen
    teen-age mother
    thermoacidurans agar modified
    total active motion
    toxoid-antitoxin mixture
    transient abnormal myelopoiesis
TAME — toluene-sulfo-trypsin-arginine methyl ester
TAMIS — Telemetric Automated Microbial Identification System
TAML — therapy-related acute myeloid leukemia
TAN —
    total adenine nucleotide
    total ammonia nitrogen
tan —
    tandem translocation
    tangent
TANI — total axial (lymph) node irradiation
TAO —
    thromboangiitis obliterans
    triacetyloleandomycin
    troleandomycin
TAP —
    tension by applanation

TAP — *(continued)*
    tonometry by applanation
    transesophageal atrial pacing
TAPS — trial assessment procedure scale
TAPVC — total anomalous pulmonary venous connection
TAPVD — total anomalous pulmonary venous drainage
TAPVR — total anomalous pulmonary venous return
TAQW — transient abnormal Q wave
TAR —
    thoracic aortic rupture
    thrombocytopenia with absence of radius
    tissue-air ratio
    total abortion rate
    total ankle replacement
    transaxillary resection
    Treatment Authorization Request
TARA —
    total articular replacement arthroplasty
    tumor-associated rejection antigen
TARS — threonyl-tRNA synthetase
TART — tumorectomy, axillary dissection, radiotherapy
TAS —
    tetanus antitoxin serum
    Therapeutic Activities Specialist
    thoracoabdominal syndrome
TASA — tumor-associated surface antigen
Tase — tryptophan synthetase
TASS — thyrotoxicosis–Addison disease–Sjögren syndrome–sarcoidosis [syndrome]
TAT —
    tetanus antitoxin
    Thematic Apperception Test
    Thematic Aptitude Test
    thrombin-antithrombin complex

TAT — *(continued)*
 thromboplastin activation test
 total antitryptic activity
 toxin-antitoxin
 transacting transcriptional
  [regulation]
 transactivator
 transaxial tomography
 tray agglutination test
 tumor activity test
 turn-around time
 tyrosine aminotransferase
TATA — tumor-associated transplantation antigen
TATBA — triamcinolone aceto-
 nide *tert*-butyl acetate
TATR — tyrosine aminotransferase
 regulator
TATST — tetanus antitoxin skin
 test
TAV — trapped air volume
TB —
 Taussig-Bing [syndrome]
 term birth
 terminal bronchiole
 terminal bronchus
 thromboxane B
 thymol blue
 toluidine blue
 total base
 total bilirubin
 total body
 tracheal bronchiolar [region]
 tracheobronchitis
 trapezoid body
 tub bath
 tubercle bacillus
 tuberculin
 tuberculosis
 tumor-bearing
T-B — Thomas-Binetti [test]
Tb —
 Tbilisi [phage]
 terbium
 tubercle bacillus
 tuberculosis
T_b —
 biological half-life

T_b — *(continued)*
 body temperature
TBA —
 tertiary butylacetate
 testosterone-binding affinity
 thiobarbituric acid
 thyroxine-binding albumin
 to be absorbed
 to be added
 to be administered
 to be admitted
 total bile acid
 total body area
 trypsin-binding activity
 tubercle bacillus
 tumor-bearing animal
TBAB — tryptose blood agar base
TBAN — transbronchial aspiration
 needle
T banding — telomere or terminal
 banding
TBB — transbronchial biopsy
TBBC — total vitamin B_{12} binding
 capacity
TBBM — total body bone minerals
TBC —
 thyroxine-binding capacity
 thyroxine-binding coagulin
 total body calcium
 total body clearance
 total body counting
Tbc — tubercle bacillus
tbc. — tuberculosis
TBD —
 total body density
 Toxicology Data Base
TBE —
 tick-borne encephalitis
 tuberculin bacillary emulsion
TBF — total body fat
TBFB — tracheobronchial foreign
 body
TBFVL — tidal breathing flow-volume loops
TBG —
 testosterone-binding globulin
 thyroglobulin
 thyroid-binding globulin

TBG — (*continued*)
   thyroxine-binding globulin
   tracheobronchography
   tris-buffered Gey's solution
TBGI — thyroxine-binding globulin index
TBGP — total blood granulocyte pool
TBH — total body hematocrit
tBHP — terbutyl hydroperoxide
TBHT — total-body hyperthermia
TBI —
   thyroid-binding index
   thyroxine-binding index
   tooth-brushing instruction
   total-body irradiation
   traumatic brain injury
TBII — thyroid-stimulating hormone–binding inhibitory immunoglobulin
T bili — total bilirubin
TBK — total body kalium (potassium)
TBLB — transbronchial lung biopsy
TBLC — term birth, living child
TBLF — term birth, living female
TBLI — term birth, living infant
TBLM — term birth, living male
TBM —
   total body mass
   tracheobronchomalacia
   tracheobronchomegaly
   trophoblastic basement membrane
   tuberculous meningitis
   tubular basement membrane
TBMN — thin basement membrane nephropathy
TBN —
   bacillus emulsion
   total body nitrogen
TBNA —
   total body neutron activation
   transbronchial needle aspiration
   treated but not admitted
TBNAA — total body neutron activation analysis

TBP —
   testosterone-binding protein
   thiobisdichlorophenol
   thyroxine-binding protein
   total body photograph
   total bypass
   tributyl phosphate
   tuberculous peritonitis
TBPA — thyroxine-binding prealbumin
TBPT — total body protein turnover
TBR —
   total bed rest
   tumor-bearing rabbit
TB-RD — tuberculosis and respiratory disease
TBS —
   total body solids
   total body solute
   total body surface
   total burn size
   tracheobronchial submucosa
   tracheobronchoscopy
   tribromosalicylanilide
   triethanolamine-buffered saline
tbsp. — tablespoonful
TBSA —
   total body surface area
   total burn surface area
TBSV — tomato bushy stunt virus
TBT —
   tolbutamide test
   tracheobronchial toilet
   tracheobronchial tree
TBTNR — Toronto Biculture Test of Nonverbal Reasoning
TBTT — tuberculin tine test
TBV —
   total blood volume
   transluminal balloon valvuloplasty
TBV_p — total blood volume predicted from body surface
TBW —
   total body washout
   total body water

TBW — *(continued)*
    total body weight
TBX —
    thromboxane
    total body irradiation
TBZ —
    tetrabenazine
    thiabendazole
TC —
    target cell
    taurocholate
    taurocholic acid
    temperature compensation
    teratocarcinoma
    tertiary cleavage
    tetracycline
    thermal conductivity
    thoracic cage
    throat culture
    thyrocalcitonin
    tissue culture
    to contain
    total calcium
    total capacity
    total cholesterol
    total colonoscopy
    total correction
    transcobalamin
    transcutaneous
    transplant center
    transverse colon
    trauma center
    Treacher Collins [syndrome]
    tropocollagen
    true conjugate
    tubocurarine
    tumor cell
    tumor of cerebrum
T&C —
    turn and cough
    type and crossmatch
$T_4(C)$ — serum thyroxine measured by column chromatography
TC_{50} — median toxic concentration
Tc —
    technetium

Tc — *(continued)*
    temporal complex
    tetracycline
    transcobalamin
T_c —
    cytotoxic T-cell
    generation time of a cell cycle
$t(°C)$ — temperature on the Celsius scale
tc —
    transcutaneous
    translational control
TCA —
    T-cell A locus
    terminal cancer
    tetracyclic antidepressant
    thyrocalcitonin
    total cholic acid
    total circulating albumin
    total circulatory arrest
    transluminal coronary angioplasty
    tricalcium aluminate
    tricarboxylic acid
    trichloroacetate
    trichloroacetic acid
    tricuspid atresia
    tricyclic antidepressant
TCAB — 3,3′,4,4′-tetrachloroazobenzene
TCABG — triple coronary artery bypass graft
TCAD — tricyclic antidepressant
TCAG — triple coronary artery graft
TCAOB — 3,3′,4,4′-tetrachloroazoxybenzene
TCAP — trimethylcetylammonium pentachlorophenate
TCAR — T-cell antigen receptor
TCB —
    tetrachlorobiphenyl
    total cardiopulmonary bypass
    transcatheter biopsy
    tumor cell burden
TCBS — thiosulfate citrate bile salts sucrose [agar]

TCC —
> terminal complement complex
> thromboplastic cell component
> transitional-cell carcinoma
> trichlorocarbanilide

Tcc — triclocarban

TCCA — transitional cell cancer-associated [virus]

TCCB — transitional cell carcinoma of bladder

TCCL — T-cell chronic lymphocytic leukemia

TC CO$_2$ — transcutaneous carbon dioxide

^{99}Tc — technetium isotope

TCD —
> T-cell depletion
> thermal conductivity detector
> tissue culture dose
> transcranial Doppler
> transverse cardiac diameter

TCD$_{50}$ — median tissue culture dose

TCDB — turn, cough, and deep breathe

TCDC — taurochenodeoxycholate

TCDD — 2,3,7,8-tetrachlorodibenzo-p-dioxin

TC detector — thermal conductivity detector

TCE —
> T-cell enriched
> tetrachlorodiphenyl ethane
> tetrachloroethylene
> trichloroethylene

TCES — transcutaneous cranial electrical stimulation

TCESOM — trichloroethylene-extracted soybean oil meal

TCET — transcerebral electrotherapy

TCF —
> tissue coding factor
> total coronary flow
> Treacher Collins-Franceschetti [syndrome]

T-CFC — T-colony–forming cell

TCFU — tumor colony–forming unit

TCGF — thymus-cell growth factor

TCH —
> tanned cell hemagglutination
> thiophene-2-carboxylic acid hydrazide
> total circulating hemoglobin
> turn, cough, hyperventilate

TChE — total cholinesterase

TcHIDA — technetium hepato-iminodiacetic acid [scan]

TCI —
> total cerebral ischemia
> transient cerebral ischemia
> tricuspid insufficiency

TCi — teracurie

TCID —
> tissue culture infective dose
> tissue culture inoculated dose

TCID$_{50}$ — median tissue culture infective dose

TCIDA — technetium iminodiacetic acid

TCIE — transient cerebral ischemic episode

TcIPA — tumor-cell induced platelet aggregation

TCL —
> thermochemiluminescence
> total capacity of the lung
> transverse carpal ligament

T-CLL — T-cell chronic lymphatic leukemia

TC$_{Lo}$ — toxic concentration low

TCM —
> tissue culture medium
> transcutaneous monitor

Tc^{99m} — technetium medronate [scan]

TCMA — transcortical motor aphasia

TCMH — tumor-direct cell–mediated hypersensitivity

TCMI — T-cell–mediated immunity

TCMP — thematic content modification program

TCMZ — trichloromethiazide

TCN — tetracycline

TcNM — tumor with lymph node metastases

TCNS —
 transcutaneous nerve stimulation
 transcutaneous nerve stimulator

TCNV — terminal contingent negative variation

T_{CO_2} — total carbon dioxide

TCOM — transcutaneous oxygen monitor

TCP —
 therapeutic continuous penicillin
 total circulating protein
 tranylcypromine
 tricalcium phosphate
 trichlorophenol
 tricresyl phosphate

$tcPCO_2$ — transcutaneous carbon dioxide pressure

$tcPO_2$ — transcutaneous (partial) oxygen pressure

TCPA — tetrachlorophthalic anhydride

2,4,5-TCPPA — 2-(2,4,5-trichlorophenoxy)-propionic acid

TCPS — total cavopulmonary shunt

TCR —
 T-cell antigen receptor
 T-cell reactivity
 T-cell receptor
 T-cell rosette
 thalamocortical relay
 total cytoplasmic ribosome

tcRNA — translation control ribonucleic acid

TCRP — total cellular receptor pool

TCRV — total red cell volume

TCS —
 T-cell supernatant

TCS — (continued)
 tethered cord syndrome
 total coronary score

TCSA — tetrachlorosalicylanilide

TCSF — T-colony–stimulating factor

TCT —
 thrombin-clotting time
 thyrocalcitonin
 tracheal cytotoxin
 transmission computed tomography

TčT — tympanostomy with tube placement

Tct — tincture

TCu — copper T

TCV —
 thoracic cage volume
 three-concept view

TCVA — thromboembolic cerebral vascular accident

TD —
 Takayasu disease
 tardive dyskinesia
 T-cell dependent
 temporary disability
 teratoma differentiated
 terminal device
 tetanus-diphtheria [toxoid]
 tetrodotoxin
 therapy discontinued
 thermal dilution
 thoracic duct
 three times per day
 threshold dose
 threshold of detectability
 threshold of discomfort
 thymus-dependent
 tidal volume
 timed disintegration
 tocopherol deficiency
 to deliver
 tolerance dose
 tone decay
 torsion dystonia
 total disability
 total discrimination
 total dose

TD — (*continued*)
    totally disabled
    toxic dose
    tracheal diameter
    transdermal
    transverse diameter
    traveler's diarrhea
    treating distance
    treatment discontinued
    tuberoinfundibular dopamin-
        ergic
    tumor dose
    typhoid dysentery
T/D — treatment discontinued
T_D —
    the time required to double
        the number of cells in a
        given population
    thermal death time
$T_4(D)$ — serum thyroxine mea-
    sured by displacement analysis
TD_{50} — median toxic dose
Td — tetanus and diphtheria tox-
    oid
t.d. — *ter die* (Lat.) three times
    daily
TDA —
    therapeutic drug assay
    thyroid-stimulating hormone-
        displacing antibody
    thyrotropin displacing activity
    tryptophan deaminase agar
TDB — Toxicology Data Bank
TDC —
    taurodeoxycholate
    taurodeoxycholic acid
    total dietary calories
TDD —
    Telecommunication Device
        for the Deaf
    tetradecadiene
    thoracic duct drainage
    total digitalizing dose
    toxic doses of drugs
    Tuberculous Disease Diploma
TDDA — tetradecadienyl acetate
TDE —
    tetrachlorodiphenylethane

TDE — (*continued*)
    total daily energy
    total digestible energy
    triethylene glycol diglycidyl
TDF —
    testis-determining factor
    thermal diffusion flowmetry
    thoracic duct fistula
    thoracic duct flow
    time-dose fractionation
    tissue-damaging factor
    tumor dose fractionation
TDH —
    threonine dehydrogenase
    total decreased histamine
TDI —
    temperature difference inte-
        gration
    three-dimensional inter-
        locking [hip]
    toluene diisocyanate
    total dose infusion
    total dose insulin
TDK — tardive dyskinesia
TDL —
    thoracic duct lymph
    thymus-dependent lympho-
        cyte
    toxic dose level
TDM — therapeutic drug monitor-
    ing
TDN —
    total digestible nutrients
    transdermal nitroglycerin
tDNA — transfer deoxyribonucleic
    acid
TDO — trichodento-osseous [syn-
    drome]
TDP —
    thermal death point
    thoracic duct pressure
    thymidine diphosphate
    total degradation products
TdP — *torsades de pointes* (Fr.)
    fringe of pointed tips
TdR — thymidine
TdR–^{3}H — titrated thymidine
TDS —
    temperature, depth, salinity

TDS — *(continued)*
    thiamine disulfide
    transduodenal sphinctero-
      plasty
t.d.s. — *ter die sumendum* (Lat.) to
    be taken three times a day
TDSD — transient digestive sys-
    tem disorder
TDT —
    tentative discharge tomorrow
    terminal deoxynucleotidyl
      transferase
    thermal death time
    tone decay test
    tumor doubling time
TDWB — touch-down weight-
    bearing
TDZ — thymus-dependent zone
TE —
    echo-time
    expiratory time
    tennis elbow
    tetanus
    tetracycline
    threshold energy
    thromboembolism
    thymus epithelium
    thyrotoxic exophthalmos
    tick-borne encephalitis
    time echo
    time estimation
    tissue-equivalent
    tonsillectomy
    tooth extracted
    total estrogen [excretion]
    totally embedded
    toxic epidermolysis
    Toxoplasma encephalitis
    trace element
    tracheoesophageal
    transepithelial elimination
    treadmill exercise
T&E —
    testing and evaluation
    training and experience
    trial and error
T_E — expiratory phase time
Te —
    effective half-life

Te — *(continued)*
    tellurium
    tetanic contraction
    tetanus
TEA —
    temporal external artery
    tetraethylammonium
    thermal energy analyzer
    thromboendarterectomy
    total elbow arthroplasty
    transient emboligenic aor-
      toarteritis
    triethanolamine
TEAB — tetraethylammonium bro-
    mide
TEAC — tetraethylammonium
    chloride
TEAE — triethylammonioethyl
TEAM — Training in Expanded
    Auxiliary Management
teasp. — teaspoonful
TEB — tris-ethylenediamine tetra-
    acetate borate
TeBG — testosterone-estradiol–
    binding globulin
TEC —
    total electron count
    total eosinophil count
    total exchange capacity
    transient erythroblastopenia
      of childhood
    transluminal extraction cathe-
      ter
T&EC — trauma and emergency
    center
TECA — technetium albumin
    study
tech. —
    technical
    technique
    technology
TECV — traumatic epiphyseal
    coxa vara
TED —
    Tasks of Emotional Develop-
      ment
    threshold erythema dose
    thromboembolic disease

TED — (continued)
tracheoesophageal dysraphism
TEDS — thromboembolic disease stockings
TEE —
thermic effect of exercise
transesophageal echocardiography
tyrosine ethyl ester
TEEM — tanned erythrocyte electrophoretic mobility
TEEP — tetraethyl pyrophosphate
TEF —
thermic effect of food
tracheoesophageal fistula
trunk extension-flexion [unit]
T_{eff} — effective half-life
TEFRA — Tax Equity and Fiscal Responsibility Act
TEFS — transmural electrical field stimulation
TEG —
thromboelastogram
triethylene glycol
TEI — transesophageal imaging
TEIB — triethyleneiminobenzoquinone
TEL —
telemetry
tetraethyl lead
TEM —
transmission electron microscope
transmission electron microscopy
transverse electromagnetic
triethylenemelamine
temp. —
temperature
temple
temporal
temporary
temp. dext. — *tempori dextro* (Lat.) to the right temple
temp. sinist. — *tempori sinistro* (Lat.) to the left temple
TEN —
total enteral nutrition

TEN — (continued)
total excretory nitrogen
toxic epidermal necrolysis
toxic epidermal necrosis
transepidermal neurostimulation
tenac. — tenaculum
TENS —
transcutaneous electrical nerve stimulation
transelectrical nerve stimulator
TEP —
tetraethylpyrophosphate
thromboendophlebectomy
tracheoesophageal puncture
transesophageal pacing
tubal ectopic pregnancy
TEPA — triethylene thiophosphoramide
TEPG — triethylphosphine gold
TEPP —
tetraethyl pyrophosphate
triethylene pyrophosphate
TEQU — test equivocal [possible low titer]
TER —
teratogen
total elbow replacement
total endoplasmic reticulum
transcapillary escape rate
ter —
terminal or end
ternary
tertiary
three times
threefold
ter. — *tere* (Lat.) rub
Terb — terbutaline
term — terminal
ter. sim. — *tere simul* (Lat.) rub together
tert. — tertiary
TES —
thymic epithelial supernatant
toxic epidemic syndrome
transcutaneous electrical stimulation

TES — (continued)

   transmural electrical stimulation

   trimethylaminoethane sulfonic acid

TESPA — triethylenethiophosphoramide (thiotepa)

TET —

   tetracycline

   tetralogy of Fallot

   total ejection time

   total exchange thyroxine

   transcranial electrostimulation therapy

   treadmill exercise test

tet. — tetanus

TETA —

   test-estrin–timed action

   triethylenetetramine

TETD — tetraethylthiuram disulfide

tet. tox. — tetanus toxoid

TEV —

   tadpole edema virus

   talipes equinovarus

TeV — tera-electron volt

TEWL — transepidermal water loss

TEZ — transthoracic electric impedance respirogram

TF —

   free thyroxine

   tactile fremitus

   tail flick [reflex]

   temperature factor

   testicular feminization

   tetralogy of Fallot

   thymidine factor

   thymol flocculation

   thymus factor

   tissue-damaging factor

   to follow

   total flow

   tracheal fistula

   transfer factor

   transferrin

   transformation frequency

   transfrontal

TF — (continued)

   tube feeding

   tuberculin filtrate

   tubular fluid

   tuning fork

t(°F) — temperature on the Fahrenheit scale

Tf — transferrin

T_f — freezing temperature

TFA —

   total fatty acids

   transverse fascicular area

   trifluoroacetic acid

TFB — trifascicular block

TFC — common form of transferrin

TFCC — triangular fibrocartilage complex

TFd — dialyzable transfer factor

TFE —

   polytetrafluoroethylene (Teflon)

   tetrafluoroethylene

TFEV — timed forced expiratory volume

TFF — tube-fed food

Tf-Fe — transferrin-bound iron

TFL — tensor fascia lata

TFM —

   testicular feminization male

   testicular feminization mutation

   total fluid movement

   transmission electron microscopy

TFMPP — 1-(trifluoromethyl-phenyl)-piperazine

TFN —

   total fecal nitrogen

   totally functional neutrophic transferrin

TFP —

   treponemal false positive

   tubular fluid plasma

TFPZ — trifluoperazine

TFR —

   total fertility rate

   total flow resistance

TFR — *(continued)*
   transferrin receptor
TFS —
   testicular feminization syndrome
   thyroid function study
   tube-fed saline
TFT —
   thrombus formation time
   thyroid function test
   tight filum terminale
   tight finger tip
   transfer factor test
   trifluorothymidine
TFX — toxic effects
TFZ — trifluoperazine
TG —
   tendon graft
   testosterone glucuronide
   tetraglycine
   thioglucose
   thioglycolate
   thioguanine
   thromboglobulin
   thyroglobulin
   total gastrectomy
   toxic goiter
   transglutaminase
   transmissible gastroenteritis
   treated group
   triacylglycerol
   trigeminal ganglion
   triglyceride
   tumor growth
   type genus
Tg —
   generation time
   thyroglobulin
   Toxoplasma gondii
   type genus
T_g — glass transition temperature
6-TG — thioguanine
tG_1 — the time required to complete the G_1 phase of the cell cycle
tG_2 — the time required to complete the G_2 phase of the cell cycle

TGA —
   taurocholate gelatin agar
   thyroglobulin activity
   total glycoalkaloids
   total gonadotropin activity
   transient global amnesia
   transposition of great arteries
   tumor glycoprotein assay
TgAb — thyroglobulin antibody
TGAR — total graft area rejected
TGC — time-gain compensation
TGD — thermal green dye
TGE —
   theoretical growth evaluation
   transmissible gastroenteritis [virus]
   tryptone glucose extract
TGF —
   T-cell growth factor
   transforming growth factor
   tuboglomerular feedback
   tumor growth factor
TGFA — triglyceride fatty acid
TGFα — transforming growth factor α
TGF-β3 — transforming growth factor beta 3
TGG — turkey gamma globulin
TGL —
   triglyceride
   triglyceride lipase
TGP — tobacco glycoprotein
TGPN — typical glossopharyngeal neuralgia
TGR — tenderness, guarding, rigidity
6-TGR — 6-thioguanine riboside
T-group — training group
TGS —
   tincture of green soap
   triglycine sulfate
TGT —
   thromboplastin generation test
   thromboplastin generation time
   tolbutamide-glucagon test
TGV —
   thoracic gas volume

TGV — *(continued)*
    transposition of great vessels
TGXT — thallium-graded exercise test
TGYA — tryptone glucose yeast agar
TH —
    Tamm-Horsfall [protein]
    tension headache
    tetrahydrocortisol
    T helper [cell]
    theophylline
    thorax
    thrill
    thyrohyoid
    thyroid hormone (thyroxine)
    thyrotropic hormone
    topical hypothermia
    torcular Herophili
    total hysterectomy
    tyrosine hydroxylase
Th —
    T-helper [lymphocyte]
    therapy
    thoracic
    thorax
    thorium
    throat
th. —
    thenar
    thermic
    thoracic
    thyroid
    transhepatic
THA —
    tetrahydroaminoacridine
    total hip arthroplasty
    total hydroxyapatite
    transient hemispheric attack
    Treponema hemagglutination
ThA — thoracic aorta
Thal. — thalassemia
THAM —
    tris(hydoxymethyl)aminomethane
    tromethamine
THAN — transient hyperammonemia of newborn

THB —
    Todd-Hewitt broth
    total heart beats
THb — total hemoglobin
THBI — thyroid hormone binding inhibitor
THBP — 7,8,9,10-tetrahydrobenzo[a]-pyrene
THC —
    terpin hydrate and codeine
    tetrahydrocannabinol
    tetrahydrocortisone
    thiocarbanidin
    transhepatic cholangiogram
    transplantable hepatocellular carcinoma
THCA — alpha-trihydroxy-5-beta-cholestannic acid
THC:YAG laser — thulium-holmium-chromium:YAG laser
THD —
    thioridazine
    transverse heart diameter
Thd — ribothymidine
THDOC — tetrahydrodeoxycorticosterone
THE —
    tetrahydrocortisone E
    tonic hind-limb extension
    transhepatic embolization
    tropical hypereosinophilia
theo. — theophylline
theor. —
    theoretical
    theory
ther. —
    therapeutic
    therapy
    thermometer
ther ex — therapeutic exercise
therm. —
    thermal
    thermometer
THF —
    tetrahydrocortisone F
    tetrahydrofluorenone
    tetrahydrofolate

THF — *(continued)*
    tetrahydrofuran
    thymic humoral factor
THFA —
    tetrahydrofolic acid
    tetrahydrofurfuryl alcohol
Thg — thyroglobulin
THH — telangiectasia hereditaria
    haemorrhagica
THI —
    transient hypogammaglobu-
        linemia of infancy
    trihydroxyindole
Thi — thiamine
THIO —
    thioglycolate
    thiopental sodium
thiotepa — triethylenethiophos-
    phoramide
THIP — tetrahydroisoxazolopy-
    ridinol
THIQ — tetrahydraisoquinolon
THM — total heme mass
TH₂O — titrated water
ThO₂ — thorium dioxide
THOR — thoracentesis
thor —
    thoracic
    thorax
thou — thousandth
THP —
    Tamm-Horsfall protein
    tetrahydropapaveroline
    tissue hydrostatic pressure
    total hip replacement
    total hydroxyproline
    trihexyphenidyl
THPA — tetrahydropteric acid
THPP —
    thiamine pyrophosphate
    trihydroxypropiophenone
ThPP — thiamine pyrophosphate
tHPT — tertiary hyperparathyroid-
    ism
THPV — transhepatic portal vein
THR —
    targeted heart rate
    threonine

THR — *(continued)*
    total hip replacement
    transhepatic resistance
Thr —
    thrill
    threonine
thr —
    thyroid
    thyroidectomy
THRF — thyrotropic hormone–
    releasing factor
thromb. —
    thrombosis
    thrombus
THS —
    tetrahydro-compound S
    thrombohemorrhagic syn-
        drome
THSC — totipotent hematopoietic
    stem cell
THTH — thyrotropic hormone
THU — tetrahydrouridine
THUG — thyroid uptake gradient
THVO — terminal hepatic vein
    obliteration
Thx — thromboxane
Thy — thymine
thy. —
    thymectomy
    thymus
THz — terahertz
TI —
    inversion time
    temporal integration
    terminal ileum
    thalassemia intermedia
    therapeutic index
    thoracic index
    thymus-independent
    thyroxine iodine
    time interval
    tissue impacted
    tissue invasiveness
    tonic immobility
    total iron
    transischial
    translational inhibition
    transverse inlet

TI — (*continued*)
　　tricuspid incompetence
　　tricuspid insufficiency
　　tumor induction
T_I — inspiration time
Ti — titanium
TIA —
　　transient ischemic attack
　　tumor-induced angiogenesis
　　turbidimetric immunoassay
TIAH — total implantation of artificial heart
TIB —
　　time in bed
　　tumor immunology bank
tib. —
　　tibia
　　tibialis
TIBC — total iron-binding capacity
TIC —
　　ticarcillin
　　Toxicology Information Center
　　trypsin-inhibitory capacity
　　tubulointerstitial cell
　　tumor-inducing complex
TID —
　　time interval difference [imaging]
　　titrated initial dose
t.i.d. — *ter in die* (Lat.) three times a day
TIDA — tuberoinfundibular dopaminergic system
TIE — transient ischemic episode
TIF —
　　tumor-inducing factor
　　tumor-inhibiting factor
TIFB — thrombin-increasing fibrinopeptide B
TIG — tetanus immunoglobulin
TIH — time interval histogram
TIL —
　　tumor-infiltrating leukocyte
　　tumor-infiltrating lymphocyte
TIM — transthoracic intracardiac monitoring

TIMC — tumor-induced marrow cytotoxicity
TIMI — Thrombolysis in Myocardial Infarction [trial]
TIMP — tissue inhibitor of metalloproteinases
TIN — tubulointerstitial nephropathy
t.i.n. — *ter in nocte* (Lat.) three times a night
tinct. —
　　tinctura
　　tincture
TINU — tubulointerstitial nephritis-uveitis [syndrome]
TIP —
　　thermal inactivation point
　　Toxicology Information Program
　　translation-inhibiting protein
　　tumor-inhibiting principle
TIPI — time-insensitive predictive instrument
TIPPS — tetraiodophenylphthalein sodium
TIQ — tetrahydroisoquinoline
TIR — terminal innervation ratio
TIS —
　　tetracycline-induced steatosis
　　transdermal infusion system
　　trypsin-insoluble segment
　　tumor in situ
TISP — total immunoreactive serum pepsinogen
TISS — Therapeutic Intervention Scoring System
TIT —
　　Treponema immobilization test
　　triiodothyronine
TIU — trypsin-inhibiting unit
TIUP — term intrauterine pregnancy
TIUV — total intrauterine volume
TIVC — thoracic inferior vena cava
TJ —
　　tendon jerk
　　tetrajoule

TJ — (continued)
    thigh junction
    triceps jerk
    Troell-Junet [syndrome]
TJA — total joint arthroplasty
TJN — twin jet nebulizer
TJR — total joint replacement
TK —
    through the knee
    thymidine kinase
    transketolase
    triose-kinase
T(°K.) — absolute temperature on
    the Kelvin scale
TKA —
    total knee arthroplasty
    transketolase activity
    trochanter, knee, ankle
TKD —
    thymidine kinase deficiency
    tokodynamometer
TKG — tokodynagraph
TKLI — tachykinin-like immuno-
    reactivity
TKO — to keep open
TKP — thermokeratoplasty
TKR — total knee replacement
TKVO — to keep vein open
TL —
    temporal lobe
    terminal latency
    terminal limen
    thermolabile
    thermoluminescence
    threat to life
    thymus lymphocyte
    thymus lymphoma
    thymus-leukemia [antigen]
    time lapse
    time-limited
    tolerance level
    total lipids
    total lung [capacity]
    transverse line
    tubal ligation
T-L — thymus-dependent lympho-
    cyte
Tl — thallium

TLA —
    tissue lactase activity
    tongue-to-lip adhesion
    translaryngeal aspiration
    translumbar aortogram
    transluminal angioplasty
TLAA — T-lymphocyte–associa-
    ted antigen
TLam — thoracic laminectomy
TLB — total lesion burden
TLC —
    tender loving care
    thin-layer chromatography
    total L-chain concentration
    total lung capacity
    total lung compliance
    total lymphocyte count
    triple-lumen catheter
^{201}TlCl — radioactive thallium
    chloride
TLD —
    thermoluminescent dosimeter
    thermoluminescent dosimetry
    thoracic lymphatic duct
    tumor lethal dose
T/LD_{100} — minimum dose causing
    100% deaths or malformation
    of 100% of fetuses
TLE —
    temporal lobe epilepsy
    thin-layer electrophoresis
    total lipid extract
T-lens — therapeutic contact lens
TLI —
    thymidine-labeling index
    total lymphoid irradiation
    translaryngeal intubation
    trypsin-like immunoactivity
TLm — median tolerance limit
TLQ — total living quotient
TLR — tonic labyrinthine reflex
TLS —
    thoracolumbosacral
    Tourette-like syndrome
    tumor lysis syndrome
TLSO — thoracolumbosacral or-
    thosis
TLSSO — thoracolumbosacral spi-
    nal orthosis

TLT — tryptophan load test
TLV —
  threshold limit value
  total lung volume
TLW — total lung water
TLX — trophoblast-lymphocyte
  cross-reactivity
TM —
  tectorial membrane
  temperature by mouth
  temporalis muscle
  temporomandibular
  tender midline
  tendomyopathy
  teres major
  thalassemia major
  Thayer-Martin [medium]
  time-motion
  tobramycin
  trabecular meshwork
  trademark
  traditional medicine
  transatrial membranotomy
  transcendental meditation
  transitional mucosa
  transmediastinal
  transmetatarsal
  transport mechanism
  transport medium
  transverse myelitis
  Tropical Medicine
  tuberculous meningitis
  tubular myelin
  twitch movement
  tympanic membrane
T-M — Thayer-Martin [medium]
T&M — type and crossmatch
Tm —
  melting temperature
  temperature midpoint
  thulium
  tubular maximum [of kidneys]
tM — the time required to complete the M phase of the cell cycle
tm —
  transport medium
  true mean

t_m — temperature midpoint
TMA —
  tetramethylammonium
  thrombotic microangiopathy
  thyroid microsomal antibody
  transcortical mixed aphasia
  transmetatarsal amputation
  trimellitic anhydride
  trimethoxyamphetamine
  trimethoxyphenyl aminopropane
  trimethylamine
TMAH — trimethylphenylammonium (anilinium) hydroxide
TMAI — trimethylphenylammonium (anilinium) iodide
TMAS — Taylor Manifest Anxiety Scale
T_{max} —
  maximum threshold
  time of maximum concentration
TMB —
  tetramethyl benzidine
  transient monocular blindness
TMBA — trimethoxybenzaldehyde
TMC —
  transmural colitis
  triamcinolone and Terramycin capsules
TMCA — trimethyl colchicinic acid
TMD — trimethadione
t-MDS — therapy-related myelodysplastic syndrome
TME —
  total metabolizable energy
  transmissible mink encephalopathy
  transmural enteritis
TMET — treadmill exercise test
TMF —
  transformed mink fibroblast
  transmitral flow
TMG — 3,3-tetramethyleneglutaric acid
Tmg — maximal tubular reabsorption of glucose

TMH — tetramethylammonium hydroxide

TM-HSA — trimellityl-human serum albumin

TMI —
testing motor impairment
threatened myocardial infarction
transmandibular implant
transmural myocardial infarction

TMIC — Toxic Materials Information Center

TMIF — tumor-cell migratory inhibition factor

TMIS — Technicon Medical Information System

TMJ —
temporomandibular joint
trapeziometacarpal joint

TMJS — temporomandibular joint syndrome

TML —
terminal midline
terminal motor latency
tetramethyl lead

TMM — torn medial meniscus

TMNG — toxic multinodular goiter

TMNST — tethered median nerve stress test

TMP —
thallium myocardial perfusion
thymidine monophosphate
thymine ribonucleoside-5'-phosphate
thymolphthalein
transmembrane potential
transmembrane pressure
trimethoprim
trimethylpsoralen

Tm_{PAH} — tubular maximum excretory capacity for paraaminohippuric acid

TMPD — tetramethyl-para-phenylenediamine

TMPDS —
temporomandibular pain and dysfunction syndrome

TMPDS — *(continued)*
thiamine monophosphate disulfide

TMP-SMX — trimethoprim-sulfamethoxazole

TMR —
tissue maximal ratio
topical magnetic resonance
trainable mentally retarded

TMS —
thallium myocardial scintigraphy
thread mate system
transcranial magnetic stimulation
trapezoidocephaly-multiple synostosis [syndrome]
trimethoprim and sulfamethoxazole
trimethylsilane
trimethylsilyl

TMST — treadmill stress test

TMT —
tarsometatarsal
Trail-Making Test
trimethyllin

TMTC — too many to count

TMTD — tetramethylthiuram disulfide

TMU — tetramethyl urea

TMV —
tobacco mosaic virus
tracheal mucous velocity

TMX —
tamoxifen
trimazosin

TMZ —
temazepam
transformation zone
talonavicular
tarsonavicular
team nursing
temperature normal
total negatives
trigeminal nucleus
trochlear nucleus
true negative

T/N — tar and nicotine

T₄N — normal serum thyroxine
Tn —
    normal intraocular tension
    transposon
TNA — total nutrient admixture
TNB —
    term newborn
    Tru-Cut needle biopsy
TNC — turbid, no creamy layer
TND — term normal delivery
t-NE — total norepinephrine
TNEE — titrated norepinephrine
    excretion
TNF —
    true negative fraction
    tumor necrosis factor
TNG — toxic nodular goiter
tng — tongue
TNH — transient neonatal hyper-
    ammonemia
TNI — total nodal irradiation
TNM —
    thyroid node metastases
    tumor node metastasis
    tumor, nodes, and metastasis
      [tumor staging]
TNMR — tritium nuclear mag-
    netic resonance
TNP —
    total net positive
    trinitrophenol
TNPM — transient neonatal pustu-
    lar melanosis
TNR —
    tonic neck reflex
    true negative rate
TNS —
    total nuclear score
    transcutaneous nerve stimula-
      tion
    tumor necrosis serum
TNT — trinitrotoluene
TNTC — too numerous to count
TNV — tobacco necrosis virus
TO —
    old tuberculin
    oral temperature
    original tuberculin

TO — (*continued*)
    target organ
    telephone order
    thoracic orthosis
    tinctura opii (Lat.) tincture of
      opium
    total obstruction
    tracheoesophageal
    tubo-ovarian
    turnover
T(O) — oral temperature
T&O — tubes and ovaries
TO₂ — oxygen transport
TOA — tubo-ovarian abscess
TOB — tobramycin
TobRV — tobacco ringspot
    virus
TOC —
    tocodynamometer
    total organic carbon
    tubo-ovarian complex
TOCP —
    tri-*o*-cresyl phosphate
    triorthocresyl phosphate
TOD —
    right eye (*oculus dexter*, Lat.)
      tension
    Time-Oriented Data [Bank]
    titanium-optimized design
      [plate]
TODS — toxic organic dust syn-
    drome
TOE — tracheoesophageal
TOES — toxic oil epidemic syn-
    drome
TOF —
    tetralogy of Fallot
    tracheoesophageal fistula
    train of four [monitor]
T of A — transposition of aorta
T of F — tetralogy of Fallot
TOGV — transposition of great
    vessels
TOH — transient osteoporosis of
    hip
TOL — trial of labor
tol. —
    tolerance

tol. — (*continued*)
   tolerated
tolb — tolbutamine
TOM —
   toxic oxygen metabolite
   transcutaneous oxygen moni-
      tor
TON — third occipital nerve
tonoc. — *to* (Engl.) plus *nocte*
   (Lat.) tonight
TOP —
   temporal, occipital, parietal
   termination of pregnancy
top — topical
TOPV — trivalent oral polio virus
   vaccine
TOR — Torkildsen [shunt]
TORCH — toxoplasmosis, other
   infections, rubella, cytomegalovirus infection, and herpes
   simplex [association]
TORP — total ossicular replacement prosthesis
torr — mm Hg pressure
TOS —
   left eye (*oculus sinister*, Lat.)
      tension
   thoracic outlet syndrome
   toxic oil syndrome
TOT —
   tincture of time
   total operating time
tot. prot. — total protein
TOV —
   thrombosed oral varix
   trial of voiding
TOWER — testing, orientation,
   work, evaluation, rehabilitation
tox —
   toxic
   toxicity
TOXICON — Toxicology Information Conversational On-Line
   Network
TOXLINE — Toxicology Information On-Line [data bank]
TOXLIT — Toxicology Literature
   [data bank]

TOXNET — Toxicology Network
   (NLM) [data bank]
TP —
   temperature and pressure
   temperature probe
   temporal peak
   temporoparietal
   terminal phalanx
   testosterone propionate
   tetanus-pertussis
   thick padding
   threshold potential
   thrombocytopenic purpura
   thrombophlebitis
   thymic polypeptide
   thymidine phosphorylase
   thymopentin
   thymus protein
   Todd paralysis
   torsades de pointes
   total positives
   total protein
   transforming principle
   transition point
   transpyloric
   transverse polarization
   transverse process
   Treponema pallidum
   triamphenicol
   trigger point
   triphosphate
   true positive
   tryptophan
   tryptophan pyrrolase
   tube precipitin
   tuberculin precipitate
T & P — temperature and pulse
6-TP — 6-thiopurine
Tp —
   Treponema pallidum
   tryptophan
T_p — physical half-life
TPA —
   tannic acid, polyphosphomo-
      lybdic acid, and amido acid
   12-O-tetradecanoyl-phorbol-
      13-acetate
   third-party administrator

TPA — *(continued)*
    tissue plasminogen activator
    tissue polypeptide antigen
    total parenteral alimentation
    total phobic anxiety
    Treponema pallidum agglutination
    tumor polypeptide antigen
t-PA — tissue-type plasminogen activator
TPB —
    tetraphenyl borate
    tryptone phosphate broth
TPBF — total pulmonary blood flow
TPBS — three-phase radionuclide bone scanning
TPC —
    thromboplastic plasma component
    total patient care
    total plasma catecholamines
    total plasma cholesterol
    treatment planning conference
    Treponema pallidum complement
TPCC — *Treponema pallidum* cryolysis–complement fixation [test]
TPCF — *Treponema pallidum* complement fixation [test]
TPCV — total packed cell volume
TPD —
    temporary partial disability
    thiamine propyl disulfide
    tripotassium phenolphthalein disulfate
    tumor-producing dose
TPDS — tropical pancreatic diabetes syndrome
TPE —
    therapeutic plasma exchange
    totally protected environment
    typhoid-parathyroid enteritis
T^{Pe} — expiratory pause time
TPEY — tellurite polymyxin egg yolk [agar]

TPF —
    thymus permeability factor
    thymus to peak flow
    true positive fraction
TPG —
    transmembrane potential gradient
    transplacental gradient
    tryptophan-peptone-glucose [broth]
TPGYT — trypticase-peptone-glucose-yeast extract-trypsin [medium]
TPH —
    thromboembolic pulmonary hypertension
    transplacental hemorrhage
    tryptophan hydroxylase
TPHA — *Treponema pallidum* hemagglutination assay
TPI —
    time period integrator
    treponema immobilization [test]
    Treponema pallidum immobilization [test]
    triose-phosphate isomerase
T^{Pi} — inspiratory pause time
TPIA — *Treponema pallidum* immobilization (immune) adherence
TPIIA — time of postexpiratory inspiratory activity
TPL —
    titanium proximal loading
    tyrosine phenol-lyase
T plasty — tympanoplasty
TPLV — transient pulmonary vascular lability
TPM —
    temporary pacemaker
    thrombophlebitis migrans
    total particulate matter
    total passive motion
    triphenylmethane
TPMT — thiopurine methyltransferase
TPN —
    thalamic projection neuron

TPN — *(continued)*
    total parenteral nutrition
    triphosphopyridine nucleotide
TPNH — reduced triphosphopyri-
    dine nucleotide
TPO —
    thrombopoietin
    thyroid peroxidase
    tryptophan peroxidase
TPP —
    tetraphenylporphyrin
    thiamine pyrophosphate
    transpulmonary pressure
    treadmill performance test
    triphenyl phosphate
TP & P — time, place, and person
TPPase — thiamine pyrophospha-
    tase
TPPD — thoracic-pelvic-phalangeal
    dystrophy
TPPN — total peripheral paren-
    teral nutrition
TPPS — tetraphenylporphin sulfo-
    nate
TPQ — Threshold Planning Quan-
    tity
TPR —
    temperature
    temperature, pulse, and respi-
        ration
    testosterone production rate
    total peripheral resistance
    total pulmonary resistance
    true positive rate
TPRI — total peripheral resistance
    index
TPS —
    trypsin
    tumor polysaccharide sub-
        stance
TPSE — 2-(p-triphenyl)sulfonyl-
    ethanol
TPST — true positive stress test
TPT —
    tetraphenyl tetrazolium
    time to peak tension
    total protein tuberculin
    treadmill performance test

TPT — *(continued)*
    typhoid-paratyphoid [vaccine]
TPTE — 2-(p-triphenyl)thio-
    ethanol
TPTHS — total parathyroid hor-
    mone secretion
TPTX — thyro-parathyroidectomy
TPTZ — tripyridyltriazine
TPUR — transperineal uretheral
    resection
TPV — tetanus-pertussis vaccine
TPVR —
    total peripheral vascular resis-
        tance
    total pulmonary vascular resis-
        tance
TPZ — thioproperazine
TQ —
    time questionnaire
    tocopherolquinone
Tq. — tourniquet
TQM — total quality management
TR —
    recovery time
    rectal temperature
    repetition time
    residual tuberculin
    terminal repeat
    tetrazolium reduction
    therapeutic radiology
    time recovery
    timed release
    total repair
    total resistance
    total response
    trachea
    transfusion reaction
    transplant recipient
    tricuspid regurgitation
    tuberculin R [new tuberculin]
    tuberculin residue
    tuberculin rest
    tubular reabsorption
    tumor registry
    turbidity-reducing
    turnover ratio
T & R — tenderness and rebound
T(°R) — absolute temperature on
    the Rankine scale

Tr. —
  tincture
  trace
  traction
  tragion
  transferrin
  trauma
  traumatic
  treatment
  tremor
  triradial
  trypsin
T_r —
  radiologic half-life
  retention time
TRA —
  total renin activity
  transaldolase
  tumor-resistant antigen
tra — transfer
TRAb — thyrotoxin receptor antibody
trach. —
  trachea
  tracheal
  tracheostomy
  tracheotomy
tract. — traction
TRAIDS — transfusion related AIDS
TRAJ — time repetitive ankle jerk
TRALT — transfusion-related acute lung injury
TRAM —
  transverse rectus abdominis myocutaneous [flap]
  Treatment Rating Assessment Matrix
  Treatment Response Assessment Method
TRAMPE — tricho-rhino-auriculo-phalangeal multiple exostoses
tranq. — tranquilizer
trans. —
  transfer
  transference
  transverse
trans D — transverse diameter

transm. —
  transmission
  transmitted
transpl. —
  transplantation
  transplanted
TRAP —
  tartrate-resistant acid phosphatase
  transport and rapid accessioning for additional procedures
trap — trapezius
TRAS — transplant renal artery stenosis
TRB — terbutaline
TRBF — total renal blood flow
TRC —
  tanned red cell
  therapeutic referral center
  therapeutic residential center
  total renin concentration
  total respiratory conductance
  total ridge count
TRCA — tanned red cell agglutination
TRCH — tanned red cell hemagglutination
TRCHI — tanned red cell hemagglutination inhibition
TRCV — total red cell volume
TRD —
  tongue-retaining device
  traction retinal detachment
TRDN — transient respiratory distress of the newborn
TRE —
  thymic reticuloendothelial
  true radiation emission
TREA — triethanolamine
treat. — treatment
Trend. — Trendelenburg [position]
Trep — *Treponema*
TRF —
  T-cell-replacing factor
  thymus-replacing factor
  thyrotropin-releasing factor
  tubular rejection fraction

TRFC — total rosette-forming cell

TRGI — triglycerides incalculable

TRH —
    tension-reducing hypothesis
    thyroid-releasing hormone
    thyrotropin-releasing hormone

TRH-ST — thyrotropin-releasing hormone stimulation test

TRI —
    tetrazolium reduction inhibition
    Thyroid Research Institute
    total response index
    Toxic Chemical Release Inventory
    trifocal
    tubuloreticular inclusion

tri — tricentric

T_3(RIA) — serum triiodothyronine radioimmunoassay

T_4(RIA) — serum thyroxine radioimmunoassay

Triac — triiodothyroacetic acid

TRIC — trachoma-inclusion conjunctivitis

triCB — trichlorobiphenyl

Trich. —
    trichinosis
    Trichomonas

Trid. — *triduum* (Lat.) three days

Trig. —
    trigger
    triglycerides
    trigonum

TRIMIS — Tri-Service Medical Information Service

TRIS — tris(hydroxymethyl)aminomethane

TRISS — Trauma and Injury Severity Score

TRIT — triiodothyronine

Trit. — *tritura* (Lat.) triturate

TRITC — tetrarhodamine isothiocyanate

TRK — transketolase

TRLP — triglyceride-rich lipoprotein

TRMC — tetramethylrhodaminoisothiocyanate

Trml. — terminal

TRN — tegmental reticular nucleus

tRNA — transfer ribonucleic acid

TRNG — tetracycline-resistant *Neisseria gonorrhoeae*

TRO — tissue reflectance oximetry

TROCA — tangible reinforcement operant conditioning audiometry

troch. — *trochiscus* (Lat.) troche

Trop — tropical

TRP —
    total refractory period
    trichorhinophalangeal
    tubular reabsorption of phosphate

Trp — tryptophan

TRPA — tryptophan-rich prealbumin

TrPl — treatment plan

TRPS — trichorhinophalangeal syndrome

TRPT — theoretical renal phosphorus threshold

TRR — total respiratory resistance

TRS —
    total reducing sugars
    tubuloreticular structure

TrS — trauma surgery

TRSV — tobacco ringspot virus

TRT — thermoradiotherapy

TRU — turbidity reducing unit

T_3RU — triiodothyronine resin uptake [test]

TRUS — transrectal ultrasonography

TRUSP — transrectal ultrasound of prostate

TRV — tobacco rattle virus

TRX — transsexual

trx — traction

Tryp — tryptophan

TRZ — triazolam

TS —
    Tay-Sachs [disease]

TS — (continued)
  temperature, skin
  temperature sensitivity
  temporal stem
  tensile strength
  Teratology Society
  terminal sensation
  test solution
  testosterone sulfate
  thermal stability
  thoracic surgery
  tissue space
  total solids [in urine]
  Tourette syndrome
  toxic substance
  toxic syndrome
  tracheal sound
  tracheal spiral
  transitional sleep
  transsexual
  transverse section
  transverse sinus
  transverse tubular system
  Trauma Score
  treadmill score
  tricuspid stenosis
  triple strength
  tropical sprue
  trypticase soy [plate]
  T-suppressor [cell]
  tuberous sclerosis
  tubular sound
  tumor-specific
  Turner syndrome
  type-specific
T + S — type and screen
T/S — thyroid to serum [ratio]
Ts —
  skin temperature
  tension, Schiotz
  tosylate
T_s — T-cell suppressor
tS — time required to complete
  the S phase of the cell cycle
TSA —
  technical surgical assistance
  Test of Syntactic Abilities
  thyroid-secreting adenoma

TSA — (continued)
  tissue-specific antigen
  toluene sulfonic acid
  Total Severity Assessment
  total shoulder arthroplasty
  total solute absorption
  toxic shock antigen
  transcortical sensory aphasia
  trypticase soy agar
  tumor-specific antibody
  tumor-specific antigen
  tumor-surface antigen
  tumor-susceptible antigen
  type-specific antibody
T_4SA — thyroxine-specific activity
TSAb — thyroid-stimulating antibody
TSAP — toxic-shock–associated
  protein
TSAS — total severity assessment
  score
TSAT — tube slide agglutination
  test
TSB —
  total serum bilirubin
  trypticase soy broth
  tryptone soy broth
TSBA — total serum bile acids
TSBB — transtracheal selective
  bronchial brushing
TSC —
  technetium sulfur colloid
  theophylline serum concentra-
    tion
  thiosemicarbazide
  total static compliance
  transverse spinal sclerosis
  tryptose-sulfite cyclosterone
TSCA — Toxic Substances Control Act
TSD —
  target-skin distance
  Tay-Sachs disease
  theory of signal detectability
TSE —
  testicular self-examination
  total skin examination
  trisodium edetate

TSEB — total skin electron beam

T sect — transverse section

TSEM — transmission scanning electron microscopy

TSES — Target Symptom Evaluation Scale

T-set — tracheotomy set

TSF —
>	testicular feminization syndrome
>	thrombopoiesis-stimulating factor
>	tissue-coding factor
>	total systemic flow
>	triceps skinfold

TSG — tumor-specific glycoprotein

TSH —
>	thyroid-stimulating hormone
>	transient synovitis of the hip

TSH-RF — thyroid-stimulating hormone-releasing factor

TSH-RH — thyroid-stimulating hormone-releasing hormone

TSI —
>	thyroid-stimulating immunoglobulin
>	triple sugar iron [agar]

TSIA —
>	total small intestinal allotransplantation
>	triple sugar iron agar

tSIDS — totally unexplained sudden infant death syndrome

TSL — terminal sensory latency

TSM — type-specific M protein

TSN — tryptophan-peptone-sulfide-neomycin [agar]

TSP —
>	thrombin-sensitive protein
>	total serum protein
>	total suspended particulate
>	tribasic sodium phosphate
>	trisodium phosphate
>	tropical spastic paraparesis

tsp — teaspoonful

TSPAP — total serum prostatic acid phosphatase

T-spica — thumb spica

T/spine — thoracic spine

TSPP —
>	technetium stannous pyrophosphate
>	tetrasodium pyrophosphate

TSR —
>	testosterone-sterilized rat
>	theophylline sustained release
>	thyroid-to-serum ratio
>	total shoulder replacement
>	total systemic resistance
>	transient situational reaction

TSRH — Texas Scottish Rite Hospital

TSS —
>	toxic shock syndrome
>	transverse spinal sclerosis
>	tropical splenomegaly syndrome

TSSA — tumor-specific cell surface antigen

TSSE — toxic shock syndrome exotoxin

TSST — toxic shock syndrome toxin

TSSU — theater sterile supply unit

TST —
>	thromboplastin screening test
>	total sleep time
>	trans-scrotal testosterone
>	treadmill stress test
>	tumor skin test

TSTA —
>	toxoplasmin skin test antigen
>	tumor-specific tissue antigen
>	tumor-specific transplantation antigen

TSU — triple sugar urea [agar]

TSV — total stomach volume

TSY — trypticase soy yeast

TT —
>	tablet triturate
>	tactile tension
>	tendon transfer
>	test tube
>	tetanus toxin
>	tetanus toxoid

TT — (continued)
 tetrathionate
 tetrazol
 thrombin time
 thymol turbidity
 tibial torsion
 tibial tubercle
 tilt table
 tine test
 tolerance test
 total thyroxine
 total time
 transferred to
 transient tachypnea
 transit time
 transthoracic
 transtracheal
 tuberculin test
 tube thoracostomy
 tumor thrombus
 turnover time
 twitch tension
 tyrosine transaminase
T&T —
 time and temperature
 touch and tone
TT_2 — total diiodothyronine
TT_3 — total triiodothyronine
TT_4 — total thyroxine
TTA —
 tetanus toxoid antibody
 timed therapeutic absence
 total toe arthroplasty
 transtracheal aspiration
TTAP — threaded titanium acetabular prosthesis
TTC —
 triphenyltetrazolium chloride
 T-tube cholangiogram
TTD —
 temporary total disability
 tissue tolerance dose
 transient tic disorder
 transverse thoracic diameter
 trichothiodystrophy
TTE — transthoracic and transesophageal color-flow Doppler echocardiography
TTFD — thiamine tetrahydrofurfuryldisulfide

TTG — tellurite, taurocholate, and gelatin [agar]
TTH —
 thyrotropic hormone
 tritiated thymidine
TTI —
 tension-time index
 time-tension index
 tissue thromboplastin inhibition [test]
 transtracheal insufflation
TTIB — tension-time index per beat
TTL —
 total thymus lymphocytes
 transistor-transistor logic
TTLC — true total lung capacity
TTLD — terminal transverse limb defect
TTM — transtelephonic arrhythmia monitoring
TTN — transient tachypnea of the newborn
TTNA — transthoracic needle aspiration
TTNB — transthoracic needle biopsy
TTO — transtracheal oxygen
TTP —
 Testicular Tumor Panel
 thrombotic thrombocytopenic purpura
 thymidine triphosphate
 time to peak
 total triose phosphate
TTPA — triethylenethiophosphoramide
TTR —
 transthoracic resistance
 transthyretin
 triceps tendon reflex
TTS —
 tarsal tunnel syndrome
 temporary threshold shift
 through the skin
 tilt table standing
 transdermal therapeutic system

TTS — *(continued)*
    twin transfusion syndrome
TTT —
    thymol turbidity test
    tolbutamide tolerance test
    total twitch time
    tuberculin time test
TTTT — test tube turbidity test
TTV —
    tracheal transport velocity
    transfusion-transmitted virus
TTVP — temporary transvenous
    pacemaker
TTX — tetrodotoxin
TU —
    thiouracil
    thyroid uptake
    Todd unit
    toxic unit
    transmission unit
    transurethral
    tuberculin unit
    turbidity unit
T_3U — T_3 (triiodothyronine) resin
    uptake [test]
TUB — tubouterine [junction]
tuberc. — tuberculosis
TUD — total urethral discharge
TUF — total ultrafiltration
TUG — total urinary gonadotro-
    pin
TUI — transurethral incision
TUIP — transurethral incision of
    the prostate
TUPAO — temporary unilateral
    pulmonary artery occlusion
TUPR — transurethral prostatic re-
    section
TUR — transurethral resection
TURB — transurethral resection of
    bladder [tumor]
turb. —
    turbid
    turbidity
    turbinate
TURP —
    transurethral prostatectomy
    transurethral resection of the
    prostate

TURS — transurethral resection
    syndrome
TURV — transurethral resection of
    valves
tus. — *tussis* (Lat.) cough
TUU — transureteroureterostomy
TV —
    talipes varus
    television
    tetrazolium violet
    thoracic vertebra
    tickborne virus
    tidal volume
    total volume
    toxic vertigo
    transvenous
    transverse
    transvestite
    trial visit
    tricuspid valve
    trivalent
    true vertebra
    truncal vagotomy
    tuberculin volutin
    tubovesicular typhoid vaccine
Tv — *Trichomonas vaginalis*
TVA — truncal vagotomy and an-
    trectomy
TVC —
    timed ventilatory capacity
    timed vital capacity
    total viable cells
    total vital capacity
    total volume capacity
    transvaginal cone
    triple voiding cystogram
    true vocal cords
TVD —
    transmissible virus dementia
    triple vessel disease
TUDALV — triple vessel disease
    with abnormal left ventricle
TVF — tactile vocal fremitus
TVG — time-varied gain
TVH —
    total vaginal hysterectomy
    transvaginal hysterectomy
    turkey virus hepatitis

TVI — temperature-viscosity index
TVL —
    tenth value layer
    tunica vasculosa lentis
TVP —
    tensor veli palatini [muscle]
    textured vegetable protein
    transvenous pacemaker
    transvesical prostatectomy
    tricuspid valve prolapse
    truncal vagotomy and pyloro-
        plasty
TVR —
    tonic vibratory reflex
    total vascular resistance
    tricuspid valve replacement
TVSS — transient voltage surge
    suppressor
TVT —
    transmissible venereal tumor
    tunica vaginalis testis
TVU — total volume of urine
TVUS — transvaginal ultrasound
TVV — transmissible venereal
    virus
TW —
    tapwater
    terminal web
    test weight
    thymic weight
    total body water
    triphasic wave
Tw — twist
TWA — time-weighted average
TWAR — Taiwan acute respiratory
TWBC —
    total white blood cells
    total white blood count
TWD — total white and differen-
    tial [cell count]
TWE —
    tapwater enema
    tepid water enema
TWG — total weight gain
TWL — transepidermal water loss
TWR — total wrist replacement
TWS — tranquilizer withdrawal
    syndrome

TWWD — tapwater wet dressing
TWZ — triangular working zone
TX —
    a derivative of contagious tu-
        berculin
    thromboxane
    thyroidectomized
    transplantation
    treatment
T&X — type and crossmatch
Tx —
    therapy
    traction
    transfuse
    transplant
    treatment
TXA_2 — thromboxane A_2
TXB_2 — thromboxane B_2
TXDS — qualifying toxic dose
ty. —
    thyroxine
    type
    typhoid
TYCO — Tylenol with Codeine
Tyl —
    Tylenol
    tyloma
TYMP —
    tympanic
    tympanicity
    tympanogram
    tympanostomy
    tympanum
TYMV — turnip yellow mosaic vi-
    rus
typ. — typical
Tyr — tyrosine
TyRIA — thyroid radioisotope
    assay
TZ —
    transition zone
    triazolam
    Tuberculin zymoplastische
        (Ger.) zymoplastic tubercu-
        lin [the dried residue that
        is soluble in alcohol]

U

U —
 congenital limb absence
 internal energy
 international unit of enzyme
  activity
 Mann-Whitney rank sum statistic
 potential difference
 ulcer
 ulna
 ultralente [insulin]
 uncertain
 unerupted
 unit
 unknown
 upper
 uracil
 uranium
 urea
 urethra
 uridine
 uridylic acid
 urinary concentration
 urine
 urologist
 urology
 uterus
 uvula
 volume velocity
U — unknown
U/ — at the umbilicus
1/U — one fingerbreadth above
  the umbilicus
U/1 — one fingerbreadth below
  the umbilicus
U/2 — upper half
U/3 — upper third
^{235}U — isotope of uranium of mass
  number 235
u —
 atomic mass unit
 ulna
 unified
u. — *utendus* (Lat.) to be used

υ — upsilon (twentieth letter of
  the Greek alphabet), lowercase
UA —
 Ulex agglutinin
 ultra-audible
 ultrasonic arteriography
 umbilical artery
 unaggregated
 unauthorized absence
 uncertain about
 unit of analysis
 unstable angina
 upper airway
 upper arm
 urethra
 uric acid
 uridylic acid
 urinalysis
 urinary aldosterone
 urinary (basement membrane)
  antigen
 urine aliquot
 urine analysis
 urocanic acid
 uronic acid
 uterine aspiration
U/A —
 uric acid
 urinalysis
 uterine activity
ua — umbilical artery
u.a. — *usque ad* (Lat.) up to, as far
  as
UAC —
 umbilical artery catheter
 underactive
 upper airway congestion
UA/C — uric acid–creatinine [ra-
  tio]
UAD — upper airway disease
UAE —
 unilateral absence of excretion

UAE — *(continued)*
  urine albumin excretion
UAG — uracil-adenine-guanine
UAI — uterine activity interval
UAL —
  umbilical artery line
  up ad lib.—up *ad libitum*
    (Lat., as desired)
UA&M — urinalysis and microscopy
U-AMY — urinary amylase
UAN — uric acid nitrogen
UAO — upper airway obstruction
UAP —
  unstable angina pectoris
  urinary acid phosphatase
  urinary alkaline phosphatase
UAR —
  upper airway resistance
  uric acid riboside
UAS —
  upper abdomen surgery
  upstream activation site
UASA — upper airway sleep apnea
UAT — up as tolerated
UAU — uterine activity unit
UAVC — univentricular atrioventricular connection
UB —
  ultimobranchial [body]
  Unna boot
  upper back
  urinary bladder
UBA — undenatured bacterial antigen
UBBC — unsaturated vitamin B_{12}–binding capacity
UBC —
  University of British Columbia [brace]
  unsaturated binding capacity
UBF —
  unknown black female
  uterine blood flow
UBG —
  ultimobranchial gland
  urobilinogen

UBI — ultraviolet blood irradiation
UBL — undifferentiated B-cell lymphoma
UBM — unknown black male
UBN — urobilin
UBO — unidentified bright object
UBP — ureteral back pressure
UBW — usual body weight
UC —
  ulcerative colitis
  Uldall catheter
  ultracentrifugal
  umbilical cholesterol
  umbilical cord
  unchanged
  unclassifiable
  unconscious
  undifferentiated cells
  unfixed cryostat
  unit clerk
  unit coordinator
  unsatisfactory condition
  untreated cell
  urea clearance
  urethral catheterization
  urinary catheter
  urine concentrate
  urine culture
  usual case
  uterine contractions
U/C — urine culture
U&C —
  urethral and cervical
  usual and customary
$U_{Ca}V$ — urinary calcium volume
UCBC — umbilical cord blood culture
UCBR — unconjugated bilirubin
UCC — urgent care center
UCD —
  urine collection device
  usual childhood diseases
UCDM — University of California, Davis, Medical Center
UCE — urea cycle enzymopathy
UCG —
  ultrasonic cardiogram

UCG — (*continued*)
    ultrasonic cardiography
    urinary chorionic gonadotropin
UCHD — usual childhood diseases
UCHI — usual childhood illnesses
UCHS — uncontrolled hemorrhagic shock
UCI —
    urethral catheter in
    urinary catheter in
    usual childhood illnesses
UCIMC — University of California, Irvine, Medical Center
UCL —
    ulna collateral ligament
    uncomfortable listening level
    uncomfortable loudness level
    upper collateral ligament
    upper confidence limit
    urea clearance [test]
UCLP — unilateral cleft of lip and palate
UCO —
    urethral catheter out
    urinary catheter out
UCP —
    United Cerebral Palsy [Association]
    urethral closure pressure
    urinary coproporphyrin
    urinary C-peptide
UCPP — urethral closure pressure profile
UCPT — urinary coproporphyrin test
UCR —
    unconditioned reflex
    unconditioned response
    usual, customary, and reasonable
UCRE — urine creatinine
UCRP — Universal Control Reference Plasma
UCS —
    unconditioned stimulus
    unconscious
    uterine compression syndrome

Ucs — unconscious
UCT — unchanged conventional treatment
UCTD — unclassifiable connective tissue disease
uCTD — undifferentiated connective tissue disease
UCU — urinary care unit
UCV — uncontrolled variable
UCX — urine culture
UD —
    ulcerative dermatosis
    ulcerative dermatitis
    ulnar deviation
    underdeveloped
    undesirable discharge
    undetermined
    unipolar depression
    unit dose
    urethral discharge
    uridine diphosphate
    uroporphyrinogen decarboxylase
    uterine delivery
    uterine distension
u.d. — *ut dictum* (Lat.) as directed
UDA — under direct vision
UDC —
    ursodeoxycholate
    usual diseases of childhood
UDCA — ursodeoxycholic acid
UDE — undetermined etiology
UDN —
    ulcerative dermal necrosis
    updraft nebulizer
UDO — undetermined origin
UDP — uridine diphosphate
UDPG — uridine diphosphoglucose
UDPGA — uridine diphosphoglucuronic acid
UDPGT — uridine diphosphoglucuronyl transferase
UdR — uracil deoxyriboside (deoxyuridine)
UDR-BMD — ultradistal radius bone mineral density
UDRP — uridine diribosyl phosphate

UDS —
  ultra-Doppler sonography
  unconditioned stimulus
  unscheduled deoxynucleic
    acid synthesis
  unscheduled deoxyribonucleic
    acid synthesis
UE —
  uncertain etiology
  under elbow
  undetermined etiology
  uninvolved epidermis
  upper esophagus
  upper extremity
  urinary energy
U/E — upper extremity
UEA — upper extremity arterial
UEG —
  ultrasonic encephalography
  unifocal eosinophilic granu-
    loma
UEL — upper explosive limit
UEM — universal electron micro-
    scope
UEMC — unidentified endosteal
    marrow cell
UER — unaided equalization refer-
    ence
UES —
  undifferentiated embryonal
    sarcoma
  upper esophageal sphincter
uE$_s$ — unconjugated estriol
UESP — upper esophageal sphinc-
    ter pressure
u/ext — upper extremity
UF —
  ultrafiltrable
  ultrafiltrate
  ultrafiltration
  ultrafine
  ultrasonic frequency
  umbrella filter
  unflexed
  universal feeder
  unknown factor
  until finished
  urea formaldehyde

UF — (continued)
  urinary formaldehyde
UFA — unesterified fatty acids
UFB — urinary fat bodies
UFC — urinary free cortisol
UFD —
  ultrasonic flow detector
  unilateral facet dislocation
UFE — uniform food coding
UFF —
  uniform-field-flicker
  unusual facial features
UFFI — urea formaldehyde foam
    insulation
UFL — upper flammable limit
UFN — until further notice
UFO —
  unflagged order
  unidentified flying object
  unidentified foreign object
UFP — ultrafiltration pressure
UFR —
  ultrafiltration rate
  urine filtration rate
uFSH — urinary follicle-stimulat-
    ing hormone
UFV — unclassified fecal virus
UG —
  until gone
  urinary glucose
  urogastrone
  urogenital
  uteroglobulin
μg — microgram
UGA — under general anesthesia
UGD — urogenital diaphragm
UGDP — University Group Diabe-
    tes Program
UGF — unidentified growth factor
UGH — uveitis-glaucoma-hyphema
  · [syndrome]
UGH + — uveitis-glaucoma-hy-
    phema plus vitreous hemor-
    rhage [syndrome]
UGI — upper gastrointestinal
UGIH — upper gastrointestinal
    hemorrhage
UGIS — upper gastrointestinal
    series

UGIT — upper gastrointestinal tract

UGK — urine glucose ketone

UGPP — uridyl diphosphate glucose pyrophosphorylase

UGS — urogenital sinus

UGT — urogenital tuberculosis

UH —
umbilical hernia
unfavorable histology
upper half

U24H — twenty-four-hour urine

UHBI — upper hemibody irradiation

UHC — ultrahigh carbon

UHD — unstable hemoglobin disease

UHDDS — Uniform Hospital Discharge Data Set

UHF — ultrahigh frequency

UHL — universal hypertrichosis lanuginosa

UHMW — ultrahigh molecular weight

UHR — underlying heart rhythm

UHSC — university health services clinic

UHT — ultrahigh temperature

UHV —
ultrahigh vacuum
ultrahigh voltage

UI —
Ulcer Index
urinary incontinence
uroporphyrin isomerase

U/I — unidentified

UIBC —
unbound iron-binding capacity
unsaturated iron-binding capacity

UICAO — unilateral internal carotid artery occlusion

UICC — Union Internationale Contre Cancer (International Union Against Cancer)

u.i.d. — *uno in die* (Lat.) once daily

UIF — undegraded insulin factor

UIP —
usual interstitial pneumonia
usual interstitial pneumonitis

UIQ — upper inner quadrant

UIS — Utilization Information Service

UJT — unijunction transistor

UK —
United Kingdom
unknown
urinary kallikrein
urine potassium
urokinase

UKA — unicompartmental knee arthroplasty

UKa — urinary kallikrein

UKAEA — United Kingdom Atomic Energy Authority

UKCCSG — United Kingdom Children's Cancer Study Group

UKM — urea kinetic modeling

U_KV — urinary potassium volume

UL —
unauthorized leave
ultrasonic
undifferentiated lymphoma
upper limb
upper limit
upper lobe
utterance length

U&L — upper and lower

U/l — units per liter

ULA — undedicated logic array

ULBW — ultralow birth weight

ULDH — urinary lactate dehydrogenase

ULL — uncomfortable loudness level

ULLE — upper lid, left eye

ULN — upper limits of normal

uln —
ulna
ulnar

ULP — ultralow profile

ULPE — upper lobe pulmonary edema

ULQ — upper left quadrant
ULRE — upper lid, right eye
ULT — ultrahigh temperature
ult. — *ultimus* (Lat.) ultimately, last
ult. praes. — *ultimum praescriptus* (Lat.) last prescribed
ULV — ultralow volume
ULYTES — urine electrolytes
UM —
　　unmarried
　　upper motor [neuron]
　　uracil mustard
　　utilization management
UMA —
　　ulcerative mutilating acropathy
　　urinary muramidase activity
Umax. — maximum urinary osmolality
UMB —
　　umbilical
　　umbilicus
UMB + #F — umbilicus plus number of fingerbreadths
umb-ven — umbilical vein
UMC — unidimensional chromatography
UMCV-TO — ulnar motor conduction velocity across thoracic outlet
UMDNS — Universal Medical Device Nomenclature System
$U_{Mg}V$ — urinary magnesium volume
UMI — urinary meconium index
UMLS — Unified Medical Language System
UMMC — University of Michigan Medical Center
UMN — upper motor neuron
UMNB — upper motor neurogenic bladder
UMNL — upper motor neuron lesion
UMP — uridine monophosphate (uridine-5′-phosphate)
UMPK — uridine monophosphatase kinase

UMS — urethral manipulation syndrome
UMT — unit of medical time
UN —
　　ulnar nerve
　　undernourished
　　unilateral neglect
　　urea nitrogen
　　urinary nitrogen
UNA — urinary nitrogen appearance
UNa — urinary sodium
U_{Na} — urinary concentration of sodium
$U_{Na}V$ — urinary sodium volume
uncomp — uncompensated
uncond — unconditioned
uncond ref — unconditioned reflex
uncor — uncorrected
UnCS — unconditioned stimulus
unct. — *unctus* (Lat.) smeared
UNCV — ulnar nerve conduction velocity
undet — undetermined
UNE — urinary norepinephrine
ung. — *unguentum* (Lat.) ointment
$U_{NH4}{}^+$ — urinary ammonium
UNID — unidentified
unil, unilat — unilateral
univ — universal
unkn — unknown
UNL — upper normal limit
UNOS — United Network of Organ Sharing
U_nS — unconditioned stimulus
uns —
　　unsatisfactory
　　unsymmetrical
unsat — unsaturated
unsym — unsymmetrical
UNT — untreated
UNTS — unilateral nevoid telangiectasia syndrome
UNX — uninephrectomy
UO —
　　under observation
　　undetermined origin
　　ureteral orifice

UO — (continued)
  urethral orifice
  urinary output
u/o — under observation
UOA — United Ostomy Association
UOP — urinary output
UOQ — upper outer quadrant
UOsm. — urinary osmolality
UOV — units of variance
UOZ — upper outer zone
UP —
  ulcerative proctitis
  ultrahigh purity
  unipolar
  Unna-Pappenheim [stain]
  upright posture
  ureteropelvic
  uridine phosphorylase
  uroporphyrin
  uteropelvic
  uteroplacental
U/P — urine-plasma ratio
UPA — unpressurized aerosol
u-PA — urinary plasminogen activator
UPC — usual provider continuity
UPD — urinary production
UPDRS — Unified Parkinson's Disease Rating Scale
UPEP — urinary protein electrophoresis
UPF — universal proximal femur
UPG — uroporphyrinogen
UPGMA — unweighted pair group method with averages
UPI —
  uteroplacental insufficiency
  uteroplacental ischemia
UPJ —
  ureteropelvic junction
  uteropelvic junction
UPL — unusual position of limbs
UPN — unique patient number
UPOR — usual place of residence
UPP —
  universal proximal (femoral) prosthesis

UPP — (continued)
  urethral pressure profile
  urethral pressure profilometry
  uvulopalatoplasty
UPPP —
  uvulopalatopharyngoplasty
  uvulopharyngopalatoplasty
UPPRA — upright peripheral plasma renin activity
UPS —
  ultraviolet photoelectron spectroscopy
  uninterruptible power supply
  uroporphyrinogen synthase
  uterine progesterone system
UPSIT — University of Pennsylvania Smell Identification Test
UPT —
  uptake
  urine pregnancy test
U_pV — urinary phosphate volume
UQ —
  ubiquinone
  upper quadrant
UQS — upper quadrant syndrome
UR —
  unconditioned reflex
  unconditioned response
  unrelated
  unsatisfactory report
  upper respiratory
  uridine
  urinal
  urine
  urology
  utilization review
ur —
  urinary
  urine
URA — uracil
ur anal — urine analysis
URC —
  upper rib cage
  utilization review committee
URC-A — uric acid
URC SP — uric acid–urine spot [test]
URD —
  undifferentiated respiratory disease

URD — *(continued)*
　　unspecified respiratory disease
　　upper respiratory disease
Urd — uridine
UREA-S — urea nitrogen–urine spot [test]
URED — unable to read
ureth — urethra
URF —
　　unidentified reading frame
　　uterine-relaxing factor
UR-FST — urine-fasting
urg — urgent
URI —
　　upper respiratory illness
　　upper respiratory infection
url — unrelated
UR&M — urinalysis, routine and microscopic
U-RNA — uridylic acid–ribonucleic acid
URO —
　　urology
　　uroporphyrin
　　uroporphyrinogen
UROBIL — urobilinogen
UROD — uroporphyrinogen decarboxylase
uro-gen — urogenital
URO-2H — urobilinogen—2 hours
Urol. —
　　urological
　　urologist
　　urology
UROS — uroporphyrinogen synthetase
URQ — upper right quadrant
URS — ultrasonic renal scanning
URSO — ursodeoxycholic acid
URT — upper respiratory tract
URTI — upper respiratory tract infection
ur-tim — urine-time
URVD — unilateral renovascular disease
ur-vol — urine-volume
US —
　　ultrasonic

US — *(continued)*
　　ultrasonography
　　ultrasound
　　unconditioned stimulus
　　unique sequence
　　unit secretary
　　unit separator
　　unknown significance
　　upper segment
　　upper strength
　　urinary space
　　urinary sugar
　　Usher syndrome
U/S — ultrasound
USA — unit services assistant
USAFH — United States Air Force Hospital
USAFRHL — United States Air Force Radiological Health Laboratory
USAH — United States Army Hospital
USAHC — United States Army Health Clinic
USAHS — United States Army Hospital Ship
USAIDR — United States Army Institute of Dental Research
USAMEDS — United States Army Medical Service
USAN — United States Adopted Names
USAP — unstable angina pectoris
USB — upper sternal border
USBS — United States Bureau of Standards
USCI — United States Catheter Instrument
USCVD — unsterile controlled vaginal delivery
USD — United States Dispensary
USDA — United States Department of Agriculture
USDHEW — United States Department of Health, Education, and Welfare
USDHHS — United States Department of Health and Human Services

USE — ultrasonic echography

USFMG — United States foreign medical graduate

USG —
ultrasonogram
ultrasonograph
ultrasonography

USH — usual state of health

USHL — United States Hygienic Laboratory

USHMAC — United States Health Manpower Advisory Council

USI — urinary stress incontinence

US/LS — upper strength/lower strength [ratio]

USMG — United States medical graduate

USMH — United States Marine Hospital

USMLE — United States Medical Licensing Examination

USN —
ultrasonic nebulizer
unilateral spatial neglect

USNCHS — United States National Center for Health Statistics

USNH — United States Naval Hospital

USO — unilateral salpingo-oophorectomy

USOGH — usual state of good health

USP — United States Pharmacopeia

USPDI — United States Pharmacopeia Drug Information

USPE — unsatisfactory specimen

USPET — Urokinase Streptokinase Pulmonary Embolism Trial

USPHS — United States Public Health Service

USPSTF — United States Preventive Services Task Force

USPTA — United States Physical Therapy Association

USR — unheated serum reagin [test]

USS — ultrasound scanning

ust. — *ustus* (Lat.) burnt

USUCVD — unsterile uncontrolled vaginal delivery

USVH — United States Veterans Hospital

USVMD — urine specimen volume measuring device

USVMS — urine specimen volume measuring system

USW — ultrashort waves

UT —
Ullrich-Turner [syndrome]
Unna-Thost [syndrome]
untested
untreated
urinary tract
urticaria
uterus

uT — unbound testosterone

ut — uterus

U_{TA} — urinary titratable acidity

UTBG —
unbound testosterone–binding globulin
unbound thyroxine–binding globulin

UTC — upper thoracic compression

UTD — up to date

ut dict. — *ut dictum* (Lat.) as directed

utend. — *utendus* (Lat.) to be used

utend. mor. sol. — *utendus more solito* (Lat.) to be used in the usual manner

UTF — usual throat flora

UTI —
urinary tract infection
urinary trypsin inhibitor

UTLD — Utah Test of Language Development

UTO —
unable to obtain
upper tibial osteotomy

UTP —
unilateral tension pneumothorax

UTP — (continued)
　uridine triphosphate
UTS —
　Ullrich-Turner syndrome
　ulnar tunnel syndrome
　ultimate tensile strength
　ultrasound
ut supr. — *ut supra* (Lat.) as above
UTZ — ultrasound
UU —
　urinary urea
　urine urobilin
　urine urobilinogen
UUN —
　urinary urea nitrogen
　urine urea nitrogen
UUO —
　unilateral urethral obstruction
　unilateral urethral occlusion
UUP — urine uroporphyrin
U$_{urea}$ — urinary urea [concentration]
UV —
　ultrafine
　ultraviolet
　umbilical vein
　ureterovesical
　urethrovesical
　urinary volume
U$_v$ — Uppsala virus
UVA —
　ultraviolet A
　ureterovesical angle

UVA — (continued)
　urethrovesical angle
UVB — ultraviolet B
UVC —
　ultraviolet C
　umbilical venous catheter
　urgent visit center
UVER — ultraviolet-enhanced reactivation
UVGI — ultraviolet germicidal irradiation
UVI — ultraviolet irradiation
UVJ —
　ureterovesical junction
　urethrovesical junction
UVL —
　ultraviolet light
　umbilical venous line
UVP — ultraviolet photometry
UVR — ultraviolet radiation
UW — unilateral weakness
UWB — unit of whole blood
UWD — Urbach-Wiethe disease
UWF — unknown white female
UWL — unstirred water layer
UWM —
　unknown white male
　unwed mother
UWSC — unstimulated whole saliva collection
UX — uranium X (protactinium)
ux. — *uxor* (Lat.) wife
UYP — upper yield point

V

V —
　coefficient of variation
　dead space
　factor V
　minute volume
　mixed venous [blood]
　tidal volume
　unipolar chest lead
　vaccinated

V — (continued)
　vaccine
　vagina
　valine
　valve
　vanadium
　variable
　variation
　varnish

V — (continued)
vector
vegetarian
vegetative
velocity
venous
ventilation
ventral
ventricle
ventricular
venule
verbal comprehension [factor]
verbalization
verbalize
vertebra
vertex
vestibular
violet
viral [antigen]
virgin
virulence
virus
vision
visitor
visual acuity
visual capacity
voice
volume
vomiting

V. — Vibrio

$\dot{V}$ —
gas volume per unit of time
ventilation

V_0 — standard volume

V_1 — volume of inspired gas [per minute]

V− — vicinal isomer

+V — positive vertical divergence

v —
specific volume
velocity
vena
venous
versus
very
virus
vitamin
voltage

v. — vide (Lat.) see

$\bar{v}$ — mixed venous [blood]

VA —
alveolar voltage
vacuum aspiration
valproic acid
vasodilator agent
venoarterial
ventricular aneurysm
ventricular arrhythmia
ventriculoatrial
ventroanterior
vertebral artery
Veterans Administration
Veterans Affairs
viral antigen
visual acuity
visual aid
visual axis
volt-ampere
volume average

V_A — alveolar ventilation per minute

Va — arterial gas volume

V&A — vagotomy and antrectomy

VAB — violent antisocial behavior

VABP — venoarterial bypass pumping

VAC —
ventriculoarterial connection
ventriculoatrial conduction
virus capsid antigen

vac. —
vaccine
vacuum

Vacc — visual acuity with correction

vacc. — vaccination

VACTERL — vertebral abnormalities, anal atresia, cardiac abnormalities, tracheoesophageal fistula and/or esophageal atresia, renal agenesis and dysplasia, and limb defects

VACURG — Veterans Administration Cooperative Urological Research Group

VAD —
        vascular access device
        venous access device
        venous admixture
        ventricular assist device
        virus-adjusting diluent
        vitamin A deficiency
        Voluntary Aid Detachment
$V_A$eff — effective alveolar ventilation
VAER — visual auditory evoked response
vag. —
        vagina
        vaginal
        vaginitis
VAG HYST — vaginal hysterectomy
VAH —
        vertebral ankylosing hyperostosis
        Veterans Administration Hospital (obsolete)
        virilizing adrenal hyperplasia
VAHS — virus-associated hemophagocytic syndrome
VAIN — vaginal intraepithelial neoplasm
VAKT — visual, association, kinesthetic, tactile
Val —
        valine
        Valium
val — value
VALE — visual acuity, left eye
VALG — Veterans Administration Lung Cancer Study Group
VAM —
        ventricular arrhythmia monitor
        visual analogue mood [scale]
VAMC — Veterans Affairs Medical Center
VAN — ventricular aneurysmectomy
VAOD — visual acuity, right eye
VAOL — visual acuity, left eye

VAP —
        vaginal acid phosphatase
        variant angina pectoris
        venous access port
vap. — vapor
V_A/Q_C — ventilation-perfusion [ratio]
VAR — visual-auditory range
var —
        variable
        variant
        variation
        variety
var. —
        varicose
        variety
VARE — visual acuity, right eye
VAS —
        vascular
        vasectomy
        vesicle attachment site
        viral analogue scale
        viral arthritis syndrome
        Visual Analogue Scale
vas. —
        vas deferens
        vasectomy
VASC —
        Verbal Auditory Screen for Children
        visual-auditory screening
VAsc — visual acuity sans (without) correction
vasc. — vascular
VASOG — Veterans Administration Surgical Oncology Group
VAS RAD — vascular radiology
vas vit. — *vas vitreum* (Lat.) a glass vessel
VAT —
        variable antigen type
        ventricular accommodation test
        ventricular activation time
        visual action time
        visual apperception test
        vocational apperception test

VATER — vertebral defects, imperforate anus, tracheoesophageal fistula, and radial and renal dysplasia

VATERL — vertebral defects, imperforate anus, tracheoesophageal fistula, and radial and renal dysplasia and limb anomalies

VATS — Veterans Affairs (Medical Center) transference syndrome

VATs — surface variable antigen

VB —
vaginal bulb
valence bond
van Buren catheter
venous blood
ventrobasal
Veronal buffer
vertebral body
vertebrobasilar
viable birth
vinblastine
virus buffer
voided bladder

VBAC — vaginal birth after cesarean section

VBAIN — vertebrobasilar artery insufficiency nystagmus

VBD —
vanishing bile duct
Veronal-buffered diluent

VBG —
vagotomy and Billroth gastroenterostomy
venoaortocoronary bypass graft
venous blood gases
venous bypass graft
Veronal-buffered gelatin
vertical-banded gastroplasty

VBI —
vertebrobasilar insufficiency
vertebrobasilar ischemia

VBJ — vertebrobasilar junction

VBL — vinblastine

VBOS — Veronal-buffered oxalated saline

VBP —
vagal body paraganglia
venous blood pressure
ventricular premature beat

VBR — ventricle-brain ratio

VBS —
Veronal-buffered saline
vertebrobasilar system

VBS:FBS — Veronal-buffered saline–fetal bovine serum

VBT — vertebral body tenderness

VC —
color vision [activity]
vascular changes
vasoconstriction
vasoconstrictor
vena cava
venereal case
venous capacitance
venous capillary
ventilatory capacity
ventral column
ventricular contraction
verbal comprehension
vertebral canal
Veterinary Corps
videocassette
vincristine
vinyl chloride
visual capacity
visual cortex
vital capacity
vitamin capsule
vocal cord
voluntary closing

V/C — ventilation/circulation [ratio]

V&C — vertical and centric [bite]

V_c — pulmonary capillary blood volume

VCA —
vancomycin, colistin, and anisomycin
viral capsid antibody
viral capsid antigen

vCBF — venous cerebral blood flow

VCC —
vasoconstrictor center

VCC — (continued)
  ventral cell column
VCCA — velocity, common carotid artery
VCD — vibrational circular dichroism
VCDQ — verbal comprehension deviation quotient
VCE — vagina, ectocervix, and endocervix
V_{CE} — velocity of contractile element
V_{CF} — velocity of circumferential fiber
VCFS — velocardiofacial syndrome
VCG —
  vectorcardiogram
  vectorcardiography
  voiding cystogram
  voiding cystography
  voiding cystourethrography
VCI — volatile corrosion inhibitor
V-cillin — penicillin V
VCIU — volatile control of involuntary utterances
VCM — vinyl chloride monomer
VCN —
  Vibrio cholerae neuraminidase
  vancomycin hydrochloride, colistimethate sodium, nystatin [medium]
V_{CO} — endogenous production of carbon monoxide
V_{CO2} —
  carbon dioxide output
  carbon dioxide production
VCP — Virus Cancer Program
VCR —
  vasoconstriction rate
  vincristine
  volume clearance rate
VCS —
  vasoconstrictor substance
  vesicocervical space
  Vocabulary Comprehension Scale
VCSA — viral cell surface antigen

VCSF — ventricular cerebrospinal fluid
VCT — venous clotting time
VCU —
  videocystourethrogram
  videocystourethrography
  voiding cystourethrogram
  voiding cystourethrography
VCUG —
  vesicoureterogram
  voiding cystourethrogram
VD —
  vapor density
  vascular disease
  vasodilation
  vasodilator
  venereal disease
  venous dilatation
  venous distension
  ventricular dilator
  ventrodorsal
  vertical deviation
  vertical divergence
  video disk
  viral diarrhea
  voided
  volume of dead space
  volume of distribution
+ VD — positive vertical divergence
V&D — vomiting and diarrhea
V_D —
  dead space
  ventilation per minute of dead space
  volume of dead air space
Vd —
  void
  voiding
V_d — apparent volume of distribution
vd — double variation
VDA —
  venous digital angiogram
  visual discriminatory acuity
V_DA —
  ventilation of alveolar dead space

V$_D$A — (*continued*)
   volume of alveolar dead space
VDAC —
   vaginal delivery after cesarean
      section
   voltage-dependent anion
      channel
V$_D$an —
   ventilation of anatomic dead
      space
   volume of anatomic dead
      space
VdB — van den Bergh [test]
VDBR — volume of distribution of
   bilirubin
VDC — vasodilator center
VDD — vitamin D–dependent
VDDR — vitamin D–dependent
   rickets
VDEL — Venereal Disease Experimental Laboratory
VDEM — vasodepressor material
VDF — ventricular diastolic frag-
   mentation
VDG — venereal disease—gonorrhea
vdg. — voiding
VDH —
   valvular disease of the heart
   vascular disease of the heart
VDL —
   vasodepressor lipid
   visual detection level
VDM — vasodepressor material
V$_{DM}$ — volume of mechanical dead
   space
VDP — ventricular premature
   depolarization
VDR — venous diameter ratio
V$_D$rb —
   rebreathing ventilation
   rebreathing volume
VDRL — Venereal Disease Research Laboratory
VDRR — vitamin D–resistant rickets
VDRS — Verdun Depression Rating Scale

VDRT — Venereal Disease Reference Test
VDS —
   vasodilator substance
   venereal disease—syphilis
   vindesine
VDT —
   vibration disappearance
      threshold
   visual display terminal
   visual distortion test
VDU — video display unit
VDV — ventricular end-diastolic
   volume
Vd/Vt — ratio of dead space ventilation to total ventilation
VE —
   vacuum extraction
   vaginal examination
   Venezuelan encephalitis
   venous emptying
   venous extension
   ventilation
   ventilatory equivalent
   ventricular elasticity
   ventricular escape
   ventricular extrasystole
   vertex
   vesicular exanthema
   viral encephalitis
   visual efficiency
   visual examination
   vitamin E
   vocational evaluation
   volume ejection
   volumic ejection
   voluntary effort
V$_E$ —
   airflow per unit of time
   environmental variance
   respiratory minute volume
   volume of expired gas
V&E — Vinethine and ether
VEA —
   ventricular ectopic activity
   ventricular ectopic arrhyth-
      mia
   viral envelope antigen

VEB — ventricular ectopic beat
VEC — vecuronium
VECG — vector electrocardiogram
VEC MRI — velocity-encoded cine-magnetic resonance imaging
VECP — visually evoked cortical potential
vect. — vector
VED —
    vacuum erection device
    ventricular ectopic depolarization
    vital exhaustion and depression
VEDP — ventricular end-diastolic pressure
VEE —
    vagina, ectocervix, endocervix
    Venezuelan equine encephalitis
    Venezuelan equine encephalomyelitis
VEF —
    ventricular ejection fraction
    visually evoked field
VEGAS — ventricular enlargement with gait apraxia syndrome
V_{EH} — extrahepatic distribution
vehic. — *vehiculum* (Lat.) vehicle
veloc. — velocity
VEM — vasoexcitor material
V_{Emax} — maximal flow per unit of time
vent. —
    ventilation
    ventilator
    ventral
    ventricle
    ventricular
vent. fib. — ventricular fibrillation
ventric. —
    ventricle
    ventricular
VEP — visual evoked potential
VER —
    ventricular escape rhythm

VER — *(continued)*
    veratridine
    visual evoked response
verc — vervet (African green monkey) kidney cells
vert. —
    vertebra
    vertebral
    vertical
VERU — verumontanum
ves. —
    vesica (Lat.) bladder
    vesicular
    vessel
vesic. — *vesicula, vesicatorium* (Lat.) a blister
vesp. — *vesper* (Lat.) evening
vest. — vestibular
ves. ur. — *vesica urinaria* (Lat.) urinary bladder
VESV — vesicular exanthema of swine virus
VET — vestigial testis
Vet. —
    veteran
    veterinarian
    veterinary
v. et. — *vide etiam* (Lat.) see also
VetMB — Bachelor of Veterinary Medicine
Vet Med — veterinary medicine
VETS — Veterans (Adjustment) Scale
Vet Sci — veterinary science
VEWA — Vocational Evaluation and Work Adjustment
VF —
    left leg [electrode]
    ventricular fibrillation
    ventricular fluid
    ventricular flutter
    ventricular fusion
    video frequency
    visual field
    vitreous fluorophotometry
    vocal fremitus
Vf — visual frequency
V_f — variant frequency

VFA — volatile fatty acid
VFC — ventricular function curve
VFD — visual feedback display
VFDF — very fast death factor
VFI — visual fields intact
VFib — ventricular fibrillation
VFL — ventricular flutter
VFP —
    ventricular filling pressure
    ventricular fluid pressure
    vitreous fluorophotometry
VFR — voiding flow rate
VFS — vascular fragility syndrome
VFT —
    venous filling time
    ventricular fibrillation thresh-
        old
    Verbal Fluency Test
VFW — velocity wave form
VG —
    van Gieson [stain]
    vein graft
    ventricular gallop
    ventrogluteal
    volume of gas
V&G — vagotomy and gastroen-
    terotomy
V_G — genetic variance
VGCC — voltage-gated calcium
    channels
VGH —
    very good health
    Veterinary General Hospital
VGM — venous graft myringo-
    plasty
VGP — viral glycoprotein
VH —
    vaginal hysterectomy
    venous hematocrit
    ventricular hypertrophy
    Veterans Hospital
    viral hepatitis
    visually handicapped
    vitreous hemorrhage
V_H —
    hepatic distribution volume
    variant domain of heavy
        chain immunoglobulin

VHD —
    valvular heart disease
    ventricular heart disease
    viral hematodepressive disease
VHDL — very high density lipo-
    protein
VHF —
    very high frequency
    viral hemorrhagic fever
    visual half-field
VHL — von Hippel-Lindau [syn-
    drome]
VHN — Vickers hardness number
VHP — viral hepatitis panel
VI —
    vaginal irrigation
    variable interval
    vastus intermedius
    virgo intacta
    virulence
    virulent
    viscosity index
    visual imagery
    visual impairment
    visual inspection
    vitality index
    volume index
Vi —
    virginium
    virulence
    virulent
VIA —
    virus inactivating agent
    virus infection–associated an-
        tigen
vib. — vibration
VIBS — vocabulary, information,
    block design similarities
VIC —
    vasoinhibitory center
    visual communication [ther-
        apy]
    voice intensity control
vic. — *vices* (Lat.) times
VICA — velocity of internal ca-
    rotid artery (blood flow)
VI-CTS — vibration-induced car-
    pal tunnel syndrome

VID —
  vaginal intraepithelial dysplasia
  video densitometry
  visible iris diameter
vid. — *vide* (Lat.) see
VIF — virus-induced interferon
VIG — vaccinia immune globulin
vig. — vigorous
VIIag — factor VII antigen
VIIIc — factor VIII clotting activity
VIII$_{vwf}$ — von Willebrand factor
VIM —
  video-intensification microscopy
  vimentin
VIN —
  vaginal intraepithelial neoplasia
  vinbarbital
  vulvar intraepithelial neoplasia
vin. —
  vinyl
  vinum (Lat.) wine
VIP —
  vasoactive intestinal polypeptide
  vasoactive intracorporeal pharmacotherapy
  vasoinhibitory peptide
  venous impedance plethysmography
  very important person
  voluntary interruption of pregnancy
VIPoma — vasoactive intestinal polypeptide-secreting tumor
VIQ — Verbal Intelligence Quotient
VIR — virology
Vir —
  viral
  virus
vir. —
  viridis (Lat.) green
  virulent

VIR AC — viral antibody, acute
VIS —
  vaginal irrigation smear
  venous insufficiency syndrome
  vertebral irritation syndrome
  visible
  visual information storage
vis. —
  vision
  visiting
  visitor
  visual
VISC — vitreous infusion suction cutter
visc. —
  viscera
  visceral
  viscosity
  viscous
VISI — volar intercalated segment instability
VISTAR — Vistaril
VIT — venom immunotherapy
vit —
  vital
  vitamin
  vitrectomy
  vitreous
vit. — *vitellus* (Lat.) yolk
vit. cap. —
  vital capacity
  vitamin capsule
vit. ov. sol. — *vitello ovi solutus* (Lat.) dissolved in egg yolk
vitr. —
  vitreous
  vitrum (Lat.) glass
viz. —
  videlicet (Lat.) namely
  visualized
VJ —
  ventriculojugular
  Vogel-Johnson [agar]
VJC — ventriculojugular cardiac
VK — vervet (African green monkey) kidney [cells]
VKC — vernal keratoconjunctivitis

VKH — Vogt-Koyanagi-Harada [syndrome]

VL —
  left arm [electrode]
  vastus lateralis
  ventralis lateralis [nucleus]
  ventrolateral
  visceral leishmaniasis
  vision, left eye

V_L —
  actual volume of lung
  expired volume per minute
  variable domain of the light chain

VLA —
  vanillactic acid
  very late appearing antigen
  virus-like agent

VLBR — very low birth rate

VLBW — very low birth weight

VLCD — very low calorie diet

VLCFA — very long chain of fatty acid

VLD — very low density

VLDL — very low density lipoprotein

VLDL-TG — very low density lipoprotein-triglyceride

VLDS — Verbal Language Development Scale

VLF — very low frequency

VLG — ventral nucleus of the lateral geniculate body

VLH — ventrolateral nucleus of the hypothalamus

VLM — visceral larva migrans

VLO — vastus lateralis obliquus

VLP —
  ventriculolumbar perfusion
  virus-like particle

VLR — vinleurosine

VLS — vascular leak syndrome

VLSI — very large scale integration

VM —
  vasomotor
  vastus medialis
  ventralis medialis

VM — (continued)
  ventromedial
  ventricular mass
  ventricular muscle
  ventriculometry
  ventromedial
  vestibular membrane
  viomycin
  viral myocarditis
  voltmeter

V_M — viomycin

VM-26 — teniposide

V/m — volts per meter

VMA —
  vanillylmandelic acid
  vanilmandelic acid

V-mask — Venturi mask

V_{max} —
  maximum flow per unit of time
  maximum velocity of an enzyme-catalyzed reaction
  peak flow velocity [Doppler]

VMC —
  vasomotor center
  void metal composite
  von Meyenburg complex

VMCG — vector magnetocardiogram

VMD — *Veterinariae Medicinae Doctor* (Lat.) Doctor of Veterinary Medicine

vMDV — virulent Marek disease virus

VMF — vasomotor flushing

VMGT — Visual Motor Gestalt Test

VMH — ventromedial hypothalamic [neurons]

VMI — visual-motor integration [test]

VMN — ventromedial nucleus

VMO — vastus medialis obliquus [muscle]

VMR — vasomotor rhinitis

VMS — visual memory span

VMSC — Vineland Measurement of Social Competence

VMST — visual motor sequencing test

VMT —
    vasomotor tonus
    ventilatory muscle training
    ventromedial tegmentum

VN —
    vesical neck
    vestibular nucleus
    virus neutralization
    visceral nucleus
    Visiting Nurse
    Vocational Nurse
    vomeronasal

VNA — Visiting Nurse Association

VNC — vesical neck contracture

VNDPT — Visual Numerical Discrimination Pretest

VNE — verbal nonemotional [stimuli]

VNO — vomeronasal organ

VNR — ventral nerve root

VNS —
    villonodular synovitis
    Visiting Nursing Service

VNTR — variable number of tandem repeats

VO —
    verbal order
    volume overload
    voluntary opening

VO_2 — volume of oxygen consumption

VO_{2max} — maximum oxygen consumption

VOC — volatile organic chemical

voc. — vocational

VOCA — Voice Output Communication Aid

VOCC — voltage-operated calcium channel

VOCTOR — void on call to operating room

VOD —
    veno-occlusive disease
    visio, oculus dexter (Lat.) vision, right eye

VOL% — volume percent

vol. —
    volar
    volatilis (Lat.) volatile
    volume
    volumetric
    voluntary
    volunteer
    volvendus (Lat.) to be rolled

vol. adm. — voluntary admission

vol/vol — volume per volume [ratio]

VOM — volt-ohm-milliammeter

vom. — vomited

VON — Victorian Order of Nurses (Canada)

v-onc — viral oncogene

VOP —
    venous occlusion plethysmography
    Viral Oncology Program

VOR — vestibulo-ocular reflex

VOS — *visio, oculus sinister* (Lat.) vision, left eye

v.o.s. — *vitello ovi solutus* (Lat.) dissolved in yolk of egg

VOT —
    Visual Organization Test
    voice onset time

VOU — *visio, oculus uterque* (Lat.) vision, each eye

voxel — volume element

VP —
    physiological volume
    vapor pressure
    variegate porphyria
    vascular permeability
    vasopressin
    velopharyngeal
    venipuncture
    venous plethysmograph
    venous pressure
    ventricular pacing
    ventricular-peritoneal
    ventricular premature [beat]
    ventriculoperitoneal
    ventroposterior
    vertex potential

VP — *(continued)*
    viral protein
    Voges-Proskauer [test]
    volume-pressure
    vulnerable period
V/P — ventilation/perfusion [ratio]
V&P —
    vagotomy and pyloroplasty
    ventilation and perfusion
      [scan]
VP-16 — etoposide
V_p —
    peak voltage
    phenotype variance
    plasma volume
    ventricular premature [beat]
vp — vapor pressure
VPA — valproic acid
VPB — ventricular premature beat
VPC —
    vapor-phase chromatography
    ventricular premature com-
      plex
    ventricular premature contrac-
      tion
    volume-packed cells
    volume percent
VPCT — ventricular premature
    contraction threshold
VPD — ventricular premature de-
    polarization
VPDF — vegetable protein diet
    and fiber
VPF — vascular permeability fac-
    tor
VPG — velopharyngeal gap
VPGSS — venous pressure gradi-
    ent support stockings
VPI —
    vapor phase inhibitor
    velopharyngeal incompetence
    velopharyngeal insufficiency
    ventral posterior inferior
VPL — ventroposterolateral
VPM —
    ventilator pressure manometer
    ventroposteromedial
vpm — vibrations per minute

VPN — ventral pontine nucleus
VPO —
    vapor pressure osmometry
    velopharyngeal opening
    vertical pendular oscillation
VPP — viral porcine pneumonia
VPR —
    Voges-Proskauer reaction
    volume/pressure ratio
VPRBC — volume of packed red
    blood cells
VPRC — volume of packed red
    cells
VPS —
    valvular pulmonic stenosis
    ventriculoperitoneal shunt
    visual pleural space
vps — vibrations per second
VPT — vibratory perception
    threshold
VQ — voice quality
$\dot{V}/\dot{Q}$ — ventilation-perfusion [ratio]
VQR — ventilation-perfusion quo-
    tient ratio
VR —
    valve replacement
    variable rate
    vascular resistance
    venous reflux
    venous return
    ventilation rate
    ventilation ratio
    ventral root
    ventricular rate
    ventricular response
    ventricular rhythm
    verbal reprimand
    vesicular rosette
    vision, right [eye]
    visual reproduction
    vital reaction
    vital records
    vocal resonance
    vocational rehabilitation
V_r —
    ventral root
    volume of relaxation
VRA —
    visual reinforcement audiome-
    try

VRA — *(continued)*
    Vocational Rehabilitation Administration
VRBC — volume of red blood cells
VRC — venous renin concentration
VR CON — viral antibody, convalescent
VRCP — vitreoretinochoroidopathy
VRD —
    ventricular radial dysplasia
    von Recklinghausen's disease
VR&E — vocational rehabilitation and education
VRG — ventral respiratory group
VRI — viral respiratory infection
VRL —
    ventral root, lumbar
    Virus Reference Library
VRNA — viral ribonucleic acid
VROM — voluntary range of motion
VRR — ventral root reflex
VRS — verbal rating scale
VRT —
    variance of resident time
    vehicle rescue technician
    ventral root, thoracic
    Visual Retention Test
VRV —
    ventricular residual volume
    viper retrovirus
VS —
    vaccination scar
    vaccine serotype
    vagal stimulation
    vasospasm
    venesection
    ventral subiculum
    ventricular septum
    verbal scale [IQ]
    very sensitive
    vesicular sound
    vesicular stomatitis
    Veterinary Surgeon
    vibration syndrome
    villonodular synovitis

VS — *(continued)*
    visual storage
    vital signs
    Vogt-Spielmeyer [syndrome]
    volatile solids
    volumetric solution
    voluntary sterilization
Vs. — *venaesectio* (Lat.) venesection
V·s — volt-second
V×s — volts by seconds
vs —
    single vibration
    vibrations per second
vs. — versus
v.s. —
    venae sectio (Lat.) cutting of vein
    vide supra (Lat.) see above
    vital signs
VSA —
    variant-specific surface antigen
    ventral spinal artery
Vs. B. — *venaesectio brachii* (Lat.) bleeding in the arm
VSBE — very short below-elbow [cast]
VSC — voluntary surgical contraception
VSCS — ventricular specialized conduction system
VSD —
    ventricular septal defect
    virtually safe dose
VSFP — venous stop flow pressure
VSG — variant surface glycoprotein
VSHD — ventricular septal heart defect
VSINC — Virus Subcommittee of the International Nomenclature Committee
VSM — vascular smooth muscle
VSMS — Vineland Social Maturity Scale
vsn. — vision
VSO — vertical subcondylar oblique

VSOK — vital signs (okay) normal
VSP — variable spine plating
VSPFT — Vitalor screening pulmonary function test
VSR — venous stasis retinopathy
VSS — vital signs stable
VST — ventral spinothalamic tract
VSULA — vaccination scar, upper left arm
VSV —
  vesicular stomatitis virus
  vesiculovirus
VSW — ventricular stroke work
VT —
  tetrazolium violet [stain]
  tidal volume
  total ventilation
  vacuum tube
  vacuum tuberculin
  vasotocin
  vasotonin
  venous thrombosis
  ventricular tachyarrhythmia
  ventricular tachycardia
  verocytotoxin
  verotoxin
  vibration threshold
V_T —
  tidal volume
  tissue volume
  total ventilation
V&T — volume and tension
VTA — ventral tegmental area
V_TA — alveolar tidal volume
Vtach — ventricular tachycardia
VTD — villous tumor of the duodenum
VTE —
  venous thromboembolism
  ventricular tachycardia event
  vicarious trial and error
VTEC — verotoxin-producing *Escherichia coli*
V-test — Voluter test [radiology]
VTG — volume thoracic gas
VTI — volume thickness index
VTM —
  mechanical tidal volume

VTM — *(continued)*
  virus transport medium
VTR —
  variable tandem repeats
  variegated translocation mosaicism
  vesicular transport [system]
  videotape recording
VTS — vesicular transport system
VTSRS — Verdun Target Symptom Rating Scale
VTVM — vacuum tube voltmeter
VTX — vertex
VU —
  varicose ulcer
  very urgent
vu — volume unit
VUR —
  vesicoureteral reflex
  vesicoureteral regurgitation
VUV — vacuum ultraviolet
VV —
  varicose veins
  venovenous [bypass]
  vesicovaginal
  viper venom
V-V — veno-venous [bypass]
V&V — vulva and vagina
vv. — *venae* (Lat.) veins
v/v — percent volume (of solute) per volume (of solvent)
VVD —
  vaginal vertex delivery
  vascular volume of distribution
VVFR — vesicovaginal fistula repair
VVI —
  ventricular inhibited [pacemaker]
  vocal velocity index
V/VI — grade five on a six-grade basis
vvMDV — very virulent Marek disease virus
VVOR — visual vestibulo-ocular reflex
VVQ — verbalizer-visualization questionnaire

VVS —
  vesicovaginal space
  vestibulo-vegetative syndrome
VVT — ventricular triggered [pace-maker]
VW —
  vascular wall
  vessel wall
  von Willebrand's [disease]
v/w — volume per weight
vWD — von Willebrand's disease
VWF —
  velocity waveform
  vibration-induced white finger
vWF — von Willebrand's factor

VWFT — variable-width forms tractor
VWM — ventricular wall motion
vWS — von Willebrand's syndrome
Vx — vertex
VY — veal yeast
V-Y — configuration of incisions in surgical procedure
VZ — varicella-zoster
VZIG — varicella-zoster immune globulin
VZL — vinzolidine
VZV — varicella-zoster virus

W

W —
  dominant spotting
  energy
  section modulus
  tryptophan
  ward
  water
  watt
  Weber's [test]
  week
  wehnelt [unit of penetration of roentgen rays]
  weight
  west
  wetting
  white
  white cell
  whole [response]
  widow
  widowed
  widower
  width
  wife
  Wilcoxon's rank sum test
  Wilcoxon's signed rank test
  Wistar [rat]
  Wolfram (Ger.) tungsten

W — (*continued*)
  wolframium (tungsten)
  word fluency
  wound
W — work
W. — wehnelt (unit of penetration of roentgen rays)
W+ — weakly positive
^{185}W — radioactive tungsten
μW — microwatt
w —
  water
  watt
  while
  white
  with
w. —
  week
  wife
ω — omega (twenty-fourth and final letter of the Greek alphabet), lowercase
WA —
  Wellness Associates
  when awake
  while awake
  white adult

WA — (continued)
  Wiskott-Aldrich [syndrome]
  Women's Auxiliary
W/A — watt/ampere
W & A — weakness and atrophy
WAADA — Women's Auxiliary of
  the American Dental Associa-
  tion
WAB — Western Aphasia Battery
WABT — Western Aphasia Bat-
  tery Test
WACH — wedge adjustable cush-
  ioned heel
WAF —
  weakness, atrophy and fascicu-
  lation
  white adult female
WAGR — Wilms' tumor, aniridia,
  genitourinary abnormalities,
  and mental retardation
WAIS — Wechsler Adult Intelli-
  gence Scale
WAIS-R — Wechsler Adult Intelli-
  gence Scale—Revised
WAK — wearable artificial kidney
WAM — white adult male
WAP — wandering atrial pace-
  maker
WAPT — Weidel's Auditory Pro-
  cessing Test
WAR —
  Wasserman antigen reaction
  without additional reagent
WARDS — Welfare of Animals
  Used for Research in Drugs
  and Therapy
WARF —
  warfarin
  Wisconsin Alumni Research
  Foundation
WAS —
  Ward Atmosphere Scale
  weekly activities summary
  Wiskott-Aldrich syndrome
  World Association for Sexol-
  ogy
WASAMA — Women's Auxiliary
  to the Student American
  Medical Association

WASP —
  Weber's Advanced Spatial
  Perception [test]
  white Anglo-Saxon Protestant
  World Association of Societies of Pathology
WASS — Wasserman [reaction,
  test]
WAT — Word Association Test
WB —
  waist belt
  washable base
  washed bladder
  water bottle
  Wechsler-Bellevue [scale]
  weight-bearing
  well baby
  Western blot [assay]
  wet-bulb
  whole blood
  whole body
  Willowbrook [virus]
  Wilson-Blair [agar]
Wb —
  weber
  weight-bearing
  well-being
WBA —
  wax bean agglutinin
  whole body activity
Wb/A — weber/ampere
WBAPTT — whole blood activated partial thromboplastin
  time
WBAT — weight-bearing as tolerated
WBC —
  weight-bearing with crutches
  well-baby care/clinic
  white blood cell
  white blood (cell) count
  white blood corpuscle
  whole blood cell count
WBC/hpf — white blood cells per
  high power field
WBCT — whole blood clotting
  time

WBDC — whole-body digital scanner

WBE — whole-body extract

WBF — whole blood folate

WBGT — wet-bulb global temperature

WBH —
whole blood hematocrit
whole-body hyperthermia

WBI — will be in

WBM — whole boiled milk

Wb/m^2 — weber per square meter

WBN —
well born nursery
whole blood nitrogen
wide-band noise

WBPTT — whole blood partial thromboplastin time

WBQC — wide-base quad cane

WBR —
whole-body radiation
whole-body retention

WBRS — Ward Behavior Rating Scale

WBRT — whole blood recalcification time

WBS —
Wechsler-Bellevue Scale
whole blood serum
whole-body scan
whole-body shower
Wiedemann-Beckwith syndrome
withdrawal body shakes
wound breaking strength

WBT — wet-bulb temperature

WBTF — Waring Blendor tube feeding

WBTT — weight-bearing to tolerance

WC —
ward clerk
ward confinement
water closet
Weber-Christian [syndrome]
wet compress
wheelchair
white cell

WC — (continued)
white cell cast
white cell count
white child
whooping cough
work capacity

WC' — whole complement

WCC —
Walker's carcinosarcoma cell
well child care
white cell count

WCD — Weber-Christian disease

WCE — work capacity evaluation

WCL —
Wenckebach cycle length
whole cell lysate

w/cm^2 — watts per square centimeter

WCOT — wall coated open tubular

WCR — Walthard's cell rest

WCS — white clot syndrome

WCST — Wisconsin Card Sorting Test

WD —
wallerian degeneration
well-developed
well-differentiated
wet dressing
Whitney Damon [dextrose]
Wilson's disease
with disease
without dyskinesia
Wolman's disease
wound
wrist disarticulation

W-D — wet-to-dry dressing

W/D —
warm and dry
withdrawal
withdrawn

W4D — Worth Four Dot [test]

w/d —
well-developed
wound
wounded

wd. —
ward

wd. — (continued)
  wound
WDCC — well-developed collateral circulation
WDF — white divorced female
WDHA — watery diarrhea, hypokalemia, achlorhydria [syndrome]
WDHH — watery diarrhea, hypokalemia, hypochlorhydria [syndrome]
WDHHA — watery diarrhea, hypochlorhydria, hypokalemia, and alkalosis
WDI — warfarin dose index
WDL — well-differentiated lymphocytic
WDLL — well-differentiated lymphocytic lymphoma
WDM — white divorced male
WDMF — wall-defective microbial form
WDS —
  watery diarrhea syndrome
  wet dog shakes [syndrome]
WDWN — well-developed, well-nourished
WE —
  wax ester
  Wernicke encephalopathy
  western encephalitis
  western encephalomyelitis
  whiskey equivalent
  wound of entry
We — weber
WEE —
  western equine encephalitis
  western equine encephalomyelitis
WEF — war emergency formula
WEG — water–ethylene-glycol
WEP — weekend pass
WER — wheal erythema reaction
WF —
  Weil-Felix [reaction]
  wet film
  white female

WF — (continued)
  Wistar-Furth [rat]
  word fluency
W/F — white female
WFE — Williams flexion exercise
WFI — water for injection
WFL — within functional limits
WFOT — World Federation of Occupational Therapists
WFR —
  Weil-Felix reaction
  wheal-and-flare reaction
WFSS — Wolpe Fear Survey Schedule
WG —
  water gauge
  Wegener's granulomatosis
  Wright-Giemsa [stain]
WGA — wheat germ agglutinin
wgt. — weight
WH —
  walking heel [cast]
  well-healed
  well-hydrated
  Werdnig-Hoffmann [disease]
  whole homogenate
  wound healing
Wh — white
wh — whispered
WHA — warmed humidified air
WHAP — Women's Health and Abortion Project
WHB — weight-bearing
WhB — whole blood
WHCOA — White House Conference on Aging
WHD — Werdnig-Hoffmann disease
WHHL — Watanabe heritable hyperlipidemic [rabbeting]
WHML — Wellcome Historical Medical Library
WHMS — well-healed midline scar
WHO —
  World Health Organization
  wrist-hand orthosis
WHOIRP — World Health Organization International Reference Preparation

WHP — whirlpool
WHPB — whirlpool bath
WHR — waist:hips girth ratio
whr. — watt-hour
WHRC — World Health Research
    Center
WHS — Werdnig-Hoffmann syn-
    drome
WHV — woodchuck hepatic virus
WHVP — wedged hepatic venous
    pressure
WI —
    walk-in [patient]
    water ingestion
    waviness index
    Wistar [rat]
W/I — within
WIA —
    walking imagined analgesia
    wounded in action
WIC — women, infants, and chil-
    dren
wid. —
    widow
    widowed
    widower
WIPI — Word Intelligibility Pic-
    ture Identification
WIQ — Waring Intimacy Ques-
    tionnaire
WIS —
    Ward Initiation Scale
    Wechsler Intelligence Scale
WISC — Wechsler Intelligence
    Scale for Children
WISC-R — Wechsler Intelligence
    Scale for Children—Revised
WIST — Whitaker Index of
    Schizophrenic Thinking
WITT — Wittenborn [Psychiatric
    Rating Scale]
WJPB — Woodcock-Johnson Psy-
    choeducational Battery
WK —
    Wernicke-Korsakoff [syn-
        drome]
    Wilson-Kimmelstiel [syn-
        drome]

wk. —
    weak
    week
    work
WKD — Wilson-Kimmelstiel dis-
    ease
WKF — well-known fact
W/kg — watts per kilogram
WKS — Wernicke-Korsakoff syn-
    drome
WKY — Wistar-Kyoto [rat]
WL —
    waiting list
    Wallenstein Laboratory
    water load [test]
    wavelength
    weight loss
    withdrawal
    working level
    workload
wl — wavelength
WLE — wide local excision
WLF — whole lymphocytic frac-
    tion
WLI — weight-length index
WLM —
    white light microscopy
    working level month [radon]
WLS — wet lung syndrome
WLT —
    water load test
    whole lung tomography
WM —
    Waldenström's macroglobulin-
        emia
    wall motion
    ward manager
    warm and moist
    Wernicke-Mann [hemiplegia]
    wet mount
    white male
    whole milk
    whole mount
    Wilson-Mikity [syndrome]
W/M —
    white male
    woman
    wound, missile

W/m² — watts per square meter
WMA —
    wall motion abnormality
    World Medical Association
WMC — weight-matched control
WME — Williams' medium E
WMF —
    white married female
    white middle-aged female
WMM —
    white married male
    white middle-aged male
WMO — ward medical officer
WMP — weight management program
WMR —
    Western Medical Review
    work metabolic rate
    World Medical Relief
WMS —
    wall motion study
    Wechsler Memory Scale
WMSC — Women's Medical Specialists Corps
WMX — whirlpool, massage, and exercise
WN — well-nourished
WND — wound
WNE — West Nile encephalitis
WNF — well-nourished female
WNL — within normal limits
WNM — well-nourished male
WNPW — wide, notched P wave
WNV — West Nile virus
WO —
    wash out
    weeks old
    will order
    without
    written order
W/O — water in oil
w/o — without
wo —
    weeks old
    without
WOB — work of breathing
WOE — wound of entry
WOFL — wound fluid

WOP — without pain
WOR — Weber-Osler-Rendu [syndrome]
WOU — women's outpatient unit
W/O/W — water/oil/water
WOWS — Weak Opiate Withdrawal Scale
WOX — wound of exit
WP —
    water packed
    weakly positive
    wedge pressure
    wet pack
    wettable powder
    whirlpool
    white pulp
    word processor
    working point
W/P —
    water/powder ratio
    whirlpool
wp — wettable powder
WPA — World Psychiatric Association
WPB — whirlpool bath
WPCU — weighted patient care unit
WPF — Wright peak flow
WPFM — Wright peak flow meter
WPk —
    Ward's (mechanical tissue) pack
    wet pack
WPPSI — Wechsler Preschool and Primary Scale of Intelligence
WPRS — Wittenborn Psychiatric Rating Scale
WPS — wasting pig syndrome
WPSI —
    Wahler Physical Symptoms Inventory
    Wittenborn Psychiatric Symptoms Inventory
WPT — warbled pure tone
WPW — Wolff-Parkinson-White [syndrome]
WR —
    washroom

WR — (continued)
  Wassermann reaction
  water retention
  weak response
  weakly reactive
  whole response
  wiping reaction
  wiping reflex
  work rate
Wr. —
  wrist
  writhe
WRAIR — Walter Reed Army Institute of Research
WRAMC — Walter Reed Army Medical Center
WRAML — Wide Range Assessment of Memory and Learning
WRAT — Wide Range Achievement Test
WRBC — washed red blood cell
WRC —
  washed red cell
  water-retention coefficient
WRE — whole ragweed extract
WRK — Woodward's reagent K
WRMT — Woodcock Reading Mastery Test
WRS — Wiedemann-Rautenstrauch syndrome
WRST — Wilcoxon's Rank Sum Test
WRVP — wedged renal vein pressure
WS —
  Waardenburg syndrome
  ward secretary
  Warkany syndrome
  Warthin-Starry [stain]
  water swallow
  water-soluble
  Werner syndrome
  West syndrome
  wet swallow
  Wilder's silver [stain]
  Williams syndrome
  Wolfram syndrome

WS — (continued)
  work simplification
WSI — Waardenburg syndrome type I
W&S — wound and skin
WSA — water-soluble antibiotic
WSB — wheat-soy blend
WSD — water deal drainage
W-sec — watt-second
WSF — white single female
WSL — Wesselsbron [virus]
WSM — white single male
WSMSA — Washington Standard Metropolitan Statistical Area
WSOJ — whole blood serum of patient with obstructive jaundice
WSP —
  wearable speech processor
  withdrawal seizure–prone
WSR —
  Westergren sedimentation rate
  withdrawal seizure–resistant
W/sr — watts per steradian
WT —
  walking tank
  wall thickness
  water temperature
  whistle tip
  wild type [strain]
  Wilms' tumor
  wisdom teeth
  work therapy
wt —
  weight
  white
WTAD — Wepman Test of Auditory Discrimination
WTD — wet tail disease
WTE — whole time equivalent
WTF — weight transferral frequency
wt/vol — weight per volume
wt/wt — weight per weight [ratio]
W/U — work-up
WV —
  walking ventilation

WV — (*continued*)
　whispered voice
W/V —
　percent weight in volume
　weight/volume
W^v — variable dominant spotting
　[mouse]
w/v —
　weight (of solute) per volume
　　(of solvent)
　weight per volume
WV-MBC — walking ventilation
　to maximum breathing capac-
　ity [ratio]
WW —
　Weight Watchers
　wet weight
W/W —
　percent weight

W/W — (*continued*)
　weight in weight
　weight-to-weight [ratio]
w/w — weight (of solute)
　per weight (of total sol-
　vent)
WWAC — walk with aid of cane
WWF — World Wrestling Federa-
　tion
WWTP — wastewater treatment
　plant
WWU — weighted work unit
WX — wound of exit
WxB — wax bite
WxP — wax pattern
WY — women years
WY/NRT — Weidel Yes/No Relia-
　bility Test
Wza — wide zone alpha

X —
　androgenic [zone]
　break
　cross or transverse
　cross section
　crossbite
　crossed with
　crossmatch
　except
　exophoria distance
　exposure
　extra
　female sex chromosome
　homeopathic symbol for the
　　decimal scale of potencies
　ionization exposure rate
　Kienböck's unit of x-ray dos-
　　age
　magnification
　multiplication symbol
　multiplied by
　number of times
　removal of
　respirations [anesthesia chart]

X — (*continued*)
　Roman numeral ten
　start of anesthesia
　times
　translocation between two X
　　chromosomes
　transverse
　unknown quantity
　xanthine
　xanthosine
　x-bite (cross bite)
　xerophthalmia
　X unit
　xylene
$\dot{X}$ — time derivative
$\ddot{X}$ — second time derivative
%X — percentage of the predicted
　normal value
X + # — xiphoid plus number of
　finger breadths
$\overline{X}$ —
　average of all Xs
　except
　mean value

$\overline{X}$ — *(continued)*
    sample mean
X. — *Xenopsylla*
X′ — exophoria
X3 — orientation as to time, place, person
x —
    abscissa
    axis
    except
    exophoria distance
    extremity
    horizontal axis of a rectangular coordinate system
    mole fraction
    multiplication symbol
    reactance
    roentgen [rays]
    sample mean
    time
    unknown factor
ξ — xi (fourteenth letter of the Greek alphabet), lowercase
XA — xanthurenic acid
X-A — xylene and alcohol
Xa —
    antifactor X
    chiasma
Xaa — unknown amino acid
Xam — examination
Xan — xanthine
Xant. — xanthochromic
Xanth. — xanthomatosis
Xao — xanthosine
X-bite — cross bite
XBT — xylose breath test
XC — excretory cystogram
XCCE — extracapsular cataract extraction
X-CGD — X-linked chronic granulomatous disease
X-chrom — female sex chromosome
XD —
    times daily
    X-linked dominant
X&D — examination and diagnosis
XDH — xanthine dehydrogenase
XDP —
    xanthine diphosphate

XDP — *(continued)*
    xeroderma pigmentosum
XDR — transducer
Xe —
    electric susceptibility
    xenon
XECT — xenon-enhanced computed tomography
XEF — excess ejection fraction
Xero — xeromammography
XES — X-ray energy spectrometry
XF — xerophthalmic fundus
Xfb — cross-linked Gibrin
Xfmr — transformer
XGP — xanthogranulomatous pyelonephritis
XH — extra high
XIP —
    x-ray induced polypeptide
    x-ray in plaster
XKO — not knocked out
XL —
    excess lactate
    X-linked [inheritance]
    xylose-lysine [agar base]
    extra large
X-LA — X-linked agammaglobulinemia
XLAS — X-linked aqueductal stenosis
XLD — xylose-lysine-deoxycholate [agar]
X-leg — cross leg
XLH — X-linked hypophosphatemia
XLI — X-linked ichthyosis
XLJR — X-linked juvenile retinoschisis
XLMR — X-linked mental retardation
XLP — X-linked lymphoproliferative [syndrome]
XLR — X-linked recessive
XLS — X-linked recessive lymphoproliferative syndrome
XM — crossmatch
X_m — magnetic susceptibility
Xm — maternal chromosome X
Xma — chiasma
X-mas — Christmas [factor]

XMM — xeromammography

XMP — xanthosine monophosphate (xanthosine-5'-phosphate)

XMR — X-linked mental retardation

XN — night blindness

XO —
    presence of only one sex chromosome
    xanthine oxidase

XOAN — X-linked (Nettleship) ocular albinism

XOM — extraocular movements

XOP — x-ray out of plaster

XOR — exclusive operating room

XP —
    xanthogranulomatous pyelonephritis
    xeroderma pigmentosum

Xp —
    paternal chromosome X
    short arm of chromosome X

Xp − — deletion of short arm of chromosome X

XPA — xeroderma pigmentosum group A

XPC — xeroderma pigmentosum group C

XPN — xanthogranulomatous pyelonephritis

X-Prep — bowel evacuation prior to radiography

XPS — x-ray photoemission spectroscopy

Xq — long arm of chromosome X

Xq − — deletion of long arm of chromosome X

XR —
    X-linked recessive [inheritance]
    x-ray

x-ray — roentgen ray

XRD — x-ray diffraction

XRF — x-ray fluorescence

XRMR — X-linked recessive mental retardation

XRS — x-ray sensitivity

XRT —
    external beam radiotherapy

XRT — (continued)
    x-ray diffraction
    x-ray technician
    x-ray therapy

XS —
    cross section
    excess
    xiphisternum

XSA —
    cross-section area
    xenograph surface area

X-sect — cross section

XS-LIM — exceeds limits of procedure

XSLR — crossed straight leg raising

XSP — xanthoma striatum palmare

XT — exotropia

X(T) — intermittent exotropia

XT′ — exotropia (near)

X_2t — chi-square test

Xta — chiasmata

Xtab — cross tabulating

XTE — xeroderma, talipes, and enamel defect [syndrome]

X-TEP — crossed immunoelectrophoresis

XTM — xanthoma tuberosum multiplex

XTP — xanthosine triphosphate

XU —
    excretory urogram
    X-unit

Xu — x-unit

XULN — times upper limit of normal

XuMP — xylulose monophosphate

XUV — extreme ultraviolet

XX —
    double strength
    normal female chromosome type
    xylocaine

XX/XY — sex karyotypes

XY — normal male chromosome type

Xyl. — xylose

Xylo — Xylocaine

Y ....

Y —
  body
  chromatin
  chromosome
  fragment Y
  male sex chromosome
  ordinate
  protein
  tyrosine
  year
  yellow
  yield
  young
  yttrium
Y. — *Yersinia*
^{90}Y — radioactive yttrium
y — wave on phlebogram
Υ, υ — upsilon (twentieth letter of
    the Greek alphabet), upper-
    and lowercase
YR — year
YA — *Yersinia* arthritis
Y/A — years of age
YACP — young adult chronic pa-
    tient
YADH — yeast alcohol dehydro-
    genase
YAG — yttrium aluminum garnet
Y/B — yellow blue
Yb — ytterbium
^{169}Yb — ytterbium-169
YBT — Yerkes-Bridges test
YCB — yeast carbon base
YCT — Yvon coefficient test
yd — yard
YDV — yeast-derived hepatitis B
    vaccine
YDYES — yin deficiency–yang ex-
    cess syndrome
YE —
  yeast extract
  yellow enzyme
YEH$_2$ — reduced yellow enzyme
YEI — *Yersinia enterocolitica* infec-
    tion

Yel — yellow
YET — youth effectiveness train-
    ing
YF — yellow fever
YFI — yellow fever immunization
YFMD — yellow fever membrane
    disease
YHMD — yellow hyaline mem-
    brane disease
YHT — Young-Helmholtz
    theory
YJV — yellow jacket venom
Yk — York [antibody]
YLC — youngest living child
YLF — yttrium lithium fluoride
YM — yeast and mannitol
YMA — yeast morphology agar
Y$_{max}$ — maximum yield
YNB — yeast nitrogen base
YNS — yellow nail syndrome
YO — year(s) old
y/o — years old
YOB — year of birth
YORA — younger-onset rheuma-
    toid arthritis
YP —
  yeast phase
  yield point
  yield pressure
YPA — yeast, peptone, and ade-
    nine sulfate
YPLL — years of potential life
    lost
YRD — Yangtze River disease
YS —
  yellow spot
  yolk sac
YSC — yolk cell carcinoma
YST —
  yeast
  yolk sac tumor
YT — yttrium
YTD — year to date
YVS — yellow vernix syndrome

Z —

 atomic number
 glutamine
 impedance
 ionic charge number
 no effect
 point formed by a line perpendicular to the nasion-
   menton line through the
   anterior nasal spine
 proton number
 section modulus
 standard score
 standardized deviate
 zero
 zone
 Zuckung (Ger.) contraction
 Zwischen- (Ger.) intermediate
   (*Zwischenscheibe*, intermediate disk or Z-band)

Z, Z′, Z″ — increasing degrees of
   contraction

z —

 algebraic unknown or space
   coordinate
 atomic number
 catalytic amount
 standard normal deviate
 standardized device
 third axis of three-dimen-
   sional rectangular coordinate system
 zero

ζ — zeta (sixth letter of the Greek
   alphabet), lowercase

ZAP — zymosan-activated plasma

ZAPF — zinc adequate pair-fed

ZAS — zymosan-activated autologous serum

ZB — zebra body

ZCP — zinc chloride poisoning

Z/D —

 zero defects
 zero discharge

Z/D — *(continued)*
 zinc deficiency

ZDDP — zinc dialkyldithiophos-
   phate

Z-DNA — zig-zag deoxyribonucleic
   acid

ZDO — zero differential overlap

ZDS —

 zinc depletion syndrome
 Zung Depression Scale

ZE — Zollinger-Ellison [syndrome]

ZEC — Zinsser-Engman-Cole [syn-
   drome]

ZEEP — zero end-expiratory pressure

ZES — Zollinger-Ellison syndrome

Z-ESR — zeta erythrocyte sedimentation rate

ZF —

 zero frequency
 zona fasciculata

ZFF — zinc fume fever

ZG — zona glomerulosa

Z/G —

 zoster immunoglobulin
 zoster serum immune globulin

ZGM — zinc glycinate marker

ZI — zona incerta

ZI^a — isotope with atomic number
   Z and atomic weight A

ZIFT — zygote intrafallopian tube
   transfer

ZIG —

 zoster immunoglobulin
 zoster serum immune globulin

ZIM — zimeldine

ZIP — zoster immune plasma

ZK — Zuelzer-Kaplan [syndrome]

ZLS — Zimmerman-Laband syndrome

Zm — zygomaxillare

ZMA — zinc meta-arsenite

ZMC —

 zygomatic

ZMC — (continued)
  zygomaticomaxillary complex
ZN — Ziehl-Neelsen [stain]
Zn — zinc
Zn fl — zinc flocculation [test]
ZnO — zinc oxide
ZnOE — zinc oxide and eugenol
ZNS — Ziehl-Neelson stain
$ZnSO_4$ — zinc sulfate
ZO —
  Zichen-Oppenheim [syn-
    drome]
  Zuelzer-Ogden [syndrome]
ZOE — zinc oxide–eugenol
Zool —
  zoological
  zoology
ZPA — zone of polarizing activity
ZPC — zero point of change
ZPG — zero population growth
ZPLS — Zimmerman Preschool
  Language Scale
ZPO — zinc peroxide
ZPP — zinc protoporphyrin
ZPT — zinc pyrithione

ZR — zona reticularis
Zr —
  zirconium
  zygomatic root
^{95}Zr — radioactive zirconium
ZS — Zellweger syndrome
ZSB — zero stool since birth
ZSR —
  zeta sedimentation rate
  zeta sedimentation ratio
ZT — Ziehen test
ZTN — zinc tannate of naloxone
ZTS — zymosan-treated serum
Z-TSP — Zephiran–trisodium
  phosphate
ZTT — zinc turbidity test
ZVT — Zellenverbindungstest (Ger.)
  cell-binding test
Zy — zygion
ZyC — zymosan complement
zyg — zygotene
Zylo — Zyloprim
zz. — zingiber (Lat.) ginger
Z.Z.'Z″ — increasing degrees of
  contraction

Medical Eponyms

Medical Eponyms

 A

Aaron's sign

Aarskog's syndrome — a hereditary syndrome marked by abnormal distances between paired organs and by a broad upper lip, anomalous scrotal fold, relaxed ligaments, and small hands; called also *faciodigito-genital dysplasia*

Aarskog-Scott syndrome — same as *Aarskog's syndrome*

Aase's syndrome — a familial syndrome characterized by mild growth retardation, hypoplastic anemia, triphalangeal thumbs, narrow shoulders, and late closure of fontanels

Abadie's clamp, sign

Abbe's operation(s) — a lateral intestinal anastomosis; division of an esophageal stricture

Abbe's condenser, flap, illuminator, ring, string, method, test plate, treatment

Abbe-Estlander operation — the transfer of a full-thickness flap from one lip to fill a defect in the other

Abbe-Estlander flap

Abbe-Zeiss apparatus, counting cell, counting chamber

Abbott's elevator, gouge, method, stain for spores, tube

Abbott-Lucas approach

Abbott-Miller tube

Abbott-Rawson tube

Abderhalden's dialysis, reaction, test

Abderhalden-Fanconi syndrome — osteomalacia, renal glycosuria, aminoaciduria, phosphaturia, and cystine deposition throughout the body

Abderhalden-Fauser reaction

Abegg's rule

Abel's expert system

Abelin's reaction, test

Abell's method, uterine suspension

Abell-Kendall method

Abelson's cannula, murine leukemia virus, oncogene

Abercrombie's syndrome — amyloid degeneration

Abercrombie's degeneration, tumor

Abernethy's fascia, sarcoma

abortus Bang ring (ABR) test

Abrahams' cannula, elevator, knife, protocol, sign

Abrami's disease — same as *Hayem-Widal syndrome*

Abramov-Fiedler myocarditis

Abrams' heart reflex, needle, punch, reflex, test

Abramson's tube

Abrikosov's (Abrikossoff's) tumor

Abt-Letterer-Siwe syndrome — a proliferation of nonlipid histiocytes in the visceral organs, causing red-to-brown, firm nodules to appear, followed by a maculopapular rash or multiple nodules that ulcerate and hemorrhage

Achard's syndrome — arachnodactyly

Achard-Castaigne method, test

Achard-Thiers syndrome — association of diabetes and hirsutism in postmenopausal women; sometimes said to involve an increased incidence of uterine cancer

Achenbach's syndrome — sudden appearance of hematomas of the hand with piercing pain and edema

Achilles bursa, bursitis, jerk, reflex, tendon

Achor-Smith syndrome — nutritional deficiency with pernicious anemia, sprue, and pellagra, due to potassium depletion

Achucárro's stain

Acosta's disease — acute mountain sickness

Acree-Rosenheim reaction, reagent, test

Acrel's ganglion

Adair's forceps, procedure

Adair-Allis forceps

Adair-Dighton syndrome — same as *van der Hoeve's syndrome*

Adamantiades-Behçet syndrome — same as *Behçet's syndrome*

Adami's theory

Adamkiewicz's demilunes, reaction, test

Adams' disease — same as *Adams-Stokes disease*

Adams' operation(s) — subcutaneous intracapsular division of the neck of the femur for ankylosis of the hip; subcutaneous division of the palmar fascia; excision of a wedge-shaped piece from the eyelid

Adams' aspirator, clasp, position, retractor, saw, test

Adams-Stokes syndrome — same as *Morgagni-Adams-Stokes syndrome*

Adams-Stokes disease — heart block with sudden unconsciousness

Adams-Stokes attack, syncope

Adasoy's procedure

Addis' count, method, test

Addison's disease — hypofunction of the adrenal glands with prostration and progressive anemia

Addison's anemia, keloid, melanoderma, planes, point, scleroderma

Addison-Biermer disease — pernicious anemia

Addison-Gull disease — vitiligines of the skin, chronic jaundice, splenomegaly and hepatomegaly

Adelmann's operation — disarticulation of a finger

Adelmann's method

Aden's fever, ulcer

Adie's syndrome — reaction in which one pupil contracts more slowly than the other

Adie's pupil

Adie-Holmes syndrome — same as *Adie's syndrome*

Adler's forceps, punch, test, theory

Adson's syndrome — same as *Naffziger's syndrome*

Adson's maneuver, test

Adson-Brown forceps

Adson-Murphy needle

Aeby's muscle, plane

African histoplasmosis, lymphoma, sleeping sickness, tick-borne fever, trypanosomiasis

Afzelius' erythema

Agazotti's mixture

Agnew's keratome, splint

Agnew-Verhoeff incision

Agostini's reaction, test

Ahlfeld's method

Ahlquist-Durham clip

Ahumada–del Castillo syndrome — amenorrhea, low gonadotropin secretion and galactorrhea, not related to pregnancy

Aicardi's syndrome — diffuse central nervous system anomalies in female infants

Åkerlund's deformity, diaphragm

Akin's bunionectomy

Akiyama's procedure

Akureyri disease — chronic fatigue syndrome

Alagille's syndrome — an autosomal dominant syndrome of neonatal jaundice, cholestasis with pulmonic stenosis and occasionally septal defects

Alajouanine's syndrome — symmetric lesions of the sixth and seventh cranial nerves with double facial paralysis and external oculomotor paralysis associated with double clubfoot and strabismus

Aland eye disease — same as *Forsius-Eriksson syndrome*

Alanson's amputation

Albarrán's disease — presence of *Escherichia coli* in the urine

Albarrán's gland, test, tubules

Albee's operation(s) — operation for ankylosis of the hip; transplantation of a portion of the tibia

Albee-Delbet operation — for fracture of the neck of the femur

Albers-Schönberg disease/syndrome — osteopetrosis—a hereditary disease characterized by abnormal density of bone

Albers-Schönberg marble bones, method

Albert's syndrome — painful inflammation of the bursa located between the os calcis and the Achilles tendon

Albert's disease — inflammation of the bursa

Albert's operation — excision of the knee to secure ankylosis

Albert's diphtheria stain, position, suture

Albert-Andrews laryngoscope

Albert-Linder bone sectioning

Albertini's treatment

Albini's nodules

Albinus' muscle

Albl's ring

Albrecht's bone

Albright's syndrome — same as *Albright-McCune-Sternberg syndrome*

Albright's dystrophy, hereditary osteodystrophy, solution

Albright-Butler-Bloomberg syndrome — vitamin D–resistant rickets

Albright-Hadorn syndrome — a disorder of potassium metabolism associated with osteomalacia and sudden hypokalemic muscular paralysis

Albright-McCune-Sternberg syndrome — fibrous dysplasia of bone with endocrine dysfunction

Alcock's canal

Alcock-Hendrickson lithotrite

Alcock-Timberlake obturator

Alden's retractor

Alder's constitutional granulation anomaly

Alder-Reilly anomaly, bodies

Aldrich's syndrome — same as *Wiskott-Aldrich syndrome*

Aldrich's mixture

Aldrich-McClure test

Aldridge-Studdefort urethral suspension

Aleutian mink disease — disease of mink caused by *Parvovirus* and marked by weight loss, lethargy, and hemorrhage

Alexander's syndrome — congenital factor VII deficiency resulting in hemophilia-like hemorrhagic diathesis with epistaxes, deep muscular hematomas, and internal hemorrhages

Alexander's disease — an infantile form of leukodystrophy

Alexander's operation(s) — shortening of the round ligaments of the uterus; ligation of the vertebral arteries for relief of epilepsy; prostatectomy

Alexander's deafness, gouge, hearing loss, incision, method, punch

Alexander-Adams operation — shortening of the round ligaments of the uterus

Alexander-Farabeuf elevator, periosteotome

Alezzandrini's syndrome — degenerative retinitis

Alfraise's test

Alibert's disease — a progressive lymphoma of the skin

Alibert's keloid, mentagra

Alibert-Bazin syndrome — a rare, usually fatal, disease of the reticuloendothelial system

Allarton's operation — median lithotomy

Allemann's syndrome — familial, hereditary double kidney and clubbed fingers

Allen's correction, fossa, maneuver, paradoxic law, rule, test, treatment

Allen-Barkan knife

Allen-Brown shunt

Allen-Doisy test, unit

Allen-Masters syndrome — pelvic pain resulting from laceration during delivery

Allesandri-Guaceni test

Allgrove's syndrome — familial, hereditary achalasia and alacrima

Allingham's operation(s) — inguinal colotomy; excision of the rectum by an incision into the ischiorectal fossae

Allingham's ulcer

Allis' clamp, forceps, inhaler, sign

Allis-Coakley forceps

Allis-Duval forceps

Allis-Ochsner forceps

Allison's atrophy, clamp, retractor

Allport's hook, retractor, searcher

Allport-Babcock retractor, searcher

Almeida's disease — South American blastomycosis

Almén's reagent, test

Alouette's operation — amputation at the hip with a semicircular outer flap to the great trochanter and a large internal flap from within outward

Alouette's amputation

Alpers' disease — degeneration of the cerebral gray matter with preservation of the white matter, manifested by progressive mental deterioration, spasticity, myoclonus, generalized convulsions, choreoathetosis, ataxia and early death

Alpers' test

Alport's syndrome — progressive sensorineural hearing loss with pyelonephritis or glomerulonephritis

Alsberg's angle, triangle

Alsever's solution

Alström's syndrome — retinal degeneration with nystagmus and loss of central vision

Alström-Hallgren syndrome — a familial syndrome characterized by obesity, diabetes mellitus, deafness, retinitis pigmentosa and mental disorders

Alström-Olsen syndrome — familial inborn visual abnormality due to genetic retinal lesions with no neurological or endocrine changes

Althausen's test

Altmann's aniline-acid fuchsin stain, fixative, fluid, granules, theory

Altmann-Gersh method

Alvarez's prosthesis

Alvarez-Rodriguez catheter

Alvegniat's pump
Alvis' curet
Alyea clamp
Alzheimer's disease/syndrome —
    presenile dementia
Alzheimer's cells, corpuscles, de-
    mentia, fibrillary degenera-
    tion, sclerosis, stain
Amalric's syndrome — deafness
    with macular dystrophy and
    central visual defects
Amann's coefficient, test
Amato's bodies
Ambard's coefficient, constant,
    equation, formula, law
Amberg's line
Ames cryostat, test
Amici's disk, line, striae
Ammon's operation(s) — bleph-
    aroplasty by a flap from the
    cheek; dacryocystotomy, resec-
    tion of a spindle-shaped piece
    of skin over the bridge of the
    nose for epicanthus
Ammon's filaments, fissure, horn,
    quick test, scleral prominence
amniotic infection syndrome of
    Blane — fetal sepsis following
    swallowing and aspiration of
    contaminated amniotic fluid
Amoss' sign
Amplatz's catheter
Amsler's charts, marker
Amsterdam's dwarf, type
Amussat's operation — a long
    transverse incision for expo-
    sure of the colon
Amussat's probe, valve
Anagnostakis' operation(s) — for
    entropion; for trichiasis
Ancell-Spiegler cylindroma
Andernach's ossicles
Anders' disease — deposit of fatty
    masses in subcutaneous tissues
    throughout the body
Anders' syndrome — same as
    Dercum's syndrome
Andersch's ganglion, nerve

Andersen's disease — glycogen-
    storage disease
Andersen's syndrome — bronchi-
    ectasis, pancreatic cystic fi-
    brosis, and vitamin A defi-
    ciency
Andersen's triad
Anderson's operation — longitu-
    dinal splitting of a tendon to
    produce lengthening of the
    tendon
Anderson's medium, phenomenon,
    procedure, splint, test
Anderson-Adson retractor
Anderson-Collip test
Anderson-Goldberger test
Andes disease — chronic moun-
    tain sickness
Andogsky's syndrome — bilateral
    cataracts involving the entire
    lens
Andrade's syndrome — a form of
    amyloidosis marked by sen-
    sory disorders and progressive
    paralysis
Andrade's indicator, type of amy-
    loidosis
Andral's decubitus, sign
André's test
André-Thomas sign
Andreasch's test
Andresen's appliance
Andrewes' test
Andrews' disease — eruptions of
    pustules on palms and soles
    due to bacterial infection else-
    where in the body
Andrews' bacterid, forceps
Andrews-Hartman forceps, retrac-
    tor, rongeur
Andrews-Pynchon tube
Anel's operation — dilation of the
    lacrimal duct followed by an
    astringent injection
Anel's probe, syringe
Angelchik's prosthesis
Angeli's sulfone
Angell's curet

Angelman's syndrome — an autosomal recessive syndrome marked by jerky puppet-like movements

Angelucci's syndrome — extreme excitability and vasomotor disturbance, associated with vernal conjunctivitis

Anghelescu's sign

Angle's classification, malocclusion, splint

Anglesey's leg

Angström's law, unit

Anichkov's (Anitschkow's) cell, myocyte

Annam ulcer

Annandale's operation(s) — the removal of the condyles of the femur; the fixation of displaced cartilages of the knee joint by stitches

Annapolis lymphoblast globulin

Ann Arbor staging classification

Anrep effect

Ansbacher's unit

Anschütz's chloroform

Anson-McVay herniorrhaphy

Anstie's limit, reagent, rule, test

Anthony's capsule, retractor, stain, tube

Anthony-Fisher balloon

Antole-Condale elevator

Anton's syndrome — same as *Anton-Babinski syndrome*

Anton's symptom, test

Anton-Babinski syndrome — denial or unawareness of blindness in cortical blindness

Antonucci's test

Antopol-Goldman lesion

Apathy's gum syrup medium

Apert's disease/syndrome — craniostenosis associated with syndactyly

Apert-Crouzon disease — a hereditary disease consisting of hand and foot malformations with craniofacial abnormalities

Apert-Gallais syndrome — same as *Cooke-Apert-Gallais syndrome*

Apgar's scale, score

Apley's grind test, maneuver, sign

Appolito's suture

Apt test

Arakawa's reaction, reagent, test

Arakawa-Higashi syndrome — hypochromic anemia with megaloblastic bone marrow

Aran's law

Aran-Duchenne disease — spinal muscular atrophy

Arantius' bodies, canal, duct, ligament, nodules, ventricle

Arbuckle's probe

Arcelin's method

Archer's forceps

Archetti's test

Arctic anemia

Arey's rule

Argand's burner

Argonz–Del Castillo syndrome — a combination of galactorrhea with amenorrhea and low urinary follicle-stimulating hormone not associated with pregnancy or acromegaly

Argyle's catheter, tube

Argyle-Salem tube

Argyll Robertson pupil, sign

Arias' syndrome — hyperbilirubinemia with jaundice of the skin, sclera and mucous membranes

Arias-Stella cells, effect, phenomenon, reaction

Aries-Pitanguy mammaplasty

Aristotle's anomaly

Arkin's disease — same as *Bayford-Autenrieth dysphagia*

Arloing-Courmont test

Arlt's disease — a contagious infection by *Chlamydia trachomatis* characterized by keratoconjunctivitis, papillary hypertrophy, follicles, and scarring, often leading to blindness

Arlt's operation — any of several operations on the eye and eye-lid

Arlt's recess, sinus, trachoma

Arlt-Jaesche operation — transplantation of the ciliary bulbs from the edge of the lid for correction of distichiasis

Armanni-Ebstein cells, change, kidney, lesion

Armanni-Ehrlich degeneration

Armstrong's disease — lymphocytic choriomeningitis

Arndt's law

Arndt-Gottron disease/syndrome — scleromyxedema

Arndt-Schulz law

Arneth's syndrome — muffled speech caused by complete hepatization of the lung tissue

Arneth's classification, count, formula, index, stages

Arning's carcinoid

Arnold's nerve reflex cough syndrome — reflex cough from irritation of the area supplied by the auricular branch of the vagus nerve

Arnold's bodies, canal, fold, ganglion, ligament, nerve, neuralgia, sterilizer, substance, test

Arnold-Chiari syndrome — malformation of the cerebellum with hydrocephalus

Arnold-Chiari deformity, malformation

Arnold and Gunning method

Arnott's bed, dilator

Aron's test

Aronson's culture medium, method

Arrhenius's doctrine, equation, formula, theory

Arrhigi's point

Arroyo's sign

Arruga's expressor, forceps, retractor, speculum

Arruga-Gill forceps

Arthus' phenomenon, reaction

Artmann's chisel

Arzberger's pear (pear-shaped vessel)

Asboe-Hansen's disease — a skin disease of newborn girls characterized by bullous, keratogenic, pigmented dermatitis

Asboe-Hansen's incontinentia pigmenti

Asch's operation — correction of deflection of the nasal septum

Asch's forceps, splint

Ascher's syndrome — relaxation of the skin of the eyelid, double lip and nontoxic thyroid gland enlargement

Ascher's glass-rod phenomenon, veins

Ascherson's membrane, vesicles

Aschheim-Zondek hormone, test

Aschner's phenomenon, reflex, sign, test

Aschner-Danini test

Aschoff's bodies, cells, node, nodules

Aschoff-Rokitansky sinus

Aschoff-Tawara node

Ascoli's reaction, test, treatment

Aselli's glands, pancreas

Ashby's agar, culture medium, differential agglutination method

Asherman's syndrome — adhesions within the endometrial cavity, often causing amenorrhea and infertility

Asherson's syndrome — dysphagia and achalasia of the cricopharyngeal sphincter

Ashford's mamilliplasty

Ashhurst's splint

Ashman's phenomenon

Asiatic cholera

Askanazy's cell

Askenstedt's method

Askin's tumor

Ask-Upmark kidney

Asperger's psychopathy

Assézat's triangle

Assmann's focus, tuberculous infiltrate

Astler-Coller rectal system

Astwood's test

Atkins' knife

Atkins-Cannard tube

Atkins-Tucker laryngoscope

Atkinson's lid block

Atkinson and Kendall test

Atlee's clamp, dilator

Aub-Dubois table

Auberger's blood group system

Aubert's phenomenon

Auchencloss-Madden mastectomy

Audouin's microsporon

Audry's syndrome — same as *Uehlinger's syndrome*

Auenbrugger's sign

Auer's bodies, phenomenon, rods

Auerbach's ganglion, plexus

Aufranc's gouge, hip prosthesis, retractor

Aufranc-Turner hip prosthesis

Aufrecht's disease — alterations of the parenchyma of the liver and kidney in infectious jaundice

Aufrecht's sign

Aufricht's retractor, speculum

Aufricht-Lipsett rasp

Auger's effect, electron spectroscopy

Augustine's nail

Aujeszky's disease — pseudorabies

Aujeszky's itch

Ault's clamp

Auricchio and Chieffi test

Auspitz's disease — same as *Alibert-Bazin syndrome*

Auspitz's dermatosis, sign

Austin's knife

Austin Flint murmur, phenomenon, respiration

Austin Moore arthroplasty, prosthesis

Austin and Van Slyke method

Australian hepatitis antigen

Australian X disease — Murray Valley encephalitis

Autenrieth and Funk method

Auvard's cranioclast, speculum

Auvard-Remine speculum

Auvray's incision

Aveline Gutierrez parotidectomy

Aveling's repositor

Avellis' syndrome — unilateral paralysis of the larynx and soft palate with loss of pain and temperature senses

Avellis' paralysis

Avellis-Longhi syndrome — same as *Avellis' syndrome*

Avery's culture medium

Avicenna's gland

Avila's approach

Avogadro's constant, law, number

Axenfeld's syndrome — congenital ocular maldevelopment

Axenfeld's anomaly, calcareous degeneration, conjunctivitis, test

Axenfeld-Krukenberg spindle

Axenfeld-Schürenberg syndrome — oculomotor paralysis alternating with spasm

Ayala's equation, index, quotient

Ayer's forceps, test

Ayer-Tobey test

Ayerst's knife

Ayerza's syndrome — pulmonary hypertension with dilatation of pulmonary arteries

Ayerza's disease — a form of polycythemia vera marked by cyanosis, dyspnea, bronchitis, bronchiectasis and hyperplasia of bone marrow and associated with sclerosis of the pulmonary artery

Ayoub-Shklar method

Ayre's brush, knife

Ayre-Scott knife

Azorean disease — a progressive degenerative disease of the central nervous system in Portuguese-Azorean families

Aztec ear, idiocy

Azua's pseudoepithelioma

B ....

Baaser's dermatostomatitis

Baastrup's disease/syndrome — a disorder in which the spinous processes of adjacent vertebrae are in contact (kissing spine)

Babbitt's metal

Babcock's operation — removal of the saphenous vein

Babcock's forceps, herniorrhaphy, needle, raspatory, test, trocar, tube

Baber's syndrome — congenital cirrhosis of the liver

Babès' node, nodule, treatment, tubercles

Babès-Ernst bodies, corpuscles, granules

Babington's disease — same as *Osler's syndrome* (skin disease)

Babinski's syndrome — association of cardiac and arterial disorders with late syphilis

Babinski's law, phenomenon, reflex, sign, test

Babinski-Fröhlich syndrome — adiposogenital dystrophy

Babinski-Nageotte syndrome — multiple lesions affecting the pyramidal and sensory tracts

Babinski-Vaquez syndrome — same as *Babinski's syndrome*

Babinski-Weil test

Babkin's reflex

Baccelli's mixture, sign

Bachman's reaction, test

Bachman-Pettit test

Bachmann's bundle

Bachmeier's test

Backhaus' clamp, dilator, forceps

Bacon's anoscope, forceps, raspatory, retractor, rongeur

Badal's operation — laceration of the infratrochlear nerve for pain of glaucoma

Badgley's nail, retractor

Baehr-Löhlein lesion

Baehr-Schiffrin disease — same as *Moschcowitz's disease*

Baelz's disease/syndrome — congenital and familial papules at the duct openings of the mucous glands of the lips with fissures radiating from the angles of the mouth

Baer's cavity, law, membrane, method, nystagmus, plane, vesicle

Baerensprung's erythrasma

Baermann's test

Baeyer's test

Bäfverstedt's syndrome — benign inflammatory hyperplasia of cutaneous lymphocytes

Baggenstoss' change

Bagot's mixture

Bahson's clamp, retractor

Bailey's cannula, clamp, dilator, forceps, Gigli-saw guide, leukotome, rongeur

Bailey-Cowley clamp

Bailey-Gibbon rib contractor

Bailey-Glover-O'Neil commissurotomy, knife, valvulotome

Bailey-Morse clamp, knife

Bailey-Williamson forceps

Baillarger's syndrome — same as *Frey's syndrome*

Baillarger's bands, layer, lines, sign, striae, striations, stripes

Bailliart's ophthalmodynamometer, tonometer

Baillière's Medical Transparencies

Bainbridge's clamp, forceps, reflex

Baird's forceps

Bakamjian's deltopectoral flap

Baker's cyst, forceps, method, test, tube, velum

Baker-Lima-Baker mask

Bakes's dilator

Bakwin-Eiger syndrome — multiple fractures in early life with bowing of all extremities

Bakwin-Krida syndrome — same as *Pyle's disease*

Balamuth's buffer solution, culture medium

Balbiani's body, chromosome, nucleus, rings

Baldwin's operation — formation of an artificial vagina by transplantation of a piece of ileum between the bladder and the rectum

Baldy's operation — for retrodisplacement of the uterus

Baldy-Webster operation — same as *Webster's operation*

Baldy-Webster uterine suspension

Balfour's disease—green cancer — a condition marked by development of localized green masses of abnormal cells

Balfour's bodies, gastrectomy, gastroenterostomy, infective granule, retractor, test, treatment

Balint's syndrome — cortical paralysis of visual fixation

Balkan grippe, nephropathy

Balkan's fracture frame, splint

Ball's method, valves

Ballance's sign

Ballantine's clamp

Ballantine-Drew coagulator

Ballantyne-Runge syndrome — prolonged gestation syndrome

Ballen-Alexander retractor

Ballenger's curet, elevator, forceps, periosteotome, urethroscope

Ballenger-Forster forceps

Ballenger-Hajek chisel, elevator

Ballenger-Lillie bur

Ballenger-Sluder tonsillectome

Ballentine's forceps

Ballentine-Peterson forceps

Baller-Gerold syndrome — craniosynostosis and radial aplasia

Ballet's disease — paralysis of one or more of the nerves supplying the extrinsic eye muscles

Ballet's sign

Ballingall's disease — maduromycosis

Balme's cough

Baló's disease — inflammation of the white substance of the brain in which demyelination occurs in concentric rings

Balser's fatty necrosis

Bamatter's syndrome — a familial syndrome marked by progeria with nanism, microcornea, corneal opacity, enlarged joints, osseous dysplasia, flabby skin and tooth discoloration

Bamberger's disease(s) — polyserositis with effusion of fluid into the pleural and peritoneal cavities; spasm or tic of the lower extremities

Bamberger's area, fluid, hematogenic albuminuria, sign

Bamberger-Marie disease — hypertrophic pulmonary osteoarthropathy

Bamby's clamp

Bamle's disease — epidemic pleurodynia

Bancroft's filarial worm, filariasis

Bancroft-Plenk gastrectomy

Bancroftian filariasis

Bandeloux's bed

Bandl's ring

Bane's forceps, rongeur

Bang's disease — undulant fever

Bang's bacillus, method, ring test

Bankart's retractor

Bankson Language Screening Test

Banner's snare

Bannister's disease — angioneurotic edema

Bannwarth's syndrome — meningopolyneuritis

Bantam's coagulator

Banti's disease/syndrome — same as *Klemperer's disease*

Banti's spleen

Banting's cure, diet, treatment

Bantu siderosis

Bar's syndrome — pain in the area of the gallbladder, ureters, and appendix with occasional fever

Bar's incision

Barach's index

Bárány's syndrome — a combination of unilateral headache, ipsilateral deafness, vertigo, tinnitus, and inability to point a finger

Bárány's apparatus, pointing test, sign, symptom

Barbados' leg

Barbara's pelvimeter

Barber's dermatosis

Barclay's niche

Barcoo disease—desert sore — a form of tropical ulceration of the face, hands, and lower extremities

Barcoo rot, vomit

Barcroft's apparatus

Bard's syndrome — pulmonary metastases in cancer of the stomach

Bard's catheter, dilator, electrode, resectoscope, sign

Bard-Parker blade, dermatome, forceps, scissors

Bardach's test

Bardam's catheter

Bardeen's disk

Bardel's serum

Bardenheuer's extension, incision

Bardet-Biedl syndrome — a recessive, heritable disorder marked by mental retardation, polydactyly and hypogenitalism

Bareggi's reaction, test

Baréty's method

Barfoed's reagent, test

Barfurth's law

Bargen's serum, streptococcus

Barger's method

Barile-Yaguchi-Eveland (BYE) agar, culture, medium

Barkan's operation — goniotomy for congenital glaucoma

Barkan's forceps, goniotomy, knife

Barker's operation(s) — excision of the hip joint; a method of excising the astragalus

Barker's needle, point

Barkman's reflex

Barkow's colliculus, ligament

Barlow's disease — infantile scurvy

Barlow's syndrome — late apical systolic murmur due to protrusion of the posterior mitralvalvular leaflet into the atrial cavity

Barlow's forceps

Barnard's carcinoma

Barnes' bag, compressor, curve, dilator, speculum

Barnes-Dormia stone basket

Barnes-Simpson forceps

Barnett-Bourne acetic alcohol silver nitrate method

Barnhill's curet

Baron's elevator, knife, retractor, tube

Barr's bodies, body analysis, body test, bolt, hook, nail, retractor, speculum

Barral's test

Barraquer's disease — any disturbance of fat metabolism marked by progressive diminution of body fat

Barraquer's operation — removal of lens in cataract by suction

Barraquer's brush, erysiphake, forceps, method, scissors, sutures, trephine

Barraquer-Colibri eye speculum

Barraquer-DeWecker scissors

Barraquer-Simons syndrome — same as *Simons' disease*

Barraquer-Zeiss microscope

Barraya's forceps

Barré's signs

Barré-Guillain syndrome — acute febrile polyneuritis

Barré-Lieou syndrome — vertigo of cervical arthrosis

Barré-Masson syndrome — glomus tumor

Barrett's syndrome — chronic peptic ulcer of the lower esophagus

Barrett's epithelium, esophagus, forceps, knife, tenaculum, ulcer

Barrett-Adson retractor

Barrett-Allen forceps

Barrett-Murphy forceps

Barrnett-Seligman method

Barron's ligation

Barroso-Moguel-Costero silver method

Barsky's operation — repair of a cleft hand

Barsky's cleft lip repair, elevator, pharyngoplasty

Bársony-Polgár syndrome — a diffuse, esophageal spasm caused by disruption of the advance of peristaltic waves by an irregular contraction

Bársony-Teschendorf syndrome — same as Bársony-Polgár syndrome

Bart's syndrome — an autosomal-dominant trait marked by absence of skin with formation of blisters

Bart's hemoglobin, vibrator

Bart-Pumphrey syndrome — a familial, hereditary syndrome consisting of knuckle pads, leukonychia, and deafness

Bartelmez's club ending

Barth's hernia

Barthelemy's disease — a symmetric eruption of papules or nodules in children and young adults with tuberculosis

Bartholin's abscess, cyst, anus, duct, foramen, glands

Bartholomew's rule of fourths

Bartlett's procedure, stripper

Barton's operation — for ankylosis, by sawing through the bone and removing a V-shaped section

Barton's bandage, dressing, forceps, fracture

Barton-Cone tongs

Bärtschi-Rochain syndrome — headache, paresthesia, scotoma, stiffness in the neck, pain on pressure of the vertebrae, and vertigo

Bartter's syndrome — primary juxtaglomerular cell hyperplasia

Baruch's law, scissors, sign

Barwell's operation — osteotomy for genu valgum

Basedow's disease — a thyroid disorder of unknown etiology, usually called Graves' disease

Basedow's goiter, paralysis, triad

Basham's mixture, solution, test

Basile's screw

Bass-Watkins test

Bassen-Kornzweig syndrome — abetalipoproteinemia

Basset's operation — dissection of the inguinal glands for cancer of the vulva

Bassini's operation — for the radical cure of inguinal hernia

Bastedo's rule

Bastian's aphasia, law

Bastian-Bruns law, sign

Bastow's raspatory

Batch-Spittler-McFadden amputation

Bateman's disease — a viral skin disease marked by formation of firm, translucent, depressed papules containing caseous matter

Bateman's prosthesis, purpura

Bates' operation — the division of a urethral stricture from within outward with a special type of urethrotome

Bather's leukemia
Batten's disease — same as *Batten-Mayou disease*
Batten-Mayou disease — a juvenile form of cerebral sphingolipidosis
Battey's disease — a tuberculosis-like lung disease caused by "Battey bacilli"
Battey bacilli-type mycobacterium
Battle's operation — for appendicitis, with retraction of the rectus muscle
Battle's incision, sign
Battle-Jalaguier-Kammerer incision
Battley's sedative
Baudelocque's operation — an incision through the posterior cul-de-sac of the vagina for removal of the ovum, in extrauterine pregnancy
Baudelocque's diameter, line
Bauer's reaction, test, valve
Bauer-Feulgen technique
Bauer-Trusler-Tondra cleft lip repair
Bauhin's gland, valve
Baum's operation — stretching of the facial nerve by an incision below the ear
Baumann's coefficient, test
Baumann-Goldmann test
Baumè's scale
Baumgarten's glands
Baumgartner's method
Baumrucker's resectoscope
Baunscheidt's treatment
Baurer's chromic acid leucofuchsin stain
Bayer's test
Bayes' rule, theorem
Bayford-Autenrieth dysphagia
Bayle's disease — paralytic dementia
Bayle's granulations
Bayliss' effect
Baylor's rapid autologous transfusion, splint

Baynton's bandage
Bayrac's test
Bazex's syndrome — lesions on the skin of the extremities in patients with carcinoma of the upper respiratory and digestive tracts
Bazin's disease — a chronic, necrotizing vasculitis of unknown origin, usually occurring on the calves of young women
Béal's conjunctivitis
Beale's ganglion cells
Beall's mitral valve prosthesis
Bean's syndrome — association of erectile, bluish, cavernous hemangiomas of the skin with bleeding hemangiomas of the gastrointestinal tract
Beard's disease/syndrome — neurasthenia
Beard's cystotome, knife, speculum, test treatment
Beardsley's dilator, forceps, tube
Bearn-Kunkel syndrome — a condition seen in young women marked by cirrhosis of the liver with hypergammaglobulinemia and increase of plasma cells in the liver
Bearn-Kunkel-Slater syndrome — same as *Bearn-Kunkle syndrome*
Beatson's operation — ovariotomy in inoperable breast cancer
Beatty-Bright friction sound
Beau's disease/syndrome — cardiac insufficiency
Beau's lines
Beaupre's forceps
Beauvais' disease — rheumatoid arthritis
Beaver's blade, curet, direct smear method, electrode, keratome, retractor
Beaver-DeBakey blade
Beccari's process
Bechtel's prosthesis, screw

Beck's disease — a disease affecting young people in Siberia, marked by swelling of the phalanges, enlargement of joints and retardation of growth

Beck I operation — an operation for supplying collateral circulation to the heart

Beck II operation — a two-stage operation for supplying collateral circulation to the heart, performed two to three weeks apart

Beck's syndrome — occlusion of the anterior spinal artery resulting in various neurological complications

Beck's cardiopericardiopexy, forceps, gastrostomy, raspatory, triad

Beck-Jianu gastrostomy

Beck-Mueller tonsillectome

Beck-Satinsky clamp

Beck-Schenck tonsillectome

Becker's disease — cardiomyopathy leading to fatal congestive heart failure

Becker's muscular dystrophy, nevus, phenomenon, retractor, scissors, sign, stain, test, trephine

Becker-Lennhoff index

Beckman's assay

Beckman-Adson retractor

Beckman-Colver speculum

Beckman-Eaton retractor

Beckman-Weitlaner retractor

Beckmann's apparatus, formula, thermometer

Beckwith's syndrome — a hereditary disorder marked by extreme cytomegaly of the fetal adrenal cortex

Beckwith-Wiedemann syndrome — a recessive, hereditary syndrome marked by exophthalmos, macroglossia, and gigantism

Béclard's amputation, hernia, nucleus, sign, triangle

Béclère's method

Becquerel's rays

Becton-Dickinson spinal needle

Bednar's aphtha, tumor

Bedson's test

Beer's operation — flap operation for cataract

Beer's collyrium, knife, law

Beevor's sign

Begbie's disease — a thyroid disorder of unknown etiology, usually called *Graves' disease*

Begg's appliance, technique

Béguez César disease — a lethal, progressive, autosomal recessive disorder marked by massive leukocytic inclusions, pancytopenia, and hepatosplenomegaly

Behçet's disease/syndrome — a complex of disorders including severe uveitis, optic atrophy, lesions of the mouth and genitalia and other symptoms suggestive of diffuse vasculitis

Behçet's aphthae

Béhier-Hardy sign, symptom

Behla's bodies

Behnken's unit

Behr's syndrome — optic atrophy-ataxia syndrome

Behr's disease — degeneration of the retinal macula in adult life

Behr's pupil, sign

Behre-Benedict test

Behring's law, tuberculin

Beigel's disease — a fungal disease of the hair in which hair shafts bear nodular masses of fungi

Beisman's sign

Békésy's audiometry

Bekhterev's (Bechterew's) disease — ankylosing spondylitis

Bekhterev's (Bechterew's) arthritis, layer, nucleus, nystagmus, reaction, reflex, sign, spondylitis, symptom, test, tract

Bekhterev-Mendel reflex

Bekhterev-Strumpell-Marie syndrome — ankylosing polyarthritis

Belfield's operation — vasotomy

Belgian Congo anemia

Bell's disease — acute delirium

Bell's delirium, law, mania, muscle, nerve, palsy, paralysis, phenomenon, sign, spasm, suture, test, treatment

Bell-Dally dislocation

Bell-Magendie law

Bellini's ducts, ligament, tubules

Bellocq's cannula, sound, tube

Bellows' cryoextractor

Bellucci's scissors

Belsey's esophagoplasty, herniorhaphy

Belsey Mark IV operation — for gastroesophageal reflux through a thoracic incision

Belzer's apparatus

Benaron's forceps

Benassi's method

Bence Jones albumin, albumosuria, bodies, cylinders, globulin, myeloma, protein, proteinuria, reaction test, urine

Benda's stain

Bender's Gestalt test

Bender's Visual-Motor Gestalt test

Bendien's test

Benditt's hypothesis

Benedict's gastroscope, method, reagent, solution, test

Benedict-Denis method, test

Benedict-Franke method

Benedict-Hitchcock method

Benedict-Hopkins-Cole reagent

Benedict-Leche method

Benedict-Murlin method, test

Benedict-Osterberg method

Benedict-Theis method

Benedikt's syndrome — ipsilateral oculomotor paralysis, contralateral hyperkinesia, paresis of the arm and leg and ataxia

Beneventi's retractor

Bengolea's forceps

Bengston's method

Béniqué's sound

Benjamin's anemia

Bennell's bandage

Bennet's syndrome — erythroblastic anemia, osteoporosis, and steatorrhea in children

Bennet's corpuscles

Bennett's disease — leukemia

Bennett's operation — for varicocele, by partial excision of the pampiniform plexus

Bennett's angle, forceps, fracture, sulfhydryl method, movement, retractor, seal

Bennhold's Congo red method, stain

Benoist's scale

Benoy's scale

Bensley's neutral gentian orange G stain

Benson's disease — spherical, calcium-containing opacities in the vitreous humor

Benson's separator

Bent's operation — shoulder excision with flap from the deltoid region

Bentley's filter

Benton's visual retention test

Benzhaf's serum

Béraneck's tuberculin

Bérard's aneurysm, ligament

Berardinelli's syndrome — congenital hyperpituitarism of hypothalamic origin

Béraud's valve

Berbecker's pliers

Berbridge's scissors

Bereitschafts' potential

Berenreuther's test

Berens' dilator, forceps, implant, keratome, retractor, scissors, speculum

Berens-Rosa eye implant

Berg's chelate removal method, stain

Bergeim's method

Bergenhem's operation — surgical implantation of the ureter into the rectum

Berger's disease — glomerulone-phritis

Berger's operation — interscapulo-thoracic amputation

Berger's method, paresthesia, rhythm, sign, symptom

Bergeron's disease — chorea of childhood marked by violent, rhythmic spasms, but running a benign course

Bergeron's chorea

Bergersen's medium

Bergey's classification

Bergh's staging system

Bergman's sign

Bergmann's syndrome — hiatus hernia in which pressure exerted on the thoracic organs produces dysphagia, tachycardia, hiccups, and discomfort and pain in the cardiac region

Bergmann's operation — incision of the tunica vaginalis, performed for hydrocele

Bergmann's cells, cords, fibers, glia, incision, rule

Bergmann-Israel incision

Bergmann-Meyer test

Bergmeister's papilla

Bergonié's method, treatment

Bergonié-Tribondeau law

Bergstrand's disease — osteoid osteoma

Berke's operation — for ptosis of the upper eyelid, with resection of the levator muscle through a skin incision

Berke-Motais operation — for ptosis of the upper eyelid, with suspension of the ptotic lid from the superior rectus muscle

Berkefeld's filter

Berlin's syndrome — a familial abnormality marked by short stature

Berlin's disease — edema of the macular region of the retina

Berlin's edema

Berlind-Auvard speculum

Berman's clamp, locator

Berman-Moorhead locator

Bermenam-Werner probe

Berna's retractor

Bernard's syndrome(s) — acute familial hemolysis; also same as *Bernard-Horner syndrome*

Bernard's canal, duct, layer, puncture

Bernard-Horner syndrome — ptosis, miosis, anhidrosis, and endophthalmos due to paralysis of the cervical sympathetic nerves

Bernard-Sergent syndrome — acute adrenocortical insufficiency

Bernard-Soulier syndrome/disease — a coagulation deficiency marked by thrombocytopenia, also called *giant platelet disease*

Bernay's retractor, sponge

Bernberg's intrauterine device

Berndt's hip ruler

Berne's forceps

Berne pain questionnaire

Bernhardt's disease — same as *Bernhardt-Roth disease*

Bernhardt's formula, paralysis, paresthesia

Bernhardt-Roth disease — tingling, itching and paresthesia in the area of distribution of the external femoral nerve

Bernheim's syndrome — right heart failure without pulmonary congestion

Bernheimer's fibers

Bernoulli's distribution

Bernstein's gastroscope, test

Bernthsen's methylene violet

Bernuth's syndrome — sporadic hemophilia

Berry's circles, clamp, forceps, ligament, raspatory
Berry-Dedrick phenomenon
Berson's test
Bertel's method
Berthelot's procedure, reaction, reagent, test
Bertin's bone, columns, ligament, ossicles
Bertini's renal columns
Bertolotti's syndrome — sacralization of the fifth lumbar vertebra with scoliosis
Bertoni-Raymondi test
Bertrand's method, reagent, test
Bertrandi's sutures
Berwick's dye
Berzelius' test
Besnier's prurigo, rheumatism
Besnier-Boeck disease — sarcoidosis
Besnier-Boeck-Schaumann disease/ syndrome — same as *Besnier-Boeck disease*
Bespaloff's sign
Besredka's antivirus, reaction
Bessey-Lowry units
Bessey-Lowry-Brock unit
Bessman's anemia calcification
Best's disease — congenital macular degeneration
Best's carmine stain, forceps, telescope
Bethe's method
Bethea's method, sign
Bethesda method, unit
Bethesda-Ballerup group of *Citrobacter*
Betke-Kleihauer test
Betke's stain
Bettendorff's test
Bettmann's test
Betz's cell area, cells
Beuren's syndrome — a congenital syndrome combining multiple cardiovascular disorders, dental abnormalities, mental retardation, peculiar facies, and a coarse, metallic voice

Beutler's test
Bevan's operation — for undescended testicle
Bevan's incision
Bevan-Lewis cells
Beyer's forceps, rongeur
Bezold's abscess, ganglion, mastoiditis, perforation, reflex, sign, triad
Bezold-Jarisch reflex
Bial's reagent, test
Bianchi's syndrome — a sensory aphasia with loss of ability to comprehend writing, seen in lesions of the left parietal lobe
Bianchi's nodules, valve
Biber-Haab-Dimmer dystrophy
Bibron's antidote
Bicek's retractor
Bichat's canal, fissure, foramen, ligament, membrane, tunic
Bickel's ring
Bickerstaff's encephalitis
Bidder's ganglia, organ
Biebrich's scarlet-picroaniline blue
Biederman's sign
Biedert's cream mixture
Biedl's disease — a hereditary disorder characterized by mental retardation, obesity, retinitis, hypogonadism, and polydactyly
Bieg's entotic sign
Bielschowsky's disease — same as *Bielschowsky-Jansky disease*
Bielschowsky's method, head-tilting test, stain, technique
Bielschowsky-Jansky disease — the late infantile form of cerebral sphingolipidosis
Bielschowsky-Lutz-Cogan syndrome — internuclear ophthalmoplegia
Biemond's syndrome — a hereditary disorder marked by mental deficiency, obesity, progressive loss of retinal response and polydactyly

Biemond's ataxia

Bier's operation — osteoplastic amputation of the leg with a bone flap cut out of the tibia and fibula above the stump

Bier's amputation, anesthesia, hyperemia, spots, treatment

Biermer's disease — pernicious anemia

Biermer's anemia, sign

Biermer-Ehrlich anemia

Biernacki's sign

Biesenberger's operation — reduction mammaplasty

Biesiadecki's fossa

Biett's disease — discoid lupus erythematosus

Biett's collar

Bietti's syndrome — xerosis conjunctivae with iridopupillary anomalies

Bietti's dystrophy

Bigelow's operation — crushing of a calculus in the bladder followed by washing out of the fragments

Bigelow's ligament, litholapaxy, lithotrite, septum

Bilderbeck's disease — acrodynia

Bilhaut-Celoquet wedge resection

Bill's traction handle

Billeau's curet

Billroth's disease — meningocele from fracture of the skull

Billroth's operation(s) — partial resection of the stomach with anastomosis; pylorogastrectomy with anterior gastroenterostomy; excision of the tongue by transverse incision below the symphysis of the jaw

Billroth's cords, forceps, hypertrophy, strands, tube

Bimler's appliance

Binda's sign

Binelli's styptic

Binet's age, staging system test

Binet-Simon test

Bing's erythroprosopalgia, test

Bing-Neel syndrome — hyperglobulinemia with involvement of the central nervous system, marked by fever, anorexia, emaciation, irritability, personality changes, and mental deterioration

Binkhorst's eye implant

Binswanger's disease — presenile dementia caused by demyelination of the subcortical white matter of the brain

Binswanger's dementia, encephalitis

Binz's test

Biondi-Heidenhain stain

Biot's breathing, respiration, sign

Birbeck's granules

Birch-Hirschfeld lamp, tumor, stain

Bird's disease — susceptibility to infection as a result of oxalic poisoning

Bird's formula, respirator, sign, treatment

Birkett's forceps, hernia

Birkhaug's test

Birnberg's bow

Birtcher's cautery, coagulator, hyfrecator

Birt-Hogg-Dubé syndrome — autosomal dominant disorder with growth of ectodermal and mesodermal components of the pilar system

Bischoff's test

Bishop's score, sphygmoscope

Bishop-Black tendon tucker

Bishop-Coop enterostomy

Bishop-DeWitt tendon tucker

Bishop-Harmon forceps, irrigator

Bishop-Peter tendon tucker

Bismarck brown

Bissell's operation — excision of a portion of the round and broad ligaments for uterine retroversion

Bitot's patches, spots

Bittner agent, virus
Bittorf's reaction
Bivine's method
Bizzarri-Guiffrida knife, laryngo-
scope
Bizzozero's cells, corpuscles, plate-
lets
Bjerrum's scotoma, scotometer,
screen, sign
Björk's drill
Björk-Shiley mitral valve prosthe-
sis
Björnstad's syndrome — congenital
cochlear deafness
Björnström's algesimeter
Black's formula, method, reagent,
test
Black-Wylie dilator
Blackberg-Wanger test
Blackett-Healy method
Blackfan-Diamond syndrome —
congenital hypoplastic anemia
Blackfan-Diamond anemia
Blackman's reaction
Blainville's ear
Blair's hook, knife, retractor
Blair-Brown operation — repair of
cleft lip
Blair-Brown graft, procedure, re-
tractor
Blake's curet, disks, forceps
Blakemore-Sengstaken tube
Blakesley's forceps, retractor, tre-
phine
Blalock's anastomosis, forceps, pro-
cedure
Blalock-Hanlon operation — the
creation of a large, atrial sep-
tal defect as a palliative proce-
dure for transpostion of the
great vessels
Blalock-Niedner clamp
Blalock-Taussig operation — anastomosis of the subclavian artery to the pulmonary artery
to shunt some systemic circulation into the pulmonary circulation

Blanchard's cryptotome, forceps,
method, treatment
Bland-White-Garland syndrome —
anomalies of the coronary artery from the pulmonary artery associated with enlargement of the heart
Blandin's ganglion, glands
Blandin-Nuhn glands
Blandy's urethroplasty
Blane's amniotic infection syndrome — fetal sepsis following
swallowing and aspiration of
contaminated amniotic fluid
Blaschko's lines
Blasius' duct
Blaskovic's operation — resection
of a semilunar piece of skin
from the canthal fold, for
blepharoptosis
Blasucci's catheter
Blatin's syndrome — the tremulous
impulse sometimes felt upon
palpation over a hydatid cyst
Blatin's sign
Blaud's pills
Blegvad-Haxthausen syndrome —
osteogenesis imperfecta and
blue sclera, with atrophy of
the skin and zonular cataract
Blencke's disease — metaepiphys-
eal osteodystrophy of the cal-
caneum
Blessig's cysts, groove, lacuna,
spaces
Blessig-Iwanoff cyst
Blinks' effects
Bloch's reaction, scale
Bloch-Stauffer dyshormonal dermatosis
Bloch-Sulzberger syndrome — a
congenital defect in females
consisting of lesions of the
skin, eyes, nails, teeth, central
nervous system, and hair
Bloch-Sulzberger incontinentia pigmenti, melanoblastosis
Block-Steiger test

Blocq's disease/syndrome — inability to stand or walk although the legs are normal—often a sign of conversion hysteria

Blondel's serum

Blondheim's test

Blondlot's rays

Bloodgood's disease — cystic disease of the breast

Bloodgood's inguinal herniorrhaphy

Bloodwell's forceps

Bloom's syndrome — congenital telangiectatic erythema

Bloor's method, test

Bloor, Pelkan, and Allen method

Blot's perforator

Blount's disease — same as *Erlacher-Blount disease*

Blount's osteotome, osteotomy, test

Blount-Barber syndrome — same as *Erlacher-Blount syndrome*

Blount-Barber disease — aseptic necrosis of the medial condyle of the tibia

Bloxam's test

Bluemel's treatment

Blum's syndrome — deficiency of sodium chloride, fixation of chlorine in tissues, and excess urea in the urine

Blum's reagent, substance, test

Blumberg's ligament, sign

Blumenau's nucleus, test

Blumenbach's clivus, plane, process

Blumenthal's disease — erythroleukemia

Blumenthal's lesion

Blumer's shelf

Blyth's test

Boari's operation — transplantation of the vas deferens, enabling emptying into the urethra

Boari's button

Boas' algesimeter, point, test

Boas-Oppler bacillus, lactobacillus

Bobroff's operation — osteoplastic operation for spina bifida

Bochdalek's duct, foramen, ganglion, gap, hernia, pseudoganglion, sinus, valve

Bock's ganglion, nerve

Bock-Benedict method

Bockhart's impetigo

Bodal's test

Bodansky's unit

Bodenheimer's anoscope, speculum

Bodian's copper-Protargol stain, method

Bodin-Gibb staging system

body of Luys syndrome — a violent form of motor restlessness, involving only one side of the body, caused by a lesion of the hypothalamic nucleus

Boeck's disease — sarcoidosis

Boeck's itch, lupoid, sarcoid, scabies

Boeck-Drbohlav culture medium

Boeck-Drbohlav-Locke egg serum

Boedeker's test

Boehm's anoscope, proctoscope, sigmoidoscope

Boehmer's hematoxylin

Boehringer Mannheim Diagnostics

Boerhaave's syndrome — spontaneous rupture of the esophagus

Boerhaave's glands

Boerner-Lukens test

Boettcher's cells, forceps, hemostat, trocar

Bogaert's disease — a rare hereditary disorder characterized by abnormal cholesterol metabolism and bile acid formation causing progressive ataxia, mental deterioration, cataracts, and multiple xanthomas

Bogdän-Buday disease — abscesses of the liver and possibly of the lungs, spleen, and joints following extrahepatic injuries

Bogg's method, reagent
Bogomolets' serum
Bogorad's syndrome — paroxysmal
    lacrimation appearing after fa-
    cial palsy
Bogros' space
Bogue's operation — multiple liga-
    tion of the veins in varicocele
Böhler's clamp, fracture frame,
    splint
Böhler-Braun splint
Bohlman's pin
Böhm's operation — tenotomy of
    an ocular muscle for strabis-
    mus
Bohmansson's test
Bohme's reagent
Bohn's epithelial pearls, nodules
Bohr's atom, effect, equation, mag-
    neton
Boies' elevator, forceps
Boley's gauge
Boling's burner
Bolk's retardation theory
Bollinger's bodies, granules
Bolton's point, triangle
Bolton-Hunter reagent
Bolton-nasion plane
Boltz's reaction, test
Boltzmann's constant
Bombay blood group, phenotype
Bomford-Rhoads anemia
Bonaccolto's forceps, scleral ring
Bonain's solution
Bonanno's test
Bonchardat's reagent
Bond's forceps, splint
Bonferroni-Holm correction
Bongiovanni-Eisenmenger syn-
    drome — a chronic liver dis-
    ease that features hyperadre-
    nalism, marked by elevation of
    serum gamma globulin and to-
    tal proteins, high urinary corti-
    costeroid level, and increased
    glycogen storage activity
Bonhoeffer's symptom
Bonina-Jacobson tube
Bonn's forceps

Bonnaire's method
Bonnano's tube
Bonner's position
Bonnet's syndrome(s) — visual hal-
    lucinations in the elderly, not
    associated with mental disor-
    ders; trigeminosympathetic
    neuralgia
Bonnet's capsule, enucleation of
    eyeball, plexus, sign
Bonnet-Dechaume-Blanc syn-
    drome — tortuosity of the ves-
    sels of the retina, with arterio-
    venous angioma of the optic
    nerve, thalamus, and mesen-
    cephalon
Bonnevie-Ullrich syndrome — a
    complex syndrome character-
    ized by webbing of the neck,
    lymphangiectatic edema of
    the hands and feet, dwarfism,
    and other anomalies
Bonney's clamp, forceps, hysterec-
    tomy
Bonnier's syndrome — a complex
    of symptoms caused by a le-
    sion of the lateral vestibular
    nucleus, involving vertigo,
    pallor, and other aural and oc-
    ular disturbances
Bonnot's gland
Bonsignore's test
Bonta's knife
Bonwill's triangle
Bonzel's operation — surgical sepa-
    ration of the external margin
    of the iris from the ciliary
    body
Böök's syndrome — a rare familial
    syndrome marked by premolar
    aplasia, excessive sweating,
    and premature grayness
Boolean algebra, factor analysis,
    function
Boothby, Lovelace, Bulbulian
    [mask]
Borchardt's test
Borchgrevink method
Borden's test

Bordet's amboceptor, phenomenon, test

Bordet-Gengou agar, bacillus, medium, phenomenon, reaction

Bordier-Fränkel sign

Börjeson's syndrome — same as *Börjeson-Forssman-Lehmann syndrome*

Börjeson-Forssman-Lehmann syndrome — mental deficiency, epilepsy, hypogonadism, and hypometabolism

Bornholm's disease — epidemic pleurodynia

Boros' esophagoscope

Borrel's blue stain, bodies

Borries' syndrome — localized encephalitis with cerebrospinal fluid changes, headache, fever, and other symptoms suggesting abscess of the brain

Borrmann's classification

Borsch's bandage

Borsieri's line, sign

Borst-Jadassohn intraepidermal basal cell epithelioma

Borthen's operation — iridotasis

Bose's operation — a type of tracheotomy

Bose's hook, tracheotomy

Bosher's knife

Bossi's dilator

Bostock's disease — hay fever

Bostock's catarrh

Boston Collaborative Drug Surveillance Program

Boston's exanthem, sign, test

Bosviel's syndrome — hemorrhage from a ruptured uvular hematoma

Bosworth's drill, retractor, speculum

Bosworth-Shawler incision

Botallo's duct, foramen, ligament

Botelho's test

Botkin's disease — infectious hepatitis

Böttcher's cells, crystals

Böttger's test

Bottini's operation — making a channel through the prostate to cure prostate enlargement

Bottu's test

Botvin's forceps

Botzmann's constant, equation

Bouchard's disease — dilatation of the stomach from inefficiency of the gastric muscles

Bouchard's coefficient, index, nodes, nodules, sign

Bouchardat's test, treatment

Boucheron's speculum

Bouchet-Gsell disease — a benign meningitis seen in people who work with swine and pork

Bouchut's respiration, tubes

Boudin's law

Bouguer's law

Bouillaud's syndrome — the coexistence of pericarditis and endocarditis in acute articular rheumatism

Bouillaud's disease — rheumatic endocarditis

Bouillaud's sign

Bouin's fluid, solution

Bouin-Ancel test

Bourdon's test

Bourgery's ligament

Bourget's test

Bourneville's disease/syndrome — tuberous sclerosis

Bourneville-Pringle syndrome — tuberous sclerosis

Bourns' respirator

Bouveret's disease/syndrome — paroxysmal tachycardia; obstruction of gastric outlet by a gallstone passed into the duodenal bulb

Bouveret's ulcer

Boveri's test

Bovie's cautery, electrosurgical unit, knife

Bovin's fixation

Bowditch's law, staircase phenomenon

Bowen's disease — intraepidermal squamous cell carcinoma

Bowen's epithelioma, osteotome, precancerous dermatosis

Bowen-Grover meniscotome

Bowers-McComb unit

Bowie's stain

Bowlby's splint

Bowman's capsule, disks, glands, lamina, layer, membrane, muscle, probe, scissors, space, theory, tubes

Bowman-Birk soybean inhibitor

Box-DeJager adenotome

Boyce's position, sign

Boyd's amputation, incision

Boyd-Stearns syndrome — rickets beginning during infancy, dwarfism, osteoporosis, and malnutrition associated with metabolic disorders

Boyden's chamber assay, sphincter, test meal

Boyer's bursa, cyst

Boyes-Goodfellow hook retractor

Boyksen's test

Boyle's law

Boyle Davis mouth gag

Boynton's needle holder

Boys-Allis forceps

Bozeman's operation — turning the cervix uteri into the bladder and suturing it for the relief of vesicouterovaginal or ureterouterine fistula

Bozeman's catheter, clamp, forceps, position, speculum, sutures

Bozeman-Frisch catheter

Bozeman-Wertheim needle holder

Bozicevich's test

Bozzi's foramen

Bozzolo's sign

Braasch's bulb catheter, cystoscope, forceps

Braastad's retractor

Brace's test

Brachet's mesolateral fold

Brachmann-de Lange syndrome — a congenital syndrome in which severe mental retardation is associated with numerous anomalies, including dwarfism, webbed neck, brachycephaly, and others

Bracht's maneuver

Bracht-Wächter bodies, lesions

Bracken's forceps

Brackett's probe

Brackin's incision

Bradbury-Eggleston syndrome — postural hypertension with visual disturbances, hypohidrosis, lowered basal metabolic rate, syncope, and slow unchanging pulse

Braden's reservoir

Bradford's forceps, frame

Bradley's disease — epidemic nausea and vomiting

Bradshaw's albumosuria, test

Bradshaw-O'Neill clamp

Bragard's sign

Bragg's curve, peak of proton beam, reflection

Bragg-Paul pulsator

Braid's effect, strabismus

Brailey's operation — stretching the supratrochlear nerve to relieve pain in glaucoma

Brailsford-Morquio disease — a rare form of mucopolysaccharidosis marked by severe dwarfism and lumbar kyphosis

Brain's reflex

Bram's test

Brand's bath

Brand-Legal nitroprusside reaction

Brande's test

Brandt's syndrome — a familial syndrome of childhood marked by diarrhea, steatorrhea, alopecia, paronychia with nail dystrophy, pustulous dermatitis and blepharitis, and conjunctivitis

Brandt's method, technique, treatment

Brandt-Andrews maneuver, method

Branham's bradycardia, sign

Bransford-Lewis dilator

Brant's splint

Brantley-Turner retractor

Brasil's alcoholic picro-formol, fixative

Brauch-Romberg symptom

Brauer's cardiolysis

Braun's anastomosis, canal, cranioclast, culture medium, forceps, graft, hook, ring, tenaculum, test

Braun-Husler reaction, test

Braun-Jaboulay gastrectomy, gastroenterostomy

Braun-Wangensteen graft

Braune's canal

Braunwald's sign

Braunwald-Cutter prosthesis

Bravais-jacksonian epilepsy

Brawley's rasp, retractor

Braxton Hicks contractions, sign, version

Brazelton behavioral scale

Brazilian trypanosomiasis

Brecher's new methylene blue technique

Brecher-Cronkite method

Breck's pin

Breda's disease — yaws

Breed's smear

Brehmer's method, treatment

Breisky's disease — atrophy of the female genitalia, most commonly occurring in older women

Breisky's pelvimeter

Breisky-Navratil speculum

Breitman's adenotome

Bremer's test

Brennemann's syndrome — mesenteric and retroperitoneal lymphadenitis

Brenner's operation — a modification of *Bassini's operation* in which the abdominal muscles are sutured to the cremaster muscle

Brenner's forceps, formula, nodules, test, tumor

Brentano's syndrome — a disorder of muscle glycogen metabolism during pregnancy, with depletion of liver glycogen and creatinuria

Breschet's canals, hiatus, sinus, veins

Brescia-Cimino arteriovenous fistula

Breslau's method

Breslow's thickness

Bret's syndrome — on radiographs one lung presents a clear picture and the other an opaque shadow

Breton's law

Bretonneau's disease — diphtheria

Bretonneau's angina, diphtheria

Breus' mole

Brewer's infarcts, point, speculum

Brewster's retractor

Bricker's operation — creation of an ileal conduit with a flat stoma for the collection of urine

Brickner's position, sign

Brieger's cachexia, reaction, test

Briggs' transilluminator

Brigham's forceps

Bright's disease — a broad term for kidney disease, usually glomerulonephritis

Bright's blindness, eye, granulations

Brighton's balloon

Brill's disease — a recurrence of typhus, sometimes occurring many years after the initial acute episode

Brill-Baehr-Rosenthal disease — same as *Brill-Symmers syndrome*

Brill-Symmers disease/syndrome —
giant follicular lymphoma

Brill-Zinsser disease — same as
Brill's disease

Brinell hardness number

Brinkerhoff's anoscope, speculum

Brinster's medium for ovum culture

Brinton's disease — diffuse fibrous
proliferation of the submucosal connective tissue of the
stomach

Brion-Kayser disease — infection
caused by *Salmonella* of all
groups except *S. typhosa*

Briquet's syndrome — shortness of
breath due to hysterical paralysis of the diaphragm

Briquet's ataxia

Brissaud's disease — habitual spasmodic movement or contraction of any part

Brissaud's dwarf, infantilism, reflex,
scoliosis

Brissaud-Marie syndrome — unilateral spasm of the tongue
and lips, usually due to hysteria

Brissaud-Marie sign

Brissaud-Sicard syndrome — spasmodic hemiplegia caused by
lesions of the cerebral commissure

Bristol's hemoglobin

Bristow's procedure

Bristowe's syndrome — a series of
symptoms characteristic of tumor of the corpus callosum

British antilewisite, thermal unit

Brittain's arthrodesis, chisel

Broadbent's apoplexy, registration
point, sign, test

Broadbent-Bolton plane

Broberger-Zetterström syndrome — idiopathic hypoglycemia in children without increase in urinary excretion of
adrenalin

Broca's amnesia, angle, aphasia,
ataxia, band, center, convolution, fissure, formula, gyrus,
motor speech area, parolfac-
tory area, plane, point, pouch,
region

Brock's syndrome — atelectasis of
the right middle pulmonary
lobe, with pneumonitis

Brock's operation — an incision
into the ventricle and dilation of the pulmonary valve

Brock's dilator, incision, infundibu-
lectomy, valvotomy, valvulotome

Brock-Suckow polyposis

Brockenborough's sign

Brockenbrough's needle

Brocq's disease — parapsoriasis

Brocq's pseudopelade

Brocq-Pautrier glossitis

Brödel's white line

Broden's methods

Broders' classification, grading system, index

Brodie's disease — chronic synovitis; hysterical pseudofracture
of the spine

Brodie's abscess, bursa, finger,
joint, knee, ligament, pain,
pile, probe, reaction, sign, tumor

Brodin's syndrome — duodenal stenosis caused by lymphadenitis
associated with appendicitis

Brodmann's areas

Brodney's cannula, clamp

Broesike's fossa

Brompton's mixture

Bronson's magnet

Bronson-Turz retractor

Brönsted-Lowry acid, base

Brook reaction test

Brooke's disease — trichoepithe-
lioma

Brooke's epithelioma, tumor

Brooks' punch, scissors

Brophy's operation — for cleft
palate

Brophy's bistoury, forceps, mouth gag, periosteotome, scissors, tenaculum

Brophy-Deschamps needle

Broviac's catheter

Brown's vertical retraction syndrome — adhesion of the ocular muscles of the fetus

Brown's applicator, clamp, dermatome, method, periosteotome, reaction, test, tonsillectome

Brown-Adson forceps

Brown-Blair dermatome

Brown-Brenn stain, technique

Brown-Buerger cystoscope, forceps

Brown-Dohlman eye implant

Brown-Pearce carcinoma, epithelioma, tumor

Brown-Pusey trephine

Brown-Roberts-Wells stereotactic system

Brown-Séquard disease/syndrome — ipsilateral paralysis due to damage of one side of the spinal cord

Brown-Séquard's epilepsy, hemiplegia, injection, lesion, paralysis, sign, treatment

Brown and Sharp sutures

Brown-Symmers disease — fatal, acute serous encephalitis in children

Brown-Vialetto-van Laere syndrome — progressive bulbar palsy with nerve deafness, facial weakness, dysarthria, and dysphagia

Browne's operation — urethroplasty for repair of hypospadias

Browne's opacity, tubes, urethral reconstruction

Brownian-Zsigmondy movement

Browning's vein

Broyles' aspirator, bronchoscope, esophagoscope, laryngoscope, nasopharyngoscope

Bruce's bundle, septicemia, tract

Bruce-Muir tract

Bruch's glands, layer, membrane

Bruck's disease — deformity of bones, ankylosis of joints, and atrophy of muscles

Bruck's reaction, test

Brücke's fibers, lens, lines, muscle, protein-free pepsin, reagent, test, tunic

Brudzinski's reflex, sign

Brudzinski, Oppenheim, Chaddock, and Guillaird reflex, sign

Brueghel's syndrome — dystonia of facial and oromandibular muscles with blepharospasm, mouth movements, and tongue protrusion

Bruening's bronchoscope, otoscope, snare, speculum

Bruening-Citelli rongeur

Brug's filaria, filariasis

Brugsch's syndrome — acropachyderma

Brugsch's index, test

Brunati's sign

Brunauer-Emmet-Teller method

Bruner's speculum

Brunetti's chisel

Brunhilde's virus

Brunn's epithelial nests, membrane, method

Brunner's chisel, forceps, glands, incision, raspatory

Brünninghausen's method

Bruns' syndrome — intermittent headache, vertigo, vomiting, and visual disturbance upon sudden movement of the head

Bruns' disease — pneumopaludism—a lung disease of malarial origin

Bruns' apraxia of gait, glucose medium, sign

Brunn's epithelial nests

Brunschwig's operation — pancreatoduodenectomy done in two stages

Brunschwig's forceps

Brunsting's syndrome — grouped vesicular lesions about the head and neck, usually occurring in older men
Brunton's otoscope
Bruser's incision
Brushfield's spots
Brushfield-Wyatt syndrome — a congenital condition marked by hemianopia, contralateral hemiplegia, cerebral angioma and mental retardation
Bruton's agammaglobulinemia
Bryan's high titer
Bryant's operation — lumbar colotomy
Bryant's line, sign, traction, triangle
Bryce's sign, test
Bryce-Teacher ovum
Bryson's sign
Buchner's bodies
Bucholz's prosthesis
Buchwald's atrophy
Buck's operation — a wedge-shaped excision of the patella and the ends of the tibia and fibula
Buck's curet, extension, fascia, osteotome, traction
Bücklers' dystrophy
Buckley's syndrome — hyperimmunoglobulinemia E
Bucknall's procedure
Buckstein's insufflator
Bucky's diaphragm, grid, ray
Bucky-Potter diaphragm
Bucy's knife, retractor
Bucy-Frazier suction tube
Bud's bar
Budd's disease — chronic hepatic enlargement
Budd's cirrhosis, jaundice
Budd-Chiari syndrome — symptomatic obstruction of the hepatic veins, usually of unknown origin
Budge's center

Budin's joint, rule
Büdinger-Ludloff-Läwen syndrome — traumatic separation of the cartilage of the patella with fissures
Buerger's disease — thromboangiitis obliterans
Buerger's bougie, symptom
Buerger-Grütz disease — idiopathic hyperlipemia
Buerger-McCarthy forceps, scissors
Buergi's theory
Bufano's test
Bugbee's electrode
Buhl's disease — an acute sepsis affecting newborn infants, marked by hemorrhages into the skin, mucous membranes, navel, and intestinal organs
Buhl's desquamative pneumonia
Buhl-Dittrich law
Bühler's baby test
Buie's cannula, electrode, forceps, hemorrhoidectomy position, tube
Buie-Hirschman anoscope, clamp, speculum
Buie-Smith retractor, speculum
Buisson's articulation
Buist's method
Buller's bandage, shield
Bullis fever
Bumke's pupil
Bumper's fracture
Bumpus' forceps, resectoscope
Bunge's amputation, law, spoon
Büngner's bands, cell cordons
Bunim's forceps
Bunnell's drill, splint, sutures
Bunsen burner, coefficient
Bunsen's solubility coefficient
Bunsen-Roscoe law
Bunts's catheter
Bunyamwera virus
Bunyan's bag
Burch's caliper, evisceration
Burch-Greenwood tendon tucker
Burchard-Liebermann reaction, test

Burckhardt's operation — incision into a retropharyngeal abscess from the outside of the neck

Burckhardt's corpuscles, dermatitis

Burdach's columns, fasciculus, fibers, fissure, nucleus, tract

Burdick's cautery, electrosurgical unit

Burdizzo's vasectomy

Bureau-Barrière disease — a nonfamilial form of Hicks' syndrome marked by pseudosyringomyelic ulcerative lesions of the foot, found chiefly in middle-aged males who have had frequent injuries

Burford's retractor, spreader

Burford-Finochietto retractor, spreader

Burger's scalene triangle, sign, test

Bürger-Grütz syndrome — hyperlipoproteinemia

Burghart's sign, symptom

Burke's syndrome — progressive pulmonary dystrophy

Burkitt's acute lymphoblastic leukemia, lymphoma, tumor

Burkitt-like lymphoma

Burks' Behavior Rating Scale

Burnam's test

Burnett's syndrome — hypercalcemia and severe renal insufficiency attributed to ingestion of milk over long periods of time

Burnett's disinfecting fluid, solution

Burnham's forceps, scissors

Burnier's syndrome — dwarfing, optic atrophy and adiposogenital dystrophy from decreased functioning of the anterior pituitary

Burns' amaurosis, chisel, ligament, space, telescope

Burow's operation — plastic operation for the removal of tumors

Burow's blepharoplasty, solution, vein

Burrow's triangle

Burton's line, sign

Buruli ulcer

Burwell's bur

Bury's disease — a chronic eruption of flattened nodules occurring on the buttocks, wrists, elbows and knees with final scarring

Busacca's floccule, nodule

Buscaino's reaction, test

Busch's scissors

Buschke's disease — cryptococcosis

Buschke's memory test, scleredema

Buschke-Löwenstein giant condyloma, tumor

Buschke-Ollendorff syndrome — dermatofibrosis

Busquet's disease — exostoses on the dorsum of the foot

Busse's saccharomyces

Busse-Buschke disease — same as *Buschke's disease*

Butchart staging system

Butcher's saw

Bütschli's emulsion, granules, nuclear spindle

Butter's cancer

Butterfield's cystoscope

Buxton's clamp

Buzzi's operation — creation of an artificial pupil by a needle passed through the cornea

Bwamba fever virus

Bychowski's test

Byford's retractor

Byler's disease — familial cholestasis with hepatosplenomegaly and dwarfism

Bywaters' syndrome — edema, oliguria and other manifestations of renal failure following a crushing injury

Cabot's ring bodies, splint
Cacchi-Ricci disease — a heredi-
    tary disorder marked by multi-
    ple cystic dilations of the re-
    nal collecting tubes—sponge
    kidney
Cache Valley virus
Caffey's disease/syndrome — infan-
    tile cortical hyperostosis
Caffey-Silverman disease/syn-
    drome — same as *Caffey's dis-
    ease*
Cagot ear
Cahn-Ingold Prelog Sequence
    Rules
Cahoon's method
Caillan's test
Cain's complex
Cairns' operation — to relieve glau-
    coma
Cairns' forceps, retractor
Cajal's cells, interstitial nucleus,
    method, solution, stain
Caldani's ligament
Caldwell's method, position,
    projection
Caldwell-Luc operation — creation
    of an opening into the maxil-
    lary antrum through the supra-
    dental fossa above the maxil-
    lary premolar teeth
Caldwell-Moloy classification,
    method
Calhoun-Merz needle
Calibri's forceps
California disease — a fungous
    disease caused by infection
    with *Coccidioides immitis* and
    marked by an acute respira-
    tory infection; the secondary
    form is a virulent granuloma-
    tous disease affecting the cen-
    tral nervous system and lungs
California encephalitis

Call-Exner bodies
Callahan's flange, forceps, method
Callander's amputation
Callaway's test
Calleja's islands, islets
Callison's fluid
Calmette's ophthalmoreaction, re-
    action, serum, test, tubercu-
    lin, vaccine
Calmette-Guérin bacillus
Calori's bursa
Calot's operation — forcible reduc-
    tion of kyphosis
Calot's node, treatment, triangle
Caltagirone's chisel, knife
Calvé's syndrome — vertebral os-
    teochondritis
Calvé's cannula
Calvé-Legg-Perthes syndrome —
    osteochondrosis of the capitu-
    lar epiphysis of the femur
Calvé-Perthes disease — same as
    Calvé-Legg-Perthes syndrome
Calvert's test
Calvin's cycle
Camera's syndrome — vertebral and
    paravertebral lumbosciatic oste-
    opathy caused by inflammatory
    lesions of the lower lumbar
    spine and sacrum
Camerer's law
Cameron's appliance, gastroscope
Cameron-Haight elevator
Cameron-Lorenz cautery
Cameroon fever
Cammann's stethoscope
Cammidge's reaction, test
Camp-Coventry method
Camp-Gianturco method
Campani's test
Campbell's catheter, cruciate sul-
    cus, forceps, ligament, osteo-
    tome, sound, test, trocar
Camper's angle, fascia, ligament, line

Camurati-Engelmann disease —
diaphyseal dysplasia

Canada-Cronkhite syndrome — familial gastrointestinal polyposis

Canavan's disease — spongy degeneration of the central nervous system

Canavan's sclerosis

Canavan-van Bogaert-Bertrand disease — same as *Canavan's disease*

Canfield's knife

Cannizzaro's reaction

Cannon's syndrome — increased adrenal epinephrine secretion during emotional stress

Cannon's nevus, point, reflex, ring

Cannon-Bard theory

Cannon-Rochester elevator

Cantani's test, treatment

Cantelli's sign

Cantlie's foot tetter

Cantor tube

Caparosa's bur, crimper

Capdepont's syndrome — hereditary disease transmitted as an autosomal dominant trait in which tooth development is marked by dark discoloration, poorly formed dentin and abnormally low mineral content

Capgras' syndrome — the schizophrenic illusion that impostors have replaced friends or relatives

Capgras' symptom

Caplan's syndrome — the presence of intrapulmonary nodules

Cappagnoli's test

Capps' sign

Capranica's test

Capuron's points

Carabelli's cusp, sign, tubercle

Carassini's spool

Carazzi's hematoxylin

Carcassonne's ligament

Cardarelli's aphthae, sign, symptom

Carden's amputation

Cardillo's retractor

Carey-Coombs murmur

Carey's Ranvier technique

Cargile's membrane, sutures

Carini's syndrome — congenital ichthyosis at birth marked by smooth, deep red skin with cracks at the flexures, followed by peeling of the scales

Carlens' catheter, forceps, mediastinoscope, tube

Carleton's spots

Carmack's curet

Carmalt's clamp, forceps, hemostat

Carman's sign

Carmel's clamp

Carmichael's crown

Carmody's aspirator, drill, forceps

Carmody-Batson operation — reduction of fractures of the zygoma and zygomatic arch

Carmody-Brophy forceps

Carnett's sign

Carney's procedure, triad

Carnochan's operation — removal of Meckel's ganglion and part of the fifth nerve for neuralgia

Carnot's test

Carnoy's fixative, solution

Caroli's disease — folding of the neck of the gallbladder, causing biliary dyskinesia and hypertonia

Carpenter's syndrome — a congenital syndrome marked by premature closing of cranial sutures and webbing of fingers

Carpenter's dissector, knife

Carpentier's anuloplasty, valve

Carpentier-Edwards valve

Carpue's operation — same as *Indian operation*

Carr's tourniquet

Carr-Price reaction, test

Carr-Purcell-Meiboom-Gill sequence

Carr-Walker method
Carrel's method, treatment, tube
Carrel-Dakin fluid, treatment
Carrell's patch
Carrez's test
Carrión's disease — South American infectious disease caused by *Bartonella bacilliformis*
Carrion's prosthesis
Carroll's elevator, osteotome
Carroll-Legg osteotome
Carroll-Smith-Petersen osteotome
Carson's catheter
Carter's operation(s) — formation of an artificial pupil by a small opening into the cornea and performing an iridotomy; reconstruction of the bridge of the nose by transplanting bone from the rib
Carter's clamp, retractor, splenectomy, splint
Cartwright's antigen, blood group, prosthesis, test
Carus' circle, curve
Cary-Blair transport medium
Casal's collar, necklace
Casalá-Mosto disease — eczematid-like purpura marked by small red maculae of the lower extremities, extending to the entire body
Casamajor's test
Casilli's test
Casman's broth
Casoni's reaction, test
Caspar's ring opacity
Caspersson's type B cells
Cassel's operation — excision of exostoses of the ear through the external auditory meatus
Casselberry's cannula, position
Casser's (Casserio's, Casserius') fontanelle, ligament, muscle
Cassidy's syndrome — intestinal carcinoma associated with a sharp rise of blood serotonin, arterial hypertension, cyanotic spots, dyspnea, colic, and diarrhea

Cassidy-Brophy forceps
Cassier's syndrome — cyanosis of the extremities with discoloration of the skin of the fingers, wrists, and ankles
Castallo's retractor, speculum
Castaneda's method, stain
Castellani's syndrome — febrile hepatosplenomegaly with arthritis, marked by malaise, fever, and arthritic pain
Castellani's disease — an infectious disease of the bronchi caused by *Spirochaeta bronchialis*
Castellani's bronchitis, mixture, paint, test, treatment
Castellani-Low symptom
Castelli-Paparella tube
Castellino's sign
Castenada technique
Castle's factor
Castleman's giant lymph node hyperplasia
Castroviejo's dermatome, dilator, forceps, keratome, punch, speculum, trephine
Castroviejo-Arruga forceps
Castroviejo-Kalt needle holder
Cathelin's method, segregator
Cattani's serum
Cattell's Infant Intelligence Scale, T-tube
Catu virus
Caulk's punch
Causse-Shea prosthesis
Cavanaugh's bur
Cavare's disease — familial periodic paralysis
Cave's incision, retractor, spatula
Cavin's osteotome, shunt
Caylor's scissors
Cazenave's disease(s) — erythematous scaly patches of the face, ears, and scalp with atrophy and scars; a chronic form of pemphigus in adults with flaccid bullae and later generalized exfoliation
Cazenave's vitiligo

Cecil's operation — a three-stage operation for urethral stricture

Cecil-Culp urethroplasty

Cederschiöld's massage

Ceelen-Gellerstedt syndrome — essential pulmonary hemosiderosis

Cegka's sign

Celebes vibrio

Celestin's prosthesis, tube

Celsius scale, thermometer

Celsus' kerion, lithotomy

Cerenkov's radiation

Cesaris Demel bodies

Céstan's syndrome — same as *Céstan-Chenais syndrome*

Céstan-Chenais syndrome — lesions of the brainstem, causing hemiplegia, hemisynergia, endophthalmia, miosis, and ptosis

Céstan-Raymond syndrome — obstruction of the basilar artery, marked by quadriplegia and nystagmus

Chabaud's mixture

Chaddock's reflex, sign

Chaffin's catheter, tube

Chaffin-Pratt tube

Chagas' disease — same as *Chagas-Cruz disease*

Chagas' disease serological test

Chagas-Cruz disease — a form of trypanosomiasis caused by *Trypanosoma cruzi*

Chagres fever, virus

Chamberlain's forceps, incision, mediastinotomy, method

Chamberland's filter

Chamberlen's forceps

Chambers' pessary

Champetier de Ribes' bag

Championière's disease — fibrinous bronchitis

Champy's fixative

Chandelier's sign

Chandler's disease — primary idiopathic nontraumatic necrosis of the femoral head, seen most often in early middle age

Chandler's felt collar splint, forceps, fusion, method, retractor

Chang's aniline-acid fuchsin method

Chantemesse's reaction

Chaoul's therapy, tube

Chapman's mixture, pill, test

Chapman-Stone agar

Chapple's syndrome — unilateral facial weakness or paralysis in the neonate, with weakness or paralysis of the vocal cord and muscles of deglutition

Chapple's sign

Chaput's method

Charcot's disease — neuropathic arthropathy

Charcot's syndrome(s) — amyotrophic lateral sclerosis; intermittent claudication; intermittent fever due to cholangitis

Charcot's arthritis, arthropathy, arthrosis, bath, cirrhosis, edema, fever, foot, gait, joint, pains, sclerosis, sign, triad, vertigo, zone

Charcot-Böttcher crystalloids

Charcot-Bouchard aneurysm

Charcot-Leyden crystals

Charcot-Marie atrophy, type

Charcot-Marie-Tooth disease — progressive neuropathic muscular atrophy

Charcot-Marie-Tooth atrophy, type

Charcot-Marie-Tooth-Hoffman syndrome — neuropathic muscular atrophy

Charcot-Neumann crystals

Charcot-Vigouroux sign

Charcot-Weiss-Barker syndrome — stimulation of a hyperactive carotid sinus causing a marked fall in blood pressure

Chardack's pacemaker
Chardack-Greatbatch pacemaker
Charles' law, needle
Charlevoix-Saguenay ataxia
Charlin's syndrome — neuritis of the nasal ciliary nerve
Charlouis' disease — yaws
Charlton's needle, trocar
Charmot's syndrome — macroglobulinemia with splenomegaly, seen in adults of the Congo region
Charnley's arthrodesis, arthroplasty, forceps, prosthesis, retractor
Charnley-Mueller arthroplasty, prosthesis
Charrière's scale
Charrin's disease — infection with *Pseudomonas aeruginosa*
Chase-Sulzberger phenomenon
Chaslin's gliosis
Chassaignac's axillary muscle, paralysis, tubercle
Chassard-Lapiné maneuver, method, position
Chatfield-Girdleston splint
Chauffard's syndrome — polyarthritis, enlargement of lymph nodes and fever, usually caused by some form of nonhuman tuberculosis
Chauffard's point
Chauffard-Still syndrome — same as *Chauffard's syndrome*
Chauffeur's fracture
Chaussé's method, procedure
Chaussier's areola, line, tube
Chautard's test
Chauveau's bacillus, bacterium
Chauvenet's method
Chavany-Brunhes syndrome — a genetic syndrome characterized by persistent headache and psychoneurotic disorders associated with calcification of the falx cerebri
Cheadle's disease — infantile scurvy

Cheatle's disease — benign cystic disease of the brest
Cheatle's forceps
Cheatle-Henry incision
Chédiak's anomaly, reaction, test
Chédiak-Higashi syndrome — abnormalities of the nuclear structure of leukocytes with cytoplasmic inclusions, and often with hepatosplenomegaly, lymphadenopathy, anemia, and thrombocytopenia. Called also *Béguez César disease*
Chédiak-Higashi anomaly
Chédiak-Steinbrinck anomaly
Chédiak-Steinbrinck-Higashi syndrome — same as *Chédiak-Higashi syndrome*
Chédiak-Steinbrinck-Higashi anomaly
Cheever's operation — complete tonsillectomy through the neck
Chelsea-Eaton speculum
Chen's test
Cheney's syndrome — osteoporosis, with changes in the skull and mandible
Chenuda virus
Cherchevski's (Cherchewski's) disease — ileus of nervous origin
Cherney's incision
Chernez's incision
Cheron's forceps, serum
Cherry's extractor, osteotome, probe, scissors
Cherry-Adson forceps
Cherry-Austin drill
Cherry-Crandall procedure
Cherry-Kerrison forceps
Chervin's method, treatment
Chester's disease — xanthomatosis of the long bones with spontaneous fractures
Chevalier Jackson bronchoscope, esophagoscope, gastroscope, laryngoscope, speculum, tube
Chevallier's glossitis
Chevassu's tumor

Cheyne's disease — hypochondria

Cheyne's dissector, elevator, nystagmus

Cheyne-Stokes asthma, nystagmus, psychosis, respiration, sign

Chiari II syndrome — elongation of the medulla and cerebellar vermis through the foramen magnum into the upper spinal canal

Chiari's syndrome — same as *Chiari-Budd syndrome*

Chiari's disease — same as *Budd-Chiari syndrome*

Chiari's malformation, network, reticulum

Chiari-Arnold syndrome — same as *Arnold-Chiari syndrome*

Chiari-Budd syndrome — thrombosis of the hepatic vein

Chiari-Frommel syndrome — abnormal prolongation of post-pregnancy lactation

Chicago disease — North American blastomycosis

Chick-Martin method, test

Chido test

Chiene's operation(s) — removal of a wedge from the inner condyle of the femur for cure of knock knee; exposure of the retropharyngeal space by lateral cervical incision

Chiene's incision, lines, test

Chievitz's layer, organ

Chiffelle-Putt method

Chilaiditi's syndrome — interposition of the colon between the liver and diaphragm

Chilcott's cannula

Child's forceps, pancreatectomy

Child-Phillips forceps, needle

Chimani-Moos test

Chinese liver fluke

Chinese restaurant syndrome

Chlumsky's button

Choix fever

Chopart's operation(s) — amputation of the foot with the calcaneus, talus, and other parts of the tarus being retained; plastic operation of the lip

Chopart's amputation, articulation, joint

Chopra's antimony test

Chorine's test

Chotzen's syndrome — a congenital disorder marked by premature closure of the cranial sutures and webbing of the fingers

Choyce's eye implant

Christ-Siemens syndrome — a congenital ectodermal dysplasia

Christ-Siemens-Touraine syndrome — same as *Christ-Siemens syndrome*

Christchurch chromosome

Christeller reaction

Christensen's phenomenon, urea agar

Christensen-Krabbe disease — progressive cerebral poliodystrophy with blindness, seizures, and deafness, usually beginning in the first year of life

Christian's disease/syndrome — a chronic idiopathic form of histiocytosis marked by bone defects, exophthalmos, and diabetes insipidus

Christian-Weber disease — a nodular, nonsuppurative form of lupus erythematosus

Christison's formula

Christmas disease — deficiency of plasma thromboplastin

Christmas factor

Christopher's spots

Chrobak's test

Church's scissors

Churchill's iodine caustic

Churg-Strauss syndrome — allergic granulomatous angiitis

Chvostek's anemia, sign, symptom, test, tremor

Chvostek-Weiss sign

Ciaccio's fluid, glands, method, positive lipids, stain

Ciamician-Magnanini's test

Ciarrocchi's disease — erosion between the interdigital webs of the fingers, caused by *Candida albicans*

Cicherelli's forceps, rongeur

Cinelli's chisel

Cinelli-McIndoe chisel

Cipollina's test

Citelli's syndrome — mental backwardness and drowsiness arising from adenoidal or sinus infection

Citelli-Meltzer punch

Civatte's disease — hyperpigmentation and telangiectasia of the skin

Civatte's body, poikiloderma

Civiale's operation — crushing of a vesical calculus within the bladder with a lithotrite

Civinini's canal, ligament, process, spine

Clado's anastomosis, band, fossa, ligament, point

Clagett's cannula, needle

Clairborne's clamp

Clapton's line

Clara cells, hematoxylin

Clark's operation — a plastic operation for urethral fistula

Clark's restiform body, electrode, level, rule, scale, test

Clark-Collip method, procedure

Clark-Guyton forceps

Clark-Lubs culture medium

Clark-Verhoeff forceps

Clarke's cells, column of spinal cord, fluid, nucleus, ulcer

Clarke-Hadfield syndrome — cystic fibrosis of the pancreas

Classon's scissors

Clauberg's agar, culture medium, test, unit

Claude's syndrome — paralysis of the third oculomotor nerve on one side and asynergia on the other

Claude's hyperkinesis sign

Claude Bernard-Horner syndrome — same as *Bernard-Horner syndrome*

Claudius' cells

Clausen's method

Clauss' method

Clawicz's chisel

Clay Adams Ultra-flow 100 Counter

Clayton's osteotome, splint

Cleaves' method

Cleeman's sign

Cleland's reagent

Cleopatra projection

Clérambault-Kandinsky syndrome — a mental disturbance in which one believes his mind is under the control of some outside influence or person

Clérambault-Kandinsky complex

Clerf's aspirator, dilator, forceps, laryngoscope

Clerf-Arrowsmith safety pin closer

Cleveland procedure

Clive's test

Cloquet's canal, fascia, ganglion, gland, hernia, ligament, needle sign, node, pseudoganglion, septum

Cloudman's melanoma

Clough-Richter's syndrome — anemia in which erythrocytes undergo severe autoagglutination

Clouston's syndrome — hidrotic ectodermal dysplasia

Cloward's blade, drill, hammer, osteotome, punch, rongeur

Cloward-Hoen retractor

Clute's incision

Clutton's joint

Coakley's operation — for frontal sinus disease

Coakley's cannula, forceps, hemostat, sutures

Coats' disease — chronic, progressive exudative retinopathy

Coats' retinitis, ring

Coban's dressing, wrap

Cobb's syndrome — a disorder of the spinal cord similar to *Sturge-Weber syndrome*

Cobb's elevator, osteotome

Cobbett's knife

Cobelli's glands

Cochin China diarrhea

Cock's operation — urethrotomy

Cockayne's syndrome — a heritable disorder marked by dwarfism, pigmentary degeneration of the retina, optic atrophy, deafness and mental retardation

Codivilla's operation — for pseudoarthrosis

Codivilla's extension

Codman's clamp, incision, sign, triangle, tumor

Cody's tack

Coe virus

Coffey's incision, technique, uterine suspension

Coffin-Lowry syndrome — mental retardation with distorted facies and digital anomalies

Coffin-Siris syndrome — hypoplasia or absence of fifth fingers and toenails associated with growth and mental deficiencies

Cogan's syndrome(s) — nonsyphilitic interstitial keratitis, followed by deafness and associated with infectious disease; congenital oculomotor apraxia

Cogan's dystrophy, oculomotor apraxia

Cohen's elevator, forceps, test

Cohen-Eder cannula, tongs

Cohn's solution, test

Cohnheim's areas, artery, fields, theory

Colcher-Sussman method

Cole's frame, hematoxylin, retractor, sign, test

Coleman's syndrome — injury of the cervical spine associated with head and shoulder injury

Coleman-Schiff reagent

Coleman-Shaffer diet

Coley's fluid, toxin

Colibri's forceps, speculum

Coller's forceps

Colles' fascia, fracture, law, ligament, mother, space

Colles-Baumès law

Collet's syndrome — same as *Collet-Sicard syndrome*

Collet-Sicard syndrome — glossolaryngoscapulopharyngeal hemiplegia

Collie phenomenon

Collier's fold

Collin's dissector, forceps, law, osteoclast, pelvimeter, speculum, tube

Collin-Duvall forceps

Collings' electrode, knife

Collip's unit

Collis' mouth gag, technique

Collison's drill, screw

Colliver's symptom

Collyer's pelvimeter

Colonna's operation(s) — a reconstruction operation for intracapsular fracture of the femoral neck; capsular arthroplasty of the hip

Colorado tick fever virus

Colt's cannula

Colton antigen, blood agar, blood group system

Colver's dissector, forceps, needle, retractor

Colver-Coakley forceps

Comel's acrorhigosis

Comessatti's test

Comly's syndrome — methemoglobinemia caused by drinking water with high concentrations of nitrates

Commando's operation — for management of oral cancer

Comolli's sign

Compere's chisel, gouge, osteotome

Compton's edge, effect, photon

Concato's disease — progressive malignant polyserositis with effusions into the pericardium, pleura, and peritoneum

Condorelli's disease — acro-osteodystrophy, amenorrhea, and parathyroid disorders

Condy's fluid

Cone's caliper, cannula, forceps, retractor, tube

Cone-Bucy cannula

Congo red test

Conn's syndrome — primary aldosteronism

Conn's tourniquet

Connell's incision, sutures

Conolly's system

Conor and Bruch disease — epidemic in the Mediterranean region and South Africa, caused by infection from *Rickettsia conorii*

Conrad-Crosby needle

Conradi's disease/syndrome — a rare, hereditary syndrome marked by multiple opacities in the epiphyses, dwarfism, cataract, general debility, and dulled mentation

Conradi's line

Conradi-Hünermann syndrome — a rare bone disease in infants, marked by manifestations of discrete calcific densities in the hyaline cartilage

Constantine's catheter

Contejean's test

Contino's epithelioma, glaucoma

Converse's chisel, curet, knife, method, osteotome, saw, scissors, speculum

Converse-MacKenty elevator

Conway's operation — partial breast amputation and transplantation of the nipples and aerolae for correction of macromastia

Conway's cell, technique

Conzett's goniometer

Cook's retractor, speculum

Cooke's count, criterion, formula, index, test

Cooke-Apert-Gallais syndrome — congenital adrenal hyperplasia in females resulting in defective synthesis of adrenocortical steroids

Cooley's disease — diminished synthesis of beta chains of hemoglobin, marked by microcytic anemia, hepatosplenomegaly, skeletal deformities, and cardiac enlargement

Cooley's anemia, clamp, dilator, forceps, graft, trait, tube

Cooley-Bloodwell-Cutter prosthesis

Cooley-Pontius blade, shears

Coolidge's tube

Coomassie brilliant blue

Coombs' serum, test

Cooper's disease — chronic cystic disease of the breast

Cooper's bougie, cannula, fascia, gouge, hernia, irritable breast, irritable testis, ligament, neuralgia

Coopernail's sign

Coors' filter

Cope's clamp, law, method bronchography, needle, sign, test

Cope-DeMartel clamp

Copeland's retinoscope

Copeman-Ackermann syndrome — painful lumbar sclerolipoma marked by hard, subcutaneous nodules

Coplin jar

Coppridge's forceps

Corbett's forceps

Corbin's technique

Corbus' disease(s) — a rapidly destructive infection producing erosion of the glans penis and often destruction of the entire external genitalia; infection thought to be due to a spirochete

Cordes' forceps, punch

Cordes-New forceps, punch

Cords' angiopathy

Corey's forceps, tenaculum

Cori's disease — glycogenosis of the liver, with muscle and heart involvement from glucosidase deficiency

Cori's cycle, ester

Corley-Denis method

Cornelia de Lange's syndrome — same as *Brachmann-de Lange syndrome*

Corner's plug, tampon

Corner-Allen test, unit

Cornet's forceps

Corning's anesthesia, method, puncture

Corper's culture medium

Correra's line

Corri's method

Corrigan's disease — aortic insufficiency

Corrigan's cautery, cirrhosis, line, pneumonia, pulse, respiration, sign

Corti's arches, canal, cells, fibers, ganglion, membrane, organ, rods, tunnel

Corvisart's disease — tetralogy of Fallot with right aortic arch; chronic hypertrophic myocarditis

Corvisart's complex, facies

Corwin's forceps, hemostat

Coryllos' elevator, raspatory, retractor, thoracoscope

Coryllos-Bethune rib shears

Coryllos-Doyen elevator

Coryllos-Moure rib shears

Coryllos-Shoemaker rib shears

Coschwitz's duct

Cosman-Roberts Wells stereotactic system

Cossio's syndrome — interauricular septal defect associated with plastic pericarditis

Costa's test

Costello-Dent syndrome — hypohyperparathyroidism

Costen's syndrome — a complex of symptoms resulting from trauma to or arthritis of the temporomandibular joint— pain, malocclusion, muscle tremor and ankylosis

Cotard's syndrome — a form of depressive insanity with delusions and suicidal impulses

Cotlove titrator

Cotte's operation — removal of the presacral nerve

Cotting's operation — for ingrown toenail

Cottle's caliper, clamp, elevator, forceps, incision, osteotome, speculum, tenaculum, tube

Cottle-Arruga forceps

Cottle-Jansen forceps

Cottle-Joseph hook

Cottle-Kazanjian forceps

Cottle-MacKenty elevator

Cottle-Neivert retractor

Cottle-Walsham forceps

Cotton's fracture, procedure

Cotugno's disease — sciatica

Cotunnius' aqueduct, canal, nerve, space

Coulomb's law

Coulter's counter, thrombocounter, whole blood lysing kit

Councill's catheter, dilator, stone basket

Councilman's bodies, lesions

Councilman-Mallory blood serum

Coupland's elevator, tube

Cournand's catheter, needle

Cournand-Grino needle

Courvoisier's gallbladder, gastroenterostomy, incision, law, sign

Courvoisier-Terrier syndrome — dilatation of the gallbladder with retention jaundice due to obstruction

Coutard's law, method

Couto's disease — fatty degeneration of the visceral organs

Couvelaire's syndrome — premature separation of a normally implanted placenta in association with albuminuria, azotemia, and shock

Couvelaire's uterus

Cova's point

Cowden's syndrome/disease — a familial syndrome involving abnormalities of the central nervous system and defects of many body structures, including hypertrophy of the breasts with fibrocystic disease and early malignant degeneration

Cowdry's bodies

Cowen's sign

Cowie's guaiac test

Cowling's rule

Cowper's cyst, gland, ligament

Cox's treatment, vaccine

Cox's proportional hazards model

Cox-Mantel log-rank test

Coxsackie virus

Cozzolino's zone

Crabtree's dissector, effect

Craford's clamp, forceps, scissors

Crafoord-Cooley tunneler

Crafts' test

Craig's culture medium, forceps, pin, scissors, test

Craig-Sheehan retractor

Craigie's tube method

Cramer's 2.5 reagent, splint, test

Crampton's muscle, test

Crandall's syndrome — hearing defects associated with hypogonadism

Crane's chisel, mallet, osteotome

Crapeau's snare

Credé's antiseptic, maneuver, method, ointment

Creevy's dilator, stone dislodger

Crenshaw's forceps

Creutzfeldt-Jakob disease — a rare, usually fatal, viral encephalopathy accompanied by degeneration of the pyramidal and extrapyramidal systems and by progressive dementia

Creyx-Lévy syndrome — a reverse form of *Sjögren's syndrome*

Crichton-Browne's sign

Crigler's evacuator

Crigler-Najjar syndrome — a congenital familial form of nonhemolytic jaundice

Crile's blade, clamp, forceps, hemostat, spatula

Crile-Crutchfield clamp

Crile-Matas operation — production of regional anesthesia by intraneural infiltration

Crimean hemorrhagic fever virus

Crippa's lead tetra-acetate method

Cripps' obturator

Crismer's test

Crisp's aneurysm

Critchett's operation — excision of the anterior part of the eyeball

Crocker's disease — chronic inflammation of the skin of the extremities

Crocq's disease — acrocyanosis

Crohn's disease — a chronic, granulomatous, inflammatory disease of unknown etiology invading any part of the gastrointestinal system, frequently leading to intestinal obstruction

Crombie's ulcer

Cronin's implant, method

Cronin-Lowe reaction, test

Cronkhite's syndrome — same as *Cronkhite-Canada syndrome*

Cronkhite-Canada syndrome — a sporadic condition of gastrointestinal polyposis

Crooke's cells, changes, hyaline degeneration

Crooke-Russell basophils, changes

Crookes' lens, space, tube

Crosby's syndrome — hereditary nonspherocytic hemolytic anemia

Crosby's capsule, knife

Crosby-Cooney operation — for drainage of fluid from the peritoneal cavity in ascites

Cross syndrome — same as *Cross-McKusick-Breen syndrome*

Cross-Bevan reagent

Cross-McKusick-Breen syndrome — oculocerebral hypopigmentation

Crotti's retractor

Crouzon's disease — craniofacial dysostosis

Crow-Fukase syndrome — a peculiar progressive polyneuritis associated with pigmentation, edema, and plasma cell dyscrasia

Crowel-Beard procedure

Crozat's appliance

Cruickshank's clamp

Crutchfield's clamp, drill, tongs

Crutchfield-Raney tongs

Cruveilhier's disease — spinal muscular atrophy

Cruveilhier's artery, atrophy, fascia, joint, ligaments, navicular fossa, nodules, paralysis, plexus, sign, tumor, ulcer

Cruveilhier-Baumgarten syndrome — cirrhosis of the liver with patent umbilical veins

Cruveilhier-Baumgarten cirrhosis, murmur

Cruz's trypanosomiasis

Cruz-Chagas disease — same as *Chagas-Cruz disease*

Cryer's elevator

Csapo's abortion

Csillag's disease — a chronic atrophic skin disease characterized by indurated papules and keratotic plugs

Cubbins' screw

Cuignet's method, test

Cullen's sign

Culley's splint

Cullom-Mueller adenotome

Culp's ureteropelvioplasty

Cummings' catheter

Cummings-Pezzer catheter

Cunisset's test

Cunningham's clamp

Curdy's knife, sclerotome

Curie's law, therapy

Curling's factor, ulcer

Curry's nail, needle, splint

Curschmann's disease — the peritoneal covering of the liver is converted into a white, undifferentiated mass

Curschmann's mask, spiral

Curschmann-Batten-Steinert syndrome — atrophic myotonia, especially in the lingual and thenar muscles

Curtis' forceps

Curtius' syndrome(s) — hypertrophy of one side of the entire body; ovarian insufficiency marked by menstrual disturbances and leukorrhea, constipation, and vasomotor disorders

Cushing's syndrome(s) — a condition occurring chiefly in women and marked by facial adiposity, osteoporosis of the spine, hypertension, amenorrhea and diabetes mellitus, resulting from hyperadrenocorticism due to neoplasm of the adrenal cortex; tumors of the cerebellopontine angle and acoustic tumors marked by impairment of hearing, cerebellar ataxia, and eventual impairment of the sixth and seventh nerve function with elevated intracranial pressure

Cushing's disease — Cushing's syndrome, in which the hyperadrenocorticism is due to excessive pituitary secretion of adrenocorticotropic hormone

Cushing's operation(s) — exposure of the gasserian ganglion and three divisions of the fifth nerve; a type of ureterorrhaphy without support

Cushing's basophilism, law, medulloblastoma, phenomenon, reflex, suture, tumor, ulcer

Cushing-Hopkins elevator

Cushing-Rokitansky ulcer

Cushman's drain

Custer's cells

Cutler's eye implant

Cutler-Beard technique

Cutler-Ederer method

Cutler-Power-Wilder test

Cutola's test

Cutting's test

Cuvier's canal, ducts, sinuses

Cyon's experiment, nerve

Cyriax's syndrome — pain similar to that of angina pectoris but caused by slipped rib cartilage pressing on the interchondral joint nerves

Czapek-Dox agar, solution

Czermak's keratome, lines, spaces

Czerny's disease — periodic hydrarthrosis of the knee

Czerny's anemia, diathesis, incision, sutures

Czerny-Lembert sutures

Da Costa's syndrome(s) — a hereditary skin disorder marked by hyperkeratotic plaques and erythrodermic areas of varying size and shape; neurocirculatory asthenia

Da Costa's disease(s) — misplaced gout; neurocirculatory asthenia

Da Fano's stain

Daae's disease — same as *Daae-Finsen disease*

Daae-Finsen disease — epidemic pleurodynia

Dabney's grippe

Daclin test

D'Acosta's syndrome — anoxia from diminished oxygen intake at high altitudes, with difficulty in breathing and giddiness

Daems' clamp

Daguet's ulceration

Dakin's antiseptic, fluid, solution

Dakin-Carrel method

Dale's phenomenon, reaction

Dale-Laidlaw capillary clotting time method

Dalen-Fuchs nodules, spots

Dalrymple's disease — inflammation of the ciliary body and cornea

Dalrymple's sign

Dalton's law

Dalton-Henry law

Dam unit

D'Amato's reaction, sign, test

Dameshek's syndrome — same as *Cooley's anemia*

Damocrates' confection

Damoiseau's curve, sign

Damshek's needle, trephine

Dana's syndrome — degenerative changes in the white matter of the spinal cord, associated with pernicious anemia

Dana's operation — posterior rhizotomy

Danberg's forceps

Danbolt-Closs syndrome — acro-dermatitis enteropathica

Dancel's treatment

Dandy's operation — destruction of part of the sensory root of the trigeminal nerve for relief of trigeminal neuralgia

Dandy's forceps, hemostat, rhizot-omy, ventriculostomy

Dandy-Walker syndrome — con-genital hydrocephalus caused by obstruction of the foram-ina of Magendie and Luschka

Dandy-Walker deformity, malfor-mation

Dane's method, particle, stain

Daniel's operation — exploration for nonpalpable lymph nodes on the scalene muscles, to de-termine the absence or pres-ence of lymphoma, metastatic tumors, and sarcoidosis

Daniels' clamp, tonsillectome

Danielssen's disease — same as *Danielssen-Boeck disease*

Danielssen-Boeck disease — lep-rosy, marked by hyperesthesia and followed by anesthesia, paralysis, ulcers, gangrene, and mutilation

Danielus-Miller modification of Lorenz's method

Danlos' disease/syndrome — same as *Ehlers-Danlos syndrome*

Danubian endemic familial ne-phropathy

Danysz's effect, phenomenon

Dar es Salaam bacterium

Dare's method

Darier's disease/syndrome — a skin disease usually beginning in childhood, marked by kera-totic papules that become crust-covered and produce vegetating tumor-like growths of the head, neck, back, chest, and groin

Darier's sign

Darier-Ferrand dermatofibroma, dermatofibrosarcoma

Darier-Roussy sarcoid

Darier-White disease — same as *Darier's disease*

Darkshevich's fibers, ganglion, nu-cleus

Darling's disease — histoplasmosis

Darling's capsulotome

Darlington's amplifier

Darrach's ulnar resection

d'Arsonval current, meter

Darwin's ear

Daubenton's angle, line, plane

Davat's operation — compressing the veins by acufilopressure for cure of varicocele

Davenport's diagram, graph, stain

David's disease(s) — tuberculosis of the spine; an unexplained form of hemorrhagic disease in women

David's speculum

Davidoff's (Davidov's) cells, knife, retractor

Davidsohn's sign, test

Davidson's anemia, forceps, sy-ringe, trocar

Daviel's operation — extraction of cataract through a corneal in-cision without cutting the iris

Daviel's spoon

Davies's disease — endomyocardial fibrosis

Davies-Colley's operation — re-moval of a wedge of bone from the outer side of the tar-sus for correction of talipes

Davies-Colley's syndrome — same as *Cyriax's syndrome*

Davis' bronchoscope, crown, for-ceps, graft, hemostat, sign, splint, stone dislodger, uterine suspension

Davis-Crowe mouth gag

Davis-Geck incision

Davy's test

Dawbarn's sign
Dawson's encephalitis
Day's factor, hook, knife, test
De Alvarez' forceps
De Azua's pseudoepithelioma
De Castro's fluid
de Clérambault's syndrome — same as *Clérambault-Kandinsky syndrome*
De Galantha's method for urates
de Gimard's syndrome — gangrenous purpura
de Grandmont's operation — for ptosis of the eyelid
de la Camp's sign
de Lange's syndrome — same as *Brachmann-de Lange syndrome*
De Martini-Balestera syndrome — same as *Burke's syndrome*
de Morsier's syndrome — septo-optic dysplasia
de Musset's sign
de Mussy's point, sign
de Pezzer's catheter
de Quervain's disease — painful tenosynovitis from narrowness of the tendon sheath
de Quervain's fracture, tenosynovitis, thyroiditis
De Ritis ratio
De Salle's line
De Sanctis–Cacchione syndrome — a hereditary condition marked by atrophic lesions of the skin, with mental retardation, retarded growth, gonadal hypoplasia, and sometimes neurologic complications
de Signeux's dilator
De Tomasi–Coleman method
De Toni–Caffey syndrome — same as *Caffey's disease*
De Toni–Fanconi syndrome — cystinosis
De Vries' syndrome — a familial congenital condition of both sexes marked by factor V deficiency with bleeding and syndactyly

De Vries' theory
De Watteville current
de Wecker's cannula, scissors, sclerotomy
de Wecker-Pritikin scissors
Dean's applicator, hemostat, periosteotome
Dean-MacDonald clamp
Dean-Webb titration
Deaver's incision, retractor, scissors, tube
DeBakey's blade, forceps, graft, implant, prosthesis, stripper, tube
DeBakey-Bahnson clamp, forceps
DeBakey-Bainbridge forceps
DeBakey-Balfour retractor
DeBakey-Cooley dilator, forceps, retractor
DeBakey-Metzenbaum scissors
Debler's syndrome — familial hemolytic anemia
Débove's disease — splenomegaly
Débove's membrane, treatment, tube
Debré's syndrome(s) — cat-scratch disease; a disease caused by an inborn error of metabolism, resulting in disturbances of carbohydrate/lipid metabolism
Debré's phenomenon
Debré-Fibiger syndrome — pseudospasm of the pylorus marked by vomiting, dehydration and early death
Debré-Marie syndrome(s) — fever followed by edema and polyneuritis, involving all four extremities; dwarfism, genital infantilism, and a disorder of water metabolism, marked by hydrophilia, oligodypsia, oliguria, retarded water elimination and high density of urine
Debré-Mollaret syndrome — same as *Debré's syndrome* (cat-scratch disease)
Debré-Paraf antigen reaction

Debré-Sémélaigne syndrome — muscular hypertrophy, weakness, cretinism, and occasionally mental retardation in children

Debye's light scatter

Decker's culdoscope, retractor

Declat's liquid

DeCourcy's clamp

Dedichen's test

Dedo-Pilling laryngoscope

Deehan's typhoid reaction

Deelman's effect

Deen's test

Dees' needle

Deetjen's bodies

Defer's method

Defourmental's forceps

Degener's test

Degnon's sutures

Degos' disease/syndrome — malignant papulosis

Degos' acanthoma malignant papillomavirus

Degos-Delort-Tricot syndrome — malignant papulosis with atrophy

Dehio's test

Dehn-Clark method

Deiters' nucleus syndrome — same as *Bonnier's syndrome*

Deiters' cells, frame, nucleus, phalanges, process, tract

DeJager's elevator

Dejean's syndrome — orbital floor lesions associated with exophthalmos, diplopia, maxillary pain and numbness along the trigeminal nerve branches

Dejerine's syndrome(s) — polyneuritis secondary to an infection with *Corynebacterium diphtheriae*; hemorrhage or thrombosis of the anterior spinal artery, causing paralysis of the tongue, arm, and leg

Dejerine's disease — progressive hypertrophic interstitial neuropathy

Dejerine's sign, type

Dejerine-Klumpke syndrome — same as *Klumpke-Dejerine syndrome*

Dejerine-Klumpke paralysis

Dejerine-Landouzy dystrophy, type

Dejerine-Lichtheim phenomenon

Dejerine-Roussy syndrome — thrombosis of the thalamogeniculate artery that produces pain, sensory disorders, hemiataxia, hemiplegia, and choreoathetoid movements

Dejerine-Sottas disease — same as *Dejerine's disease*

Dejerine-Sottas syndrome — progressive, hypertrophic interstitial neuropathy

Dejerine-Thomas syndrome — olivopontocerebellar atrophy

Dejerine-Thomas atrophy

Dejust's test

del Castillo's syndrome — galactorrhea-amenorrhea not associated with pregnancy

Del Toro's operation — destruction of the apex of a conical cornea

Delaborde's dilator

Delafield's fluid, hematoxylin

Delaney's retractor

Delaye's paralysis

Delbet's sign

DeLee's catheter, forceps, maneuver, pelvimeter, speculum, tenaculum

DeLee-Breisky pelvimeter

DeLee-Hillis obstetric stethoscope

DeLee-Perce perforator

DeLee-Simpson forceps

DeLee-Zweifel cranioclast

Delff's test

Delgado's electrode

Delmege's sign

Delore's method

Delorme's operation — pericardiectomy

Delpech's abscess

Delphian node

Delves' cup technique

Demarest's forceps

Demarquay's sign

Demarquay-Richet syndrome — a congenital orofacial abnormality marked by cleft lip, cleft palate, fistula of the lower lip and progeria facies

DeMartel's clamp, forceps, scissors

DeMartel-Wolfson clamp, forceps

Demel's forceps

Demianoff's sign

Deming's nephropexy

Demme's method

Demoivre's formula

Demons-Meigs syndrome — same as *Meigs' syndrome*

DeMorgan's spots

Demours' membrane

Deneke's spirillium

Denhardt-Dingman mouth gag

Denigès's reagent, test

Denis' method

Denis Browne operation — same as *Browne's operation*

Denis Browne forceps, needle, procedure, splint

Denis-Leche method

Denker's trocar, tube

Denker-Kahler approach

Denman's method, spontaneous evolution, version

Dennie's sign

Dennie-Marfan syndrome — spastic paralysis and mental retardation associated with congenital syphilis

Dennis' anastomosis, clamp, forceps, technique

Dennis-Silverman test

Denny-Brown syndrome — hereditary sensory radicular neuropathy

Denonvilliers' operation — plastic correction of a defective ala nasi by transferring a triangular flap from the adjacent side of the nose

Denonvilliers' aponeurosis, fascia

Denucé's ligament

Denver classification

Denys' tuberculin

Denys-Leclef phenomenon

Depage's position

Depage-Janeway gastrostomy

DePalma's hip prosthesis

Depaul's tube

Depuy's arthroplasty, awl, extractor, frame, prosthesis, retractor, rongeur, splint

DePuy-Pott splint

DePuy-Weiss needle

Derbyshire's neck

Dercum's disease/syndrome — pain and tenderness with paresthesia in menopausal women from subcutaneous deposits of fat and pressure on cutaneous nerves

Derf's needle holder

Derlacki's chisel, gouge, knife, punch

Derlacki-Shambaugh chisel, microscope

Derra's clamp, knife, valvulotome

D'Errico's bur, drill, forceps, elevator, trephine

D'Errico-Adson retractor

Derrien's test

Desault's apparatus, bandage, ligation, sign

Descartes' law

Descemet's membrane, posterior lamina

Deschamps' carrier, compressor, needle

Deschamps-Navratil needle

Deseret's angiocatheter, drain

Desilet's catheter

Desjardin's forceps, point, probe, scoop

Desmarres' clamp, dacryolith, elevator, forceps, law, scarifier

d'Espine's sign

Detakats-McKenzie forceps

Determann's syndrome — intermittent myasthenia of muscles as a result of arteriosclerosis

Detre's reaction

Deutschländer's disease — tumor of the metatarsal bones; march foot [fracture]

Deutschman's knife

DeVega's annuloplasty

Deventer's diameter

Devereux's method

Devergie's disease — a chronic inflammatory disease of the skin marked by scaling macules and follicular papules

Devergie's attitude

Devic's disease/syndrome — encephalomyelopathy with demyelination of the optic nerves and spinal cord causing progressive blindness in both eyes

Devic-Gault syndrome — same as *Devic's syndrome*

Devine's tube

Devonshire's catheter, colic, knife

Dew's sign

Dewar's flask, procedure

Dewey's forceps

Deyerle's drill, pin, punch

d'Herelle's phenomenon

Di Guglielmo disease — a malignant blood dyscrasia marked by progressive anemia, myeloid dysplasia, hepatosplenomegaly, and hemorrhagic tendency; erythroleukemia

Di Guglielmo's test, tube

Diamond-Blackfan syndrome — a rare hypoplastic anemia of young infants with deficiency of nucleated erythrocytes in the bone marrow

Diamond-Blackfan anemia

Diana complex

Dick's dilator, reaction, serum, test, toxin

Dicken's test

Dickinson's syndrome — same as *Alport's syndrome*

Dickinson's method

Dide-Botcazo syndrome — bilateral calcarine lesions causing visual disorders, spatial agnosia and amnesia

Dieffenbach's operation(s) — amputation at the hip; plastic closure of triangular defects by displacing a quadrangular flap toward one side of the triangle

Dieffenbach's amputation, forceps

Diego antigen, blood group system

Diertz's shears

Dieter's forceps

Dieterle's method, stain

Diethrich's clamp

Dietl's crisis

Dietlen's syndrome — cardiac flutter and diaphragmatic tension on inspiration in patients with cardiopericardial and cardiodiaphragmatic adhesions and adhesions at the apex of the heart

Dietrich's syndrome — aseptic epiphyseal necrosis of the metacarpal bone

Dietrich's apparatus

Dieudonné's culture medium

Dieulafoy's aspirator, erosion, theory, triad, ulcer

DiGeorge's syndrome — congenital absence of the thymus and parathyroid glands, with delayed development and marked susceptibility to infection

DiGeorge's anomaly

Dighton-Adair syndrome — same as *van der Hoeve's syndrome*

Dimitri's disease — a congenital syndrome marked by angiomas, glaucoma, intracranial calcification, hemiplegia and epilepsy

Dimitry's erysiphake, trephine

Dimitry-Bell erysiphake

Dimitry-Thomas erysiphake

Dimmer's keratitis

Dingman's abrader, forceps, mouth gag, osteotome
Dingman-Denhardt mouth gag
Dingman-Senn retractor
Dioscorides' granule
Dirck's fibrils
Disse's spaces
Dittel's operation — enucleation of the lateral lobes of an enlarged prostate
Dittel's sound
Dittrich's plugs, stenosis
Dix's gouge, needle, spud
Dixon's blade, tuberculin, test
Dixon-Mann's sign
Dixon-Thomas-Smith clamp
Dobbie-Trout clamp
Dobell's solution
Dobie's globule, layer, line
Dochez's serum
Dochez-Avery reaction
Docktor's forceps, needle
Döderlein's bacillus
Dogiel's corpuscle
Dogliotti's valvulotome
Dogliotti-Guglielmini clamp
Doherty's eye implant
Döhle's disease — syphilitic aortitis
Döhle's inclusion bodies
Döhle-Amato bodies
Döhle-Heller aortitis
Dohlman's hook
Dold's reaction, test
Doleris' operation — for retrodeviation of the uterus
Döllinger's ring
Dollinger-Bielschowsky syndrome — early juvenile ganglioside lipidosis
Dollo's law
Dolman's test
Domagk's method
Dombrock's antigens, blood group
Donald's clamp
Donaldson's test, tube
Donath's phenomenon, test

Donath-Landsteiner syndrome — hemoglobinuria due to hemolysis, caused by an autohemolysin in the blood uniting the erythrocytes at low temperatures
Donath-Landsteiner antibody, cold hemolysis, phenomenon, test
Donders' glaucoma, law, pressure, test
Donnan's equilibrium, potential
Donné's bodies, corpuscles, test
Donogany's test
Donohue's syndrome — a rare and lethal familial condition marked by slow physical and mental growth, elfin facies, and severe endocrine disorders
Donovan's bodies
Dooley's nail
Doppler's operation — injection of phenol into tissues around the sympathetic nerve leading to the gonads to increase hormone production and sexual rejuvenation
Doppler's apparatus, echocardiography, effect, monitor, phenomenon, principle, shift, ultrasonography, unit
Doppler-Cavin monitor
Dopter's serum
Dorello's canal
Dorendorf's sign
Dorn-Sugarman test
Dorner's stain
Dorno's rays
Dorothy Reed cells
Dorset's egg culture medium
Dorset-Niles serum
Dorsey's cannula, forceps, leukotome, spatula
Dos Santos' needle
Dott's mouth gag, retractor
Doubilet's sphincterotome
Dougherty's irrigator

Douglas' abscess, bag, cry, cul-de-sac, fold, forceps, graft, ligament, line, mechanism, method, pouch, space, septum, speculum, trocar

Dourmashkin's bougie

Dover's powder

Dowell's hernia repair

Down's syndrome — retarded growth, mongoloid features, and moderate-to-severe mental retardation, associated with chromosomal abnormality

Downes' cautery

Downey's cells

Downey-type lymphocyte

Downing's clamp, knife, retractor

Downs' analysis

Doyen's operation — eversion of the sac for relief of hydrocele

Doyen's clamp, forceps, raspatory, retractor, scissors, speculum

Doyen-Jansen mouth gag

Doyère's eminence, hillock

Doyle's vein stripper

Doyne's familial colloid degeneration, familial honeycomb choroiditis, honeycomb degeneration, iritis

Drabkin's reagent

Dragendorff's solution, test

Draper's law

Drapier's needle

Drash syndrome — familial syndrome consisting of Wilms' tumor with glomerulopathy and male pseudohermaphroditism

Drechsel's test

Dresbach's syndrome — the presence of elliptical erythrocytes in normal persons and in patients with some types of anemia

Dresbach's anemia

Dreser's formula

Dressler's disease — intermittent hemoglobinuria

Dressler's syndrome(s) — a condition occurring after myocardial infarction, marked by leukocytosis, chest pain, fever, pleurisy, and pneumonitis; intermittent hemoglobinuria

Drew-Smythe catheter

Dreyer's test

Dreyfus' syndrome — congenital flattening of the vertebrae followed by development of kyphoscoliosis, ankylosis of the spine, short neck, dwarfism, and muscular weakness and atonia

Drinker's respirator

Drosin's postures

Drummond's artery, sign

Drysdale's corpuscles

Du Noüy's phenomenon

Du Vries' hammer toe repair

Duane's syndrome — a hereditary syndrome in which ocular muscle function is severely impaired

Duane's test

Duane-Hunt relation

Dubin-Johnson syndrome — chronic or intermittent jaundice, marked by hyperbilirubinemia and amorphous, granular, brown pigment in the liver

Dubin-Sprinz disease/syndrome — same as *Dubin-Johnson syndrome*

Dubini's disease — a violent and fatal form of chorea caused by acute infectious disease of the central nervous system

Dubini's chorea

Dubois' disease — multiple abscesses of the thymus gland in congenital syphilis

Dubois' abscess, formula, method, sign, treatment

DuBois-Reymond's law

Dubos' crude crystals, culture medium, enzyme, lysin

Duboscq's colorimeter

Dubovitz's syndrome — intra-uterine dwarfism

Dubreuil-Chambardel's syndrome — dental caries of the incisors, usually appearing in early adolescence

Dubreuilh's melanosis

Duchenne's syndrome — the collective signs of bulbar paralysis

Duchenne's disease(s) — spinal muscular atrophy; bulbar paralysis; tabes dorsalis

Duchenne's muscular dystrophy, paralysis, sign, trocar, type

Duchenne-Aran disease — spinal muscular atrophy

Duchenne-Erb syndrome — paralysis of the upper roots of the brachial plexus caused by destruction of the fifth and sixth cervical roots

Duchenne-Griesinger disease — pseudohypertrophic muscular dystrophy

Duchenne-Landouzy dystrophy, type

Duckworth's phenomenon, sign

Ducrey's disease — infection of the genitalia with *Haemophilus ducreyi*, marked by soft pustules that rupture and form ulcers on the genital organs

Ducrey's bacillus

Duddell's membrane

Dudley's hook

Dudley-Klingenstein syndrome — tumors of the small intestine, with melena and ulcer-like symptoms

Dudley-Smith speculum

Duffield's scissors

Duffy's antibodies, antigens, blood group system

Dufourmental's rongeur

Dugas' sign, test

Duhamel's operation — for Hirschsprung's disease, by modification of the pull-through procedure and establishment of a longitudinal anastomosis between the proximal ganglionated segment of the colon and the rectum

Duhot's line

Duhring's disease — chronic dermatitis marked by erythematous, papular, vesicular, eczematous, or bullous lesions occurring in successive combinations

Duhring's pruritus

Dührssen's operation — vaginofixation of the uterus

Dührssen's incisions

Dujarier's clasp

Duke's method

Dukes' disease — a febrile disease of childhood, probably a mild form of scarlet fever

Dukes' cannula, cell counter, classification, method of bleeding time, staging system, test, tube

Dukes-Filatov disease — same as *Dukes' disease*

Dulbecco's modified Eagle's medium

Dulong-Petit law

Dumdum fever

Dumont's retractor, scissors

Dumontpallier's test

Dunbar's serum

Duncan's syndrome — X-linked lymphoproliferative syndrome

Duncan's folds, mechanism, method, placenta, position, ventricle

Duncan-Bird sign

Duncan-Hoen method

Dunfermline's scale

Dungern's test

Dunham's cones, fans, triangles

Dunhill's forceps, hemostat

Dunlap, Swanson, and Penner method

Dunlop's stripper, traction

Dunn's tongue depressor

Dunning's elevator

Dunphy's sign

Duplay's disease — subacromial or subdeltoid bursitis

Duplay's operation — plastic procedures for a congenitally deformed penis

Duplay's bursitis, fibroma, hook, method, procedure, speculum, tenaculum

Duplay-Lynch speculum

Dupont's test

Dupré's disease/syndrome — symptoms of meningeal irritation associated with acute febrile illness but without infection of the meninges

Dupuis' cannula

Dupuy's syndrome — same as *Frey's syndrome*

Dupuy-Dutemps operation — blepharoplasty of the lower lid with tissue from the opposite lid

Dupuytren's disease — plantar fibromatosis

Dupuytren's operation — amputation of the arm at the shoulder joint

Dupuytren's abscess, amputation, contraction, contracture, enterotome, fibromatosis, fracture, hydrocele, phlegmon, sign, splint, suture, tourniquet

Duran-Reynals' permeability factor

Durand's disease — a viral disease marked by upper respiratory, meningeal and gastrointestinal symptoms

Durand-Nicolas-Favre disease — venereal lymphogranuloma

Durand-Zunin syndrome — an association of the agenesis of the septum pellucidum with various structural abnormalities

Durant's disease — an inherited condition, transmitted as an autosomal dominant trait, in which bones are abnormally brittle and susceptible to fracture

Dürck's granuloma, nodes

Duret's hemorrhage, lesion

Durham's culture medium, decision, rule, trocar, tube

Duroziez's disease — congenital mitral stenosis

Dutcher body

Dutton's disease — trypanosomiasis

Dutton's relapsing fever, spirochete

Duval's nucleus

Duval-Allis forceps

Duval-Coryllos rib shears

Duval-Crile forceps

Duvergier's sutures

Duverney's foramen, fracture, gland

Dwyer's instrumentation

Dyggve-Melchior-Clausen syndrome — osteochondrodysplasia with mental retardation, short stature and deformities of long bones

Dyke-Davidoff-Masson syndrome — a condition, possibly due to neonatal injury, affecting one side of the brain and marked by mental retardation, hemiplegia, and neurological impairment

Dyke-Young syndrome — macrocytic hemolytic anemia

Dzierzynsky's syndrome — a form of craniomandibulofacial dysostosis

E ....

Eadie-Hofstee equation, plot

Eagle syndrome — facial pain from an elongated styloid process

Eagle's medium, test

Eagle-Barrett syndrome — a condition in which lower parts of abdominis and oblique muscles are absent, bladder and ureters are dysplastic, and testes are undescended; the abdomen protrudes; known as *prune-belly syndrome*

Eales' disease/syndrome — recurrent hemorrhage into the retina and vitreous

Earle's clamp, probe, solution

Earle L fibrosarcoma, sarcoma

Eastman's clamp, forceps, retractor

Eaton agent pneumonia, pneumonia

Eaton's speculum

Eaton-Lambert syndrome — myasthenia-like syndrome associated with oat-cell carcinoma of the lung

Ebbinghaus' test

Eber's forceps

Eberth's disease — typhoid fever

Eberth's lines, epithelium

Ebner's fibrils, glands, lines, reticulum

Ebola virus disease — a fatal hemorrhagic fever caused by the Ebola virus occurring in the Sudan and adjacent areas of Zaire

Ebstein's disease(s) — hyaline degeneration and necrosis of the epithelial cells of the renal tubules; a malformation of the tricuspid valve

Ebstein's angle, anomaly, lesion, malformation, treatment

Eck's fistula

Ecker's fissure, fluid, plug

Ecklin's syndrome — a usually fatal form of normoblastic myelocytic anemia of newborn infants, marked by splenomegaly, hepatomegaly, low hemoglobin level, reticulocytosis, erythroblastosis, moderate leukocytosis, and jaundice

Ecklin's anemia

Economo's disease — lethargic encephalitis

Economo's encephalitis

Eddowes' syndrome — blue sclera associated with abnormal brittleness and fragility of bone

Edebohls' operation — decapsulation of the kidneys for Bright's disease

Edebohls' incision, position

Edelmann's syndrome(s) — a form of chronic infectious anemia; chronic pancreatitis with secondary involvement of the nervous system and skin

Edelmann's anemia, cell

Edelmann-Galton whistle

Eder's forceps, gastroscope, laparoscope

Eder-Chamberlin gastroscope

Eder-Hufford esophagoscope, gastroscope

Eder-Palmer gastroscope

Eder-Puestow dilator

Edinburgh's retractor, sutures

Edinger's fibers, law, nucleus

Edinger-Westphal nucleus

Edlefsen's reagent, test

Edman's reaction

Edsall's disease — a form of heat exhaustion accompanied by pain, muscular spasm, and weak pulse

Edwards' syndrome — a condition caused by an extra chromosome 18, marked by mental retardation, cranial deformities, micrognathia, corneal opacities, ventricular septal defects, and other abnormalities

Edwards' generator, implant, patch, prosthesis

Edwards-Carpentier aortic valve brush

Effler's tack

Eggers' plate, screw, splint

Eggleston's method

Eglis' glands

Egyptian splenomegaly

Ehlers-Danlos disease/syndrome — a congenital syndrome marked by hyperelasticity of the skin, fragility of blood vessels, excessive susceptibility of the skin to trauma, hematomas, loose joints, and pigmented, granulomatous pseudotumors

Ehrenfried's disease — hereditary deforming chondrodysplasia

Ehrenritter's ganglion

Ehret's syndrome — paralysis developing after a painful injury

Ehrhardt's forceps

Ehrlich's acid hematoxylin, biochemical theory, diazo reaction, granules, hemoglobinemic bodies, line, postulate, reagent, side-chain theory, stains, test, tumor, unit

Ehrlich-Hata preparation, remedy, treatment

Ehrlich-Heinz granules

Ehrlich-Türck line

Ehrlich-Weigert formula

Ehrmann's test

Eicher's chisel, hip prosthesis

Eichhorst's disease — neuritis affecting the nerve sheath and interstitial muscle tissue

Eichhorst's atrophy, corpuscles, neuritis, type

Eichstedt's disease — a chronic superficial dermatomycosis caused by *Malassezia furfur*, marked by desquamating macules on the chest and shoulders

Eicken's method

Eijkman's lactose broth, test

Einarson's gallocyanin-chrome method, stain

Einhorn's dilator, saccharimeter, string test, tube

Einstein-Starck law

Einthoven's formula, galvanometer, law, triangle

Eiselt's test

Eisenberg's milk-rice culture medium

Eisenlohr's syndrome — numbness and weakness of the extremities with paralysis of the lips, tongue, and palate

Eisenmenger's syndrome — ventricular septal defect with pulmonary hypertension and cyanosis

Eisenmenger's complex, tetralogy

Eitelberg's test

Ekbom's syndrome — a sense of uneasiness or restlessness on going to bed that leads to involuntary twitching of the legs

Ekman-Lobstein syndrome — same as *Lobstein's disease*

El Tor's vibrio

Eldridge-Green lamp

Electra complex

Elek immunodiffusion test

Elkind's recovery

Ellermann-Erlandsen method, test

Ellik's evacuator, meatotome, sound, stone basket

Ellinger's method

Elliot's operation — trephining the sclerocornea for relief of increased tension in glaucoma

Elliot's forceps, position, sign, trephine

Elliott's law

Ellis' curve, line, needle holder, sign, spud

Ellis' glomerulonephritis, nephritis

Ellis-Garland curve, line

Ellis–van Creveld syndrome — polydactyly, chondrodysplasia with acromelic dwarfism, hidrotic ectodermal dysplasia, and congenital heart defects

Ellman's reagent

Ellsner's gastroscope

Ellsworth-Howard test

Eloesser's flap

Elsberg's cannula, incision, test

Elschnig's syndrome — extension of the palpebral fissure laterally, displacement of the lateral canthus and ectropion of the lower eyelid and lateral canthus

Elschnig's bodies, conjunctivitis, forceps, pearls, retractor, scoop, spatula, spots

Elschnig-O'Brien forceps

Elschnig-O'Connor forceps

Elsner's asthma

Ely's operation — skin grafting on granulating surfaces in chronic suppurative otitis media

Ely's sign, test

Elzholz's bodies, mixture

Emanuel-Cutting test

Embden's ester

Embden-Meyerhof cycle, pathway

Embden-Meyerhof-Parnas pathway

Emerson's agar, bronchoscope, effect, stripper, suction tube

Emmens' test

Emmert-Gellhorn pessary

Emmet's operation(s) — repair of a lacerated perineum; trachelorrhaphy; surgical creation of a vesicovaginal fistula

Emmet's forceps, retractor, scissors, sutures, tenaculum, trocar

Engel's syndrome — anaphylactic edema of the lungs, with eosinophilia and cough

Engel's alkalimetry, saw

Engel-Lysholm maneuver

Engel-May nail

Engel-Recklinghausen disease — osteitis with fibrous degeneration and formation of cysts

Engel-von Recklinghausen syndrome — same as *Recklinghausen's disease* (of bone)

Engelmann's disease — same as *Camurati-Engelmann disease*

Engelmann's disk, splint

English disease — rickets

English forceps, position, rhinoplasty

English sweating disease — a deadly pestilential fever that ravaged England during the Middle Ages

Engman's syndrome — same as *Zinsser-Cole-Engman syndrome*

Engman's disease — dermatitis marked by erythematous, crusted, scaling lesions and oozing spots

Engstrom's respirator

Ennis' forceps

Enroth's sign

Enslin's triad

Entner-Doudoroff pathway

Envacor test

Epstein's syndrome — a kidney disorder marked by edema, albuminuria, hypoalbuminemia, hyperlipemia, and great susceptibility to infection

Epstein's disease — pseudodiphtheria

Epstein's blade, method, needle, nephrosis, osteotome, pearls, rasp, symptom

Epstein-Barr nasopharyngeal carcinoma, nuclear antigen, virus (EBV)

Equen's magnet

Equen-Neuffer knife

Eranko's fluorescent stain

Eraso's method

Erb's disease — muscular dystrophy

Erb's syndrome — the aggregate of signs of myasthenia gravis

Erb's atrophy, dystrophy, palsy, paralysis, phenomenon, point, sclerosis, sign, spastic paraplegia, syphilitic spastic paraplegia, waves

Erb-Charcot disease/syndrome — spastic spinal paralysis

Erb-Duchenne paralysis

Erb-Goldflam disease/syndrome — myasthenia gravis

Erb-Landouzy disease — muscular dystrophy

Erb-Oppenheim-Goldflam syndrome — same as *Erb-Goldflam syndrome*

Erb-Zimmerlin type

Erben's phenomenon, reflex, sign

Erdheim's syndrome — acromegaly with bone and cartilage hypertrophy of the clavicle, vertebral bodies and intervertebral disks

Erdheim's disease — cystic medial necrosis

Erdheim's cystic medial necrosis, rest, tumor

Erdmann's reagent, test

Erhard's test

Erhardt's clamp, forceps, speculum

Erich's arch bar, forceps, splint

Erichsen's disease — traumatic neurosis following spinal injury

Erichsen's ligature, sign, spine, test

Erlacher-Blount syndrome — bowleg in children, not caused by rickets

Erlanger's sphygmomanometer

Erlenmeyer's flask

Erni's sign

Ernst's radium application

Esbach's method, reagent, test

Escamilla-Lisser syndrome — hypothyroidism in adults, associated with ascites; cardiac, intestinal and bladder atony; anemia; menorrhagia; and carotinemia

Escat's phlegmon

Escherich's bacillus, reflex, sign, test

Escudero's test

Esmarch's bandage, probe, scissors, tourniquet, tubes

Espildora-Luque's syndrome — blindness in one eye, with contralateral hemiplegia

Esser's operation — a method of securing epithelialization of an unhealed deep wound

Esser's graft

Essex-Lopresti maneuver, method, technique

Essig's splint

Essrig's forceps, scissors

Estes' operation — implantation of an ovary into a uterine cornu, performed when the tubes are absent

Estlander's operation — resection of one or more ribs in empyema; rotation of a triangular flap from lower lip to fill a defect in the upper lip

Estlander's cheiloplasty, flap

Estren-Dameshek syndrome — a familial type of hypoplastic anemia marked by pancytopenia, pallor, weakness, and a tendency to bleed

Estren-Dameshek anemia, familial aplasia

Eternod's sinus

Ethridge's forceps

Eulenburg's disease — a congenital hereditary disease marked by tonic spasm and muscular rigidity

European blastomycosis, hookworm, rat flea

Eustace Smith's murmur, sign

Evans' syndrome — autoimmune hemolytic anemia, leukopenia, thrombocytopenia and purpura

Evans' disease — familial cardiomegaly

Evans' blue, forceps, staging system

Evans–Lloyd-Thomas syndrome — suspended heart

Eve's method

Everett's forceps

Everitt's salt

Eversbusch's operation — for correction of ptosis

Eves' snare

Ewald's evacuator, forceps, law, node, test, tube

Ewart's phenomenon, sign

Ewing's angioendothelioma, endothelial sarcoma, sign, tumor

Exner's plexus

Exton's reagent, test

Exton-Rose glucose tolerance test

F

Faber's syndrome — hypochromic anemia

Faber's anemia

Fabre's test

Fabricius' bursa

Fabry's disease — a hereditary sphingolipidosis in which glycolipids are deposited in tissues, especially the kidneys, causing edema, enlargement of the heart, and hypertension

Faget's law, sign

Fahey's method, pin

Fahr's disease — progressive calcific deposition in the walls of cerebral blood vessels

Fahr-Volhard disease — malignant nephrosclerosis

Fahraeus' method, phenomenon, reaction, test

Fahraeus-Lindqvist effect

Fahrenheit's scale, thermometer

Fairbank's disease — idiopathic familial osteophytosis

Fajans' law

Fajans-Conn criteria

Fajersztajn's crossed sciatic sign

Falcon assay

Falconer-Weddell syndrome — intermittent compression of the subclavian artery and vein between the clavicle and first thoracic rib, with vascular disorders in the upper limbs

Falk's clamp, forceps, retractor

Falk-Tedesco's test

Fallopio's foramen

Fallopius' aqueduct, ligament

Fallot's disease/syndrome — tetralogy of Fallot

Fallot's pentalogy, tetrad, tetralogy, trilogy

Falope's ring

Falret's disease — manic-depressive psychosis

Falta's syndrome — polyglandular insufficiency, usually combining hypofunction of the anterior gland and myxedema

Falta's coefficient, triad

Fañaná's cell, glia

Fanconi's syndrome — a rare hereditary disorder with poor prognosis, marked by pancytopenia and hypoplasia of bone marrow with accompanying musculoskeletal and genitourinary anomalies

Fanconi's anemia, pancytopenia

Fanconi-Albertini-Zellweger syndrome — a congenital disease of bone characterized by a heart defect and other abnormalities

Fanconi-Hegglin syndrome — pulmonary infiltrations with positive Wassermann reactions in nonsyphilitic patients

Fanconi-Petrassi syndrome — hereditary hemolytic anemia with macrocytosis and hyperchromia

Fanconi-Schlesinger syndrome — dwarfism, mental retardation, convergent strabismus, hypercalcemia, azotemia, hypertension, and other anomalies

Fanconi-Türler syndrome — a congenital, probably familial, syndrome characterized by cerebellar ataxia associated with uncoordinated eye movement, nystagmus, and mental retardation

Fansler's anoscope, proctoscope, speculum

Fantus' antidote, test

Farabeuf's amputation, forceps, raspatory, retractor, saw, triangle

Farabeuf-Lambotte clamp, forceps

Faraday's constant, dark space, effect, law

Farber's syndrome — same as *Farber-Uzman syndrome*

Farber's disease — a rare, hereditary disorder of ceramide metabolism marked by loss of voice; desquamating dermatitis; foam cell infiltration of bones and joints; granulomatous reaction in the heart, lung, and kidneys; and psychomotor retardation

Farber's lipogranulomatosis, test

Farber-Uzman syndrome — a progressive form of hereditary lipidosis marked by nodular erythematous swellings and cardiopulmonary and central nervous system involvement, usually leading to death within the first two years of life

Farlow's tongue depressor

Farlow-Boettcher snare

Farnham's forceps

Farr's law, retractor, test

Farrant's medium, mounting fluid, solution

Farre's tubercles, white line

Farrington's forceps

Farrior's forceps, speculum

Farris' forceps

Fauchard's disease — periodontitis

Faught's sphygmomanometer

Faulkner's chisel, curet, trocar

Faulkner-Browne chisel

Fauser's reaction

Faust's method, zinc sulfate flotation procedure

Fauvel's forceps, granules

Favoloro's retractor

Favre's disease — night blindness and microcystic edema of the macula retinae, associated with development of macular retinoschisis

Favre's bodies

Favre-Durand-Nicholas disease — lymphogranuloma venereum

Favre-Racouchot syndrome — nodular elastosis

Fazio-Londe disease — progressive bulbar palsy of childhood

Fazio-Londe atrophy, type

Fearon's test

Fechner's law

Fede's disease — granuloma of the frenum of the tongue, occurring in children

Federici's sign

Federoff's splenectomy

Federov's eye implant
Feer's disease — acrodynia
Fehland's clamp
Fehleisen's streptococcus
Fehling's solution, test
Feilchenfeld's forceps
Fein's needle, trocar
Feingold's diet
Feiss' line
Feitis' flecked spleen
Feldman's retractor
Feleky's instrument
Felix Vi serum
Felix-Weil reaction
Fell-O'Dwyer apparatus
Felton's paralysis, phenomenon, serum, unit
Felty's syndrome — a combination of rheumatoid arthritis, splenomegaly, leukopenia, anemia, and thrombocytopenia
Fenger's forceps
Fenton's bolt, reaction
Fenwick's disease — idiopathic atrophic gastritis
Fenwick's ulcer
Fenwick-Hunner ulcer
Féré-Langmead lipomatosis
Féréol's nodes
Féréol-Graux paralysis
Ferguson's angiotribe, forceps, method, retractor, scissors, stone basket
Ferguson-Metzenbaum scissors
Ferguson-Moon retractor
Ferguson-Smith epithelioma
Fergusson's operation — an incision for surgical removal of the upper jaw
Fergusson's incision, speculum
Fergusson and Critchley's ataxia
Fernandez's reaction
Fernbach's flask
Ferrata's cell
Ferrein's canal, cords, foramen, ligament, pyramid, tubes, tubules
Ferrier's method, treatment
Ferris' dilator, forceps

Ferris-Robb knife
Ferris Smith forceps, knife, retractor, rongeur
Ferris Smith–Gruenwald rongeur
Ferris Smith–Halle bur
Ferris Smith–Kerrison forceps, rongeur
Ferris Smith–Sewal retractor
Ferris Smith–Takahashi rongeur
Ferry-Porter law
Feuerstein-Mims syndrome — a condition marked by hamartomas of the scalp, face, or neck with progressive changes throughout life
Feulgen's reaction, stain, test
Feulgen-Schiff reaction
Fevold's test
Févre-Languepin syndrome — a familial syndrome marked by popliteal webbing associated with cleft lip, cleft palate, fistula of the lower lip, syndactyly, onychodysplasia, and deformity of the foot
Feyrter's disease — pulmonary plasmocytosis in premature infants
Fichera's method, treatment
Fick's bacillus, equation, first law of diffusion, formula, halo, method, phenomenon, principle, veil
Ficker's diagnosticum
Ficoll-Hypaque separation, technique
Fiedler's disease — leptospiral jaundice; same as *Weil's syndrome*
Fiedler's myocarditis
Fielding's membrane
Fields' rapid stain
Fiessinger's syndrome — a severe form of erythema multiforme
Fiessinger-Leroy-Reiter syndrome — nongonococcal urethritis, followed by conjunctivitis and arthritis

Fieux's test

Figueira's syndrome — weakness of the neck muscles, with spasticity of the muscles of the lower extremities

Filatov's disease — infectious mononucleosis

Filatov-Dukes disease — same as *Dukes' disease*

Fildes' culture medium, law

Filhos' caustic

Filipovitch's (Filipowicz's) sign

Fillauer's splint

Finckh's test

Finikoff's method, treatment

Fink's curet, forceps, laryngoscope, retractor, tendon tucker

Fink-Heimer stain

Fink-Jameson forceps

Finkelstein's albumin milk, feeding

Finkler-Prior spirillium

Finn chamber test

Finney's operation — enlargement of the pyloric canal and establishment of an anastomosis between the stomach and duodenum

Finney's gastroenterostomy, pyloroplasty

Finnoff's transilluminator

Finochietto's forceps, retractor, scissors, stirrup

Finsen's apparatus, bath, lamp, light, rays, treatment

Finsen-Reya lamp

Finsterer's sutures

Fisch-Renwick syndrome — congenital deafness, hypertelorism, ocular heterochromia, and white forelock

Fischer's syndrome — a familial congenital syndrome, with keratosis of the palms and feet, clubbing of the distal phalanges of the toes and fingers, and various other anomalies

Fischer's needle, projection formula sign, test

Fischler's method

Fish's forceps

Fishberg's concentration test, method

Fishberg-Friedfeld test

Fisher's syndrome — paralysis of one or more of the ocular motor nerves

Fisher's autocytometer, cannula, forceps, knife, procedure, retractor

Fisher-Arlt forceps

Fisher-Nugent retractor

Fisher-Race system, theory

Fishman-Doubilet test

Fishman-Lerner unit

Fisk's method

Fiske's method

Fiske-Subbarow method

Fite's method

Fitz's syndrome — a series of symptoms indicative of acute pancreatitis, epigastric pain and vomiting, followed by collapse

Fitz's law

Fitz Gerald method, treatment

Fitzgerald's factor, forceps

Fitzgerald-Williams-Flaujeac factor

Fitz-Hugh–Curtis syndrome — perihepatitis as a complication of gonorrhea in women, marked by fever and upper abdominal pain and spasm

Fitzpatrick's suction tube

Fitzwater's forceps

Flack's node, test

Flagg's laryngoscope

Flajani's disease — exophthalmic goiter

Flajani's operation — separation of the external margin of the iris from the ciliary body

Flanagan's gouge

Flannery's speculum

Flatau's law

Flatau-Schilder disease — a subacute or chronic form of leukoencephalopathy of children and adolescents. Symptoms include blindness, deafness, and progressive mental deterioration

Flaujeac's factor

Flechsig's areas, column, cuticulum, fasciculus, field, law, primordial zones, tract

Fleck's phenomenon

Flegel's disease — a hereditary skin disorder marked by red or brown scaly papules on the extremities and usually keratoses on palms and soles

Fleig's test

Fleischer's dystrophy, line, keratoconus ring, vortex

Fleischer-Strümpell ring

Fleischl's test

Fleischmann's bursa, follicle, hygroma

Fleischner's syndrome — horizontal linear atelectasis

Fleischner's disease — osteochondritis affecting the middle phalanges of the hand

Fleischner's method

Fleitmann's test

Fleming's conization of cervix

Flemming's body, center, fixing fluid, mass, solution, substance, triple stain

Fletcher's afterloading tandem, factor, medium

Fletcher–Van Doren forceps

Flexner's bacillus, dysentery, serum

Flexner-Jobling carcinoma, carcinosarcoma, tumor

Flexner-Strong bacillus

Flexner-Wintersteiner rosette

Flieringa's scleral ring

Fliess's therapy, treatment

Flint's arcade, law, murmur

Floegel's layer

Flood's ligament

Florence's crystals, flask, reaction, test

Florentine's iris

Florey's unit

Florschütz's formula

Flourens' doctrine, law, theory

Flower's index

Floyd's needle

Fluhmann's test

Flynn-Aird syndrome — a familial syndrome marked by muscle wasting, ataxia, dementia, epidermal atrophy, and ocular anomalies

Flynt's needle

Fochier's abscess

Focker's test

Foerster — see also *Förster*

Foerster's syndrome — generalized amyotonia

Fogarty catheter, clamp, probe

Foix's syndrome — paralysis of the oculomotor nerves, paresis of the sympathetic nerves and neuroparalytic keratitis

Foix-Alajouanine syndrome — subacute necrotizing myelitis

Foley bag, catheter, forceps

Foley's pyeloplasty, Y-type ureteropelvioplasty

Foley-Alcock catheter

Folin's method, reagent, test

Folin-Bell method

Folin-Benedict-Myers method

Folin-Berglund method

Folin-Cannon-Denis method

Folin-Ciocalteu reagent

Folin-Denis method, test

Folin-Farmers method

Folin-Flander method

Folin-Hart method

Folin-Looney test

Folin-Macallum method

Folin-McEllroy test

Folin-McEllroy-Peck method

Folin-Peck method

Folin-Pettibone method

Folin-Shaffer method

Folin-Wright method

Folin-Wu method, test

Folin-Youngburg method

Folius' muscle, process

Fölling's disease — phenylketonuria

Follmann's balanitis

Foltz's valve

Fomon's knife, periosteotome, retractor, scissors

Fonio's solution

Fontan's procedure

Fontana's markings, spaces, stain

Fontana-Mason staining method

Foot's method, reticulin impregnation stain

Forbes' disease — glycogen storage disease

Forbes' amputation

Forbes-Albright syndrome — a condition in which a pituitary tumor secretes excessive amounts of prolactin and produces persistent lactation

Fordyce's disease — a developmental anomaly marked by ectopic sebaceous glands that appear as papules on the oral mucosa

Fordyce's angiokeratoma, granules, lesion, spots

Foregger's bronchoscope, laryngoscope

Forel's areas, commissure, decussation, field

Forestier disease — hypertrophy of the vertebral column in the thoracic region

Forestier-Certonciny syndrome — senile rheumatic gout

Forestier and Rotés-Querol syndrome — ankylosing vertebral hyperostosis

Forget-Fredette agar

Formad's kidney

Fornet's reaction, ring test

Forney's syndrome — familial mitral insufficiency

Forrester's clamp, splint

Forrester-Brown head halter

Forschheimer's spots

Forsius-Eriksson syndrome — a familial syndrome transmitted as a recessive X-linked trait and marked by albinism, hypoplasia, nystagmus, astigmatism, and myopia; called also *Aland eye disease*

Forssell's syndrome — polycythemia associated with kidney diseases

Forssell's sinus

Forssman's antibody, antigen, lipoid

Förster's atonic-astatic syndrome — atonic-astatic diplegia

Förster's disease — central choroiditis in which the spots are at first black and then become enlarged and white

Förster's operation(s) — intradurally cutting the seventh, eighth, and ninth dorsal nerve roots on both sides in locomotor ataxia; an operation to produce rapid artificial ripening of a cataract

Förster's choroiditis, forceps, photometer, snare, uveitis

Förster-Penfield operation — excision of scar tissue in the epileptogenic cortical area in traumatic epilepsy

Fort Bragg fever

Foshay's reaction, serum, test

Fosler's splint

Foss' clamp, forceps, retractor

Foster's frame

Foster-Ballenger speculum

Foster Kennedy syndrome — retrobulbar optic neuritis, with atrophy on one side of the lesion and papilledema on the other, occurring in frontal lobe tumor of the brain

Fothergill's disease — scarlet fever associated with painful pharyngitis or peritonsillar abscess

Fothergill's operation — for uterine prolapse

Fothergill's neuralgia, pill, sore throat

Fouchet's reagent, stain, test

Foulis' cells

Fourier's analysis

Fourmentin's thoracic index

Fournier's disease — fulminating gangrene of the scrotum

Fournier's gangrene, sign, teeth, test, tibia, treatment

Foville's syndrome — a form of hemiplegia affecting alternate sides

Foville's fasciculus

Fowler's incision, maneuver, position, solution, sound

Fowler-Murphy treatment

Fowler-Weir incision

Fox's disease — a rare skin disease marked by bullous and vesicular eruptions brought on by trauma

Fox's blepharoplasty, eye implant, eye shield, impetigo, speculum, splint

Fox-Fordyce disease — a persistent, itching papular eruption from inflammation of the apocrine sweat glands

F. R. Thompson hip prosthesis, rasp

Frackelton's needle

Fraenkel's nodules, symptom

Frahur's clamp, scissors

Fraley's syndrome — dilation of the renal calices caused by stenosis of the upper infundibulum

Franceschetti's syndrome — mandibulofacial dysostosis

Franceschetti's disease — retinal dystrophy marked by multiple yellow-white lesions of the retina

Franceschetti's dystrophy

Franceschetti-Jadassohn syndrome — a hereditary condition of reticular skin pigmentation with keratosis of the palms and soles; called also *Naegeli's syndrome*

Francis' disease — tularemia

Francis forceps, test

Franck's plethysmograph

Francke's needle

Franco's operation — suprapubic cystotomy

François' syndrome — a complex syndrome characterized chiefly by brachycephaly, mandibular hypoglossia, hypotrichosis, and bilateral congenital cataracts

François' dysencephaly, dystrophy

François-Haustrate syndrome — otomandibular dysostosis

Frangenheim's forceps

Frank's operation — a method of performing a gastrostomy

Frank-Starling curve, mechanism, relation

Franke's operation — removal of the intercostal nerves for the visceral crises of tabes

Franke's triad

Frankel's disease — indurative pneumonia

Fränkel's appliance, sign, speculum, test, treatment

Fränkel-Voges asparagin culture medium

Franken's test

Frankenhäser's ganglion

Frankfeldt's forceps, sigmoidoscope

Frankfort's horizontal plane

Frankl-Hochwart's disease — the symptom complex of cochlear, vestibular, facial and trigeminal nerve irritation occurring in early syphilis

Franklin's disease — plasma proteinemia, characterized by abnormal globulins and associated with malignant disorders of plasmacytic and lymphoid cells

Franklin's glasses, retractor

Franklin-Silverman curet, needle

Franz's syndrome — cessation of vibration after ligation of the vein proximal to an arteriovenous fistula

Franz's retractor

Fraser's syndrome — congenital absence of eyelids with multiple anomalies, including ear malformation, digital deformities, and renal maldevelopment

Fraser's forceps

Fraser-Lendrum stain for fibrin

Frater's retractor

Fraunhofer's lines

Frazier's osteotome, retractor, scissors, tube

Frazier-Adson clamp

Frazier-Paparella suction tube

Frazier-Sachs clamp

Frazier-Spiller operation — a subtemporal trigeminal rhizotomy

Fredal's test

Frederick's syndrome — auricular fibrillation associated with complete atrioventricular block

Frederick's needle

Fredet-Ramstedt operation — pyloromyotomy

Fredrickson's dyslipoproteinemia classification, phenotype

Freeman's clamp, leukotome

Freeman-Sheldon syndrome — craniocarpotarsal dystrophy

Freeman-Swanson prosthesis

Freer's elevator, knife, periosteotome, retractor

Freer-Gruenwald forceps

Frégoli's phenomenon

Frei's disease — lymphogranuloma venereum

Frei's antigen, bubo, test

Freiberg's disease — osteochondrosis of the head of the second metatasal

Freiberg's infarction, infraction, knife, retractor, traction

Freiburg's method

Frei-Hoffman reaction

Freimuth's curet

Frejka's pillow splint

French flap, scale

Frenkel's syndrome — ocular contusion syndrome

Frenkel's movements, treatment

Frerichs' theory

Fresnel's fringe, zone plate

Freud's cathartic method

Freund's operation — chondrotomy for congenital funnel breast

Freund's adjuvant, anomaly, dermatitis, reaction

Freund-Kaminer reaction

Frey's syndrome — localized flushing and sweating of the ear and cheek in response to eating

Frey's eye implant, hairs

Frey-Freer bur

Frey-Gigon method

Freyer's operation — suprapubic enucleation of the hypertrophied prostate

Freyer's drain

Fricke's bandage, dressing

Friderichsen's test

Friderichsen-Waterhouse syndrome — same as *Waterhouse-Friderichsen syndrome*

Fridericia's method

Fried's rule

Friedenwald's syndrome — lifting of a ptosed eyelid on turning the eyes to the right, opening the mouth wide, and sticking out the tongue

Friedenwald's ophthalmoscope

Friedländer's disease — inflammation of the innermost coat of an artery, by which smaller vessels become constricted or obliterated

Friedländer's bacillus, pneumobacillus, pneumonia, stain

Friedman's retractor, test, vein stripper

Friedman-Lapham test

Friedman-Otis bougie

Friedman-Roy syndrome — the association of mental deficiency, strabismus, extensor plantar reflexes, speech defects, and clubfoot

Friedmann's syndrome(s) — a cycle of symptoms caused by progressive, subacute encephalitis, including headache, vertigo, insomnia, debility, and defective memory; a form of petit mal epilepsy in children

Friedmann's vasomotor syndrome — postconcussional syndrome

Friedmann's disease — recurrent spastic paralysis in children, resulting from congenital syphilis

Friedreich's disease(s) — a disorder marked by rapid muscle contractions occurring simultaneously or consecutively in various unrelated muscles; facial hemihypertrophy

Friedreich's ataxia, foot, phenomenon, sign, tabes

Friedrich's syndrome — a rare, aseptic form of epiphyseal necrosis of the sternal ends of the clavicles

Friedrich's clamp, raspatory

Friedrich-Petz clamp

Friend's catheter, leukemia

Friesner's knife

Friess-Pierrou syndrome — filariasis with eosinophilia, adenopathies, and pneumopathies

Frisch's bacillus

Fritsch's catheter, retractor

Fritsch-Asherman syndrome — amenorrhea or hypomenorrhea, dysmenorrhea, habitual abortion, and sterility following puerperal or postabortal infection or curettage

Fritz's aspirator

Fröhde's reagent, test

Fröhlich's disease/syndrome — adiposogenital dystrophy caused by adenohypophyseal tumor

Frölich's dwarfism

Frohn's reagent, test

Froin's syndrome — lumbar spinal fluid with presence of large amounts of protein, rapid coagulation, and progressive absence of cells

Froment's paper sign

Frommann's lines

Frommel's disease — same as *Chiari-Frommel syndrome*

Frommel's operation — shortening of the uterosacral ligaments for retrodeviation of the uterus

Frommel-Chiari syndrome — same as *Chiari-Frommel syndrome*

Frommer's dilator, test

Froriep's ganglion, induration, law

Fröschel's symptom

Frost's sutures

Frost-Lang operation — insertion of a gold ball to replace an enucleated eyeball

Fruehjahr's catarrh

Frugoni's syndrome — thrombophlebitic splenomegaly

Frugoni's disease — infectious eosinophilia

Frye's test

Fuchs' syndrome — a progressive ocular disease of unknown cause, marked by heterochromia of the iris, iridocyclitis, and cataracts

Fuchs' adenoma, atrophy, coloboma, crypts, dellen, dimple, dystrophy, forceps, heterochromia, keratitis, lamella, method, position, spot, test

Fuchs-Rosenthal chamber, hemocytometer

Fuhrman's grading system

Fujiwara reaction

Fukala's operation — removal of the lens of the eye for treatment of myopia

Fukuyama's syndrome — congenital muscular dystrophy

Fulci's spherules

Fuld's test
Fuld-Goss test
Fülleborn's method
Fuller's operation — incision and
    drainage of the seminal vesi-
    cles
Fuller's cell, dressing, tube
Fulton's retractor, rongeur, scis-
    sors
Funkenstein's test
Fürbringer's sign, test

Furniss' anastomosis, catheter,
    clamp, forceps, incision
Furniss-Clute clamp, pin
Furniss-McClure-Hinton clamp
Furst-Ostrum syndrome — platy-
    basia associated with congeni-
    tal synostosis of the neck and
    Sprengel's deformity
Fürstner's disease — pseudospastic
    paralysis with tremor
Furth's tumor

Gaboon ulcer
Gabriel's proctoscope
Gabriel Tucker bougie, forceps
Gad's hypothesis
Gaddum-Schild test
Gaenslen's sign, test
Gaffky's scale, table
Gaillard-Arlt suture
Gailliard's syndrome — location of
    the heart in the right hemi-
    thorax
Gairdner's disease — cardiac dis-
    tress without apprehension
Gairdner's coin test
Gaisböck's disease/syndrome —
    stress polycythemia
Galassi's pupillary phenomenon
Galbiati's ischiopubiotomy
Gale's formula
Galeati's glands
Galeazzi's fracture, sign
Galen's anastomosis, bandage, fora-
    men, pore, veins, ventricle
Galezowski's dilator
Gall's body, craniology
Gallego's differentiating solution
Galli-Mainini test
Gallie's herniorrhaphy, needle,
    transplant
Gallois' test
Galt's trephine

Galton's delta, law, whistle
Gambee's sutures
Gambian trypanosomiasis
Gamgee's tissue
Gamna's disease — a form of sple-
    nomegaly with thickening of
    the splenic capsule
Gamna's nodules
Gamna-Favre bodies
Gamna-Gandy nodules
Gamstorp's disease/syndrome — a
    hereditary, familial syndrome
    marked by attacks of periodic
    paralysis, with hyperkalemia
    and normal urinary potassium
    during the attacks
Ganassini's test
Gandhi's knife
Gandy's clamp
Gandy-Gamna bodies, nodules,
    spleen
Gandy-Nanta disease — siderotic
    splenomegaly
Gangi's reaction
Gangolphe's sign
Gannetta's dissector
Gannther's test
Ganser's syndrome — amnesia, dis-
    turbances of consciousness,
    hallucinations, and sensory

Ganser's syndrome — (*continued*) changes, usually of hysterical origin

Ganser's diverticulum, ganglion, symptom

Gänsslen's disease — familial form of constitutional leukopenia, transmitted as a dominant trait

Gant's operation — division of the femoral shaft for hip joint ankylosis

Gant's clamp, line

Garceau's catheter

Garcin's syndrome — unilateral global involvement of cranial nerves

Gardiner-Brown test

Gardner's syndrome — familial polyposis of the large bowel, with supernumerary teeth, fibrous dysplasia of the skull, osteomas, and fibromas

Gardner's headrest, needle

Gardner-Diamond syndrome — a reaction syndrome occurring principally in young women, in which spontaneous, painful ecchymoses occur without trauma — possibly of emotional origin

Gardner-Wells tongs

Gardos' phenomenon

Garel's sign

Garfield-Holinger laryngoscope

Gariel's pessary

Garland's clamp, curve, forceps, triangle

Garré's disease — sclerosing nonsuppurative osteomyelitis

Garré's osteitis, osteomyelitis

Garretson's bandage

Garrett's dilator

Garriga's test

Garrigue's forceps, speculum

Garrison's forceps, rongeur

Garrod's pads, test

Gärtner's bacillus, duct cyst, phenomenon, tonometer

Gartner's canal, cyst, duct

Garven-Gairns method

Gaskell's bridge, clamp

Gasser's syndrome — a rare syndrome of unknown cause occurring in young children, consisting of renal failure, hemolytic anemia, and severe thrombocytopenia

Gasser's ganglion

Gasser-Karrer syndrome — fatal hemolytic anemia

Gastaut's syndrome — unilateral convulsions associated with hemiplegia and epilepsy in young children

Gatch's bed

Gatellier's incision

Gaucher's disease — familial splenic anemia

Gaucher's cell, splenomegaly

Gaul's pits

Gaule's spots

Gault's cochleopalpebral reflex, test

Gauran's test

gaussian curve

Gaustad's syndrome — reversible attacks of confusion, stupor and coma with personality changes and motor disturbances, associated with cirrhosis of the liver

Gauvain's brace, fluid

Gavard's muscle

Gavin-Miller clamp, forceps

Gawalowski's test

Gay's glands

Gay-Force test

Gay-Lussac's law

Gayer's test

Gaylor's forceps, punch

Gaynor-Hart method

Gaza's operation — cutting the appropriate rami communicantes of the sympathetic nervous system

Gee's disease — same as *Gee-Herter-Heubner disease*

Gee-Herter disease — same as *Gee-Herter-Heubner disease*

Gee-Herter-Heubner syndrome — the infantile form of nontropical sprue

Gee-Herter-Heubner disease — childhood celiac disease

Gee-Thaysen disease — adult celiac disease

Gegenbaur's cell, sulcus

Gehrung pessary

Geigel's reflex

Geiger counter

Geiger-Downes cautery

Geiger-Müller counter

Geissler's test, tube

Geissler-Pluecker tube

Gélineau's syndrome — narcolepsy

Gell-Coombs classification

Gellé's test

Gellhorn's forceps, pessary, punch

Gelman's filter

Gelpi's forceps, retractor

Gelpi-Lowrie forceps

Gély's suture

Gemini's clamp, forceps

Gendre's fixative, fluid

Genga's bandage

Gengou's phenomenon

Gennari's band, layer, line, stria, stripe

Gensoul's disease — diffuse, purulent inflammation of the floor of the mouth, spreading to the soft tissues of the upper neck, sometimes causing airway obstruction

Gentele's test

Georgi's test

Geraghty's test

Gerald's forceps

Gérard-Marchand fracture

Gerbasi's anemia

Gerbich's blood group system

Gerbich's-negative red cell

Gerbode's defect, dilator

Gerdy's fibers, fontanelle, hyoid fossa, interauricular loop, ligament, tubercle

Gerhardt's syndrome — bilateral abductor paralysis of the vocal cords

Gerhardt's disease — a condition chiefly affecting the extremities, marked by paroxysmal vasodilation with burning pain and rise in skin temperature

Gerhardt's dullness, phenomenon, reaction, sign, test, triangle

Gerhardt-Semon law

Gerlach's network, tonsil, valve

Gerlier's disease — a disease of the nerves and nerve centers characterized by pain, paresis, vertigo, ptosis, and muscular contractions, usually found among farm laborers and stablemen

German measles

Germistan virus

Gerota's capsule, fascia, fasciitis, method

Gerrard's test

Gerson-Herrmannsdorfer diet

Gerstmann's syndrome — a combination of right-left disorientation, inability to express thoughts in writing, and inability to do simple calculations

Gerstmann-Sträussler disease — same as *Gerstmann-Sträussler-Scheinker disease*

Gerstmann-Sträussler-Scheinker disease — a rare neurologic disorder characterized by progressive speech disturbances, cerebellar ataxia, slow physical and mental responses, and dementia

Gerzog's knife, speculum

Gerzog-Ralks knife

Gesvelst's network

Getsowa's adenoma

Ghilarducci's reaction

Ghon's complex, focus, primary lesion, tubercle

Ghon-Sachs bacillus

Giacomini's band

Gianelli's sign

Giannuzzi's bodies, cells, crescents, demilunes

Gianotti-Crosti syndrome — eruptive papulous dermatitis of the extremities

Gibbon's hernia, hydrocele

Gibbon-Landis test

Gibbs' theorem

Gibbs-Donnan equilibrium, law

Gibert's disease — pityriasis rosea

Gibert's pityriasis

Gibney's disease — painful inflammation of the spinal muscles

Gibney's bandage, boot, perispondylitis, strapping

Gibson's disease — a rare disease that may be familial, marked by a decrease in the rate of methemoglobin reduction in the presence of glucose or lactate

Gibson's bandage, glioma, incision, murmur, rule, splint, sutures, vestibule

Gibson-Balfour retractor

Gibson-Cooke sweat test

Giemsa's stain

Gierke's disease — glycogen storage disease

Gierke's cells, corpuscles

Giertz-Shoemaker rib shears

Gies' biuret reagent, biuret test

Gifford's operation(s) — delimiting keratotomy; destruction of the lacrimal sac by trichloracetic acid

Gifford's curet, forceps, keratotomy, maneuver, reflex, retractor, sign

Gifford-Galassi reflex

Gigli's operation — lateral section of the os pubis with Gigli's wire saw, performed in difficult labor

Gigli's pubiotomy, wire saw

Gilbert's syndrome — constitutional hepatic dysfunction, constitu-

Gilbert's syndrome — (continued) tional hyperbilirubinemia, familial nonhemolytic jaundice

Gilbert's disease — a familial, benign elevation of bilirubin levels without liver damage

Gilbert's catheter, cholemia, forceps, sign

Gilbert-Dreyfus syndrome — a familial form of pseudohermaphroditism, marked by male phenotype, hypospadias, gynecomastia, scanty axillary hair, absent beard, and nearly normal testes

Gilbert-Graves speculum

Gilbert-Lereboullet syndrome — hereditary nonhemolytic jaundice

Gilchrist's disease — North American blastomycosis

Gilchrist's mycosis

Giliberty's prosthesis

Gill's operation — insertion of a wedge of bone for dropfoot or pes equinus

Gill's blade, forceps, knife, scissors

Gill-Fuchs forceps

Gill-Hess forceps

Gill-Manning decompression laminectomy

Gill-Safar forceps

Gill-Thomas-Cosman relocatable stereotactic localizer

Gilles de la Tourette's syndrome — motor incoordination, with involuntary repetition of another's words and involuntary utterance of obscenities

Gillespie's syndrome — aniridia, cerebellar ataxia, and mental retardation

Gillespie's operation — excision of the wrist by a lengthwise dorsal incision

Gilliam's operation — retroversion of the uterus

Gillies' operation(s) — for correction of ectropion utilizing a

Gillies' operation(s) — (*continued*)
split-skin graft; a technique
for reducing fractures of the
zygoma and zygomatic arch

Gillies' elevator, flap, forceps,
graft, incision, scissors

Gillies-Dingman hook

Gillmore's needle

Gilman-Abrams tube

Gilmer's intermaxillary fixation,
method, splint, wiring

Gilmore's probe

Gilson's solution

Gilvernet's retractor

de Gimard's syndrome — gangrenous purpura

Gimbernat's ligament, reflex ligament

Gimenez' stain

Gimmick's elevator

Ginsberg's forceps

Giordano's sphincter

Giordano-Giovannetti diet

Giovannini's disease — a fungus infection that produces a nodular disease of the hair

Giraldés' organ

Girard's forceps, method, probe, reagent, treatment

Giraud-Teulon law

Girdlestone operation — removal
of the femoral head and neck
in cases of severe hip infection

Girdner's probe

Giuffrida-Ruggieri stigma

Givens' method

Gjessing's syndrome — periodic
catatonic stupor and excitement, coinciding with nitrogen retention and responding
to thyroid therapy

Glanzmann's syndrome — congenital hemorrhagic thrombocytic dystrophy

Glanzmann's disease — a platelet
abnormality characterized by
defective clot formation and
prolonged bleeding

Glanzmann's thrombasthenia

Glanzmann-Naegeli thrombasthenia

Glanzmann-Riniker syndrome —
X-linked hypogammaglobulinemia, with susceptibility to
pyogenic infection

Glanzmann-Saland syndrome —
severe polyneuritic paralysis
following diphtheria

Glaser's retractor

Glasgow's sign

Glassman's basket, clamp, forceps

Glassman-Allis clamp, forceps

Glatzel's mirror

Glauber's salt

Gleason's score, tumor grade

Glénard's disease/syndrome — prolapse or downward displacement of the viscera that may
be associated with neurasthenic manifestations

Glenn's operation — anastomosis
of the superior vena cava to
the right pulmonary artery for
congenital cyanotic heart disease

Glenn's anastomosis, procedure

Glenner's forceps, retractor

Glenner-Lillie stain

Gley's cells, glands

Glisson's disease — rickets

Glisson's capsule, cirrhosis, sling

Glover's clamp, forceps, organism,
rongeur

Gluck's shears

Gluge's corpuscles

Gluzinski's test

Gmelin's reaction, test

Godélier's law

Godfried-Prick-Carol-Prakken
syndrome — a familial syndrome consisting of multiple
neurofibromatoses, with atrophoderma vermiculatum,
mongoloid facies, mental retardation, and heart abnormalities, including congenital
heart block

Godtfredsen's syndrome — cavernous sinus–nasopharyngeal tumor syndrome

Godwin's tumor

Goeckerman's treatment

Goelet's retractor

Goethe's suture

Goetsch's skin reaction, test

Goffe's colporrhaphy

Gofman's test

Goggia's sign

Gohrbrand's dilator, valvulotome

Golaski's graft

Goldbacher's anoscope, proctoscope, speculum

Goldberg's syndrome — galactosialidosis

Goldberg-Maxwell syndrome — male pseudohermaphroditism characterized, when complete, by female external genitalia

Goldblatt's clamp, hypertension, kidney, phenomenon

Golden-Kantor syndrome — steatorrhea associated with the roentgenological picture of "moulage sign," dilation and segmentation of the small intestine

Goldenhar's syndrome — oculoauriculovertebral dysplasia

Goldflam's disease — same as Goldflam-Erb disease

Goldflam-Erb disease — myasthenia gravis

Goldie-Coldman hypothesis

Goldman's curet, knife, punch

Goldman-Fox knife

Goldman-Kazanjian forceps

Goldmann's applanation tonometer

Goldmann-McNeill blepharostat

Golds' forceps

Goldscheider's disease — the epidermis is loosely attached to the corium, giving rise to blisters that usually heal without scarring

Goldscheider's percussion, test

Goldstein's syndrome — a disease of the cerebellum marked by disorders of equilibrium and associated with distorted perception of space, time, and weight

Goldstein's disease — hereditary hemorrhagic telangiectasia

Goldstein's cannula, curet, hematemesis, hemoptysis, heredofamilial angiomatosis, irrigator, rays, sign, speculum

Goldthwait's fracture frame, sign, symptom

Golgi's alterations, apparatus, body, cells, complex, corpuscles, cycle, fibril, law, organ, stain, theory, types I and II neurons, zone

Golgi-Mazzoni corpuscles

Golgi-Rezzonico apparatus, spiral, threads

Goll's column, fasciculus, fibers, nucleus, tract

Golonbov's sign

Goltz's syndrome — same as Goltz-Gorlin syndrome

Goltz's experiment, theory

Goltz-Gorlin syndrome — focal dermal hypoplasia

Gombault's degeneration, neuritis

Gombault-Philippe triangle

Gomori's method, stains

Gomori-Jones periodic acid–methenamine-silver stain

Gomori-Takamatsu procedure, stains

Gomori-Wheatley stain

Gompertz's equation, law

Gonin's operation — treatment of retinal detachment by thermocautery of the retinal fissure

Gonin-Amsler marker

Gooch's filter, splint

Good's syndrome — immunodeficiency with thymoma

Good's forceps, rasp, scissors

Goodale-Lubin catheter

Goodell's dilator, law, sign

Goodenough draw-a-man test, draw-a-person test

Goodenough-Harris drawing test

Goodfellow's cannula

Goodhill's forceps, retractor

Goodman's syndrome — acrocephalopolysyndactyly, type IV

Goodpasture's syndrome — glomerulonephritis, usually progressing to death from renal failure

Goodpasture's stain

Goodwin's clamp

Goormaghtigh's apparatus, cells

Gopalan's syndrome — severe burning and aching of the feet associated with hyperesthesia, raised skin temperature, and vasomotor changes

Gordon's disease — protein-losing gastroenteropathy

Gordon's agent, elementary body, forceps, reflex, sign, splint, stethoscope, test

Gordon-Overstreet syndrome — ovarian agenesis, mild virilization, primary amenorrhea, lack of development of the breast, growth retardation, and increased excretion of gonadotropins

Gordon-Sweet silver impregnation method, stain

Gordon-Taylor amputation

Gorham's syndrome — massive osteolysis

Gorham's disease — extensive decalcification of a single bone without known cause

Goriaew's rule

Gorlin's syndrome — multiple nevoid basal-cell epitheliomas, jaw cysts and bifid ribs

Gorlin's cyst

Gorlin-Chaudhry-Moss syndrome — craniofacial dysostosis, dental

Gorlin-Chaudhry-Moss syndrome — (continued) and eye abnormalities, and patent ductus arteriosus

Gorlin-Goltz syndrome — a hereditary disorder consisting of multiple basal cell carcinomas, multiple anomalies of bone and other defects; also called *basal cell nevus syndrome*

Gorlin-Psaume syndrome — a condition occurring only in females, marked by mental retardation and anomalies of the mouth, tongue, face, and fingers

Gosselin's fracture

Gosset's retractor

Göthlin's index, test

Gott's prosthesis, valve

Gott-Daggett valve

Gottinger's line

Gottlieb's epithelial attachment

Gottron's syndrome — a familial form of progeria affecting the hands and feet

Gottron's papule, sign

Gottschalk's aspirator, saw

Gottstein's basal process, fibers

Gougerot's syndrome — erythematous papular lesions, purpuric macules, and dermal or dermohypodermal macules

Gougerot-Blum syndrome — pigmented, purpuric, lichenoid dermatitis

Gougerot-Carteaud syndrome — confluent and reticulated papillomatosis

Gougerot-Nulock-Houwer syndrome — a symptom complex of unknown etiology occurring in women, marked by keratoconjunctivitis and enlargement of the parotid glands; called also *Sjögren's syndrome*

Gougerot-Ruiter syndrome — allergic vasculitis

Gougerot-Sjögren disease — same as *Sjögren's syndrome*

Goulard's extract, lotion, water

Gould's sutures

Gouley's catheter, sound

Goutz's catheter

Govons' curet

Gowers' syndrome(s) — a paroxysmal condition marked by slow pulse, fall in blood pressure and sometimes convulsions; hereditary distal myopathy; irregularity of the pupillary light reflex seen in tabes dorsalis

Gowers' column, contraction, dystrophy, fasciculus, hemoglobin, maneuver, phenomenon, sign, solution, tract

Goyrand's hernia, injury

graafian follicle

Graber-Duvernay operation — boring minute channels to the center of the head of the femur for modifying circulation within the bone in chronic arthritis

Gracey's curet

Gradenigo's syndrome — paralysis of the sixth cranial nerve, with or without involvement of the ophthalmic branch of the fifth nerve, associated with lesions of the apex of the petrous bone and mastoiditis

Gradle's electrode, forceps, trephine

Graefe's disease/syndrome — gradual paralysis of the eye muscles, affecting first one muscle and then another

Graefe's operation — removal of a cataractous lens by a scleral cut, with laceration of the capsule and iridectomy

Graefe's cystotome, forceps, incision, knife, needle, sign, speculum, spots, test

Graefe-Sjögren syndrome — a hereditary, familial syndrome consisting of retinitis pigmentosa, congenital deafness and spinocerebellar ataxia

Gräfenberg's ring

Graffi's leukemia, mouse chloroleukemia

Graham's cells, elevator, hook, law, scissors, test

Graham-Cole test

Graham-Kerrison punch

Graham Little syndrome — lichen planus associated with acuminate follicular papules

Graham Steell's murmur

Gram's syndrome — juxta-articular adiposis dolorosa

Gram's iodine, method, solution, stain

Gram-Weigert stain

Grancher's disease — pneumonia with splenization of the lung

Grancher's sign, system, triad

Grandeau's test

Grandry's corpuscles

Grandry-Merkel corpuscles

Grandy's method

Granger's line, method, sign

Grant's operation — excision of tumors of the lip

Grant's retractor, separator

Grantham's electrode, needle

Graser's diverticulum

Grashey's aphasia, method

Grasset's law, phenomenon, sign

Grasset-Bychowski sign

Grasset-Gaussel phenomenon

Grasset-Gaussel-Hoover sign

Gratiolet's optic radiation, radiating fibers

Graves' disease — a thyroid disorder of unknown cause, oc-

Graves' disease — (continued)
curring principally in women
and marked by exophthalmos,
enlarged thyroid gland, nervous tremor, psychic disturbances, and emaciation

Graves' scapula, speculum

Gravindex test

Gravlee jet wash

Grawitz's basophilia, granules, tumor

Gray's clamp, forceps, resectoscope

Grayton's forceps

Green's caliper, mouth gag, resectoscope, scoop, trephine

Green-Armytage forceps

Green-Sewall mouth gag

Greene's sign

Greenfield's disease — a form of
leukoencephalopathy marked
by sphingolipid accumulations
in neural tissue and by loss of
myelin in the central nervous
system

Greenhow's disease — excoriation
and discoloration of the skin
in pediculosis, caused by
scratching

Greenhow's incision

Greenhow-Rodman incision

Greenough's microscope

Greenwald's method

Greenwald-Lewman method

Greenwood's forceps, trephine

Gregerson-Boas test

Gregg's syndrome — congenital abnormalities, including cataract, microphthalmia, heart
defects, and deafness, caused
by maternal rubella in pregnancy

Gregory's mixture

Greig's syndrome — extreme width
between the eyes due to enlargement of the sphenoid
bone, often associated with
mental retardation

Greiling's tube

Greither's syndrome — a familial
disorder marked by nonscal-
ing hyperkeratosis

Grenet's cell

Greville's bath

Grey Turner's sign

Gridley's stain

Grieshaber's extractor, forceps, keratome, trephine

Griesinger's disease — hookworm
infestation

Griesinger's sign, symptom

Griess' test

Griffith's method, sign

Grigg's test

Grignard's compound, reaction, reagent

Grimelius' argyrophic method

Grindon's disease — inflammation
of the hair follicles

Gringolo's syndrome — ankylo-
poietic spondylarthritis, hypo-
pyon, iritis, uveitis, polymorphic exudative erythema, and
ankylosis

Griscelli syndrome — hypopig-
mentation-immunodeficiency
disease

Grisolle's sign

Gritti's operation — amputation of
the leg through the knee, using the patella as an osteoplastic flap over the end of the femur

Gritti's amputation

Gritti-Stokes amputation

Grob's syndrome — partial alopecia, epicanthus, cleft lip and
cleft palate, multiple ridges in
the mucous membrane of the
jaws, fissures of the tongue,
brachydactyly, clinodactyly of
the small fingers, and mental
deficiency

Grocco's sign, test, triangle, triangular dullness

Grocott's adaptation of Gomori's
methenamine-silver stain

Grocott-Gomori method, stain
Groenholm's retractor
Groenouw's type I, type II dystrophy
Groffith's degeneration
Grönblad-Strandberg syndrome — angioid streaks of the retina with pseudoxanthoma elasticum of the skin
Grondahl-Finney operation — esophagogastroplasty, allowing enlargement of the orifice between the esophagus and the stomach
Groshong's catheter
Gross' disease — encysted rectum with dilation of the anal wall
Gross' clamp, forceps, leukemia, method, retractor, spatula, spud, test, virus antigen
Gross-Pomeranz-Watkins retractor
Grossich's method
Grossman's principle, sign
Grossmann's operation — treatment of retinal detachment by aspiration of subretinal fluid and injection of warm salt solution into the vitreous
Grotthus' law
Grove's cell
Grover's disease — transient acantholytic dermatosis
Gruber's syndrome — a malformation syndrome, lethal in the perinatal period, characterized by intrauterine growth retardation, ocular anomalies, cleft palate, polydactyly, polycystic kidney and other malformations; called also *Meckel-Gruber syndrome*
Gruber's bougies, fossa, hernia, reaction, speculum, suture, test
Gruber-Landzert fossa
Gruber-Widal reaction, test
Gruby's disease — tinea capitis in children caused by fungus infection

Grudziński's osteochondropathy
Gruentzig's balloon catheter
Gruenwald's forceps, punch, retractor, rongeur
Gruenwald-Bryant forceps
Gruft's medium
Grünbaum-Widal test
Grünfelder's reflex
Grüning's magnet
Gruskin's test
Grynfeltt's hernia, triangle
Grynfeltt-Lesshaft triangle
Gsell-Erdheim syndrome — necrotic disintegration of the medial layer of the aorta without inflammatory changes
Guama virus
Guarnieri's bodies, corpuscles, inclusions
Guaroa virus
Guatamahri's nodules
Gubler's syndrome — a form of alternating hemiplegia with ipsilateral facial paralysis
Gubler's hemiplegia, line, paralysis, reaction, sign, tumor
Gubler-Robin typhus
Gudden's atrophy, commissure, law
Gudebrod's sutures
Gudmand-Hoyer lactose tolerance test
Guedel's airway, blade, laryngoscope
Guelpa's treatment
Guéneau de Mussy's point
Guepar's prosthesis
Guérin's epithelioma, fold, fracture, glands, sinus, tumor, valve
Guérin-Stern syndrome — congenital contractures of extremities
Guggenheim's forceps, scissors
Guglielmo's detachable coil
Guibor's chart
Guidi's canal
Guild-Pratt speculum
Guilford's syndrome — congenital absence of teeth, inability to

Guilford's syndrome — *(continued)* smell or taste, hypotrichosis and anhidrosis

Guilford's stapedectomy

Guilford-Schuknecht scissors

Guilford-Zimmerman personality test

Guillain-Barré syndrome — a disease affecting the peripheral nervous system and cranial nerves, marked by demyelination, inflammation, edema, and nerve root decompression; called also *Landry's paralysis*

Guillain-Barré polyneuritis

Guilland's sign

Guinard's method, treatment

Guinon's disease — same as *Gilles de la Tourette's syndrome*

Guisez's tube

Guist's eye implant, forceps, scissors, speculum

Guist-Black speculum

Guldberg and Waage's law

Gull's disease — myxedema with atrophy of the thyroid

Gull's renal epistaxis

Gull-Sutton disease — arteriolar nephrosclerosis

Gull-Toynbee law

Gullstrand's law, ophthalmoscope, slit lamp

Gumprecht's shadow

Gun Hill hemoglobin

Gundelach's punch

Gunn's syndrome — unilateral ptosis of the eyelid

Gunn's dots, law, phenomenon, sign

Gunning's mixture, reaction, splint, test

Gunson's method

Günther's disease — congenital erythropoietic porphyria

Gunther's syndrome — an obscure form of myositis associated with myoglobinuria

Günz's ligament

Günzberg's reagent, test

Gusberg's curet, punch

Gussenbauer's operation — cutting an esophageal stricture through an opening above the stricture

Gussenbauer's artificial larynx, suture

Gutglass' forceps

Guthrie's bacterial inhibition assay, formula, muscle, test

Gutierrez's syndrome — abdominal pain in the epigastric or umbilical region, with a history of chronic constipation associated or unassociated with urinary disorders and early signs of chronic nephritis

Gutman's unit

Guttmann's retractor, sign, speculum

Gutzeit's test

Guy's gouge, knife, pill

Guye's sign

Guyon's operation — amputation above the malleoli

Guyon's amputation, bougie, clamp, dilator, sign, sound

Guyon-Benique sound

Guyon-Péan clamp

Guyton's scissors

Guyton-Friedenwald sutures

Guyton-Lundsgaard sclerotome

Guyton-Maumenee speculum

Guyton-Noyes forceps

Guyton-Park speculum

Gwathmey's hook, oil-ether anesthesia, suction tube

Gynefold's pessary

H ••

Haab's degeneration, magnet, reflex

Haagensen's test

Haagensen-Stout criteria

Haas' method

Haase's rule

Haber's syndrome — an autosomal dominant, inherited trait marked by permanent flushing and telangiectasia of the face, accompanied by keratotic lesions of the trunk

Haber-Weiss reaction

Habermann's disease — sudden onset of a polymorphous skin eruption composed of macules, papules, and vesicles

Hackenbruch's experience

Hacker's operation — for balanitic hypospadias

Haden's syndrome — hereditary hemolytic jaundice without spherocytosis

Hadfield-Clarke syndrome — same as *Clarke-Hadfield syndrome*

Haeckel's law

Haenel's syndrome — absence of pain on pressure to the eye in late stages of neurosyphilis

Haenel's symptom

Haferkamp's syndrome — a variant of *Gorham's syndrome*, marked by generalized malignant hemangiomatosis and osteolysis

Hagedorn's needle

Hagedorn-Jensen method

Hageman's factor

Hager's reagent, test

Hagie's pin

Haglund's syndrome — fracture of the bony nucleus of the calcaneus at its junction with the Achilles tendon

Haglund's disease — bursitis in the region of the Achilles tendon, caused by a disturbance of gait

Hagner's disease — symmetrical osteitis of the four limbs

Hagner's operation — drainage of gonorrheal epididymitis through an incision into the epididymis

Hagner's bag, catheter

Hague's lamp

Hahn's operation — gastrotomy with distal dilation of the pylorus

Hahn's cannula, gastrotomy, method, oxine, reagent, sign

Haidinger's brushes

Haig Ferguson forceps

Haight's elevator, retractor

Haik's eye implant

Hailey-Hailey disease — benign familial pemphigus

Haines' coefficient, formula, reagent, test

Hajek's forceps, mallet, retractor, rongeur

Hajek-Ballenger dissector, elevator

Hajek-Koffler forceps, punch

Hajek-Skillern punch

Hajna's gram-negative broth medium

Hakim's syndrome — same as *Hakim-Adams syndrome*

Hakim-Adams syndrome — normal-pressure hydrocephalus

Hakin-Cordis pump

Hakion's catheter

Halban's disease — benign ovarian tumors in young women with persistence of the corpus luteum, with amenorrhea and symptoms resembling pregnancy but no true pregnancy

Halberstaedter-Prowazek bodies

Halbrecht's syndrome — jaundice of newborn infants related to maternal-fetal ABO incompatibility

Haldane's apparatus, chamber

Hale's forceps, iron stain

Hales' piesimeter

Hall's disease — spurious hydrocephalus in children

Hall's antidote, band, dermatome, facies, intrauterine device, method, neurotome, sign

Hall-Stone ring

Hallauer's glasses

Hallberg's effect

Hallé's chisel, curet, needle, point, speculum

Hallé-Tieck speculum

Haller's ansa, arches, circle, cones, crypts, duct, frenum, glands, habenula, isthmus, layer, line, membrane, plexus, rete, tripod

Hallermann-Streiff syndrome — bony abnormalities of the face and jaw, with multiple eye defects, including cataract

Hallermann-Streiff-François syndrome — same as *Hallermann-Streiff syndrome*

Hallervorden's syndrome — complete demyelinization of certain nerve fibers

Hallervorden-Spatz syndrome — same as *Hallervorden's syndrome*

Hallgren's syndrome — vestibulocerebellar ataxia, retinal dystrophy, congenital deafness, and cataract

Halliday's hyperostosis

Hallion's test

Hallopeau's disease — an inherited disorder in which blisters are present at birth, scarring is severe, mucous membranes are involved, and death from infection often occurs in youth

Hallopeau's acrodermatitis, pemphigus

Hallopeau-Siemens syndrome — same as *Hallopeau's disease*

Hallpike's maneuver

Hallwach's effect

Halpin's operation — removal of the lacrimal gland through the middle of the eyebrow

Halsey's needle

Halsted's operation(s) — for inguinal hernia; radical mastectomy

Halsted's clamp, forceps, incision, inguinal herniorrhaphy, maneuver, radical mastectomy, sutures

Halsted-Meyer incision

Halsted–Willy Meyer incision

Ham's test

Hamberger's schema

Hamburger's interchange, law, phenomenon, test

Hamby's forceps, retractor

Hamby-Hibbs retractor

Hamdi's solution

Hamel's test

Hamilton's bandage, forceps, method, pseudophlegmon, test

Hamilton-Stewart formula

Hamm's electrode

Hamman's disease/syndrome — interstitial emphysema of the lungs from spontaneous rupture of the alveoli

Hamman's murmur, sign

Hamman-Rich syndrome — interstitial fibrosis of the lung, giving rise to right-sided heart failure

Hammar's myoid cells

Hammarsten's reagent, test

Hammer's test

Hammerschlag's method, phenomenon, test

Hammersmith's hemoglobin, prosthesis

Hammond's disease — continuous sinuous, writhing movements, especially severe in the hands

Hammond's splint

Hampson's unit

Hampton's line

Hamrick's elevator

Hamstorn's syndrome — familial intermittent adynamia

Hanafee's catheter

Hanart's disease — familial spastic paraplegia, associated with congenital mental deficiency, transmitted as a recessive trait

Hanau's laws of articulation

Hancock's operation — amputation of the foot at the ankle, with a part of the astragalus being retained in the flap, the lower surface sawed off, and the cut surface of the calcaneus brought into contact with it

Hancock's amputation, valve replacement

Hand's disease — same as *Hand-Schüller-Christian disease*

Hand-Schüller-Christian disease — a chronic form of histiocytosis with accumulation of cholesterol, characterized by defects in the membranous bones, exophthalmos, and diabetes insipidus

Handley's incision, lymphangioplasty, method

Hanes' equation

Hanganatziu-Deicher reaction, test

Hangar-Rose skin test antigen

Hanger's test

Hanhart's syndrome — a congenital syndrome marked primarily by severe micrognathia, high nose root, small eyelid fissures, low-set ears, and variable absence of digits or limbs

Hanhart's nanism

Hank's dilator

Hanke-Koessler test

Hanker-Yates reagent

Hanks-Bradley dilator

Hann's disease — an association of posterior pituitary lesions with diabetes insipidus

Hanna's splint

Hannon's curet

Hannover's canal, intermediate membrane

Hanot's disease/syndrome — biliary cirrhosis

Hanot-Chauffard syndrome — hypertrophic cirrhosis with diabetes mellitus

Hanot-Kiener syndrome — diffuse mesenchymal hepatitis with nodular lymphomatosis

Hanot-MacMahon-Thannhauser syndrome — pericholangiolitic biliary cirrhosis

Hanot-Rössle syndrome — non-obstructive extrahepatic cholangitis with obstructive intrahepatic cholangitis

Hansel's secretion stain

Hansemann's macrophage

Hansen's disease — leprosy

Hansen's bacillus

Hansen-Street nail, pin

Hanson's unit

Hantaan virus

Hapsburg's disease — hemophilia

Hapsburg's jaw, lip

Harada's disease — same as *Vogt-Koyanagi-Harada syndrome*

Harbitz-Müller disease — familial hypercholesterolemia

Harden-Young equation, ester

Harder's glands

Harding-Passey melanoma

Harding-Ruttan test

Hardy's speculum

Hardy-Weinberg equation, equilibrium, law, rule

Hare's syndrome — tumor near the apex of the lung, with neuritic pain and atrophy of the muscles of the upper extremity. Called also *Pancoast's syndrome*

Hargin's trocar

Hargraves' cell

Harkavy's syndrome — the occurrence in periarteritis nodosa of asthma, recurrent pulmonary infiltrations, eosinophilic polyserositis, pleurisy, pericar-

Harkavy's syndrome — *(continued)* ditis, and neurological symptoms

Harken's forceps, prosthesis, valve, valvulotome

Harley's disease — intermittent hemoglobinuria

Harmon's incision

Harnasch's disease — acro-osteolysis of the phalangeal diaphyses of the hand and foot with involvement of the jaws, acromion, and clavicle

Harrington's clamp, erysiphake, forceps, solution, tonometer

Harrington-Carmalt clamp

Harrington-Mayo forceps

Harrington-Mixter clamp, forceps

Harrington-Pemberton retractor

Harris' syndrome — hyperinsulinism due to a functional disorder of the pancreas

Harris' band, dissector, forceps, hematoxylin, hip prosthesis, lines, migrainous neuralgia, segregator, separator, staining method, sutures, tube

Harris-Ray test

Harrison's curve, groove, knife, prosthesis, scissors, speculum, spot test, sulcus

Harrison-Shea curet

Harrower's hypothesis

Hart's syndrome — an autosomal recessive disorder of amino acid transport, marked by a skin rash on exposure to sunlight, temporary cerebellar ataxia, and renal aminoaciduria without evident dysfunction

Hart's method, splint, test

Hartel's method, technique, treatment

Hartigan's foramen

Harting's bodies

Hartley's implant

Hartley-Krause operation — excision of the gasserian gan-

Hartley-Krause operation — *(continued)* glion and its roots for relief of trigeminal neuralgia

Hartmann's operation — resection of a diseased part of the colon, with the proximal end of the colon brought out as a colostomy and the distal stump being closed by suture

Hartmann's apraxia, catheter, colostomy, curet, forceps, fossa, point, pouch, procedure, punch, rongeur, speculum

Hartmann-Citelli forceps, punch

Hartmann-Dewaxer speculum

Hartmann-Gruenwald forceps

Hartmann-Herzfeld rongeur

Hartnup's disease — a hereditary, pellagra-like skin rash with cerebellar ataxia, renal aminoaciduria and other bizarre biochemical abnormalities

Hartridge's reversion spectroscope

Hartstein's retractor

Haseltine's clamp

Häser's coefficient, formula

Hasharon's hemoglobin

Hashimoto's disease — a progressive disease of the thyroid gland, with degeneration of its epithelial elements and replacement by lymphoid and fibrous tissue

Hashimoto's struma, thyroiditis

Haslinger's bronchoscope, electroscope, esophagoscope, laryngoscope, tracheoscope

Hasner's fold, valve

Hass' disease — disseminated neonatal herpes

Hassall's bodies, corpuscles

Hassall-Henle bodies, warts

Hasselbalch's equation

Hassin's syndrome — protrusion of the ear on the side of the lesion, combined with *Bernard-Horner syndrome*

Hata's phenomenon, preparation
Hatch's catheter
Hatchcock's sign
Hatcher's pin
Haudek's niche, sign
Haultaim's operation — modification of Huntington's operation for replacement of inverted uterus
Hauschka-Klein ascites tumor
Haverfield's cannula, retractor
Haverfield-Scoville retractor
Haverhill's clamp, fever
Hawk's test
Hawkins' forceps, fracture, keloid
Hawks-Dennen forceps
Hawley's chart, retainer
Haworth's formula
Haxthausen's syndrome — hyperkeratosis
Hay's test
Hay-Wells syndrome — ectodermal dysplasia, cleft lip and palate, and ankyloblepharon filiforme adnatum
Hayden's curet, elevator
Hayem's corpuscles, encephalitis, hematoblast, icterus, jaundice, solution
Hayem-Widal syndrome — acquired hemolytic anemia marked by a low erythrocyte count, icterus, spherocytosis, and splenomegaly
Hayes' clamp, retractor
Hayes-Olivecrona forceps
Hayflick's limit
Haygarth's nodes, nodosities
Haynes' operation — draining the cisterna magna for acute meningitis
Haynes' cannula, pin
Haynes-Griffin splint
Hayton-Williams forceps
Hazen's theorem
Head's zones
Heaf's test
Healy's forceps

Heaney's clamp, curet, forceps, hysterectomy, sutures
Heaney-Ballentine forceps
Heaney-Kantor forceps
Heaney-Rezek forceps
Heaney-Simon retractor
Hearson's capsule
Heath's operation — division of the ascending rami of the lower jaw for ankylosis — performed within the mouth
Heath's curet, dissector, forceps, scissors
Heaton's operation — for inguinal hernia
Heberden's disease(s) — rheumatism of the smaller joints accompanied by nodules around the distal interphalangeal joints; angina pectoris
Heberden's asthma, nodes, rheumatism, sign
Hebra's syndrome — a chronic skin disorder, usually beginning in infancy, marked by pruritic papules that eventually become covered with blood-colored crust
Hebra's disease — a mucocutaneous form of erythema with fever, cough, and pharyngitis; iris lesions occur, and sometimes papules, purpura, and vesiculobullous lesions may be present
Hebra's pityriasis, prurigo
Hecht's phenomenon, pneumonia, test
Hecht-Weinberg test
Hecht-Weinberg-Gradwohl reaction, test
Heck's disease — focal epithelial hyperplasia
Hector's tendon
Hedblom's syndrome — acute primary diaphragmitis
Hedblom's elevator, raspatory, retractor

Heerfordt's disease/syndrome — sarcoidosis marked by chronic inflammation of the parotid gland and the uvea

Heerman's chisel, incision

Heffernan's speculum

Hefke-Turner sign

Hegar's dilator, perineorrhaphy, sign

Hegar-Goodell dilator

Hegenbarth's forceps

Hegglin's syndrome — cardiac insufficiency during diabetic coma

Hegglin's anomaly

Hehner's number, value

Heiberg-Esmarch maneuver

Heidenhain's syndrome — a progressive, degenerative disease marked by cortical blindness, presenile dementia, ataxia, and generalized rigidity of muscle

Heidenhain's cells, demilunes, iron hematoxylin stain, law, pouch, rods

Heifitz's retractor

Heilbronner's sign, thigh

Heilmeyer-Schöner erythroblastosis

Heim-Kreysig sign

Heimlich's maneuver, tube

Heine's operation — cyclodialysis in glaucoma

Heine-Medin disease — poliomyelitis, with involvement of the central nervous system and paralysis

Heineke's operation — resection of the colon to remove tumors, done in multiple stages

Heineke-Mikulicz operation — reconstruction of the pyloric channel by incising the pylorus longitudinally and suturing the incision transversely

Heineke-Mikulicz's gastroenterostomy, herniorrhaphy, pyloroplasty

Heintz's method

Heinz's bodies, granules, stain, test

Heinz-body anemias

Heinz-Ehrlich bodies

Heise's forceps

Heisrath's operation — excision of the tarsal folds for trachoma

Heister's diverticulum, fold, valve

Heitz-Boyer clamp

Hektoen's medium, phenomenon

Hektoen, Kretschmer, and Welker protein

HeLa cells

Helanca's prosthesis

Helbing's sign

Held's end-feet, limiting membrane, space

Helfrick's retractor

Heliodorus' bandage

Hellat's sign

Hellendall's sign

Heller's syndrome — progressive infantile dementia

Heller's disease — dystrophic, median, canaliform depressions of the fingernails without apparent organic cause

Heller's operation — esophagocardiomyotomy

Heller's dementia, plexus, procedure, test

Heller-Döhle disease — syphilitic aortitis

Heller-Döhle mesoaortitis

Heller-Nelson syndrome — a variant of *Klinefelter's syndrome*, marked by atrophic testes, hyalinization of the seminiferous tubules, and elevation of urinary gonadotropins

Hellerström's disease — erythema characterized by edematous pinkish-red rings, associated with meningitis following a tick bite

Hellin's law

Hellin-Zeleny law

Helly's formol–Zenker fixative, fluid

Helmholtz's ligament, line, theory

Helmholz-Harrington syndrome — congenital clouding of the cornea associated with various abnormalities

Helweg's bundle, tract

Helweg-Larssen syndrome — a familial disease with neurolabyrinthitis developing in the fourth or fifth decade

Helwig's disease — inverted follicular keratosis

Hench-Aldrich index, test

Hench-Rosenberg syndrome — rheumatism with repeated episodes of arthritis, without fever and without irreversible damage to joints

Henderson's chisel, retractor

Henderson-Hasselbalch equation

Henderson-Jones disease — osteochondromatosis; same as *Reichel's syndrome*

Hendren's clamp, forceps

Hendrickson's drain, lithotrite

Henke's forceps, space, triangle, trigone

Henle's ampulla, ansa, band, canal, cell, fibers, fibrin, fissures, glands, incisure, layer, ligament, loop, membrane, reaction, restiform process, sheath, sinus, sphincter, spine, trapezoid bone, tubercle, tuberosity, tubule

Henle-Coenen sign, test

Hennebert's syndrome — nystagmus and vertigo on air compression of the auditory meatus, seen in congenital syphilis

Hennebert's sign, test

Henner's elevator, retractor

Henning's sign

Henny's rongeur

Henoch's disease — chronic progressive chorea of children

Henoch's chorea, purpura

Henoch-Schönlein syndrome — an eruption of purpuric

Henoch-Schönlein syndrome — (*continued*) lesions, associated with joint pains, vomiting of blood, passage of bloody stools, and sometimes glomerulonephritis

Henoch-Schönlein purpura

Henriques-Sörensen's method

Henrotin's forceps, speculum

Henry's femoral herniorrhaphy, incision, law, melanin reaction, melanin test, splenectomy

Henschen's method

Hensen's body, canal, cells, disk, duct, knot, line, node, plane, stripe

Henshaw's test

Hensing's fold, ligament

Henton's hook, needle

Hepp's osmometer

Herbert's operation — displacement of a wedge-shaped flap of sclera for formation of a filtering cicatrix in glaucoma

Herbert's pits, prosthesis

Herbert Adams clamp

Herbst's corpuscles

d'Herelle's phenomenon

Herff's clamp

Hering's canals, law, nerve, phenomenon, test, theory

Hering-Breuer reflex

Hering-Hellebrand deviation

Herlitz's syndrome — a familial, congenital and fatal variant of *Fox's disease*, marked by blisters on the skin and mucous membranes, epidermal defects, nail dystrophy, and, sometimes, skeletal atrophy

Herman's syndrome — pyramidal and extrapyramidal disorders with disturbances of speech and mentation, occurring after closed head injuries

Herman-Taylor gastroscope

Hermann's fixative

Hermann-Perutz reaction, test

Hermansky-Pudlak syndrome —
albinism, pseudohemophilia,
and pigmented macrophages
in the bone marrow

Herrenschwand's syndrome — a
difference in color of the irides, caused by sympathetic lesions

Herrick's syndrome — sickle-cell
anemia

Herrick's anemia, clamp

Herring's bodies, test

Herring-Binet test

Herrmann's syndrome — an inherited disorder of the nervous
system beginning in childhood, characterized by deafness, diabetes mellitus,
progressive dementia, pyelonephritis, and glomerulonephritis

Herrmannsdorfer's diet

Hers' disease — glycogen storage
disease

Hershell's culture medium

Hersman's disease — idiopathic
progressive enlargement of
the hands

Hertel's exophthalmometer

Herter's disease — same as *Herter-
Heubner disease*

Herter's infantilism, test

Herter-Foster method

Herter-Heubner disease — the infantile form of nontropical
sprue

Hertig-Rock ova

Hertwig's sheath

Hertwig-Magendie syndrome —
dissociation of gaze, marked
by downward and inward rotation of the eyes on the side of
a cerebellar lesion and upward and outward deviation
on the contralateral side

Hertwig-Magendie phenomenon,
sign

Hertwig-Weyers syndrome —
aplasia of the ulna with

Hertwig-Weyers syndrome —
(*continued*)
abnormalities of the sternum,
kidneys, spleen, and jaws

Herxheimer's disease — a chronic,
progressive disease of the extremities, marked by visibility
of blood vessels through a bluish, atrophic, wrinkled skin resembling tissue paper

Herxheimer's fever, fibers, reaction, spiral

Heryng's sign

Herz's triad

Herzberg's test

Heschl's convolution, gyrus

Hess' capillary test, forceps, scoop,
spoon

Hess-Barraquer forceps

Hess-Gill forceps

Hess-Horwitz forceps

Hesselbach's hernia, ligament, triangle

Hesseltine's umbiliclip

Heublein's method

Heubner's disease — syphilitic endarteritis of the cerebral vessels

Heubner's recurrent artery

Heubner's specific endarteritis

Heubner-Herter disease — the infantile form of nontropical
sprue, or celiac disease

Heuser's membrane

Hey's operation — separation of
the metatarsus from the tarsus
with removal of part of the
medial cuneiform bone

Hey's amputation, derangement,
hernia, ligament, saw

Heyd's syndrome — renal disorder
associated with diseases of the
biliary tract or the liver

Heyer-Schulte prosthesis

Heyman's capsules, forceps, law

Heyman-Paparella scissors

Heymann's glomerulonephritis, nephritis

Heyns' decompression

Heynsius' test

Hibbs' operation — fracturing the spinous processes of the vertebrae in Pott's disease

Hibbs' chisel, curet, forceps, frame, mouth gag, osteotome, retractor

Hibbs-Spratt curet

Hickey's method

Hickey-Hare test

Hickman's catheter

Hicks' syndrome — hereditary sensory radicular neuropathy

Hicks' contractions, sign, version

Hicks-Pitney thromboplastin generation test

Higbee's speculum

Higgins' catheter, incision

Highman's Congo red stain, method

Highmore's antrum, body

Higouménaki's sign

Hikojima antigen

Hildebrandt's test

Hildenbrand's disease — typhus

Hildreth's cautery

Hilger's syndrome — pain in the head and neck regions caused by vasodilation of the carotid artery and its branches

Hilger's stimulator, tube

Hill's cell, equation, reaction, sign

Hill-Ferguson retractor

Hillis' perforator, retractor

Hilsinger's knife

Hilton's law, muscle, sac, white line

Himmelstein's retractor, valvulotome

Hinckle-James speculum

Hindenlang's test

Hine-Duley phantom

Hines-Anderson pyeloureteroplasty

Hines-Bannick syndrome — intermittent attacks of low temperature

Hines-Brown test

Hinman's reflux

Hinton's test

Hippel's disease — same as *von Hippel's disease*

Hippel's trephine

Hippel-Lindau disease — retinocerebral angiomatosis; also called *von Hippel-Lindau disease*

Hippocrates' bandage

Hirand's bodies

Hirsch's syndrome — osteitis fibrosa of the ribs, sternum, and metacarpus

Hirsch-Pfeiffer stain

Hirschberg's magnet, method, reflex, sign

Hirschfeld's disease — acute diabetes mellitus

Hirschfeld's canals

Hirschfeld-Klinger reaction

Hirschfelder's tuberculin

Hirschfeldt's test

Hirschman's anoscope, forceps, proctoscope

Hirschman-Martin proctoscope

Hirschowitz's fiberscope, gastroscope

Hirschsprung's disease — congenital megacolon

Hirschtick's splint

Hirst's test

Hirst-Emmet forceps

Hirst-Hare test

His' disease — same as *His-Werner disease*

His' band, bundle, bundle electrogram, bursa, canal, duct, isthmus, space, spindle, tubercle, zones

His-Werner disease — a self-limited, louse-borne, rickettsial disease with intermittent fever, generalized aches and pains, vertigo, malaise, and multiple relapses

Hiss' capsule stain, serum water

Hitchens-Hansen antigen

Hittorf's number, tube

Hitzig's syndrome — unintentional movement of the orbicularis and other muscles innervated by the seventh cranial nerve

Hitzig's girdle, test

Hoboken's gemmules, nodules, valves

Hoche's bandelette

Hochenegg's operation — excision of the rectum, preserving the anal sphincter

Hochenegg's ulcer

Hochsinger's phenomenon, sign

Höchst's peptone

Hodara's disease — trichorrhexis of the scalp

Hodge's forceps, maneuver, pessary, planes

Hodgen's apparatus, method, splint

Hodgkin's disease — a malignant neoplasm of transformed lymphocytes, marked by painless, progressive enlargement of the lymph nodes, spleen and general lymphoid tissue

Hodgkin's cells, cycle, granuloma, lymphoma, paragranuloma, sarcoma

Hodgson's disease — aneurysmal dilatation of the aorta

Hodgson's hypospadias repair

Hoehne's sign

Hoen's elevator, forceps, hook, raspatory, scissors

Hoesch's test

Hoet-Abaza syndrome — postpartum diabetes mellitus and obesity

Hofacker-Sadler law

Hofbauer's cells

Hoff's law

Hoffa's disease — traumatic proliferation of fatty tissue in the knee joint

Hoffa's operation — same as *Lorenz's operation*

Hoffa-Kastert syndrome — chronic synovitis of the knee joint

Hoffa-Kastert syndrome — *(continued)* resulting in tumor-like lesions and adhesions that restrict joint motility

Hoffa-Lorenz operation — same as *Lorenz's operation*

Hoffmann's syndrome — muscular hypertrophy, painful spasms, pseudomyotonia, and hypothyroidism in adults

Hoffmann's anodyne, atrophy, drops, duct, forceps, phenomenon, reflex, serum, sign, test

Hoffmann-Werdnig syndrome — a hereditary, progressive form of muscular atrophy resulting from degeneration of the anterior horn cells of the spinal cord, usually followed by death in infancy or childhood

Hoffmann-Zurhelle syndrome — a lipomatous nevus of the gluteal region, marked by yellowish nodules that may become large plaques

Hofmann's bacillus, violet

Hofmeister's gastrectomy, gastroenterostomy, series, test

Hofmeister-Billroth gastrectomy

Hogben test

Hoguet's maneuver

Högyes' treatment

Hohmann's retractor

Hoke's incision, osteotome

Holden's curet, line

Holger Nielsen method

Holinger's applicator, bougie, bronchoscope, esophagoscope, forceps, laryngoscope, needle, telescope, tube

Holinger-Garfield laryngoscope

Holinger-Hurst bougie

Holinger-Jackson bronchoscope

Hollander's test

Hollenhorst's plaques

Hollerith's code

Holman's retractor

Holman-Mathieu cannula

Holman-Miller sign

Holmblad's method

Holmes' syndrome — space perception disorders caused by brain injuries, marked by inability to recognize the position, distance, and size of objects in space; impaired fixation; and absence of the blinking reflex

Holmes' disease — progressive familial ataxia with cerebello-olivary degeneration

Holmes' operation — excising the os calcis

Holmes' alkaline buffer, degeneration, forceps, method, nasopharyngoscope, phenomenon, sign, stain

Holmes-Adie syndrome — same as *Adie's syndrome*

Holmes-Stewart phenomenon

Holmgren's skeins, test

Holmgren-Golgi canals

Holt-Oram syndrome — hereditary heart disease, usually an atrial or ventricular septal defect

Holten's test

Holter's monitor, shunt, tube, valve

Holtermüller-Wiedemann syndrome — a rare, congenital form of hydrocephalus

Holth's operation — excision of the sclera by punch operation

Holth's cystotome, forceps, sclerectomy

Holthouse's hernia

Holtz's curet, machine

Holz's phlegmon

Holzer's method, stain

Holzknecht's chromoradiometer, space, stomach, unit

Homans' sign

Homén's syndrome — a genetically determined disease of the nervous system, marked by vertigo, ataxia, dysarthria, in-

Homén's syndrome — *(continued)* creasing dementia and rigidity of the body

Homer-Wright pseudorosette, rosette

Hong Kong toe

Honore-Smathers tube

Hood's dermatome

Hood-Graves speculum

Hood-Kirkland incision

Hooft's syndrome — familial hypolipidemia

Hooke's law

Hooker-Forbes test

Hooper's scissors

Hoorweg's law

Hoover's sign

Hope's resuscitator, sign

Hopf's keratosis

Hopkin's clamp, forceps, raspatory, telescope, thiophene test

Hopkins-Cole test

Hopmann's papilloma, polyp

Hopp's blade, laryngoscope

Hoppe Seyler's test

Hoppe-Goldflam disease — myasthenia gravis

Horgan's blade

Hörlein-Weber disease — chronic familial methemoglobinemia

Horn's degeneration, sign

Horner's syndrome — same as *Bernard-Horner syndrome*

Horner's law, muscle, ptosis, pupil, sign, teeth

Horner-Bernard syndrome — same as *Bernard-Horner syndrome*

Horner-Trantas spots

Horsley's operation — excision of an area of motor cortex for relief of convulsive movements of the upper extremities

Horsley's elevator, forceps, putty, pyloroplasty, sign, sutures, test, trephine, wax

Horsley-Clarke apparatus

Hortega's cell, cell tumor, method, neuroglia stain

Horton's syndrome(s) — cluster
headache; giant cell arteritis
Horton's disease(s) — migrainous
neuralgia; cluster headache; gi-
ant cell arteritis
Horton's arteritis, headache, neu-
ralgia
Hosford's dilator, spud
Hosford-Hicks forceps
Hotchkiss' operation — resection
of part of the mandible and
maxilla for epithelioma of the
cheek, with plastic restoration
of the defect
Hotchkiss-McManus technique
Hotis' test
Hottentot apron, veil
Hotz's curet, probe
Hotz-Anagnostakis procedure
Hough's forceps, hoe, method, os-
teotome
Houghton's law of fatigue, test
Hounsfield's numbers, unit
Hourin's needle
House's bur, dissector, excavator,
forceps, hammer, irrigator,
knife, prosthesis, retractor,
scissors, stapedectomy, wire
House-Barbara needle
House-Bellucci scissors
House-Dieter nipper
House-Metzenbaum scissors
House-Paparella curet
House-Rosen needle
House-Wullstein forceps
Houssay's syndrome — amelioration
of diabetes mellitus by a de-
structive lesion of the pitu-
itary gland
Houssay's animal, phenomenon
Housset-Debray gastroscope
Houston's muscle, valves
Houtz's curet
Hovius' canal, circle, membrane,
plexus
Howard's abrader, forceps, method,
stone basket, test
Howel-Evans' syndrome — pal-
moplantar keratoderma oc-

Howel-Evans' syndrome —
(continued)
curring between the ages of 5
and 15 and associated with
development of esopha-
geal cancer in later life
Howell's bodies, method, test, unit
Howell-Jolly bodies
Howorth's elevator, osteotome, re-
tractor
Howship's lacuna
Howship-Romberg syndrome —
neuralgic pain in the leg
caused by obturator hernia
Hoxworth's forceps
Hoyle's medium
Hoyne's sign
Hoyt's forceps
Hryniuk's dose-intensity hypothesis
Hryntschak's catheter
Hsieh's method
Hubbard's bolt, electrode, forceps,
tank
Hubbenet's spots
Hubell's meatoscope
Hübl number
Huchard's disease — continued ar-
terial hypertension; a possible
cause of arteriosclerosis
Huchard's sign, symptom
Hucker-Conn crystal violet solu-
tion, stain
Huckman's number
Huddleson's test
Hudgins' cannula
Hudson's brace, clamp, drill, for-
ceps, lactone rule, line, ron-
geur
Hudson-Stähli line
Huebener-Thomsen-Friedenreich
phenomenon
Hueck's ligament
Huët-Pelger nuclear anomaly
Hueter's bandage, line, maneuver,
sign
Huey's scissors
Huffman's speculum, vaginoscope
Huffman-Graves speculum

Hufnagel's clamp, forceps, prosthesis, valve

Hufner's equation

Huggins' operation — castration for cancer of the prostate

Huggins' test

Hugh-Leifson medium

Hughes' eye implant, reflex

Hughes-Stovin syndrome — pulmonary arterial thrombosis, pulmonary arterial aneurysm, and peripheral venous thrombosis

Hughes-Young adrenalectomy, incision

Hughston's method

Huguenin's edema

Huguier's canal, circle, sinus

Huguier-Jersild syndrome — lymphedema of the rectal and external genital regions, often with stricture of the anus and introitus vaginae, caused by syphilis, gonorrhea, ulcers, or lymphogranuloma venereum

Huhner's test

Huldshinsky's radiation

Human's sign

Humby's knife

Hume's clamp

Humphrey's tubercle

Humphries' clamp

Humphry's ligament

Hünermann's disease — a hereditary condition marked by multiple opacities of the epiphyses, dwarfism, cataract, shortened digits, dulled mentation, and general debility; usually a cause of death in the first year of life

Hunner's cystitis, stricture, ulcer

Hunt's syndrome — facial paralysis accompanied by otalgia and vesicular eruption of the external canal of the ear, caused by herpes zoster virus infection; called also *Ramsay Hunt syndrome*

Hunt's disease — generalized tremor due to disturbance of muscle tone and of muscular coordination associated with myoclonic epilepsy

Hunt's atrophy, clamp, epilepsy, forceps, method, neuralgia, paradoxical phenomenon, paralysis, reaction, sound, test, tremor, trocar

Hunt-Lawrence pouch

Hunt-Transley procedure

Hunter's syndrome — same as *Hunter-Hurler syndrome*

Hunter's operation — ligation of an artery for aneurysm

Hunter's canal, chancre, curet, glossitis, gubernaculum, ligament, line, separator

Hunter-Given method

Hunter-Hurler syndrome — an error of mucopolysaccharide metabolism, similar to *Hurler's syndrome* but distinguished by less severe skeletal effects

Hunter-Schreger bands, lines

Huntington's disease — a rare, hereditary disease marked by chronic, progressive chorea and severe mental deterioration

Huntington's operation — replacement of a chronically inverted uterus through an opening in the abdominal wall below the umbilicus

Huntington's chorea, sign

Hupp's retractor

Huppert's test

Huppert-Cole test

Hurd's dissector, elevator, forceps, retractor

Hurler's syndrome — a defect of mucopolysaccharide metabolism, with accumulation of abnormal cellular material in the urine and with severe abnormalities of skeletal bone

Hurler's syndrome — (continued) and cartilage, including dwarfism, and marked by deformity of limbs and mental retardation

Hurler's polydystrophy

Hurler-Pfaundler syndrome — same as *Hurler's syndrome*

Hurler-Scheie syndrome — allelic disorder of mucopolysaccharidosis characterized by receding chin with mental retardation, dwarfism, corneal clouding, deafness, claw hand, and valvular heart disease

Hurler-Scheie compound

Hurst's disease — an acute, fatal disease marked by cerebral hemorrhage, leukocytic infiltrations, and vascular degeneration

Hurst's bougie, dilator

Hürthle cell adenoma, cell carcinoma, cell metaplasia, cell nodule, cell tumor

Hurtig's dilator

Hurtley's test

Hurwitz's clamp, trocar

Huschke's auditory teeth, canal, foramen, ligaments, valve

Huse's cannula

Husks' rongeur

Hutch's diverticulum, evacuator

Hutchins' needle

Hutchinson's disease — a papular form of polymorphous benign eruption; Tay's choroiditis

Hutchinson's facies, freckle, incisor, mask, patch, prurigo, pupil, sign, teeth, triad, -type neuroblastoma

Hutchinson-Boeck disease/syndrome — sarcoidosis

Hutchinson-Gilford disease/syndrome — progeria

Hutchison's syndrome — neuroblastoma with cranial metastases

Hutinel's disease(s) — tuberculous pericarditis with cirrhosis of the liver in children; erythema due to an infection

Huxley's layer, membrane

Hyams' clamp

Hyde's syndrome — a form of severe, pruritic, nodular, and verrucous skin eruption consisting of lesions of the back, extremities, and thighs, usually in adult women

Hyde's disease — an eruption of hard nodules in the skin, accompanied by intense itching

Hynes' pharyngoplasty

Hyrtl's anastomosis, canal, loop, recess, sphincter

Iceland disease — chronic fatigue syndrome

Ide's reaction, test

Iglesias's resectoscope

Ihle's paste

Ilfeld-Gustafson splint

Ilfeld-Holder deformity

Ilheus encephalitis, virus

Iliff's trephine

Ilimow's test

Ilosvay's reagent, test

Imerslund syndrome — same as *Imerslund-Gräsbeck syndrome*

Imerslund-Gräsbeck syndrome — a chronic, relapsing, familial form of megaloblastic anemia

Imerslund-Gräsbeck syndrome —
(continued)
in children, with onset between the ages of five months
and four years; principal signs
and symptoms are pallor,
weakness, irritability, dyspnea,
fever, gastrointestinal problems with diarrhea and vomiting, lack of appetite, glossitis, jaundice, heart murmurs,
and proteinuria
Imerslund-Najman-Gräsbeck
syndrome — same as Imers-
lund-Gräsbeck syndrome
Imhoff's tank
Imlach's fat plug
Immergut's tube
Inaba antigen
Indian operation — reconstruction
of a nose by a flap of skin
from the forehead; also called
Carpue's operation
Indian childhood cirrhosis, rat
flea
Indianapolis hemoglobin
Ingals' speculum
Inge's procedure
Ingersoll's curet, needle
Ingrassia's apophysis, process,
wings
Inikawa-Ogura method
Ionescu's method
Ionescu-Shiley valve
Irvine's syndrome — macular
edema that occasionally fol-
lows cataract surgery
Irvine's scissors
Irving's sterilization operation —
tubal ligation in which the

Irving's sterilization operation —
(continued)
uterine tubes are ligated and
severed
Isaacs' syndrome — same as Isaacs-
Mertens syndrome
Isaacs' syringe
Isaacs-Ludwig arteriole
Isaacs-Mertens syndrome — pro-
gressive muscle stiffness and
spasms
Isambert's disease — acute miliary
tuberculosis of the larynx and
pharynx
Isherwood's methods
Ishihara's plate, test
Israel's dissector, familial jaundice,
retraction, shunt
Israëls-Wilkinson anemia
Israelson's reaction, test
Italian operation — reconstruction
of the nose by a flap of skin
taken from the arm
Itaqui virus
Itard's catheter
Itard-Cholewa sign
Ito's nevus
Ito-Reenstierna reaction, test
Itsenko-Cushing syndrome — same
as Cushing's syndrome due to
hyperadrenocorticism
Ivalon's implant, patch, sutures
Ivemark's syndrome — imperfect
splenic development and car-
diac malformation
Iverson's dermabrader
Ives' speculum
Ivy's method, rongeur
Iwanoff's (Iwanow's) cysts
Izar's reagent

J

Jaboulay's operation — interpelviabdominal amputation

Jaboulay's amputation, button

Jaccoud's syndrome — chronic arthritis occurring after rheumatic fever

Jaccoud's arthritis, arthropathy, fever, sign

Jackson Personality Inventory

Jackson Vocational Interest Survey

Jackson's syndrome — paralysis of the tenth, eleventh, and twelfth cranial nerves, soft palate, larynx, and one half of the tongue and the sternomastoid and trapezius muscles

Jackson's bronchoscope, clamp, dilator, epilepsy, forceps, incision, laryngoscope, law, membrane, rule, safety triangle, scissors, sign, tube, veil

Jackson-MacKenzie syndrome — same as *Jackson's syndrome*

Jackson-Moore shears

Jackson-Mosher dilator

Jackson-Plummer dilator

Jackson-Pratt drain

Jackson-Trousseau dilator

Jacob's disease — permanent constriction of the mandible, with inability to open the mouth

Jacob's clamp, forceps, membrane, ulcer

Jacobaeus' operation — thoracoscopy and cauterization for treatment of adhesions

Jacobi's disease — a form of poikiloderma characterized by telangiectasia, pigmentation and atrophy of the skin and oral mucosa

Jacobs' syndrome — a deficiency disease characterized by exfoli-

Jacobs' syndrome — (continued) ating dermatitis of the scrotum, stomatitis, and conjunctivitis

Jacobs-Palmer laparoscope

Jacobson's anastomosis, canal, cartilage, clamp, forceps, nerve, organ, plexus, retinitis, retractor, scissor, sulcus

Jacobsthal's test

Jacoby's test

Jacod's syndrome — complete paralysis of the eye muscles, blindness, and trigeminal neuralgia

Jacod's triad

Jacquart's angle

Jacquemin's test

Jacquet's biokinetic treatment, dermatitis, erythema

Jadassohn's disease — a skin disorder marked by slightly elevated, red papules that appear first at the elbow area and later spread to other parts of the arm and forearm and hand

Jadassohn's anetoderma, macular atrophy, sebaceous nevus, test

Jadassohn-Bloch test

Jadassohn-Lewandowsky syndrome — a rare congenital disorder, marked by abnormal thickening of the nails that progresses to hyperkeratosis of the palms, soles, knees, and elbows and leukoplakia of the oral mucous membranes

Jadassohn-Pellizari anetoderma

Jadassohn-Tièche nevus

Jadelot's furrows, lines

Jaeger's keratome, knife, lid retractor, test type 1, 2, and 3

Jaeger-Whiteley catheter

Jaffé's assay, reaction, test

Jaffe-Lichtenstein disease/syndrome — fibrous dysplasia of bone

Jaffe-Lichtenstein-Uehlinger syndrome — same as *Jaffe-Lichtenstein disease/syndrome*

Jahnke's syndrome — congenital angiomas of the leptomeninges and choroid, often associated with intracranial calcification, hemiplegia, and epilepsy; a variant of the *Sturge-Kalischer-Weber syndrome* without glaucoma

Jahnke-Cook-Seeley clamp

Jako's knife, laryngoscope

Jakob's disease — same as *Creutzfeldt-Jakob disease*

Jakob's pseudosclerosis

Jakob-Creutzfeldt disease — same as *Creutzfeldt-Jakob disease*

Jakob-Creutzfeldt pseudosclerosis

Jakobson's malignancy grading system

Jaksch's disease — deficiency of hemoglobin, poikilocytosis, erythroblastosis, severe leukocytosis, and hepatomegaly in infants and children

Jaksch's anemia, test

Jaksch-Hayem syndrome — same as *Jaksch's disease*

Jaksch-Hayem-Luzet syndrome — same as *Jaksch's disease*

Jalaguier's incision

Jamaican neuropathy, vomiting sickness

Jamar's dynamometer

James' fiber

James-Lange theory

Jameson's forceps, hook, needle

Jamestown Canyon virus

Jamshidi's needle

Janbon's syndrome — a gastrointestinal syndrome resembling cholera, produced by oxytetracycline

Janet's disease(s) — functional neurosis marked by morbid fears, obsessions and a sense of inadequacy and self-accusation; feelings of unreality and depersonalization

Janet's test

Janeway's gastroscope, gastrostomy, lesion, pills, sphygmomanometer, spots

Janin's tetanus

Jannetta's procedure, retractor

Janosik's embryo

Jansen's disease — metaphyseal dysostosis

Jansen's operation — for disease of frontal sinus

Jansen's forceps, periosteotome, raspatory, retractor, test

Jansen-Gifford retractor

Jansen-Gruenwald forceps

Jansen-Middleton forceps

Jansen-Newhart probe

Jansen-Struycken forceps

Jansen-Wagner retractor

Janský's classification, screening index

Jansky-Bielschowsky disease — juvenile form of cerebral sphingolipidosis

Janus' syndrome — same as *Bret's syndrome*

Japanese B encephalitis virus

Jaquet's apparatus

Jarcho's syndrome — metastatic carcinoma of the bone marrow associated with thrombocytopenia and purpura

Jarcho's cannula, pressometer

Jarcho-Levin syndrome — spondylothoracic dysplasia

Jarisch-Herxheimer reaction

Jarjavay's muscle

Jarotzky's (Jarotsky's) treatment

Jarvis' operation — removal of a portion of the lower turbinate bone

Jarvis' clamp, snare

Javal's ophthalmometer
Javid's clamp, shunt, tube
Jaworski's bodies, corpuscles, test
Jayle-Ourgaud syndrome — ataxic nystagmus
Jeanselme's nodules
Jeddah ulcer
Jefferson's syndrome — edema of the conjunctiva, upper lid, and root of the nose with paralysis of the third, fourth, and sixth cranial nerves and involvement of the ophthalmic branch of the fifth cranial nerve
Jefferson's retractor
Jegher's syndrome — same as *Peutz-Jeghers syndrome*
Jelanko's splint
Jelks' operation — incision of fibrous tissue around the rectum performed for stricture of the rectum
Jellinek's sign, symptom
Jelm's catheter
Jendrassik's maneuver, sign
Jendrassik-Grof method
Jenkins' Activity Survey
Jenner's stain
Jenner-Giemsa blood-smear staining
Jenner-Kay test, unit
Jennings' mouth gag, test
Jennings-Skillern mouth gag
Jensen's disease — a condition marked by a small area of inflammation on the fundus close to the papilla, usually seen in young healthy persons
Jensen's classification, retinitis, sarcoma, tumor
Jergesen's reamer, tube
Jerne's plaque assay, plaque technique
Jerry-Slough virus
Jersild's syndrome — same as *Huguier-Jersild syndrome*
Jervell and Lange-Nielsen syndrome — attacks of syncope

Jervell and Lange-Nielsen syndrome — *(continued)* and sudden death in persons congenitally deaf and with cardiac anomalies
Jesberg's bronchoscope, esophagoscope, forceps, tube
Jesionek's lamp
Jesness' Behavior Checklist
Jesse-Stryker saw
Jeune's syndrome — asphyxiating thoracic dystrophy
Jewett's nail, prosthesis, sound
Jewett-Strong staging system
J. Howard Mueller virus
Jirásek-Zuelzer-Wilson syndrome — congenital neurogenic ileus
Job's syndrome — a chronic granulomatous disease affecting girls with red hair and fair skin, marked by recurrent staphylococcal abscesses and eczema
Jobert's fossa, sutures
Jobert de Lamballe sutures
Jobst's pump
Jocasta complex
Jochmann's test
Joel-Baker anastomosis, tube
Joest's bodies
Joffroy's reflex, sign
John Milton Hagen antibody
John Milton Society for the Blind
Johne's disease — a lethal form of chronic enteritis caused by *Mycobacterium paratuberculosis*, usually affecting mammals other than humans
Johne's bacillus
Johns Hopkins University
Johnson's syndrome — pseudoparalysis of lateral or superior rectus muscles
Johnson's forceps, knife, modification method, retractor, stone basket, test, twin wire appliance
Johnson-Kenney screening test

Johnson-Kerrison punch

Johnson-Stevens disease — a severe form of erythema multiforme, with involvement of the oronasal and anogenital mucosa, eyes, and viscera; also called *Stevens-Johnson syndrome*

Johnson-Tooke knife

Johnston's clamp, dilator

Jolles' test

Jolliffe's syndrome — an almost always fatal condition thought to be caused by nicotinic acid deficiency, characterized by clouding of consciousness, cogwheel rigidity of the extremities, and uncontrollable grasping and sucking reflexes

Jolly's bodies, reaction

Jonas' symptom

Jonas-Graves speculum

Jonell's splint

Jones' disease — familial fibrous dysplasia of the jaws

Jones' albumosuria, clamp, criteria, cylinder, dilator, forceps, method, nasal splint, position, protein, scissors

Jones-Campbell staging system

Jones-Cantarow test

Jones-Mote reactivity

Jonge's position

Jonnesco's operation — sympathectomy

Jonnesco's fold, fossa

Jonston's arc

Joplin's forceps, toe prosthesis

Jordan's tartrate culture medium

Jordan-Day bur, drill

Jorgenson's retractor, scissors

Jorissen's test

Joseph's syndrome — an inborn defect of amino acid metabolism, characterized by a high protein level in the cerebrospinal fluid; excessive amounts

Joseph's syndrome — *(continued)* of glycine, proline, and hydroxyproline in the urine; and convulsions

Joseph's disease — same as *Azorean disease*

Joseph's clamp, elevator, periosteotome, raspatory, scissors

Joseph-Killian elevator

Joseph-Maltz saw, scissors

Josephs-Diamond-Blackfan anemia

Joslin Diabetes Center

Joubert's syndrome — a congenital disorder marked by partial or complete absence of the cerebellar vermis, mental retardation and abnormal eye movements

Joule's equivalent, law

Jourdain's disease — suppurative inflammation of the gums and alveolar processes

Judd's clamp, forceps, method, trocar

Judd-Allis clamp, forceps

Judd-DeMartel forceps

Judd-Masson retractor

Judet's dissector, prosthesis

Juers' forceps

Juers-Derlacki holder

Juers-Lempert forceps, rongeur

Juhel-Rénoy's syndrome — bilateral renal cortical necrosis

Jukes family

Julian's forceps, needle holder

Julian-Fildes clamp

Jung's method, muscle

Jungbluth's vessels

Jüngling's disease — sarcoidosis

Jüngling's polycystic osteitis

Junin virus

Junker's apparatus, bottle, inhaler

Junkman-Schoeller unit

Junod's boot

Jurasz's forceps

Jürgen's syndrome — hemorrhagic diathesis

Jürgensen's sign

Juri's flap
Juster's reflex
Justus' test
Jutte's tube
Juvara's fold

juvenile Paget's disease — a hereditary condition marked by abnormally high serum alkaline phosphatase levels and abnormal enlargement of the skull

• **K**

Kabatschnik's test
Kabuki make-up syndrome — a congenital or inherited syndrome of mental retardation, dwarfism, scoliosis, and cardiovascular abnormalities
Kader's operation — same as *Kader-Senn operation*
Kader's needle
Kader-Senn operation — gastrostomy, allowing a feeding tube to be introduced through a valvelike flap that closes when the tube is withdrawn
Kaes' feltwork, line
Kaes-Bekhterev layer
Kafka's reaction, test
Kahlbaum's disease — catatonic schizophrenia
Kahler's disease — multiple myeloma
Kahler's forceps, law
Kahn's albumin A reaction, cannula, dilator, scissors, tenaculum, test
Kahn-Graves speculum
Kaiser's nuclei
Kaiserling's fixative, fluid, method, solution
Kaiser-Permanente diet
Kaiserstuhl disease — arsenic poisoning
Kalischer's disease — same as *Dimitri's disease*
Kallikak family
Kallmann's syndrome — hypogonadism with olfactory anesthesia

Kalmuk idiocy, type
Kalt's forceps, needle, sutures
Kaminer's reaction
Kammerer's incision
Kanagawa's phenomenon
Kanavel's cannula, cock-up splint, conductor, sign, triangle
Kandel's method
Kane's clamp
Kanner's syndrome — a severe emotional disturbance of childhood, marked by inability to form meaningful interpersonal relationships
Kansas hemoglobin
Kantor's clamp, forceps, sign
Kantor-Geis test
Kantrowicz's clamp, forceps
Kaplan's lymphoma, needle, test
Kaplan-Meier method, stratification, survival curve, technique
Kaposi's disease(s) — a skin disease marked by numerous whitish punctiform papules and brownish macules arranged in a necklace-like pattern; a chronic, exfoliative disease of the skin marked by dry, acuminate papules surrounding the hair follicles; a rare variant of lichen planus
Kaposi's angiomatosis, dermatitis, dermatosis, sarcoma, varicelliform eruption, xeroderma
Kaposi-Irgang disease — a variation of discoid lupus erythematosus

Kapp's clamp
Kapp-Beck clamp
Kappeler's maneuver
Kaproski's antigen
Kapsinow's test
Kara's erysiphake
Karapandzic's flap
Karell's cure, diet, treatment
Karmen's unit
Karnofsky's performance score,
    scale, stain
Karplus' sign
Karr's method
Karras' needle
Kartagener's syndrome — a heredi-
    tary disorder of dextrocardia,
    bronchiectasis, and sinusitis
Kartagener's disease — a mild form
    of pulmonary infiltration oc-
    curring in eosinophilia
Kartagener's triad
Kasabach's method
Kasabach-Merritt syndrome — giant
    hemangiomas of the skin and
    spleen in infants
Kasai's operation — surgical anasto-
    mosis of the jejunum to a de-
    capsulated area of liver and to
    the duodenum
Kashida's sign
Kashin-Beck disease — same as
    Kashin-Bek disease
Kashin-Bek disease — a slowly pro-
    gressive, chronic, disabling,
    degenerative disease of the pe-
    ripheral joints and spine, oc-
    curring chiefly in children
Kashiwado's test
Kaslow's tube
Kast's syndrome — enchondro-
    matosis associated with multi-
    ple cutaneous or visceral hem-
    angiomas; usually called
    Maffucci's syndrome
Kasten's fluorescent Feulgen stain,
    fluorescent PAS stain, fluo-
    rescent Schiff reagent
Kastle's test

Kastle-Meyer test
Katayama's disease — acute sys-
    temic schistosomiasis caused
    by heavy infection from *Schis-*
    tosoma japonicum marked by
    fever, chills, nausea, and vom-
    iting, cough, headache, hepa-
    tosplenomegaly, and lymph-
    adenopathy
Katayama's fever, test
Kathrein's test
Kato's thick smear technique, test
Katsch's chisel
Katz's formula, scale
Katzin's scissors
Katzin-Barraquer forceps
Kauffman-White classification,
    scheme
Kaufman's forceps, pneumonia,
    prosthesis, syringe, vitrector
Kaufman-McKusick syndrome — a
    rare disorder marked by a col-
    lection of watery fluid in the
    uterus and vagina accompa-
    nied by post axial polydactyly,
    congenital cardiac defects,
    and sometimes bilateral hydro-
    nephrosis
Kaufmann-Peterson base
Kaufman's Developmental Scale
Kaup's index
Kawasaki disease — an erythema-
    tous febrile disease of un-
    known etiology accompanied
    by conjunctivitis, pharyngitis,
    cervical lymphadenopathy,
    vasculitis, and other signs of
    toxic systemic involvement
Kay's annuloplasty
Kay-Bodansky method
Kay-Shiley valve prosthesis
Kay-Suzuki valve prosthesis
Kayser's disease — hepatolenticular
    degeneration
Kayser-Fleischer ring
Kazanjian's operation(s) — surgical
    extension of the buccal vestib-
    ular sulcus of edentulous

Kazanjian's operation(s) —
    (*continued*)
    ridges; extraskeletal fixation
    for support in zygomaticomax-
    illary fractures
Kazanjian's forceps, scissors, splint,
    T bar
Kazanjian-Cottle forceps
Kearns' syndrome — pigmentary
    retinal dystrophy and cardio-
    myopathy
Kearns' dilator
Kearns-Sayre syndrome — pro-
    gressive ophthalmoplegia,
    degeneration of the retina,
    myopathy, ataxia, and cardio-
    myopathy
Keating-Hart fulguration, method,
    treatment
Kedani disease — scrub typhus
Keegan's operation — a modifica-
    tion of the Indian rhinoplasty
    for reconstructing the nose
Keeler's cryophake
Keeley's cure, vein stripper
Keen's operation — omphalectomy
Keen's point, sign
Kehr's incision, sign, tube
Kehrer's reflex
Keidel's tube
Keith's bundle, drain, low ionic
    diet, needle, node, scissors
Keith-Flack node
Keith-Wagener classification, reti-
    nopathy
Keith-Wagener-Barker classifica-
    tion
Keith-Welti-Ernst method
Keitzer's urethrotome
Kell antigen, factor blood group
Kell-Cellano blood group
Keller's bunionectomy, cresyl echt
    violet stain
Keller-Blake splint
Keller-Killian reaction
Kelley's gouge
Kelling's gastroscope, test
Kellock's sign

Kelly's operation(s) — for correc-
    tion of urinary incontinence
    in women; surgical fixation of
    arytenoid cartilage or muscle
Kelly's adenotome, cystoscope, en-
    doscope, forceps, hemostat,
    proctoscope, sigmoidoscope,
    sign, speculum, sphinctero-
    scope, sutures
Kelly-Gray curet
Kelly-Murphy forceps
Kelly-Sims retractor
Kelman pharmacoemulsification
Kelman's cryostylet, cystotome,
    extractor, forceps
Kelsey's clamp
Kelvin's scale, thermometer
Kemerova virus
Kemp Harper method
Kempf's disease — acute homosex-
    ual panic
Kempner's diet
Kempson's grading system
Ken's plate
Kendall's compound A., B., E. and
    F., culture medium, method
Kendrick's extrication device
Kennedy's syndrome — same as
    Foster Kennedy syndrome
Kennedy's bar, classification, for-
    ceps
Kenner fecal medium
Kenny's syndrome — a familial syn-
    drome marked by intrauterine
    dwarfism, late closure of the
    anterior fontanel, thickening
    of the tubular bones, myopia
    and transient hypocalcemia,
    and hyperphosphatemia
Kenny's method, treatment
Kent's bundle, forceps
Kent-His bundle
Kentmann's test
Kenya hemoglobin
Kerandel's sign, symptom
Kerckring's folds, nodules, ossicles,
    valves
Kergaradec's sign

Kerley's lines
Kern's isotypic determinant, forceps, plasma relation theory
Kernan-Jackson bronchoscope
Kernechtrot's method
Kerner's test
Kernig's sign
Kerr's cesarean section, rongeur, sign, splint
Kerrison's forceps, retractor, rongeur
Kerry's reducing substance test
Kershner-Adams syndrome — chronic, nonspecific, suppurative pneumonitis
Keshan disease — a fatal, congestive cardiomyopathy due to deficiency of essential elements in the diet, affecting children and women of childbearing age
Kessel's plate
Kessler's sutures
Kestenbach-Anderson procedure
Kestenbaum's sign
Kety-Schmidt method
Kevorkian's curet, forceps
Kevorkian-Young curet, forceps
Ken Gardens spotted fever — a mild febrile disease transmitted by a mite from a house mouse, marked by lesions, rash, headache, and backache
Key's operation — the lateral operation of lithotomy done with a straight staff
Key's elevator
Key-Retzius connective tissue sheath, foramen, lateral aperature
Keyes' chisel, lithotrite, punch
Kezerian's chisel, curet, gouge, osteotome
Kidd's antibody, antigen blood group, cystoscope, tube
Kidde-Robbins tourniquet
Kiel's classification, graft
Kielland's (Kjelland's) forceps

Kielland-Luikart forceps
Kienböck's disease — slowly progressive osteochondrosis of the carpal lunate bone
Kienböck's atrophy, dislocation, luxation, phenomenon, syringomyelia, unit
Kienböck-Adamson points
Kiernan's spaces
Kiersley Temperament Sorter
Kiesselbach's area, space
Kilian's line, pelvis
Killan's triangle
Killgren's treatment
Killian's operation — excision of the anterior wall of the frontal sinus, with removal of diseased tissue and formation of a permanent communication with the nose
Killian's bronchoscope, forceps, incision, knife, speculum, test, tube
Killian-Eichen cannula
Killian-Freer operation — submucous resection of the nasal septum
Killian-King retractor
Killian-Reinhard chisel
Kilner's hook, scissors
Kilner-Dott mouth gag
Kiloh-Nevin syndrome — ocular myopathy in persons with ptosis and paralysis of the external ocular muscles
Kimball's catheter, hook
Kimmelstiel-Wilson syndrome — glomerulosclerosis associated with diabetes, albuminuria, hypertension, and nephrotic edema
Kimmelstiel-Wilson lesion
Kimpton-Brown tube
Kimura's disease — angiolymphoid hyperplasia
Kinberg's test
King's operation — surgical fixation of arytenoid cartilage or muscle

King's syndrome — malignant hyperthermia, with physical abnormalities including short stature, curvature of the spinal column, progressive myopathy, and cardiovascular defects

King's brace, retractor, traction, unit

King-Armstrong method, unit

King-Hurd dissector, retractor

King-Prince forceps

King-Steelquist amputation

Kingsley's forceps, splint

Kinnier Wilson disease — hepatolenticular degeneration

Kinsbourne syndrome — myoclonic encephalopathy of childhood

Kinsella's elevator

Kinsella-Buie clamp

Kinyoun's carbolfuchsin stain

Kirby's keratome, knife, scissors, sutures

Kirby-Bauer agar diffusion test

Kirchoff's law

Kirchner's diverticulum

Kirk's amputation, mallet

Kirkland's disease — acute infection of the throat with regional lymphadenitis

Kirkland's knife, retractor

Kirkpatrick's forceps

Kirmisson's operation — transplantation of the Achilles tendon to the peroneus longus muscle in clubfoot

Kirmisson's elevator, raspatory

Kirschner's apparatus, wire, wire splint

Kirstein's method

Kirsten murine sarcoma

Kisch's reflex

Kisselbach's area

Kistner's button, dissector, probe, tube

Kitasato's broth, filter, glucoseformate gelatin

Kite's method, sign

Kitner's dissector, forceps

Kittel's treatment

Kittrich's stain

Kitzmiller's test

Kiwisch's bandage

Kjeldahl's method, technique, test

Klaff's speculum

Klapp's creeping treatment

Klatskin's needle, tumor

Klauder's syndrome — congenital maldevelopment of organs of ectodermal derivation — nervous system, retina, eyeball and skin

Klebs' disease — glomerulonephritis

Klebs' tuberculin

Klebs-Löffler bacillus

Kleihauer's stain, technique, test

Kleihauer-Betke test

Klein's bacillus, punch, reaction, test

Klein-Gumprecht nuclei

Klein-Waardenburg syndrome — same as *Waardenburg's syndrome*

Kleine-Levin syndrome — periodic somnolence, morbid hunger, and motor unrest, often associated with psychosis; usually occurs in adolescent boys.

Kleinert's sutures

Kleinschmidt's syndrome — influenzal infection resulting in laryngeal stenosis, suppurative pericarditis, pleuropneumonia, and, sometimes, suppurative meningitis

Kleinschmidt's technique

Kleist's apraxia, sign

Klemm's sign, tetanus

Klemme's hook, retractor

Klemperer's disease — disease of the spleen secondary to portal hypertension; also called *Banti's disease*

Klemperer's tuberculin

Klenow's fragment

Kliger's iron agar

Klimow's test

Kline's test

Kline-Young test

Klinefelter's syndrome — a chromosomal anomaly characterized by small testes, glassy seminiferous tubules, azospermia, infertility, and elevated urinary gonadotropins

Klinger-Ludwig acid-thionin stain

Klippel's disease — arthritic general pseudoparalysis

Klippel-Feil syndrome — a congenital defect marked by fusion of the cervical vertebrae and abnormalities of the brain stem and cerebellum

Klippel-Feil deformity, sign

Klippel-Feldstein syndrome — simple familial cranial hypertrophy

Klippel-Trenaunay syndrome — a rare condition affecting only one extremity, marked by hypertrophy of bone and soft tissues, large cutaneous hemangiomas, and varices

Klippel-Trenaunay-Weber syndrome — same as *Klippel-Trenaunay syndrome*

Kloepfer's syndrome — complete blindness beginning at two months of age, with blistering after exposure to sunlight, cessation of growth at the age of five or six years, and progressive mental retardation

Klondike bed

Klotz's syndrome — primary amenorrhea, genital infantilism, aplasia of the labia minora, small nonovulating ovaries and progressive sclerosis, male chromosomal sex, slight mongoloid facies, and, sometimes, hypertrichosis

Klumpke's palsy, paralysis

Klumpke-Dejerine syndrome — atrophic paralysis of the muscles of the arm and hand from a lesion of the eighth cervical and first dorsal nerves; called also *Klumpke's paralysis*

Klüver-Barrera method, Luxol fast blue stain

Klüver-Bucy syndrome — bizarre behavioral disturbances following bilateral temporal lobectomy

Knapp's operation — the formation of a peripheral opening in the capsule behind the iris, without iridectomy

Knapp's cystotome, forceps, knife, law, retractor, scissors, speculum, streaks, striae, test

Knie's sign

Kniest's syndrome — a type of dwarfism marked by short limbs, round face, stiffness of joints, contracture of fingers, and often cleft palate, scoliosis and deafness

Knight's brace, forceps, scissors

Knight-Sluder forceps

Knoepfelmacher's butter meal

Knoop hardness number

Knops' antigen

Knott's technique, test

Knowles's pin, scissors

Knudsen number

Kobak's needle

Kobelt's cyst, tubes, tubules

Kober's reagent, test

Kobert's test

Köbner's response

Koby's cataract

Kobyashi's hook

Koch's bacillus, ileostomy reservoir, law, lymph, node, phenomenon, postulates, reaction, test, triangle, tuberculin

Koch-Mason dressing

Koch-McMeekin method

Koch-Weeks bacillus, hemophilus

Kocher's operation(s) — a method of excising the ankle joint; a method of reducing a subcoracoid dislocation of the humerus; excision of the tongue; a method of mobilizing the duodenum; a method of pylorectomy

Kocher's syndrome — leukopenia resulting from granulocytopenia, occasionally accompanying thyrotoxicosis

Kocher's clamp, dilation ulcer, forceps, incision, maneuver, method, point, reflex, retractor, sign, spoon, symptom

Kocher-Crotti retractor

Kocher-Debré-Sémélaigne syndrome — same as *Debré-Sémélaigne syndrome*

Kock procedure

Kocks' operation — shortening of the base of the broad ligament by the vaginal route for uterine retroversion or prolapse

Koeberlé's forceps

Koebner's phenomenon

Koeffler Golde-1 cell line

Koenecke's reaction, test

Koenen's tumor

Koenig's syndrome — alternating attacks of constipation and diarrhea, sometimes symptomatic of cecal tuberculosis

Koenig-Wichman disease — chronic pemphigus

Koeppe's disease(s) — epithelial punctate keratitis; corneal dystrophy with a clearly defined grayish-white band on the cornea, visible to the naked eye

Koeppe's lens, nodules

Koerber-Salus-Elschnig syndrome — irregular oscillation

Koerber-Salus-Elschnig syndrome — (*continued*) of the eyeballs, either horizontal, lateral, or rotatory, with retraction of the eye backward into the orbit when the direction of sight changes

Kofferath's syndrome — obstetric diaphragmatic paralysis

Koffler's forceps

Koffler-Lillie forceps

Koga's treatment

Kogan's endospeculum

Kogoj's abscess, pustule

Köhler's bone disease — either osteochondrosis of the tarsal navicular bone in children or a disorder of the second metatarsal bone with thickening of its shaft and changes about its articular head, the latter often called *Köhler's second bone disease*

Köhler's illumination

Köhler-Pellegrini-Stieda disease — same as *Pellegrini-Stieda disease*

Köhlmeier-Degos disease — a cutaneovisceral syndrome characterized by pathognomonic papules followed by development of intestinal ulcers that perforate, causing peritonitis

Kohlrausch's folds, valves, veins

Kohn's needle, pores, technique

Kohnstamm's phenomenon

Kokka disease — epidemic hemorrhagic fever

Kolb's forceps, trocar

Koler's reaction

Kölliker's column, interstitial granules, membrane, nucleus

Kollmann's dilator

Kolmer's test with Reiter protein

Kolmer, Kline, Kahn test

Köln hemoglobin

Kolodny's forceps, hemostat

Kolomnin's operation — cauterization of the diseased tissues in hip joint disease by ignipuncture

Kondo's test

Kondoleon's operation — treatment of elephantiasis by removal of strips of subcutaneous tissue

Konew's test

König's syndrome — local infection of the cecum and terminal ileum, associated with abdominal distention, hyperperistalsis, intermittent constipation and diarrhea, colic stimulating intestinal obstruction, and intestinal spasms

König's disease — osteochondrolysis

König's operation — for congenital dislocation of hip

König's rods

Konjetzny's gastritis

Kono's procedure

Konsuloff's reaction, test

Kopetzky's bur

Koplik's sign, spots

Kopp's asthma

Kopper-Reppart medium

Korányi's auscultation, percussion, sign, treatment

Korányi-Grocco triangle

Korean hemorrhagic fever

Korff's fibers

Körner's septum

Korotkoff's method, sounds, test

Korovnikov's disease — splenomegaly with thrombocytosis and gastrointestinal hemorrhage, beginning between the ages of 20 and 37

Korsakoff's (Korsakov's) disease/syndrome — a syndrome encountered in chronic alcoholics, characterized by confusion and severe impairment of memory; delirium tremens may often precede onset of the syndrome

Korsakoff's (Korsakov's) psychosis

Körte-Ballance operation — anastomosis of the facial and hypoglossal nerves

Kortzeborn's operation — relief of ape hand caused by median nerve paralysis

Kos' cannula

Koser's citrate broth

Koshevnikoff's (Koschewnikow's, Kozhevnikov's) disease/syndrome — continuous clonic movements of a part of the body

Koshevnikoff's (Koschewnikow's, Kozhevnikov's) epilepsy

Kossa stain

Kossel's test

Köster's nodule

Kostmann's syndrome — infantile genetic agranulocytosis

Koszewski's syndrome — congenital osteosclerosis

Kottmann's reaction, test

Kovács's method, reagent

Kovalevsky's canal

Kovat's index

Kowarsky's test

Koyter's muscle

Kozowski's degeneration

Krabbe's disease — infantile familial sclerosis—a metabolic leukoencephalopathy with progressive cerebral degeneration

Krabbe's syndrome — a congenital form of generalized muscular hypoplasia beginning in infancy with irritability and rigidity

Krabbe's leukodystrophy

Kraepelin's classification

Kraft's point

Krämer's disease — suppurative scleritis

Kramer's speculum, telescope

Kramer-Gittleman method

Kramer-Pollnow disease — sudden onset of progressive hyperkinesia between the ages of one and four years, reaching a peak at age six years, followed

Kramer-Pollnow disease —
(*continued*)
by mental retardation, retro-
gression of speech ability, and
anxiety

Kramer-Tisdall method

Krankenhaus' Information System

Kraske's operation — removal of
the coccyx and part of the sacrum for access to a carcinoma of the rectum

Kraske's approach, position, retractor

Krause's syndrome — a retinopathy
associated with prematurity
and combined with cerebral
dysplasia

Krause's operation — extradural excision of the gasserian ganglion for trigeminal neuralgia

Krause's cannula, corpuscles, end
bulb, forceps, glands, ligament, line, membrane, suture,
valve

Krause-Wolfe graft

Krawitz's technique

Krebs' 2 carcinoma, cycle, leukocyte index, 2 tumor

Krebs-Henseleit buffer, solution cycle

Krebs-Ringer bicarbonate buffer,
phosphate, solution

Kreibig's opticomalacia

Kreischer's chisel

Kreiselman's incubator

Kreissl's knife

Kretschmann's space

Kretschmer's syndrome — semicoma
following unconsciousness of
several days or weeks in patients with acute brain
injuries

Kretschmer's types

Kretz's granules, paradox

Kreuscher's scissors

Kreutzmann's cannula, trocar

Kreysig's sign

Krimer's operation — plastic reconstruction of the palate, in
which mucoperiosteal flaps

Krimer's operation — (*continued*)
from each side of the palatal
cleft are sutured together at
the median line

Krishaber's disease — a neurosis
characterized by tachycardia,
insomnia, vertigo, and hyperesthesia; also called *cerebrocar-
diac syndrome*

Krisovski's (Krisowski's) sign

Kristeller's expression, method, retractor, speculum, technique

Kristiansen's screw

Kroener's fimbriectomy

Krogh's method

Krokiewicz's test

Kromayer's burn, lamp, treatment

Krompecher's carcinoma, tumor

Kron's dilator, probe

Kronecker's center, needle, puncture, stain

Kroner's tubal ligation

Kronfeld's electrode, forceps, retractor

Krönig's area, cesarean section,
field, isthmus, percussion

Krönlein's operation(s) — exposure
of the third branch of the trigeminal nerve for facial neuralgia; resection of the outer
wall of the orbit for removal
of orbital tumor without excising the eye

Krönlein's hernia

Krönlein-Berke orbital decompression

Krueger-Schmidt method

Krukenberg's amputation, arm,
hand, spindle, tumor, veins

Krull's knife

Krumwiede's triple sugar agar

Kruse's brush

Kruskal-Wallis test

Krwawicz's cryoextractor, extractor

Kuchendorf's method

Kuder's test

Kufs' disease — a juvenile form of
sphingolipidosis

Kugel-Stoloff syndrome — congenital idiopathic hypertrophy of
the heart

Kugelberg-Welander disease — a hereditary, juvenile form of muscular atrophy affecting the proximal muscles of the lower extremities

Kuhlman's brace, traction

Kuhlmann's test

Kuhn's mask, tube

Kühne's methylene blue, muscular phenomenon, spindle, terminal plates

Kuhnt's forceps, gouge, illusion, intermediary tissue, meniscus, postcentral vein

Kuhnt-Junius disease — macular degeneration

Kulchitsky's cell carcinoma, cells

Kulenkampff's anesthesia

Kulenkampff-Tarnow syndrome — spasmodic tension of the muscles of the neck, tongue, floor of the mouth, and pharynx; respiratory disorders; speech disorders; tachycardia; and hypertension, following the first few days of chlorpromazine therapy

Kulp's culture medium

Kulvin-Kalt forceps

Külz's cast, cylinder, test

Kumba virus

Kümmell's disease — vertebral compression fracture, characterized by spinal pain, intercostal neuralgia, and motor disturbances

Kümmell's kyphosis, spondylitis

Kümmell-Verneuil disease — same as *Kümmell's disease*

Kundrat's disease — lymphosarcoma

Kunitz pancreatic trypsin inhibitor

Kunkel's syndrome — lupoid hepatitis

Kunkel's test

Küntscher's nail, pin, rod

Kupffer's cells, cell sarcoma

Kupressoff's center

Kurloff's (Kurlov's) bodies

Kurnick's methyl green–pyronine Y method

Kurosaka's screw

Kurten's vein stripper

Kurz's syndrome — congenital blindness, with a high degree of axial hypermetropia, enophthalmos, pupillary areflexia and searching eye movements

Kurzbauer's method

Kurzrok-Miller test

Kurzrok-Ratner test

Kushner-Tandatnick curet

Küss' disease — stenosis of the rectum and sigmoid from inflammatory processes

Küss' experiment

Kussmaul's disease — same as *Kussmaul-Maier disease*

Kussmaul's aphasia, breathing, coma, paralysis, pulse, respiration, sign, symptom

Kussmaul-Kien respiration

Kussmaul-Landry paralysis

Kussmaul-Maier disease — polyarteritis nodosa

Küster's hernia

Küstner's operation — replacement of an inverted uterus through an incision made in the cervix and uterus

Küstner's incision, law, sign

Kutler's amputation

Kutlik's ferric iron method

Küttner's ganglion

Kveim antigen, reaction, test

Kveim-Siltzbach antigen, test

Kwilecki's method

Kyasanur Forest disease virus

Kyle's applicator, knife, speculum

Kyoto-Barrett-Boyes technique

Kypher's sutures

Kyrle's disease — a rare follicular disease characterized by discrete, keratotic patches in the hair follicles and eccrine ducts

L

La Crosse virus
La Porte's treatment
La Roque's sign, sutures, technique
Laband's syndrome — gingival fibromatosis associated with lysis of the distal phalanges
Labarraque's solution
Labbé's syndrome — intermittent hypertension associated with adrenal tumors
Labbé's neurocirculatory syndrome — an anxiety neurosis associated with tachycardia
Labbé's triangle, vein
Laborde's forceps, method, sign, test
Ladd's syndrome — congenital obstruction of the duodenum caused by peritoneal bands
Ladd's band, caliper, knife, raspatory
Ladd-Franklin theory
Ladd-Gross syndrome — icterus neonatorum associated with atresia of the bile ducts
Ladendorff's test
Ladin's sign
Laennec's disease(s) — cirrhosis of the liver associated with chronic excessive intake of alcohol; dissecting aneurysm
Laennec's catarrh, cirrhosis, pearls, sign, thrombus
Lafora's disease — myoclonic epilepsy
Lafora's bodies, sign
Laforce's adenotome, tonsillectomy
Laforce-Grieshaber adenotome
Laforce-Stevenson adenotome
Lagrange's operation — sclerectoiridectomy
Lahey's drain, forceps, osteotome, scissors, tube
Lahey-Babcock forceps

Lahey-Péan forceps
Lahore ulcer
Laidley's cystoscope
Laimer-Haeckerman area
Lake's pigment
Laki-Lorand factor
Lallemand's bodies
Lallemand-Trousseau bodies
Lalouette's pyramid
Lamarck's theory
Lamaze's method
Lambda's pacemaker
Lambert's canal, cosine law, treatment
Lambert-Berry raspatory
Lambert-Eaton syndrome — same as Eaton-Lambert syndrome
Lambert-Lowman clamp
Lambl's excrescences
Lambling's syndrome — postgastrectomy malabsorption associated with extreme thinness, anemia, hypoproteinemia, edema, and diarrhea
Lambotte's clamp, forceps, osteotome, treatment
Lambotte-Henderson osteotome
Lambrinudi's splint
Lamm's incision
Lamont's rasp, saw
Lancaster's keratome, magnet, sclerotome
Lancaster-O'Connor speculum
Lancefield's classification, grouping, precipitation test
Lancereaux's diabetes, nephritis
Lancereaux-Mathieu disease — leptospiral jaundice; also called Weil's syndrome
Lancet coefficient
Lancisi's nerves, stria
Landau's color test, reaction, reflex
Landau-Kleffner syndrome — a childhood disorder character-

Landau-Kleffner syndrome —
    (*continued*)
    ized by epileptic seizures, psy-
    chomotor abnormalities, and
    aphasia progressing to mutism
Landeker-Steinberg light
Landing-Oppenheimer syndrome —
    ceroid storage disease
Landolfi's caustic
Landolt's operation — formation of
    a lower eyelid with a bridge
    flap of eyelid skin taken from
    the upper lid
Landolt's bodies, keratome
Landouzy's syndrome — muscular
    atrophy associated with sciat-
    ica
Landouzy's disease — infectious
    jaundice; also called *Weil's syn-
    drome*
Landouzy's dystrophy, purpura,
    type
Landouzy-Dejerine atrophy, pro-
    gressive muscular dystrophy,
    type
Landouzy-Grasset law
Landry's disease/syndrome — acute,
    febrile polyneuritis
Landry's palsy, paralysis
Landschutz's tumor
Landsteiner's blood group system
Landsteiner-Donath test
Landsteiner-Miller method
Landsteiner-Wiener antigen
Landström's muscle
Landzert's fossa
Lane's disease — small bowel ob-
    struction in chronic constipa-
    tion
Lane's operation — dividing the il-
    eum near the cecum, closing
    the distal portion and anasto-
    mosing the proximal end with
    the upper part of the rectum
    or lower part of the sigmoid
Lane's bands, dissector, kink,
    method, mouth gag, plates,
    raspatory

Lang's dissector, fluid, knife, solu-
    tion, speculum, test
Langat virus
Langdon Down's disease — same as
    Down's syndrome
de Lange's syndrome — same as
    Brachmann-de Lange syndrome
Lange's operation — artificial ten-
    don transplantation with
    strands of silk
Lange's position, reaction, solu-
    tion, speculum, test
Langenbeck's amputation, incision,
    pedicle mucoperiosteal flap,
    triangle
Langenbeck-O'Brien raspatory
Langer's axillary arch, lines, mus-
    cle
Langer-Giedion syndrome — an in-
    herited disorder marked by
    mental retardation, character-
    istic facies with bulbous nose,
    and other anomalies
Langerhans' cells, cell granuloma-
    tosis, cell histiocytosis, giant
    cell, corpuscles, granules, is-
    lets, islands, layer
Langhans' cells, layer, stria
Langley's ganglion, granules,
    nerves
Langmuir's expression
Langoria's sign
Lannois-Gradenigo syndrome —
    same as *Gradenigo's syndrome*
Lansing's virus
Lantermann's clefts, incisures
Lantermann-Schmidt incisures
Lanz's operation — for elephantia-
    sis of the leg
Lanz's point, tube
Lapicque's constant, law
Lapides' catheter, needle, proce-
    dure
Lapidus' operation — wedge resec-
    tion and fusion of the cu-
    neometatarsal joint, establish-
    ing a bridge between the
    bases of the first and second
    metatarsals

Laplace's forceps, law, retractor

Laquer's stain

Laquerriere-Pierquin method

Larat's treatment

Larcher's sign

Lardennois' button

LaRocca's tube

Laron's dwarfism

Larrey's operation — disarticulation of the humerus at the shoulder joint

Larrey's amputation, bandage, cleft, dressing, spaces

Larrey-Weil disease — infectious jaundice caused by a species of *Leptospira*

Larry's director, probe

Larsen's disease — same as *Larsen-Johansson disease*

Larsen's syndrome — cleft palate and flattened facies, with multiple congenital dislocations and foot deformities

Larsen-Johansson syndrome — juvenile osteopathia patellae

Larsen-Johansson disease — presence of an accessory center of ossification in the lower pole of the patella

Lasègue's disease — persecution mania

Lasègue's sign

Lash's casein hydrolysate–serum medium

Lash-Löffler implant

Lassa fever virus

Lassar's betanaphthol paste, plain zinc paste

Lassueur-Graham Little triad

LaTarjet's angle, nerve, vein

Latham's circle

Lathbury's applicator

Latino virus

Latrobe's retractor

Latzko's operation(s) — cesarean section; a method of repairing a vesicovaginal fistula

Latzko's cesarean section, colpocleisis, radical hysterectomy

Lauber's disease — a disorder in which gray mottling of the fundus of the eyes is associated with night blindness

Laubry-Soulle syndrome — abnormal accumulations of gas in the colon and stomach following acute myocardial infarction

Lauenstein's method

Laufe-Barton-Kielland forceps

Laufe-Piper forceps

Laugier's hernia, sign

Laumonier's ganglion

Launois' syndrome — gigantism due to excessive pituitary secretion before puberty

Launois-Cléret syndrome — adiposogenital dystrophy caused by adenohypophyseal tumor; also called *Fröhlich's syndrome*

Laurell's electroimmunoassay, technique

Lauren's operation — a plastic operation for closure of a cicatricial opening following mastoid operation

Lauren's classification

Laurence-Biedl syndrome — same as *Biedl's disease*

Laurence-Moon syndrome — same as *Biedl's disease*

Laurence-Moon-Bardet-Biedl syndrome — same as *Biedl's disease*

Laurence-Moon-Biedl syndrome — same as *Biedl's disease*

Laurer's canal

Lauth's canal, ligament, sinus, violet

Lautier's test

Lavdovski's nucleoid

Laveran's bodies, corpuscles

Law's method, position

Läwen-Roth syndrome — dwarfism with thyroid deficiency and usually cretinism

Lawford's syndrome — a form of *Dimitri's disease*, consisting of

Lawford's syndrome — *(continued)*
angiomas of face and choroid
only, with late glaucoma

Lawless' stain

Lawrence's syndrome — lipoatrophic diabetes

Lawrence's forceps, method

Lawrence-Seip syndrome — loss of subcutaneous fat, associated with hepatomegaly, excessive bone growth, and insulin-resistant diabetes

Lawson-Thornton plate

Lawton's forceps, scissors

Le Dentu's suture

Le Dran's sutures

Le Fort's operation — same as *Le Fort-Neugebauer operation*

Le Fort's amputation, bougie, fracture, osteotomy, sound, suture

Le Fort-Neugebauer operation — repair of prolapse of the uterus

Le Grand-Geblewics phenomenon

Le Nobel's test

Leach's test

Leadbetter-Politano ureteroneocystotomy

Leader's forceps, hook

Leader-Kollmann dilator

Lear complex

Lebbin's test

Leber's disease(s) — a hereditary disorder of males, characterized by bilateral progressive optic atrophy; congenital amaurosis

Leber's cells, congenital amaurosis, corpuscles, optic atrophy, plexus

Leboyer's method, technique

Lebsche's forceps, knife, raspatory, shears

Lecat's gulf

Lechini's test

Leclanché's cell

Ledbetter's maneuver

Ledderhose's syndrome — plantar aponeurositis and fibrous

Ledderhose's syndrome —
(continued)
nodules of the flexor tendons, resulting in clawfoot

Lederberg's replica plating technique

Lederer's anemia

Leduc's current

Lee's ganglion, polyp, test

Lee-Cohen elevator, knife

Lee-White whole blood clotting time method

Leede-Rumpel phenomenon

Lees' clamp

Leff's stethoscope

Leffmann-Beam test

Legal's disease — a disease affecting the pharyngotympanic region, marked by headache and localized inflammation

Legal's test

Legg's disease — same as *Legg-Calvé-Perthes disease*

Legg's osteotome

Legg-Calvé-Perthes disease — osteochondrosis of the capital epiphysis of the femur

Legg-Calvé-Waldenström disease — same as *Legg-Calvé-Perthes disease*

Legueu's retractor

Lehman's catheter, syringe

Leibovitz's medium

Leichtenstern's encephalitis, phenomenon, sign, type

Leifson's staining method

Leigh's disease — necrotizing encephalomyelopathy

Leighton's tube technique

Leinbach's osteotome, prosthesis

Leiner's disease — a condition affecting chiefly newborn breast-fed infants, characterized by generalized exfoliative dermatitis and marked erythroderma

Leiner's dermatitis, test

Leipert's method

Leishman's anemia, cells, nodules, stain

Leishman-Donovan bodies

Leiter's cystoscope, tube

Leitner's syndrome — pulmonary tuberculous eosinophilic syndrome

Lejeune's syndrome — cri du chat (crying cat syndrome)

Lejeune's forceps, scissors

Leksell's forceps, rongeur

Leland-Jones forceps

Lell's esophagoscope, tube

Leloir's disease — discoid lupus erythematosus

Lem-Blay clamp

Lembert's suture

Lemesurier's cleft lip repair

Lemieux-Neemeh syndrome — an autosomal dominant syndrome consisting of muscular atrophy with progressive deafness

Lemmon's retractor, spreader

Lempert's fenestration operation — for otosclerosis

Lempert's excavator, incision, perforator, retractor, rongeur

Lempert-Colver retractor, speculum

Lempka's vein stripper

Lenard's rays

Lendrum's inclusion body stain, phloxine-tartrazine stain

Lendrum-McFarlane-Mayer hemalum

Lenegre's disease — acquired complete heart block due to primary degeneration of the conduction system

Lennarson's tube

Lennert's classification, lesion, lymphoma

Lennhoff's index, sign

Lennox syndrome — a childhood atypical form of absence epilepsy which may persist into adulthood; also called *petit mal variant*

Lennox-Gastaut syndrome — same as *Lennox syndrome*

Lenoble-Aubineau syndrome — hereditary congenital nystagmus associated with tremor of the head and arms, fasciculation of the muscles, vasomotor disorders, and overactive reflexes

Lente's probe

Lentulo's drill

Lenz's syndrome — a hereditary syndrome marked by abnormal smallness of the eyes, digital and skeletal anomalies, and sometimes urogenital and cardiovascular defects

Leo's sugar, test

Leon's virus

Leonard's forceps, tube

Leonard-George method

Leonardo's band

Leopold's law, maneuvers

Léopold-Lévi's syndrome — paroxysmal thyroid instability

Leotta's syndrome — perivisceritis on the right side in the subhepatic area

Lepehne-Pickworth benzidine technique, stain

Lepley-Ernst tube

Lepore's hemoglobin, thalassemia

Lerch's percussion

Leredde's syndrome — severe dyspnea on exertion, combined with emphysema and bronchiectasis

Leri's disease — thickening of the shafts of the long bones, with hyperostoses protruding into the medullary canal and from the external surface of the bone

Léri's pleonosteosis, sign

Léri-Weill syndrome — a form of dyschondroplasia

Lerich's treatment

Leriche's syndrome — obstruction of the terminal aorta causing

Leriche's syndrome — *(continued)*
fatigue, absence of pulse in
the femoral artery, and impotence
Leriche's disease — post-traumatic
osteoporosis
Leriche's forceps
Lermoyez's syndrome — tinnitus
and hearing loss prior to an
attack of vertigo
Lermoyez's punch
Leroy's disease — mucolipidosis
Les' culture medium
Lesch-Nyhan syndrome — a rare
hereditary disorder of purine
metabolism, marked by self-
mutilation, spastic cerebral
palsy, and excessive urinary secretion of uric acid
Leschke's syndrome — congenital
pigmentary dystrophy
Leser-Trélat sign
Lesgaft's space, triangle
L'Esperance's erysiphake
Lespinasse's sutures
Lesser's test, triangle
Letterer-Siwe disease — heritable
reticuloendotheliosis of early
childhood, marked by hemor-
rhagic tendency, hepato-
splenomegaly, and progressive
anemia
Leuckhart's embedding irons
Leudet's bruit, sign, tinnitus
Leunbach's paste
Lev's disease — acquired complete
heart block caused by sclero-
sis of the cardiac skeleton
Levaditi's method, stain
Levant's stone dislodger
Levasseur's sign
LeVeen's shunt
Lever's adenocanthoma
Levey-Jennings control chart
Lévi's syndrome — paroxysmal hy-
perthyroidism
Levi-Lorain dwarf, infantilism,
type
Levin's tube
Levine's eosin-methylene blue
(EMB) agar

Levinson's test
Levinthal-Coles-Lillie bodies
Levis' splint
Levitt's eye implant
Levret's forceps, law
Lévy-Roussy syndrome — progressive neuropathic muscular atrophy, with scoliosis and cerebral ataxia
Levy-Rowntree-Marriott method
Lewandowsky's nevus, periporitis,
tuberculid
Lewandowsky-Lutz disease — a viral disease marked by numerous warts that have a tendency to become malignant
Lewin's dissector, forceps
Lewin-Stern splint
Lewis' disease — familial congenital hepatic glycogenosis
caused by a deficiency in hepatic glycogen synthetase, associated with convulsions and
hypoglycemia following over-
night fasting
Lewis' acid, antibodies, antigens,
base, blood group, carcinoma,
cystometer, gene, hemostat,
leukotome, loupe, method,
mouth gag, phenomenon, procedure, reaction, secretor status, substance, tube
Lewis-Benedict method
Lewis-Lobban modified Schultz reaction
Lewis-Pickering test
Lewisohn's method
Lewkowitz's forceps
Lewy's bodies, laryngoscope
Lewy-Rubin needle
Lexer's chisel, scissors
Leyden's disease — periodic vomiting of uncertain cause
Leyden's ataxia, crystals, β-hemo-
philia neuritis, paralysis
Leyden jar
Leyden-Möbius syndrome — a
slowly progressive form of
muscular dystrophy in the
shoulder or pelvic girdle,
marked by wasting

Leydig's cell tumor, cells, cylinders, duct, hypoplasia, nodule

Leydig-Sertoli cell tumor

Leyro-Diaz forceps

Lhermitte's syndrome — oculomotor paralysis, with nystagmus and paralysis of abduction during attempted lateral deviation of the eye

Lhermitte's sign

Lhermitte-Cornil-Quesnel syndrome — progressive pyramidopallidal degeneration

Lhermitte-McAlpine syndrome — disease of combined pyramidal and extrapyramidal systems

Lhermitte-Trelles syndrome — lymphoblastic infiltrations of the peripheral nervous system, with paresis and amyotrophia

Liacopoulos phenomenon

Lian-Siguier-Welti syndrome — diaphragmatic hernia or eventration with venous thrombosis

Libman's sign

Libman-Sacks disease/syndrome — atypical vegetative endocarditis

Lichtenberg's keratome, trephine

Lichtenstern's syndrome — pernicious anemia in tabes dorsalis

Lichtheim's disease/syndrome — subacute degeneration of the spinal cord

Lichtheim's aphasia, plaques, sign, test

Lichtstein's sign

Lichtwicz's needle, trocar

Liddel-Sherrington reflex

Liddle's syndrome — a disorder that simulates aldosteronism marked by severe hypertension and hypokalemia with little secretion of aldosterone

Lieben's reaction, test

Lieben-Ralfe test

Lieberkühn's ampulla, crypts, follicles, glands

Lieberman's proctoscope, sigmoidoscope

Liebermann's test

Liebermann-Burchard reaction, reagent, test

Liebermeister's furrows, grooves, rule

Liebig's test, theory

Liebreich's symptom

Liepmann's apraxia

Liesegang's phenomenon, rings, striae, waves

Lieutaud's body, luette, triangle, uvula

Li-Fraumeni syndrome — a hereditary syndrome of early breast cancer associated with soft tissue sarcomas and other tumors

Liga's clip

Ligat's test

Light-Veley apparatus, drill, headrest

Lightwood's syndrome — renal tubular acidosis

Lightwood-Albright syndrome — rickets with renal tubular acidosis

Lignac's syndrome — cystine storage disease

Lignac-Fanconi disease — same as *Lignac's syndrome*

Lignières' reaction, test

Liley's three-zone chart, test

Lilienfeld's method

Lilienthal's guillotine, incision, probe

Lilienthal-Sauerbruch retractor

Lillie's alcoholic lead nitrate formalin, Biebrich scarlet picroaniline blue, method, procedure, retractor, scissors, sulfuric acid Nile blue stain speculum

Lillie-Killian forceps

Lillie Mayer hemalum

Limberg's cone

Lincoff's eye implant

Lincoln's scissors

Lindau's disease — same as *von Hippel-Lindau disease*

Lindau's tumor

Lindau-von Hippel disease — same as *von Hippel-Lindau disease*

Lindbergh's pump

Lindblom's method

Linde's walker

Lindeman's hysteroflator

Lindeman-Silverstein tube

Lindemann's cannula, method, test

Linder's sign

Lindner's initial bodies, sign, spatula, test

Lineweaver-Burk plot for enzyme reaction, equation

Links' test

Linnartz's clamp, forceps

Linser's method

Linton's incision, retractor, tourniquet, tube

Linton-Blakemore needle

Lippes' loop

Lippman's hip prosthesis

Lipps' test

Lipschütz's disease — a nonvenereal, rapidly progressing lesion of the vulva, possibly due to *Bacillus crassus*, a normally nonpathogenic organism

Lipschütz's bodies, cell, erythema, ulcer

Li-Rivers' culture medium

Lisch's nodules

Lisfranc's amputation, dislocation, joint, ligament, tubercle

Lison-Dunn method, stain

Lissauer's atrophy, column, dementia, marginal zone, paralysis, tract

Lister's antiseptic, dressing, forceps, scissors, tubercle

Lister-Burch speculum

Listing's law, plane

Liston's operation — for excision of the upper jaw

Liston's forceps, knives, scissors, splint

Liston-Stille forceps

Littauer's forceps, scissors

Littauer-Liston forceps

Litten's diaphragm phenomenon, sign

Little's syndrome — a skin disorder marked by a follicular, spinous eruption involving the scalp, trunk, and extremities

Little's disease — spastic paralysis of corresponding parts on both sides of the body

Little's area, retractor, scissors

Littlewood's amputation

Littman's agar

Littre's operation — inguinal colostomy

Littre's crypts, foramina, gland, hernia, sutures

Littre-Richter hernia

Litwak's scissors

Litwin's scissors

Litzmann's obliquity

Livermore's trocar

Livi's index

Livierato's reflex, sign

Livingston's bar, forceps, triangle

Lizars' operation — excision of the upper jaw

Lloyd's syndrome — adenoma of the pituitary, with adenomatoid enlargements of the parathyroid glands and islands of Langerhans

Lloyd's catheter, reagent, sign, tube

Lobo's disease — a chronic, localized mycosis of the skin, resulting in fibrous nodules or keloids

Lobstein's disease — an inherited condition in which bones are abnormally brittle and subject to fracture

Lobstein's ganglion

Locke's fluid, solution

Locke-Ringer solution

Lockwood's clamp, forceps, ligament

Lockwood-Allis forceps

Loeb's decidual reaction, deciduoma

Loebisch's coefficient, formula

Loevit's cell

Loewe's test

Loewenthal's purpura

Loewi's reaction, symptom, test

Löffler's disease/syndrome — transient infiltrations of the lungs associated with increased eosinophilic leukocytes in the blood

Löffler's agar, blood serum, endocarditis, eosinophilia, fibroplastic endocarditis, medium, method, methylene blue, myocarditis, pneumonia, stains, sutures

Löfgren's syndrome — bilateral hilar lymphoma syndrome

Logan's bow, procedure

Löhlein's diameter, nephritis

Löhlein-Baehr lesion

Lohmann's reaction

Lohnstein's saccharimeter

Löhr-Kindberg syndrome — eosinophilic pneumopathy

Lombard's test

Lombard-Beyer forceps, rongeur

Lombard-Boies rongeur

Lombardi's sign

Long's coefficient, formula

Long-Lukens animal

Longdwel's catheter, needle

Longmire's valvulotome

Longuet's operation — extraserous transplantation of the testicle for varicocele and hydrocele

Longuet's incision

Looser's transformation zones

Looser-Milkman syndrome — a generalized bone disease marked by multiple stripes of absorption in the long and flat bones

Lorain's disease — idiopathic infantilism

Lorain's infantilism, type

Lorain-Lévi syndrome — pituitary dwarfism

Lord-Blakemore tube

Lordan's forceps, hook

Lore's forceps, tube

Lore-Lawrence tube

Lorenz's operation — for congenital dislocation of the hip, with reduction of dislocation

Lorenz's method, osteotomy, sign, tube

Lorenzo's prosthesis

Loreta's operation — gastrotomy, with distal dilatation of the pylorus

Loreta's method

Lorfan's anesthesia

Lorie's retractor, trephine

Loring's ophthalmoscope

Lorrain Smith blood serum, stain

Lortat-Jacob disease — benign mucosal pemphigoid

Lortet's lamp

Lorthiore's method

Loschmidt's number

Lossen's law, rule

Lostorfer's bodies, corpuscles

Lotheissen's herniorrhaphy

Lothrop's dissector, forceps, retractor

Lottes' nail, pin, reamer

Loughnane's hook

Louis' angle, law

Louis-Bar syndrome — familial progressive cerebellar ataxia with oculocutaneous telangiectases

Lounsbury's curet

Loutit's anemia

Love's leukotome, retractor, splint

Love-Adson elevator

Love-Gruenwald forceps, rongeur

Love-Kerrison forceps, rongeur

Lovelace's forceps

Lovén's reflex

Lovset's maneuver, method

Low's preactivated papain technique

Löw-Beer method, projection

Lowe's syndrome — oculocerebrorenal syndrome

Lowe's disease — a hereditary disorder occurring only in males, characterized by vitamin D–resistant rickets, congenital glaucoma and cataracts, mental retardation, and tubule reabsorption dysfunction

Löwe's ring

Lowe-Breck knife

Lowe-Terrey-MacLachlan syndrome — same as *Lowe's disease*

Lowell's knife

Löwenberg's canal, forceps, scala

Löwenstein's culture medium, lithotrite, ointment

Löwenstein-Jensen culture medium

Löwenstein-Jensen-Gruft medium

Löwenthal's sclerosis, test, tract

Lower's forceps, rings, sacs, tubercle

Löwitt's bodies, lymphocytes

Lowman's balance board, clamp

Lown-Ganong-Levine syndrome — a short P-R interval (atrial activity) and normal duration of the QRS complex (ventricular activity), often associated with paroxysmal tachycardia

Lowry's assay

Lowsley's operation — repair of epispadias

Lowsley's forceps, nephropexy, tractor, urethroscope

Lowsley-Peterson cystoscope

Lowy's test

Loyez's myelin stain

Lubarsch's syndrome — primary systematized amyloidosis, marked by macroglossia and large deposits of amyloid in the skin, tongue, heart, stomach, intestine, and skeletal muscle

Lubarsch's crystals

Lubs' syndrome — a familial form of male pseudohermaphroditism

Luc's operation — same as *Caldwell-Luc operation*

Lucae's forceps, probe

Lucas' sign

Lucas-Championnière disease — fibrinous bronchitis

Lucatello's sign

Lucey-Driscoll syndrome — retention jaundice occurring in infants as a result of bilirubin dysfunction

Lucherini's syndrome — juvenile rheumatoid arthritis associated with iridocyclitis

Lucherini-Giacobini syndrome — familial endocrine osteochondropathy

Luciani's triad

Lucio's leprosy, phenomenon

Luck's fasciotome, saw

Lucké's renal adenocarcinoma, test, tumor

Luder-Sheldon syndrome — a familial, congenital disorder of renal tubular reabsorption of glucose and amino acids associated with dwarfism

Ludloff's operation — osteotomy of the first metatarsal bone for correction of hallux valgus

Ludloff's incision, osteotomy, sign

Ludovici's angulus

Ludwig's angina, angle, ganglion, labyrinths, plane, theory

Luebert's test

Luedde's exophthalmometer

Luer's syringe

Luer-Hartman rongeur

Luer-Korte scoop

Luer-Lok syringe

Luer-Whiting forceps

Luetscher's syndrome — secondary hyperaldosteronism associated with heart, kidney and liver diseases

Luft's disease — a disorder of striated muscle characterized by excessive mitochondria, abnormally increased basal metabolic rate, and debility

Luft's potassium permanganate fixative

Lugol's caustic, solution

Luikart's forceps

Luikart-Bill traction handle

Luikart-Kielland forceps

Luikart-McLane forceps

Luikart-Simpson forceps

Luke's antigen

Lukes-Butler classification

Lukes-Collins classification

Lukens' aspirator, enterotome, retractor, tube

Lumsden's center

Lund's operation — removal of the astragalus for correction of talipes

Lundsgaard's blade, knife, sclerotome

Lundsgaard-Burch knife, rasp, sclerotome

Lundvall's blood crisis

Lundy's laryngoscope, needle

Lundy-Irving needle

Lunyo virus

Luongo's cannula, elevator, needle, retractor

Luria-List learning test

Luschka's body, bursa, cartilage, crypts, duct, fibers, foramen, fossa, ganglion, gland, joint, ligament, muscle, nerve, tonsil, tubercle

Luse's bodies

Lusskin's drill

Lust's phenomenon, reflex, sign

Lutembacher's syndrome — a congenital abnormality of the heart, consisting of interatrial septal defect, mitral stenosis and right atrial hypertrophy

Lutembacher's complex

Lütkens' sphincter

Lüttke's test

Lutz's forceps

Lutz-Jeanselme nodules

Lutz-Miescher disease — a skin disease usually affecting males in their twenties, marked by ker-

Lutz-Miescher disease — (continued) atotic papules forming an eruption on the neck near the hairline

Lutz-Splendore-Almeida disease — South American blastomycosis

Luys' body syndrome — a violent form of motor restlessness, involving only one side of the body, caused by a lesion of the hypothalamic nucleus

Luys' body, nucleus, segregator, separator

Lyell's disease/syndrome — an exfoliative skin disease in infants and children that rapidly spreads over the entire body and is followed by skin scaling and separation

Lygidakis' procedure

Lyle's syndrome — blindness with normal fundus oculi, often resulting from hysteria and neurasthenia

Lyle-Curtman test

Lyman's method, rays

Lyman-Smith brace

Lyme disease — a multisystemic disorder caused by the tick *Ixodes dammini* and marked by myalgia and arthritis of the large joints with nervous system and cardiovascular system involvement

Lyme arthritis, borreliosis

Lynch's dissector, incision, laryngoscope, scissors

Lyon's effect, forceps, hypothesis, method, test, tube

Lyser's trapezoid bone

Lysholm's method

Lyster's bag, tube

Lytle's splint

Macalister's ethmoidal spine, ligament, process, triangular fascia, valve
MacAusland chisel, retractor
MacAusland-Kelly retractor
MacCallum's patch
Macchiavello's stain
MacConkey's agar, broth, medium
MacDonagh's test
Macdonald's index, test
MacDougal's theory
Macdowel's frenum
Macewen's operation(s) — supracondylar division of the femur for genu valgum; for the radical cure of hernia
Macewen's osteotomy, sign, triangle
MacFee's incision
Mach's syndrome — hyperaldosteronism with adrenal hyperplasia; retention of sodium chloride; and edema affecting the extremities and sometimes the brain, larynx, and eyes
Machado's reaction, test
Machado-Guerreiro reaction, test
Machado-Joseph disease — same as *Azorean disease*
Mache's unit
Macht's test
Machupo virus
MacIntosh's laryngoscope, prosthesis
Mack's tonsillectome
MacKay's retractor
MacKay-Marg electronic tonometer
Mackenrodt's operation — vaginal fixation of the round ligaments for retrodisplacement of the uterus
Mackenrodt's incision, ligament
MacKenty's forceps, scissors, tube

Mackenzie's syndrome — associated paralysis of the tongue, soft palate and vocal cord on the same side
Mackenzie's disease — a complex of symptoms of unknown cause, consisting of malaise with sensitivity to cold, dyspepsia, intestinal disorder, and disturbances of respiration and heart action
Mackenzie's amputation, point
Mackler's prosthesis
MacLachlan's method, process
Maclagan's thymol turbidity test
Maclay's scissors
MacLean's test
MacLean–de Wesselow test
MacLean-Maxwell disease — a chronic condition of the heel bone marked by enlargement and pain on pressure
Macleod's syndrome — a syndrome of unknown cause in which an affected lung is underventilated and underperfused with blood and in which associated obstruction of the bronchioles occurs
MacLeod's capsular rheumatism
MacMunn's test
MacNeal's tetrachrome blood stain
MacQuarrie's test
MacWilliam's test
Madden's clamp, hook
Maddox's prism, rods
Madelung's disease(s) — diffuse lipomas of the neck; radial aberration of the hand from overgrowth of the distal ulna or shortening of the radius
Madelung's deformity, neck, subluxation
Madlener's operation — female sterilization

Madura foot

Maeder-Danis dystrophy

Maffucci's syndrome — same as *Kast's syndrome*

Magendie's foramen, law, phenomenon, sign, solution, space, symptom

Magendie-Hertwig sign

Magielski's curet, forceps, needle

Magill's forceps, laryngoscope, tube

Magitot's disease — osteoperiostitis of the dental alveoli

Magnan's movement, sign, symptom

Magnus–de Kleijn neck reflexes

Magnuson's saw, splint, valve

Magovern's prosthesis

Magovern-Cromie prosthesis

Magpie's test

Magrassi-Leonardi syndrome — eosinophilic pneumopathy marked by monocytic-histiocytic cells in the blood, followed by eosinophilia

Mahaim's fibers

Maher's disease — inflammation of the vaginal tissues

Mahler's sign

Mahoney's dilator, speculum

Maier's forceps, sinus

Maillard's coefficient

Maingot's hemostat

Mainz's pouch

Maisler's treatment

Maisonneuve's amputation, bandage, sign, urethrotome

Maissiat's band, ligament, tract

Maixner's cirrhosis

Majocchi's disease — a rare, purpuric eruption beginning on the lower extremities and becoming generalized, often followed by atrophy of the affected skin and loss of hair

Majocchi's granuloma, purpura

Makeham's hypothesis

Makka's operation — for ectopia of the bladder, using the cecum

Makka's operation — *(continued)* as a bladder and the appendix as a ureter

Makonde virus

Malabar leprosy, ulcer

Malacarne's antrum, pyramid, space

Malassez's disease — testicular cyst

Malassez's rest

Malayan filariasis, pit viper venom

Maldonado–San Jose stain

Malecot's catheter

Malerba's test

Malfatti's method

Malgaigne's amputation, apparatus, fossa, fracture, hook, luxation, pad, triangle

Malherbe's disease — a benign tumor of the skin and subcutis resembling basal cell carcinoma

Malherbe's calcifying epithelioma, tumor

Malherbe-Chenantais epithelioma

Malibu disease — surfers' nodules

Malin's syndrome — anemia in which red blood cells are ingested by leukocytes; also called *autoerythrophagocytosis*

Malis' forceps, scissors

Mall's formula, ridge

Mallory's acid fuchsin, bodies, orange G and aniline blue stain, phosphotungstic acid–hematoxylin stain, triple stain

Mallory-Weiss syndrome — laceration of the lower end of the esophagus, usually caused by severe retching or vomiting

Mallory-Weiss lesion, tear

Malm-Himmelstein valvulotome

Malmejde's test

Maloney's bougies

Malot's test

Malpighi's pyramids, vesicles

Malta fever

Maltz's knife, retractor, saw

Maltz-Lipsett rasp

Maly's test
Manchester brown
Manchester's operation — same as
    Fothergill's operation
Manchester's colporrhaphy, uterine
    suspension
Mancini's method
Mandelin's reagent
Mangoldt's epithelial grafting
Mangus' sign
Mankowsky's syndrome — familial
    dysplastic osteopathy, marked
    by clubbing of the fingers and
    toes secondary to various
    chronic diseases
Mann's syndrome — contusion of
    the brain accompanied by gen-
    eralized disorders of coordina-
    tion
Mann's forceps, sign, methyl blue–
    eosin stain
Mann-Bollman fistula
Mann-Whitney rank sum statistic,
    test
Mann-Whitney-Wilcoxon test
Mann-Williamson ulcer
Mannkopf's sign, symptom
Mannkopf-Rumpf sign
Manoiloff's (Manoilov's) reaction
Manson's disease — infection with
    flukes of *Schistosoma mansoni*
    living in the mesenteric veins
    but depositing their eggs in
    venules of the large intestine
Manson's hemoptysis, schistosomia-
    sis, test
Mantel-Cox method
Mantoux's conversion, diameter,
    pit, reaction, reversion, test
Mantz's dilator
Manz's glands
Manzullo's test
Maragliano's body, tuberculin
Marañon's syndrome — scoliosis
    with ovarian insufficiency
Marañon's lipomatosis, reaction,
    sign
Marburg disease — a severe, often
    fatal, viral disease character-

Marburg disease — *(continued)*
    ized by skin lesions, conjunc-
    tivitis, enteritis, hepatitis, en-
    cephalitis, and renal failure
Marburg's agent, fever, variant of
    multiple sclerosis, virus
March's disease — same as *Graves'
    disease*
Marchal's bodies
Marchand's adrenals, adventitial
    cell, organ, rest
Marchesani's syndrome — a heredi-
    tary syndrome of abnormally
    small lens, short stature, and
    brachydactyly
Marchi's balls, globules, fixative, re-
    action, stain, tract
Marchiafava's hemolytic anemia
Marchiafava-Bignami disease —
    progressive degeneration of
    the corpus callosum, marked
    by intellectual deterioration,
    emotional disturbances, hallu-
    cinations, tremor, rigidity, and
    convulsions
Marchiafava-Micheli disease — an
    uncommon form of hemolysis
    of unknown cause, marked by
    episodic nocturnal hemoglo-
    binuria and often associated
    with leukopenia or thrombo-
    cytopenia
Marchiafava-Micheli anemia
Marcks' knife
Marcus Gunn's syndrome — same
    as *Gunn's syndrome*
Marcus Gunn's pupillary phenome-
    non, sign
Marcy agent
Maréchal's test, tuberculin
Maréchal-Rosin test
Marey's law
Marfan's syndrome — a congenital
    disorder of connective tissue,
    marked by abnormal length of
    extremities, cardiovascular ab-
    normalities, and other deform-
    ities

Marfan's abiotrophy, epigastric puncture, method, sign

Marfan-Madelung syndrome — a combination of *Marfan's syndrome* and *Madelung's deformity*

Margolis' syndrome — sex-linked deaf-mutism with albinism

Margulles' coil

Marian's operation — for stone in the bladder

Marie's anarthria, ataxia, hypertrophy, quadrilateral space, sclerosis, sign, three-paper test

Marie's disease(s) — acromegaly; hypertrophic pulmonary osteoarthropathy

Marie's syndrome — a hereditary disease of the nervous system beginning in young adulthood or middle age with spastic-ataxic gait, poor coordination, tremor, impaired deep sensibility, pain, cramps, paresthesia, and dysarthric speech

Marie-Bamberger disease/syndrome — hypertrophic pulmonary osteoarthropathy

Marié-Davy cell

Marie-Foix sign

Marie-Léri syndrome — osteolysis of the articular surfaces of the fingers, resulting in mobility of the joints so that the fingers can be elongated or shortened

Marie-Robinson syndrome — melancholia, insomnia and impotence associated with the presence of fructose in the urine

Marie-Sée syndrome — a benign type of hydrocephalus in infants, caused by large doses of vitamin A

Marie-Strümpell disease — ankylosing spondylitis

Marie-Tooth disease — progressive neuropathic muscular atrophy

Marín Amat's syndrome — closure of the eye when the mouth is widely or forcibly opened

Marinesco's sign, succulent hand

Marinesco-Garland syndrome — a rare, hereditary disorder marked by degeneration of tissues of the brain and lens with mental retardation

Marinesco-Radovici reflex

Marinesco-Sjögren's syndrome — same as *Marinesco-Garland syndrome*

Marion's disease — congenital obstruction of the posterior urethra due to muscular hypertrophy of the bladder neck or absence of the dilator fibers in the urinary tract

Mariotte's blind spot, experiment, law

Marituba virus

Marjolin's ulcer

Markham-Meyerding retractor

Markoe's abscess

Marlow's test

Marme's reagent

Marochetti's blisters

Maroteaux-Lamy syndrome — an error of mucopolysaccharide metabolism, marked by growth retardation and hepatosplenomegaly but without mental retardation

Marquardt's test

Marquis' reagent, test

Marriott's method

Marsden's paste

Marsh's disease — same as *Graves' disease*

Marsh's factor, test

Marsh-Bendall factor

Marshall's syndrome — a rare syndrome of hypoplasia, cataract, and sensorineural hearing loss

Marshall's fold, method, oblique vein, test

Marshall Hall's facies

Marshall-Marchetti operation —
   for the correction of stress incontinence
Marshall-White syndrome —
   chronic vasoconstrictor spots
   associated with insomnia and
   tachycardia
Marshik's forceps
Martel's clamp
Martin's disease — periosteoarthritis
   of the foot, usually due to prolonged walking
Martin's operation — for cure of
   hydrocele
Martin's bandage, broth, depila-
   tory, speculum
Martin-Albright syndrome —
   familial pseudohypoparathyroidism
Martin-Davy speculum
Martin du Pan–Rutishauser disease — laminar osteochondritis that occurs during adolescence, marked by pain, ankylosis, and destruction of
   cartilage
Martin-Lester agar
Martinez's technique
Martinotti's cells
Martius-scarlet-blue stain
Martorell's syndrome — progressive
   obliteration of the brachio-
   cephalic trunk and left ca-
   rotid arteries, leading to loss
   of pulse in both arms and ca-
   rotids and to transient hemi-
   plegia, transient blindness, ret-
   inal atrophy, and muscular
   atrophy of the arms
Marwedel's gastrostomy
Maryan's forceps
Maschke's test
Masini's sign
Mason's incision, splint
Mason-Allen splint
Mason-Auvard speculum
Mason Pfizer monkey virus
Masselon's spectacles

Masset's test
Masshoff's syndrome — abscess-
   forming reticulocytic lymph-
   adenitis of the mesentery,
   thought to be caused by Pas-
   teurella pseudotuberculosis
Massie's nail
Massier's solution
Masson's bodies, method, pseudo-
   angiosarcoma, stain
Masson-Fontana stain
Masson-Judd retractor
Master's "2-step" exercise test
Masterson's clamp
Mastin's clamp
Masuda-Kitahara disease — an exu-
   dative disorder of the macula
   lutea seen in Japan and Indo-
   nesia, probably caused by a vi-
   rus
Masugi's nephritis
Masugi-type nephrotoxic serum ne-
   phritis
Matas' operation — for aneurysm
   by opening the aneurysmal
   sac and closing the internal
   orifices
Matas' band, test, treatment
Matchett-Brown prosthesis
Mateer-Streeter ovum
Mátéfy's reaction, test
Mathes' mastitis
Mathews' speculum, test
Mathieu's disease — leptospiral
   jaundice
Mathieu's forceps, retractor
Matson's elevator, raspatory
Mattioli-Foggia and Raso syn-
   drome — a progressive, recur-
   rent, muscular disorder
   marked by the presence of
   hard, painless tumors
Mattis' scissors
Matuhasi-Ogata phenomenon
Matzenauer's speculum
Matzenauer-Polland syndrome — a
   skin disease marked by in-
   flammatory lesions and fol-

Matzenauer-Polland syndrome —
(continued)
lowed by attacks of erythema
and urticarial edema
Mauchart's ligaments
Maugeri's syndrome — mediastinal
silicotic lesions causing laryngeal and respiratory disturbances
Maumené's test
Maumenee's erysiphake, forceps
Maumenee-Park speculum
Maunier-Kuhn disease — slackness
of the eyelids and ears in
childhood, followed by tra-
cheomegaly and bronchomeg-
aly
Maunoir's hydrocele, scissors
Maunsell's sutures
Maurer's clefts, dots, spots, stippling
Mauriac's syndrome(s) — an erythematous, nodular eruption
on the legs, and sometimes
on other parts of the body,
seen in syphilis; hepatomeg-
aly, dwarfism, and obesity
with juvenile diabetes melli-
tus
Mauriceau's lance, maneuver
Mauriceau-Levret maneuver
Mauriceau-Smellie-Veit maneuver
Mauthner's cell, fiber, membrane,
sheath, test
Maxcy's disease — a rickettsial in-
fection endemic in southeast-
ern United States
Maximow's fixative, staining
method
Maxwell's ring, spot
Maxwell-Boltzmann distribution
law
May's method, spore stain
May-Grünwald stain
May-Grünwald-Giemsa stain
May-Hegglin anomaly, body
Mayaro virus
Maydl's operation(s) — colostomy;
insertion of the ureters into

Maydl's operation(s) — (continued)
the rectum for exstrophy of
the bladder
Maydl's hernia
Mayer's albumin, glycerin-albumin
mixture, hemalum, ligament,
method, mucihematein stain,
pessary, position, reagent, reflex, stain, test, waves
Mayer-Gross apraxia
Mayer-Rokitansky-Küster-Hauser
syndrome — lack of development of the embryonic tubes
from which the vagina and
uterus are derived, with conse-
quent lack of vagina and rudi-
mentary development of the
uterus
Mayerhofer's test
Mayfield's forceps, osteotome, spat-
ula
Maylard's incision
Mayo's operation(s) — excision of
the pyloric end of the stom-
ach; radical cure of umbilical
hernia; removal of varicose
veins
Mayo's anemic spot, sign
Mayo-Adams retractor
Mayo-Blake forceps
Mayo-Boldt inverter
Mayo-Collins retractor
Mayo-Guyon clamp
Mayo-Harrington forceps, scissors
Mayo-Kelly inverter
Mayo-Lovelace retractor
Mayo-Ochsner forceps
Mayo-Péan forceps, hemostat
Mayo-Robson forceps, incision, po-
sition
Mayo-Simpson retractor
Mayor's hammer, scarf
May-White syndrome — a rare au-
tosomal dominant syndrome
of myoclonus, cerebellar
ataxia, and deafness
Mazzini's test
Mazzoni's corpuscles

Mazzotti's reaction, test
McAllister's scissors
McArdle's disease — same as *Mc-Ardle-Schmid-Pearson disease*
McArdle-Schmid-Pearson disease — glycogen-storage disease with hepatophosphorylase deficiency
McArthur's incision, method
McAtee's apparatus
McBride's bunionectomy
McBride-Moore prosthesis
McBurney's operation — for the radical cure of inguinal hernia
McBurney's incision, point, sign
McCallum's plaque
McCarthy's cystoscope, electrotome, panendoscope, reflex, resectoscope
McCarthy-Alcock forceps
McCarthy-Campbell cystoscope
McCarthy-Peterson cystoscope
McCaskey's catheter
McCleery-Miller clamp
McClintock's soap
McClure's scissors
McClure-Aldrich test
McCollough's effect
McCollum's tube
McConckey's cocktail
McCormac's reflex
McCoy's forceps
McCrea's cystoscope
McCrudden's method
McCullough's forceps
McCune-Albright syndrome — same as *Albright-McCune-Sternberg syndrome*
McCurdy's needle
McDermott's clip
McDonald's operation — for incompetent cervix in which the cervical os is closed
McDonald's cerclage, clamp, maneuver, rule
McDowall's reflex
McDowell's mouth gag
McElroy's curet

McEwen's point
McGannon's forceps, retractor
McGee's forceps
McGee-Caparosa wire crimper
McGhan's eye implant, prosthesis
McGill's operation — suprapubic transvesical prostatectomy
McGill's forceps, retractor
McGinn-White sign
McGivney's ligator
McGoey-Evans cup
McGraw's ligature, sutures
McGuire's forceps, scissors
McHenry's forceps
McIndoe's colpocleisis, forceps, scissors
McIntire's splint
McIntosh's forceps
McIvor's mouth gag
McKay's forceps
McKee-Farrar prosthesis
McKeever's knife, prosthesis
McKenzie's clamp, drill, forceps, leukotome
McKinnon's test
McKissock's incision, sutures
McKittrick-Wheelock syndrome — adenoma of the colon and rectum, associated with electrolyte imbalance
McLane's forceps
McLane-Tucker-Luikart forceps
McLaughlin's incision, nail, speculum
McLean's formula, index, tonometer
McLean-VanSlyke method
McLeod's blood group system, phenotype
McLetchie-Aikens disease — fever followed by tumors of the thigh and, several months later, of the biceps
McManus method
McMaster's technique
McMurray's maneuver, sign, test
McNaught's prosthesis
McNealy-Glassman-Babcock forceps

McNeer's classification
McNeill-Goldmann scleral ring
McPhail's test
McPheeters' treatment
McPherson's forceps, scissors, speculum
McPherson-Castroviejo scissors
McPherson-Vannas scissors
McPherson-Wheeler knife
McPherson-Ziegler knife
McQuigg's clamp
McReynolds' keratome, knife, scissors
McVay's herniorrhaphy, incision
McWhinnie's electrode
McWhirter's technique
McWhorter's hemostat
Mead's rongeur
Means' sign
Mecke's reagent
Meckel's syndrome — same as *Meckel-Gruber syndrome*
Meckel's band, cartilage, cavity, diverticulum, ganglion, ligament, plane, rod, scan, space, tubercle
Meckel-Gruber syndrome — a malformation syndrome, lethal in the perinatal period, marked by intrauterine growth failure, ocular anomalies, cleft palate, polydactyly, polycystic kidney, and other defects; called also *Gruber's syndrome*
Medin's disease — acute anterior poliomyelitis
Medinger-Craver irradiation
Mediterranean disease — hereditary hemolytic anemia
Meeh's formula
Meeker's forceps
Mees' lines, stripes
Meesmann's dystrophy
Méglin's point
Mehlis' gland
Méhu's test
Meiboom-Gill sequence
Meige's disease/syndrome — congenital hereditary lymph-

Meige's disease/syndrome — *(continued)* edema of the legs, caused by lymphatic obstruction
Meigs' syndrome — serous fluid in the abdominal cavity, and watery fluid in the pleural cavity associated with ovarian fibroma or other pelvic tumor
Meigs' capillaries, test
Meinicke's reaction, test
Meirowsky's phenomenon
Meissner's corpuscles, ganglion, plexus
Meleda disease — a hereditary disorder marked by the formation of keratin on the palms and soles with painful lesions from fissuring of the skin
Meleney's gangrene, ulcer
Melkersson's syndrome — same as *Melkersson-Rosenthal syndrome*
Melkersson-Rosenthal syndrome — a rare, hereditary triad of recurrent facial paralysis, facial edema and fissured tongue, most often beginning in childhood or adolescence
Meller's operation — excision of the tear sac
Meller's retractor, spatula
Mellinger's speculum
Melnick-Needles syndrome — a hereditary disease marked by generalized skeletal dysplasia and constrictions of the ribs and tubular bones
Melnick-Needles osteodysplasty
Melotte's metal
Meltzer's anesthesia, law, method, nasopharyngoscope, sign
Meltzer-Lyon method, test
Mencière's mixture, solution
Mende's syndrome — a congenital familial disorder combining abnormalities of pigmentation with mongoloid characteristics and deaf mutism

Mendel's law, reflex, test

Mendel-Bekhterev reflex, sign

Mendeléeff's (Mendeléev's) law, table, test

Mendelsohn's test

Mendelson's syndrome — acid pulmonary aspiration syndrome, occurring during labor under general anesthesia

Ménétrier's disease — giant hypertrophic gastritis

Menge's pessary

Mengert's shock syndrome — a condition in the late antepartum period, resembling shock, from pressure of the uterus on the vena cava

Mengert's index

Menghini's needle

Mengo encephalomyelitis, virus

Ménière's disease — hearing loss, tinnitus, and vertigo resulting from nonsuppurative disease of the labyrinth

Menkes' syndrome(s) — a congenital metabolic defect, manifest in sparse, kinky hair, associated with mental and physical retardation and progressive deterioration of the brain; an inborn error of leucine, isoleucine, and valine metabolism, associated with gross mental deficiency

Mennell's sign

Menzel's disease — genetically transmitted, progressive ataxia of young adults

Menzies' method

Mercier's operation — prostatectomy

Mercier's bar, catheter, valve

Mercurio's position

Meretoja's syndrome — Finnish-type familial amyloid polyneuropathy

Merindino's procedure

Merkel's cells, corpuscles, disks, filtrum, muscle, tactile cells

Merkel-Ranvier cells

Merrifield's knife

Merz's serum

Merzbacher-Pelizaeus disease — same as *Pelizaeus-Merzbacher disease*

Messinger-Huppert method

Mester's test

Metchnikoff's (Mechnikov's) law, phenomenon, theory

Mett's method, test tubes

Metzenbaum's forceps, knife, scissors

Metzenbaum-Lipsett scissors

Metzenbaum-Tydings forceps

Meulengracht's diet, icterus, method

Meunier's sign

Mexican hat cell, hat corpuscle

Meyenburg's disease — same as *Meyenburg-Altherr-Uehlinger syndrome*

Meyenburg's complex

Meyenburg-Altherr-Uehlinger syndrome — relapsing polychondritis

Meyer's disease — adenoid vegetations of the pharynx

Meyer's hockey stick incision, law, line, loop, mastectomy, method, organ, reagent, sign, sinus, test

Meyer-Betz disease — a rare, familial disease marked by the presence of myoglobin in the urine, resulting in tenderness, swelling, paralysis, muscular pain and weakness, and sometimes renal failure

Meyer-Halsted incision

Meyer-Schwickerath and Weyers syndrome — anomalies of the iris, associated with malformed teeth and deformities

Meyer-Schwickerath and Weyers syndrome — *(continued)* of the fingers, including syndactyly or absent phalanges

Meyerding's curet, gouge, osteotome, retractor

Meyerding-Deaver retractor

Meyers-Kouvenaar bodies

Meyhoeffer's curet, knife

Meynert's amentia, bundle, cells, commissure, decussation, fasciculus, layer, tract

Meynet's nodes

Mezei's granules

Mibelli's disease — a rare dermatosis marked by progressive thickening of the corneal epidermis and progressive atrophy

Mibelli's angiokeratoma, porokeratosis

Michaelis' constant, rhomboid, stain, veronal acetate buffer

Michaelis-Gutmann bodies

Michaelis-Menten equation, kinetics, law

Michailow's test

Michel's clamp, deafness, forceps

Michelson's bronchoscope

Michelson-Weiss sign

Middeldorpf's splint, triangle, tumor

Middlebrook's agar, broth, media

Middlebrook-Cohn agar medium

Middlebrook-Dubos hemagglutination test

Middleton's curet

Mie's light scatter

Miehlke-Partsch syndrome — thalidomide-induced ear deformity and facial paralysis

Mielke's template method

Mierzejewski's effect

Miescher's disease — degeneration of elastic tissue, occurring alone or in association with other disorders such as *Down's syndrome* or *Marfan's syndrome*

Miescher's cheilitis, corpuscles, elastoma, granulomatosis, trichofolliculoma, tubes, tubules

Miescher-Leder granulomatosis

Mignon's eosinophilic granuloma

Migula's classification

Mikulicz's syndrome — bilateral hypertrophy of the lacrimal, parotid, and salivary glands, often accompanied by chronic lymphocytic infiltration

Mikulicz's disease — a benign, self-limited, lymphocytic infiltration of the lacrimal and salivary glands, usually affecting older women; similar to *Sjögren's syndrome*

Mikulicz's operation(s) — enterectomy; removal of the sternocleidomastoid muscle for torticollis; pyloroplasty; tarsectomy

Mikulicz's angle, aphthae, cells, clamp, drain, incision, pack, pad, pyloroplasty

Milch's method

Miles' operation — abdominoperineal resection for cancer of the lower sigmoid and rectum, which includes permanent colostomy

Miles' clamp, proctosigmoidectomy

Milian's erythema, sign

Milkman's syndrome — same as *Looser-Milkman syndrome*

Milkman's fracture

Milkman-Looser syndrome — same as *Looser-Milkman syndrome*

Millar's asthma

Millard's test

Millard-Gubler syndrome — same as *Gubler's syndrome*

Millard-Gubler paralysis

Miller's syndrome — a hereditary disorder marked by vitamin D–resistant rickets, hydrophthalmia, congenital glaucoma,

Miller's syndrome — (continued) mental retardation, and tubule reabsorption dysfunction

Miller's disease — osteomalacia

Miller modification of Welin's technique

Miller's collutory, curet, forceps, laryngoscope, method, ovum, speculum

Miller-Abbott tube

Miller-Fisher syndrome — same as Fisher's syndrome

Miller-Kurzrok test

Miller-Senn retractor

Milligan's trichrome stain

Millikan's rays

Millikan-Siekert syndrome — intermittent insufficiency of the basilar arterial system

Millin's clamp, forceps, retractor, tube

Millin-Bacon retractor

Millin-Read operation — correction of stress incontinence

Millipore filter

Millon's reaction, reagent, test

Millon-Nasse test

Millonig's fixative

Mills' disease — ascending hemiplegia, eventually developing into quadriplegia

Mills' forceps, test

Mills-Reincke phenomenon

Milroy's disease — congenital hereditary lymphedema of the legs, caused by lymphatic obstruction; also called Meige's disease

Milroy's edema

Miltenberger antigen

Milton's disease — angioneurotic edema

Milton's edema, urticaria

Minamata disease — a severe, neurologic disorder caused by alkyl mercury poisoning, leading to critical permanent

Minamata disease — (continued) neurologic and mental disabilities or death

Miner's osteotome

Minerva cast, jacket

Ming's classification

Mingazzini-Förster operation — same as Förster's operation

Minin's light

Minkowski's figure, method

Minkowski-Chauffard syndrome — congenital hemolytic icterus

Minor's disease — hemorrhage into the spinal cord, usually caused by trauma, marked by sudden onset of flaccid paralysis with sensory disturbances

Minor's sign, starch-iodine test, triangle

Minot's law

Minot-Murphy diet, treatment

Minot–von Willebrand syndrome — a congenital tendency to hemorrhage, characterized by a deficiency of coagulation and prolonged bleeding

Minsky's circles

Mira's photocoagulator, unit

Mirchamp's sign

Mirizzi's syndrome — hepatic duct stenosis

Miskiewicz's method

Mitchell's disease — a disease affecting the extremities of the body, marked by paroxysmal vasodilatation with burning pain and increased skin temperature

Mitchell's operation — resection of the medial prominence of the first metatarsal head with distal osteotomy

Mitchell's fluid, knife, stone basket, treatment

Mitchell-Diamond forceps

Mitchison's medium

Mitscherlich's test
Mitsuda's antigen, reaction, test
Mittelmeyer's test
Mittendorf's dot
Mixter's clamp, forceps, tube
Mixter-McQuigg forceps
M'Naghten (McNaughten) rule
Moberg's arthrodesis
Mobin-Uddin filter
Mobitz's block, heart block
Möbius' syndrome — developmental
    bilateral facial paralysis, usu-
    ally associated with other neu-
    rological disorders
Möbius' disease — periodic oculo-
    motor paralysis
Möbius' sign
Moe's plate
Moehle's forceps
Moeller's glossitis, reaction
Moeller-Barlow disease — subperi-
    osteal hematoma in rickets
Moerner-Sjöqvist method, test
Moersch's bronchoscope, esophago-
    scope, forceps
Moersch-Woltmann syndrome —
    prodromal tightness of the
    axial muscles progressing to
    generalized stiffness and par-
    oxysmal attacks of agonizing
    pain and tachycardia
Mohr's syndrome — orodigitofacial
    dysostosis
Mohr's method, pipette, test
Mohrenheim's fossa, space
Mohs' technique
Molisch's reaction, test
Moll's gland
Mollaret's meningitis
Möller's fluid, glossitis
Möller-Barlow disease — infantile
    scurvy
Mollison's retractor
Moloney's leukemia, reaction, test,
    virus
Molt's guillotine, mouth gag
Molteno's implant

Moltz-Storz tonsillectome
Monakow's syndrome — hemiplegia
    on the side opposite the le-
    sion in occlusion of the ante-
    rior choroidal artery
Monakow's bundle, fasciculus, nu-
    cleus, theory, tract
Monaldi's drainage
Mönckeberg's arteriosclerosis, calci-
    fication, degeneration, mesar-
    teritis, sclerosis
Moncrieff-Wilkinson syndrome — a
    combination of sucrosuria,
    mental retardation, and hia-
    tus hernia
Moncrieff's cannula, irrigator
Mondini's deafness, malformation
Mondonesi's reflex
Mondor's disease — inflammation
    of the subcutaneous veins of
    the chest wall and breast
Monge's disease — chronic moun-
    tain sickness
Monias-Shapiro's method
Monks-Esser flap
Monneret's pulse
Monro's abscesses, bursa, fissure, fo-
    ramen, line, sulcus
Monro-Kellie doctrine
Monro-Richter line
Monroe-Kerr incision
Monsel's solution
Monson's curve
Monsur's agar
Montague's abrader, proctoscope,
    sigmoidoscope
Monte Carlo method
Montefiore's tube
Monteggia's dislocation, fracture
Montenegro reaction, test
Monteverde's sign
Montevideo units
Montgomery's cups, follicles,
    glands, straps, tapes, tubercles
Montigne's test
Moon's molars, teeth
Moore's syndrome — paroxysmal
    abdominal pain expressing an

Moore's syndrome — (continued) abnormal neuronal discharge from the brain, sometimes causing convulsions

Moore's operation — introduction of a coil of wire into the sac of an aortic aneurysm for coagulation

Moore's button, extractor, forceps, fracture, osteotome, prosthesis, retractor, test, thoracoscope

Moore-Blount driver, extractor

Moore-Corradi operation — Moore's operation in which a strong galvanic current is passed through the wire

Moorehead's clamp, dissector, periosteotome, retractor

Mooren's ulcer

Moorhead's foreign body locator

Mooser's bodies, cell

Moots-McKesson ratio

Morand's foot, foramen, spur

Morawitz's theory

Morax's diplobacillus

Morax-Axenfeld bacillus, conjunctivitis, diplococcus, hemophilus

Morch's tube

Morel's syndrome — thickening of the inner table of the frontal bone

Morel's ear

Morel-Fatio blepharoplasty

Morel-Kraepelin disease — schizophrenia

Morel-Wildi syndrome — disseminated nodular dysgenesis of the frontal cerebral cortex

Morelli's reaction, test

Moreno's clamp

Moreschi's phenomenon

Morestin's operation — disarticulation of the knee with intracondyloid division of the femur

Morestin's method

Moretti's test

Morgagni's disease/syndrome — thickening of the inner table of the frontal bone

Morgagni's appendix, caruncle, column, crypt, cyst, foramen, fossa, fovea, frenula, frenum, glands, globules, hernia, hydatid, hyperostosis, lacunae, liquor, nodules, prolapse, sinus, sphere, tubercle, valves, ventricle

Morgagni-Adams-Stokes syndrome — sudden attacks of syncope in severe bradycardia or prolonged asystole accompanying heart block, with or without convulsions

Morgagni-Stewart-Morel syndrome — same as Morgagni's syndrome

Morgan's bacillus, line

Morison's incision, method, paste, pouch

Morita's therapy

Moritz's reaction, test

Moritz-Schmidt forceps

Morley's peritoneocutaneous reflex

Mörner's body, reagent, test

Moro's embrace reflex, reaction, test, tuberculin

Moro-Heisler diet

Morquio's syndrome — a lysosomal storage disease affecting the skeletal and nervous systems

Morquio's sign

Morquio-Ullrich disease — same as Morquio's syndrome

Morris' syndrome — a form of male pseudohermaphroditism characterized, when complete, by female external genitalia

Morris' catheter, hepatoma, retractor

Morrison-Hurd dissector, retractor

Morrow-Brooke syndrome — a skin disease resembling keratosis follicularis, in children

Morse-Andrews suction tube

Morse-Ferguson suction tube

Morson's forceps

Mortensen's disease — a hematologic disorder marked by prolonged bleeding time despite a permanent increase in blood platelet count

Mortimer's disease — a skin disease marked by raised, red patches that spread into a symmetrical pattern

Mortimer's malady

Morton's syndrome — a congenital insufficiency of the first metatarsal segment of the foot, causing pain and often associated with some degree of syndactylism

Morton's cough, current, fluid, foot, metatarsalgia, neuralgia, neuroma, plane, test, toe

Morvan's syndrome — edema and cyanosis with recurring felons of the hands, a condition seen in syringomyelia and sometimes in *Hansen's disease*

Morvan's chorea

Moschcowitz's disease — thrombotic thrombocytopenic purpura

Moschcowitz's operation — repair of femoral hernia by the inguinal approach

Moschcowitz's sign, test

Mosenthal's test

Moser's serum

Mosetig-Moorhof bone wax

Mosher's drain, esophagoscope, forceps, speculum, tube

Mosler's diabetes, sign

Mosny-Beaufume lipomatosis

Moss' classification

Mossbauer's spectrometer

Mosse's syndrome — polycythemia rubra vera with cirrhosis of the liver

Mossé-Marchand-Mallory cirrhosis

Mosso's ergograph, plethysmograph, sphygmomanometer

Mossuril virus

Motais' operation — for ptosis, by transplanting the middle portion of the tendon of the superior rectus muscle of the eyelid into the upper lid

Mott's bodies, cell, law of anticipation

Motulsky's dye reduction test

Mouchet's syndrome — remote paralysis of the cubital nerve caused by fracture of the external condyle of the humerus

Moult's curet

Mounier-Kuhn's syndrome — dilation of the trachea and bronchi, associated with chronic respiratory infection

Mount's syndrome — a hereditary disorder marked by attacks similar to those of *Huntington's chorea*

Mount-Mayfield forceps

Mount-Reback syndrome — a rare familial disorder marked by paroxysmal attacks of choreoathetosis and dystonic movements

Moure's esophagoscope

Movat's pentachrome method

Mowry's colloidal iron stain

Moyer's line

Moynihan's syndrome — progressive cardiomyopathic lentiginosis

Moynihan's clamp, cream, forceps, gastrojejunostomy, position, test

Moynihan-Navratil forceps

Mozambique ulcer

Mozart's ear

Mozer's disease — adult myosclerosis

Much's granules, reaction

Much-Holzmann reaction

Mucha's disease — same as *Mucha-Habermann disease*

Mucha-Habermann disease/syndrome — a cutaneous disease marked by vesicles, papules, and crusted lesions that are self-limiting but likely to recur and to leave smallpox-like scars

Muck's forceps

Muckle-Wells syndrome — familial amyloidosis involving the kidneys, marked by progressive hearing loss and periods of febrile urticaria

Mueller's arteries, prosthesis, speculum, tonometer, trephine

Mueller-Balfour retractor

Mueller-Frazier tube

Mueller-Hinton agar medium, broth

Mueller-Laforce adenotome

Mueller-Pynchon tube

Mueller-Yankauer tube

Muer's anoscope

Muir's clamp

Muir-Torre syndrome — same as *Torre's syndrome*

Muirhead's treatment

Mulder's angle, test

Muldoon's dilator, tube

Mules' operation — evisceration of the eyeball and insertion of artificial vitreous

Mules' eye implant, scoop

Müller's operation(s) — vaginal hysterectomy; cesarean section; resection of the sclera for detachment of the retina

Müller's canal, capsule, cells, duct, dust, experiment, fibers, fluid, ganglion, law, liquid, maneuver, muscle, radial cells, reaction, sign, test, tubercle

Müller-Haeckel law

Müller-Hillis maneuver

Müller-Jochmann test

Müller-Weiss disease — malacia of the navicular bone

Mulligan's prosthesis

Mumford Gigli-saw guide

Munchausen's syndrome — habitual presentation by a patient for medical treatment of an apparent acute illness, clinically convincing but all false

Münchmeyer's disease — a progressive inflammatory disease of the skeletal muscles, marked by weakness of the limbs, neck and pharynx

Mundie's forceps

Munk's disease — lipid nephrosis

Munro's abscess, microabscess, point

Munro Kerr maneuver

Munsell's colors

Munson's sign

Münzer-Rosenthal syndrome — a combination of hallucinations, anxiety, and catalepsy

Murat's sign

Murchison-Pel-Ebstein fever

Murchison-Sanderson syndrome — same as *Hodgkin's disease*

Murdock-Wiener speculum

Murphy's button, drip, kidney punch, method, percussion, sign, test, treatment

Murphy-Pattee test

Murphy-Sturm lymphosarcoma

Murray Valley encephalitis virus

Murri's disease — intermittent hemoglobinuria

Museholdt's forceps

Musken's tonometer

Musset's sign

Mussy's point

Mustard's operation — correction of a hemodynamic fault in transposition of the great vessels

Mustarde's otoplasty
Myà's disease — congenital dilation of the colon
Myers' method, punch, retractor
Myers-Fine test
Myers-Wardell method
Myerson's electrode, forceps, punch, sign

Myhrman-Zetterholm disease — an infectious renal disease marked by sudden onset of chills, fever, headache, abdominal symptoms, and vomiting
Myles' adenotome, clamp, curet, forceps, speculum, tonsillectome
Mylius' test

N

Nabatoff's vein stripper
Naboth's cysts, follicles, glands, ovules, vesicles
Nachlas' tube
Nadi reaction
Naegeli's syndrome — a hereditary disorder in which early vesicular and later bizarre pigmented lesions of the skin are associated with developmental defects of the eyes, bones and nervous system
Naegeli's culture medium, incontinentia pigmenti, law, macroblast, chromatophore nevus, solution
Naegeli's-type monocytic leukemia
Naffziger's syndrome — pain over the shoulder and extending to the arm, due to compression of nerves between a cervical rib and an anterior scalene muscle
Naffziger's operation — excision of the superior and lateral walls of the orbit for exophthalmos
Naffziger's test
Naffziger–Poppen Crain orbital decompression
Nagamatsu's incision
Nagel's test
Nägele's obliquity, pelvis, rule
Nägeli's maneuver, method, treatment

Nageotte's bracelets, cells
Nager's syndrome — same as *Nager-de Reynier* syndrome
Nager's acrofacial dysostosis
Nager–de Reynier syndrome — hypoplasia of the mandible, with abdominal implantation of the teeth, deformities of the pinna, and atresia of the external auditory meatus
Nagler's effect, reaction, test
Nakanishi's stain
Nakayama's test
Nakiwogo virus
Nance's leeway space
Napier's formol-gel test, serum test
Narath's operation — to establish collateral circulation in portal obstruction by fixing the omentum to the subcutaneous tissue of the abdominal wall
Narath's omentopexy
Narsaroff's phenomenon
Nasmyth's membrane
Natelson's pipette
Nathan's pacemaker, test
Nauheim's bath, treatment
Naunyn-Minkowski method
Nauta's stain
Neal's cannula, catheter
Nebécourt's syndrome — diabetes mellitus, pituitary dwarfism, and genital infantilism
Nebenthau's factor

Neef's hammer

Neer's prosthesis

Neftel's disease — a burning sensation of the head and neck and extreme discomfort except in a recumbent position

Nègre antigen

Negri-Jacod syndrome — unilateral blindness and paralysis of the eye muscles and one side of the body, or trigeminal neuralgia resulting from damage to cranial nerves, often from a tumor or lesion behind the sphenoid bone

Negro's phenomenon, sign

Negus' bronchoscope, telescope

Neill's medium

Neill-Dingwall syndrome — a familial syndrome allied to progeria and characterized by dwarfism

Neill-Mooser body, reaction

Neisser's diplococcus, reaction, staining method, syringe

Neisser-Doering phenomenon

Neisser-Wechsberg leukocidin, phenomenon, test

Neivert's knife, retractor

Neivert-Eves snare

Nélaton's disease — a central tumor of bone

Nélaton's operation — excision of the shoulder joint

Nélaton's catheter, dislocation, fibers, fold, line, probe, sphincter, tumor, ulcer

Nelson's syndrome — hyperpigmentation and nerve damage caused by development of a pituitary tumor after adrenalectomy

Nelson's ascites, forceps, method, scissors, trocar, tumor

Nelson-Bethune rib shears

Nelson-Roberts stripper

Nencki's test

Neri's sign

Neri-Barré syndrome — same as *Barré-Lieou syndrome*

Nernst's equation, law

Nesbit's cystoscope, resectoscope

Nessler's reagent, solution, test

Netherton's syndrome — a hereditary syndrome consisting of lamellar ichthyosis and atopic dermatitis, associated with fracturing and splitting of the cortex of hair shafts

Nettleship's syndrome — a chronic skin disease of early childhood characterized by pigmented macules or nodules

Nettleship-Wilder dilator

Neubauer's artery, hemocytometer, ruling

Neubauer-Fischer test

Neubeiser's splint

Neuber's operation — filling a cavity in bone with skin flaps taken from the sides of the wound

Neuber's treatment, tubes

Neuberg's ester

Neuendorf's treatment

Neufeld's nail, phenomenon, plate, reaction, screw, test

Neuhauser-Berenberg syndrome — cardioesophageal relaxation resulting in vomiting in infants, marked by nonfunction of the cardioesophageal sphincter, dilation of the esophagus and lack of gastric contractions

Neukomm's test

Neumann's syndrome — a benign, tender, pedunculated tumor of newborn infants, usually attached to the oral mucosa

Neumann's disease — a condition in which vegetations develop on the eroded surfaces of ruptured bullae and new bullae develop

Neumann's aphthosis, cells, law, method, pemphigus, sheath

Neusser's granules

Neve's cancer

Nevin's syndrome — subacute encephalopathy occurring between the ages of 50 and 70, marked by blindness, motor paralysis, speech disorders, cerebellar symptoms, mental disorders and myoclonus epilepsy

NeVTA virus

New's forceps, needle, scissors, tube

Newcastle disease — an influenza-like disease of birds that can be transferred to humans by contact with infected birds

Newcastle virus disease

Newcastle-Manchester bacillus

Newcomer's fixative

Newland's law

Newman's forceps, knife, proctoscope, tenaculum

Newton's alloy, disk, law, rings

New Zealand mice

Nezelof's syndrome — cellular immunodeficiency with abnormal immunoglobulin synthesis

Nezelof's T-cell deficiency

Nezelof-type thymic alymphoplasia

Nichol's clamp, method, reagent, speculum

Nickerson-Kveim test

Nickles' test

Nicol prism

Nicola's clamp, gouge, raspatory

Nicoladoni's sign

Nicolas-Favre disease — lymphogranuloma venereum

Nicolas-Moutot-Charlet syndrome — a familial, congenital, pemphigoid mucocutaneous disease, marked by a single bulla or vesicle followed by ulcerovegetative lesions

Nicolau's septineuritis

Nicolau-Hoigne syndrome — a nonallergic reaction to drugs

Nicolau-Hoigne syndrome — (continued) introduced into an artery, resulting in hearing and visual disorders, vertigo, paresthesia and anxiety

Nicolle's stain for capsules

Nidoko disease — epidemic hemorrhagic fever

Niebauer's prosthesis

Nieden's syndrome — multiple telangiectases of the face, arms and hands, with cataract and aortic stenosis

Niedner's clamp, forceps, knife, valvulotome

Nielsen's syndrome — weakness and muscular atrophy and fascicular twitching caused by extreme exhaustion

Nielsen's method

Niemann's disease — same as *Niemann-Pick disease*

Niemann's splenomegaly

Niemann-Pick disease — a hereditary disease marked by massive hepatosplenomegaly; nervous system involvement; and pressure in the liver, spleen, lung and bone marrow of phospholipid-storing histiocytes

Niemann-Pick cells

Niemann-Pick–type histiocyte

Nierhoff-Hübner syndrome — a variant of dysostosis enchondralis, marked by faulty ossification of the skull, vertebrae, ribs, and long bones in newborn infants

Nievergelt's syndrome — hereditary malformation of an extremity

Nievergelt-Erb syndrome — same as *Nievergelt's syndrome*

Niewenglowski's rays

Nikiforoff's method

Nikolsky's sign

Nimeh's method
Nippe's test
Nirenstein-Schiff method
Nisbet's chancre
Nissen's operation — mobilization of the lower end of the esophagus and plication of the fundus of the stomach around it
Nissen's forceps, gastrectomy, sutures
Nissl bodies, degeneration, granules, stain, substance alteration
Nitabuch's layer, stria, zone
Nithsdale's neck
Noack's syndrome — hereditary acrocephalosyndactyly with polydactyly
Nobel's test
Nobis' aortic occluder
Noble's forceps, position, scissors, stain
Nocard's bacillus
Noguchi's culture medium, lutein reaction, reagent, test
Noland-Budd curet
Nolke's method
Nomarski's microscope
Nonne's syndrome — hereditary cerebellar ataxia
Nonne's test
Nonne-Apelt phase, reaction, test
Nonne-Froin syndrome — same as *Froin's syndrome*
Nonne-Marie syndrome — same as *Marie's syndrome*
Nonne-Milroy syndrome — same as *Nonne-Milroy-Meige syndrome*
Nonne-Milroy-Meige syndrome — a familial form of lymphedema of the legs caused by lymphatic obstruction
Nonne–Pierre Marie syndrome — same as *Marie's syndrome*
Nonnenbruch's syndrome — oliguric kidney disease without organic renal changes

Noonan's syndrome — a symptom complex of short stature, webbed neck, ptosis, low-set ears, low nuchal hairline and deviated elbow with valvular pulmonary stenosis
Noorden treatment
Nordach's treatment
Nordau's disease — a general term for a condition of deterioration of the powers of mind and body
Norman-Wood syndrome — a congenital form of amaurotic idiocy
Norrie's disease — a hereditary disorder consisting of bilateral blindness, mental retardation, and deafness, transmitted as an X-linked trait
Norris' corpuscles
North American blastomycosis, coral snake antivenin
North Asian tick typhus
Norton's endotracheal tube
Norton-Simon hypothesis
Norum's disease — a genetic disorder, transmitted as an autosomal recessive trait, in which an absolute enzyme deficiency leads to hemolytic anemia in young adulthood, as well as liver and kidney failure, vascular degeneration, and lens opacities
Norum-Gjone disease — deficiency of lecithin and cholesterol acyltransferase
Norwalk agent, virus
Norwegian scabies
Norwood's forceps
Nothnagel's syndrome — dizziness, staggering, irregular oculomotor paralysis and often nystagmus — the symptoms of a midbrain tumor
Nothnagel's acroparesthesia, bodies, type

Nott's speculum
Nott-Guttmann speculum
Nourse's syringe
Novak's curet
Novikoff's hepatoma
Novy's rat disease — viral disease found in Novy's stock of experimental rats
Novy, McNeal, and Nicolle's medium
Noyes' forceps, rongeur, scissors, speculum
Noyes-Shambaugh scissors
Nuck's canal, diverticulum, hydrocele
Nuel's spaces
Nugent's forceps, hook
Nugent-Gradle scissors
Nugent-Green-Dimitry erysiphake
Nuhn's glands

Nunez's clamp, tube
Nunez-Nunez knife
Nunn's gorged corpuscles
Nürnberg's gold
Nussbaum's bracelet, clamp, experiment, narcosis
Nuttall's retractor
Nygaard-Brown syndrome — essential thrombophilia
Nyiri's test
Nylander's reagent, test
Nyssen–van Bogaert syndrome — the adult form of metachromatic leukodystrophy, which begins after age sixteen, presents as dementia and behavioral disturbances, and progresses to motor and postural disturbances
Nysten's law

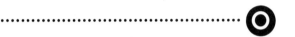

Oakley-Fulthorpe test
Obal's syndrome — amblyopia in severe malnutrition, associated with retrobulbar neuritis, scotoma, and visual disturbances
O'Beirne's experiment, sphincter, tube, valve
Ober's operation — dissection of a ligament for clubfoot
Ober's sign, tendon passer, test
Oberhill's retractor
Obermayer's reagent, test
Obermeier's spirillum
Obermüller's test
Oberst's method
Obersteiner-Redlich area, space, zone
O'Brien's akinesia, block, cataract, forceps
Obwegeser's incision, osteotomy, retractor

Ochsner's clamp, forceps, muscle, position, ring, scissors, treatment
Ochsner-Dixon forceps
Ockerblad's clamp
O'Connor's clamp, forceps, hook, operation, retractor
O'Connor-O'Sullivan retractor
O'Connor-Peter operation
Oddi's muscle, sphincter
Odelberg's disease — same as *Van Neck's disease*
Odman-Ledin catheter
O'Donaghue's splint
O'Dwyer's tube
Oedipus complex
Oehler's symptom
Oertel's treatment
Oertli's knife
Oestreicher's reaction
Ogata's method
Ogawa antigen

Ogilvie's syndrome — persistent contraction of intestinal musculature without evidence of organic disease of the colon, but simulating colonic obstruction and occurring as a result of a defect in the sympathetic nerve supply. Also called *false colonic obstruction*

Ogilvie's herniorrhaphy

Ogino-Knaus method

Ogston's operation(s) — removal of the inner condyle of the femur for knock knee; excision of the wedge of the tarsus for restoring the arch in flat feet

Ogston's line

Ogston-Luc operation — for frontal sinus disease

Oguchi's disease — a form of congenital night blindness occurring principally in Japan

O'Hanlon's forceps

Ohara's disease — occurring chiefly in Japan, probably identical with tularemia

O'Hara's forceps

O'Higgins' disease — an anicteric condition associated with leukopenia, blood platelet deficiency with retarded blood coagulation, hypocholesterolemia, hypocalcemia, capillaritis, and equilibrium disturbances

Ohm's law

Ohngren's line

Okazaki's segments

Oken's body, canal, corpus

Oldberg's dissector, forceps, retractor

Oldfield's syndrome — familial polyposis of the colon with extensive sebaceous cysts

Oliver's retractor, sign, test

Ollier's disease/syndrome — the presence of irregular fragments of nonossified cartilage

Ollier's disease/syndrome — (*continued*) in the metaphyses and diaphyses of the long bones

Ollier's incision, law, layer, raspatory, retractor

Ollier-Klippel-Trenaunay syndrome — same as *Klippel-Trenaunay syndrome*

Ollier-Thiersch graft

Olmer's disease — endemic in the Mediterranean area, caused by *Rickettsia conorii* and marked by chills, fever, and skin lesions

Olshausen's operation — for the cure of retroversion by suturing the uterus to the abdominal wall

Olshevsky's tube

O'Malley's knife

Ombrédanne's operation(s) — for hypospadias; trans-scrotal orchiopexy

Ombrédanne's syndrome — postoperative hyperthermia and pallor in children, caused by anesthesia

Ombrédanne's method

Omeliansky's nutritive culture medium

Omenn's syndrome — familial histiocytic reticulosis

Ommaya's reservoir

Omodei-Zorini syndrome — bronchial dilation caused by a broncholith

Omsk hemorrhagic fever virus

Ondine's curse

Ondiri disease — bovine infectious petechial fever

O'Neill's clamp, scissors

O'nyong-nyong fever, virus

Oort's bundle

Opalski's syndrome — a combination of hypoesthesia of pain and temperature in the face and paralysis of the extremi-

Opalski's syndrome — (continued) ties on one side of the body, associated with hypoesthesia of pain and temperature in the trunk and extremities

Opie's paradox

Opitz's syndrome — same as Opitz-Frias syndrome

Opitz's disease — enlargement of the spleen due to thombosis of the splenic vein

Opitz-Frias syndrome — a hereditary syndrome marked by hypertelorism and hernias. In males the disorder presents as hypospadias, cryptorchidism, and bifid scrotum

Oppenheim's syndrome — sclerosis of the spinal cord and tumor of the pituitary

Oppenheim's disease — a pseudoparalysis of congenital origin, observed principally in children, characterized by deficiency in tone of muscles innervated by the spinal nerves

Oppenheim's brace, gait, reflex, sign

Oppenheim-Urbach syndrome — a skin disorder observed in female diabetic patients, with multiple red or yellowish papules that later develop into round or oval scleroderma-like plaques

Optochin disk, susceptibility test

Orbeli's effect, phenomenon

Orbinsky's syndrome — abdominal muscle deficiency

Ord's operation — for breaking up joint adhesions

Ordóñez's melanosis

Oriboca virus

Oriental lung fluke disease — parasitic hemoptysis

Ormond's disease/syndrome — retroperitoneal fibrosis

Oropouche virus

Oroya fever

Orr's incision, method, technique, treatment

Orsi-Grocco method

Orth's fixative, fluid, solution, stain

Orthmann's tumor

Orticochea's flap

Ortner's syndrome — heart disease associated with laryngeal paralysis

Ortolani's click, sign

Ortved's stone dislodger

Osborne-Folin method

Osgood-Haskins test

Osgood-Schlatter disease — osteochondrosis of the tuberosity of the tibia

O'Shaughnessy's clamp, forceps

Osler's syndrome(s) — the presence in the diverticulum of Vater of a free-moving gallstone that blocks the outflow of bile from the common duct; multiple telangiectatic lesions of the face and body

Osler's disease(s) — polycythemia vera; hereditary hemorrhagic telangiectasia

Osler's erythema, maneuver, nodes, phenomenon, sign, triad

Osler-Libman-Sacks disease — same as Libman-Sacks syndrome

Osler-Vaquez disease — polycythemia vera

Osler-Weber-Rendu disease — hereditary hemorrhagic telangiectasia

Osterberg's test

Österreicher's syndrome — same as Österreicher-Turner syndrome

Österreicher-Turner syndrome — a hereditary syndrome transmitted as a dominant trait and marked by anomalies of the patellae, nails, and elbows and by iliac horns

Ostertag's streptococcus
Ostrum-Furst syndrome — congenital abnormal union of adjacent bones of the neck, deformity of the occipital bone and upper end of the cervical spine and elevation of the scapula
Ostwald's viscosimeter
O'Sullivan's retractor
O'Sullivan-O'Connor retractor, speculum
Ota's nevus
Ott's test
Ottenheimer's dilator
Otto's syndrome — same as *Guérin-Stern syndrome*
Otto's disease — osteoarthritic protrusion of the acetabulum
Otto's pelvis
Otto-Chrobak syndrome — protrusion of the acetabulum

Ottonello's method
Ouchterlony immunodiffusion, line, method, technique, test
Oudin current, immunodiffusion, resonator, test
Ovenstone factor
Overholt's elevator, forceps, raspatory, retractor
Overholt-Finochietto rib spreader
Overholt-Jackson bronchoscope
Overstreet's forceps
Owen's lines, position, spaces, sutures
Owren's syndrome(s) — hemolytic crisis; labile factor deficiency
Owren's disease — deficiency of calcium, with consequent impairment of coagulation
Owren's crisis
Oxford unit
Ozzard's filariasis

P

Paas' disease — a familial disorder marked by skeletal deformities, such as shortening of phalanges, scoliosis, and spondylitis
Pacchioni's foramen
Pace's knife
Pachon's test
Paci's operation — a modification of Lorenz's operation for congenital dislocation of the hip
Pacini's corpuscles
Padgett's dermatome, graft
Padgett-Hood electrodermatome
Padykula-Herman stain
Pagano's reaction
Page's syndrome — hypertensive diencephalic syndrome
Page's forceps, knife

Pagenstecher's circle, linen thread, ointment, scoop, sutures
Paget's disease(s) — increased bone resorption resulting in weakened and deformed bones; inflammatory cancerous affection of the areola and nipple, usually associated with carcinoma of the lactiferous ducts
Paget's disease, extramammary — a counterpart of Paget's disease of the breast, usually involving the vulva and sometimes the perianal and axillary regions
Paget's disease, juvenile — a bowing deformity of the legs, with elevated levels of blood

Paget's disease, juvenile —
(*continued*)
alkaline phosphatase, cortical
thickening of all bones, and
muscular weakness
Paget's abscess, cancer, carcinoma,
cells, nipple, quiet necrosis of
bone, test
Paget-Eccleston stain
Paget-Schroetter syndrome — intermittent venous claudication; also called *effort thrombosis*
Paget–von Schroetter syndrome —
same as *Paget-Schroetter syndrome*
Pai's culture medium
Paigen test
Paine's syndrome — microcephaly,
arthrogryposis, spastic diplegia, convulsions, mental retardation, aminoaciduria, irregular dental arches, abnormal
skin ridges, and congenital
heart defects
Pajot's hook, law, maneuver,
method
Pal's stain
Palade's buffered fixative
Palfyn's sutures
Palmar-Schatz stent implantation
Palmer's dilator
Palmgren's silver impregnation
stain
Paltauf's dwarf, nanism
Panas' operation — for ptosis, by
attaching the upper eyelid to
the occipitofrontalis muscle
Panas' technique
Pancoast's syndrome — tumor of
the apex of the lung as shown
by roentgenographic shadow,
with neuritic pain and muscle
weakness of the upper extrem-
ity caused by tumor pressure
on the brachial plexus
Pancoast's suture, tumor
Pander's islands, layer, nucleus

Paneth's cells
Pang's forceps
Panizza's plexuses
Panner's disease — osteochondrosis
of the distal end of the lateral
epicondyle of the humerus
Pansch's fissure
Panton-Valentine (P-V) leukoci-
din
Panum's area
Panzer's scissors
Pap's silver method
Papanicolaou's smear, stain, test
Paparella's catheter, curet, fenes-
trometer, retractor, scissors,
tube
Papez's circuit
Papillon-Léage and Psaume syn-
drome — orodigitofacial
dysostosis
Papillon-Lefèvre syndrome — a
congenital hyperkeratosis of
the palms and soles, with pro-
gressive destruction of alveolar bone about the teeth
Papin's digester
Pappenheim's lymphoid hemoblast,
stain
Pappenheimer's bodies
Paquelin's cautery
Paré's suture
Parenti's disease — a type of osteogenesis imperfecta marked
by absence of normal ossification and abnormal smallness
of limbs
Parhad-Poppen needle
Parham's band
Parham-Martin band, clamp
Parietti's broth
Parinaud's syndrome — a paralysis
of conjugate upward move-
ment of the eyes without paralysis of convergence, associated with lesions of the
midbrain, such as a tumor of
the pineal gland
Parinaud's oculoglandular syndrome — a general term for

Parinaud's oculoglandular syndrome — (continued) conjunctivitis, usually unilateral and follicular, often caused by infection with *Leptothrix*, or associated with other infections

Parinaud's conjunctivitis, conjunctivoadenitis, ophthalmoplegia

Paris classification, green, yellow

Parish's reaction

Park's aneurysm

Park-Guyton speculum

Park-Maumenee speculum

Park-Williams chocolate culture medium, fixative

Parker's fluid, incision, method, retractor

Parker-Heath cautery

Parker-Kerr forceps, stitch, sutures

Parker-Mott retractor

Parkinson's disease — a disease of the central nervous system of unknown etiology, characterized by masklike facies, tremor of the muscles, decreased motor power and control, postural instability, and muscular rigidity

Parkinson-dementia complex

Parkinson's facies, mask, position, sign

parkinsonian syndrome — a form of parkinsonism resulting from idiopathic degeneration of the striate body of the basal ganglia. It is slowly progressive and marked by masklike facies, tremor, slowing of voluntary movement, short accelerating steps in walking, uncertain posture, and muscle weakness

Parnum's test

Parona's space

Parrot's disease(s) — pseudoparalysis of one or more extremities of

Parrot's disease(s) — (continued) an infant, caused by syphilitic osteochondritis; short-limb dwarfism transmitted as an autosomal dominant trait

Parrot's atrophy of the newborn, cicatrix, node, pseudoparalysis, sign, ulcer

Parry's disease — same as *Graves' disease*

Parry-Romberg syndrome — facial hemiatrophy

Parson's disease — same as *Graves' disease*

Parsonage-Turner syndrome — severe pain across the shoulder and upper arm with atrophic paralysis of muscles of the shoulder girdle, usually following infection or minor surgery

Partipilo's clamp

Partsch's operation — marsupialization of a dental cyst

Pascal's law

Pascheff's conjunctivitis, folliculoma

Paschen's bodies, corpuscles, granules

Paschutin's degeneration

Pasini's syndrome — a type of epidermolysis bullosa, occurring at an early age and characterized by bullae that rupture, leaving scars and areas of pigmentation

Pasini-Pierini syndrome — progressive idiopathic atrophy of the skin, usually occurring in young women

Pasqualini's syndrome — eunuchoidism with spermatogenesis and normal secretion of follicle-stimulating hormone

Passavant's bar, cushion, pad, ridge

Passovoy's defect, factor

Passow's syndrome — essentially the same as *Bernard-Horner*

Passow's syndrome — *(continued)* *syndrome* but with color difference in the irides

Pasteur's culture medium, effect, fluid, liquid, method, pipet, reaction, solution, therapy

Pasteur-Chamberland filter

Pastia's lines, sign

Patau's syndrome — failure of cleavage of the prosencephalon, due to an extra chromosome 13, in which central nervous system defects are associated with mental retardation, cleft lip, polydactyly, and abnormalities of the heart, viscera and genitalia

Patein's albumin

Patella's disease — pyloric stenosis in tuberculosis

Paterson's syndrome — same as *Plummer-Vinson syndrome*

Paterson's bodies, cannula, corpuscles, forceps, nodules

Paterson-Brown-Kelly syndrome — same as *Plummer-Vinson syndrome*

Paterson-Kelly syndrome — same as *Plummer-Vinson syndrome*

Paterson-Kelly webs

Patey's operation — modified radical mastectomy

Paton's forceps, knife, spatula, trephine

Patrick's sign, test

Patterson's test

Patton's dilator, speculum

Paufique's knife, trephine

Paul's test, treatment

Paul-Bunnell antibodies, reaction, test

Paul-Bunnell-Barrett test

Paul-Bunnell-Davidsohn differential test

Paul-Mixter tube

Pauly's point

Paunz's test

Pautrier's abscess, microabscess

Pautrier-Woringer syndrome — lipomelanotic deposits in enlarged lymph nodes in association with various types of skin disease

Pauzat's disease — periostitis of the metatarsal bones

Pavlov's method, pouch, stomach

Pavy's disease — cyclic proteinuria

Pavy's test

Pawlik's triangle, trigone

Pawlow's method

Paxton's disease — same as *Beigel's disease*

Payne-Ochsner forceps

Payne-Péan forceps

Payne-Rankin forceps

Payr's disease — constipation, with upper quadrant pain from kinking of an adhesion between the transverse and descending colon with obstruction

Payr's clamp, method

Peabody's splint

Péan's operation(s) — vaginal hysterectomy bit by bit; hip joint amputation with ligation of vessels

Péan's amputation, forceps, hysterectomy, incision, position

Pearsall's sutures

Pearson's coefficient, method

Pecquet's cistern, duct, reservoir

Pedersen's speculum

Pel's crisis

Pel-Ebstein disease — a cyclic fever seen in Hodgkin's disease

Pel-Ebstein fever, pyrexia, symptom

Pelger's nuclear anomaly

Pelger-Huët nuclear anomaly, phenomenon

Pelizaeus-Merzbacher disease — familial centrolobar sclerosis

Pellegrini's disease — same as *Pellegrini-Stieda disease*

Pellegrini-Stieda disease — formation of a semilunar body in the upper portion of the medial lateral ligament of the knee, resulting from trauma

Pellizzi's syndrome — precocious development of external genitalia and sexual function, linked with abnormal growth of long bones and signs of internal hydrocephalus

Pélouse-Moore test

Pemberton's clamp, forceps, retractor, sign

Pende's syndrome — thymic hyperfunction associated with adiposity, genital dystrophy, and retarded mental and physical development

Pende's sign

Pendinski ulcer

Pendred's syndrome — a hereditary syndrome of congenital bilateral nerve deafness associated with goiter

Penfield's syndrome — epilepsy caused by a tumor pressing on the hypothalamus

Penfield's clip, elevator, forceps, modification of Rio-Hortega's method

Penjdeh sore, ulcer

Penn's seroflocculation reaction

Pennington's forceps, speculum

Penrose drain, tube

Penzoldt's reagent, test

Penzoldt-Fisher test

Pepper's disease/syndrome — neuroblastoma of the adrenal gland, with metastases to the liver

Pepper's tumor

Percy's cautery, forceps, retractor

Percy-Wolfson retractor

Perdrau's staining method

Perenyi's solution

Pereyra's operation — for correction of stress incontinence

Pereyra's bladder suspension, cannula, needle

Perez's sign

Peria's test

Perkins' tractor

Perlia's nucleus

Perlmann's tumor

Perls' anemia bodies, reaction, stain, test

Perrin-Ferraton disease — a condition marked by slippage of the hip joint with an audible snap

Perritt's forceps

Perroncito's apparatus, spirals

Perry's bag

Persian Gulf syndrome

Persian ulcer

Perthes' disease — osteochondrosis of the femoral epiphyses

Perthes' incision, test

Perthes-Calvé-Legg-Waldenström syndrome — same as *Calvé-Legg-Perthes syndrome*

Perthes-Jüngling disease — a progressive form of polycystic osteitis involving the surrounding soft tissue

Pertik's diverticulum

Peterman's test

Peters' anomaly, method, ovum

Petersen's operation — modification of high lithotomy

Petersen's bag

Petges-Cléjat syndrome — poikiloderma marked by extensive telangiectasia, pigmentation, atrophy of the skin and muscles, and myositis

Petit's syndrome — an oculopupillary syndrome caused by irritation of the sympathetic nervous system

Petit's canal, hernia, law, ligament, sinus, triangle

Petragnani's culture medium

Petrén's diet, treatment

Pétrequin's ligament

Petri's dish, plate, reaction, test
Petroff's synthetic culture medium
Petroff-Hauser counting chamber
Petruschky's culture medium, litmus whey, spinalgia
Pette-Döring disease — subacute sclerosing inflammation of the brain
Pette-Döring encephalitis, panencephalitis
Pettenkofer's test, theory
Petz's clamp
Petzetakis' reaction, test
Petzetakis-Takos syndrome — superficial keratitis, edema of the eyelids and bulbar conjunctiva, hypoesthesia of the cornea, diminished reflexes of the iris, xerophthalmia, and lesions of the corneal and precorneal layers
Peutz's syndrome — same as *Peutz-Jeghers syndrome*
Peutz-Jeghers syndrome — generalized multiple polyposis of the intestinal tract associated with excessive melanin pigmentation of the skin and mucous membranes
Peutz-Jeghers polyp
Peyer's follicles, glands, insulae, patches, plaques
Peyronie's disease — of unknown cause, marked by formation of dense fibrous tissue about the corpus cavernosum of the penis, causing deformity and painful erection
Peyrot's thorax
Peyton's brain spatula
Pezzer's catheter
Pfannenstiel's syndrome — hemolytic anemia of the neonate
Pfannenstiel's incision
Pfau's forceps, punch
Pfaundler-Hurler syndrome — same as *Hurler's syndrome*
Pfeiffer's syndrome — craniostenosis with polydactyly

Pfeiffer's disease — infectious mononucleosis
Pfeiffer's bacillus, blood agar, glandular fever, law, phenomenon, reaction
Pfeiffer-Comberg method
Pfiffner-Myers method
Pfister-Schwartz stone basket
Pflüger's cords, law, tubes
Pfuhl's sign
Pfuhl-Jaffé sign
Phalen's maneuver, sign
Phaneuf's clamp, forceps
Pheifer-Young retractor
Phelps' operation — an incision through the sole and inner side of the foot for talipes
Phelps' splint
Phelps-Gocht osteoclast
Phemister operation — onlay graft of cancellous bone without internal fixation, for treatment of ununited fracture
Phemister's bone graft, incision, punch, reamer
Philip's glands
Philippe-Gombault tract
Philippson's reflex
Phillips' bougie, catheter, muscle
Phipps-Bird water bath
Phocas' disease — chronic glandular mastitis
Physick's operation — removal of a circular piece of iris to create an artificial pupil
Physick's pouches
Piazza's fluid, reaction, test
Picchini's syndrome — a form of polyserositis caused by presence of a trypanosome
Pick's disease(s) — lobar atrophy of the brain with progressive intellectual deterioration, loss of memory, disorientation, and apathy; ascites and fibrotic liver disease associated with pericarditis
Pick's bodies, cells, cirrhosis, convolutional atrophy, hallucina-

Pick's bodies (continued)
tions, retinitis, testicular adenoma, tubular adenoma,
vision
Pickerill's imbricating lines
Pickrell's method, solution, spray
pickwickian syndrome — obesity,
somnolence, hypoventilation,
and erythrocytosis
Picot's retractor, speculum
Pictet's chloroform
Pictou's disease — liver cirrhosis in
livestock due to ragwort ingestion
Pierce's cannula, elevator, forceps,
syringe, tube
Pierce-Hoskins forceps
Pierre Robin syndrome — micro-
gnathia and abnormal
smallness of the tongue, with
cleft palate and often with bi-
lateral eye defects; also called
Robin's syndrome
Piersol's point
Pietrantoni's syndrome — mucosal
and cutaneous areas of anes-
thesia and neuralgia of the
face and oral cavity
Piffard's curet, paste
Pignet's formula, index, standard
Pike's streptococcal broth
Pilcher's catheter, hemostatic bag
Pillat's dystrophy
Pilling's bronchoscope, tube
Piltz's reflex, sign
Piltz-Westphal phenomenon
Pinard's maneuver
Pinaud's triangle
Pincus' test
Pindborg's tumor
Pinel's system
Pinkerton-Moorer reaction
Pinkus' disease — a rare skin erup-
tion marked by minute, flat,
sharply marginated, discrete
papules barely raised above
the skin surface
Pinkus' fibroepithelioma, tumor

Pins' sign
Piotrowski's sign, test
Piper's forceps
Piria's test
Pirie's bone, method
Piringer's lymphadenitis
Piringer-Kuchinka's syndrome —
benign cervical lymphadenitis
marked by epithelioid reticu-
lum cells in the lymph nodes
Pirogoff's amputation, angle,
edema, triangle
Pirquet's cutireaction, index, reac-
tion, test
Piry virus
Pisano's method
Pischel's electrode, elevator, for-
ceps
Piskacek's sign
Pitfield's fluid
Pitha's forceps
Pitkin's needle, solution
Pitres' sections, sign
Pittsburgh pneumonia agent
Piulachs-Hederich syndrome —
acute dilation of the colon
Pizzolato's peroxide-silver method
Placido's disk
Planck's constant, theory
Platner's crystallized bile, crystals
Plaut's angina, ulcer
Plaut-Vincent stomatitis
Playfair's treatment
Plesch's percussion, test
Pley's forceps
Plimmer's bodies, salt
Plimmer-Skelton method
Plugge's test
Plummer's disease — toxic multi-
nodular goiter
Plummer's adenoma, sign
Plummer-Vinson syndrome —
dysphagia with glossitis, ane-
mia, splenomegaly, and atro-
phy of the mouth, pharynx,
and esophagus; also called *sid-
eropenic dysphagia*
Plummer-Vinson applicator, dilator

Plunket's caustic

Pohl's mark, test

Poirier's glands, line

Poiseuille's equation, law, space

Poisson's distribution

Poisson-Pearson formula

Poitou's colic

Poland's syndrome — unilateral absence of the sternocostal head of the greater pectoral muscle; also called *Poland's deformity*

Poland's anomaly, deformity, syndactyly

Polenske number

Polhemus-Schafer-Ivemark syndrome — same as *Ivemark's syndrome*

Polisar-Lyons tube

Politzer's operation(s) — creation of an artificial opening in the membrana tympani; division of the anterior ligament of the malleus

Politzer's bag, cone, otoscope, speculum, test, treatment

Pollacci's test

Polley-Bickel trephine

Pollock's operation — amputation at the knee joint, preserving the patella

Polya's operation — anastomosis of the transected end of the stomach to the side of the jejunum following subtotal gastrectomy

Pomeroy's operation — female sterilization

Pompe's disease — glycogen storage disease

Poncet's disease — tuberculous rheumatism

Poncet's operation(s) — lengthening of the Achilles tendon for talipes equinus; perineotomy; perineal urethrostomy

Poncet's rheumatism

Pond's splint

Ponfick's shadow

Pongola virus

Pool's phenomenon, tube

Pool-Schlesinger sign

Poppen's coagulator, forceps, rongeur

Poppen-Blalock clamp

Porak-Durante syndrome — same as *Vrolik's syndrome*

Porcher's method

Porges-Hermann-Perutz reaction

Porges-Meier reaction, reagent, test

Porges-Salomon test

Porret's phenomenon

Porro's cesarean section

Porter's syndrome — a form of benign pericarditis that does not belong to the rheumatic, bacterial, or uremic group

Porter's sign, test

Porter-Silber chromogen test, reaction

Porteus' maze test

Portland hemoglobin

Portuguese-Azorean disease — same as *Azorean disease*

Porzett's splint

Posada's mycosis

Posada-Wernicke disease — coccidioidomycosis

Posey's belt

Posner's reaction, test

Posner-Schlossman syndrome — benign paroxysmal ocular hypertension

Post-Harrington erysiphake

Potain's apparatus, sign

Poth's keratosis

Pott's disease — tuberculosis of the spine

Pott's abscess, aneurysm, caries, clamp, curvature, fracture, gangrene, paralysis, paraplegia, puffy tumor

Pottenger's sign

Potter's syndrome — a rare lethal disease of infancy, marked by

Potter's syndrome — (continued)
renal agenesis or hypoplasia
with skeletal abnormalities
and characteristic facies
Potter's facies, treatment, version
Potter sequence
Potter-Bucky diaphragm, grid
Potts' operation — anastomosis be-
tween the descending aorta
and left pulmonary artery for
congenital pulmonary stenosis
Potts' dissector, periosteotome, val-
vulotome
Potts-Neidner clamp
Potts-Riker dilator, valvulotome
Potts-Satinsky clamp
Potts-Smith scissors, tenaculum,
valvulotome
Potts-Smith-Gibson operation —
anastomosis between the
aorta and the pulmonary ar-
tery in congenital pulmonary
stenosis
Poulet's disease — rheumatic osteo-
periostitis
Poupart's ligament, line
Poutasse's clamp, forceps
Pouteau's fracture
Powassan's encephalitis, virus
Power's operation — removal of a
corneal leukoma, followed by
insertion of a rabbit's cornea
Power-Wilder method
Pozzi's senile pseudorickets, tenaculum
Prader's orchidometer
Prader-Willi syndrome — a congenital disease of unknown etiology, marked by short stature,
marked obesity, mental retardation, severe muscle hypotonia, and sexual infantilism
Prague's maneuver, pelvis
Pratesi's syndrome — intermittent
claudication of the lower extremities, with cold feet

Pratt's anoscope, director, forceps,
sign, sound speculum, symp-
tom, test
Pratt-Smith forceps
Prausnitz-Küstner antibodies, reac-
tion, test
Pregl's test
Prehn's sign
Preiser's disease — osteoporosis and
atrophy of the carpal scaph-
oid from trauma or from frac-
ture that has not been kept
immobilized
Preisz-Nocard bacillus
Prendergast's test
Preshaw's clamp
Prévost's law, sign
Preyer's reflex, test
Price's precipitation reaction
Price-Jones curve, method
Price-Thomas clamp, forceps
Priessnitz's bandage, compress
Priestley's mass
Prieur-Trénel syndrome — the asso-
ciation of monilethrix and cat-
aract
Prigge's toxin
Prince's cautery, forceps, rongeur,
scissors
Prince-Potts scissors
Pringle's disease — a cutaneous
malformation or benign tu-
morlike nodule of the face, in-
volving blood vessels and con-
nective tissue
Pringle's incision
Prinzmetal's angina
Prinzmetal-Massumi syndrome —
pain and tenderness of the
anterior chest wall, which
may occur weeks or months
after myocardial infarct but
may also occur in the ab-
sence of history of coronary
disease
Pritchard's cannula, syringe
Pritikin's punch

Prochownick's diet, method
Proctor's elevator, retractor
Proetz's position, test, treatment
Profeta's immunity, law
Profichet's syndrome — growth of calcareous nodules in the subcutaneous tissues, especially about the joints, with a tendency to ulceration
Proneze's pad
Proskauer-Beck medium
Proust's law
Prowazek's bodies
Prowazek-Greeff bodies
Prower's factor
Pruitt's anoscope, proctoscope
Prussak's fibers, pouch, space
Prussian blue reaction, stain
Pryor-Péan retractor
Puchtler's method
Puchtler-Sweat stain
Pudenz's shunt, tube, valve
Pugh's nail
Purcell's retractor
Purdy's method, test
Purkinje's cells, corpuscles, effect, fibers, figures, images, layer, network, neurons, phenomenon, shadows, shift, vesicle
Purkinje-Sanson mirror images

Purmann's method
Purtscher's disease — angiopathy of the retina, with edema and hemorrhage, usually following crush injuries of the chest
Purtscher's angiopathic retinopathy
Pusey's emulsion
Pusto's dilatation
Putnam's acroparesthesia
Putnam-Dana syndrome — subacute degeneration of the spinal cord
Putti's syndrome — sciatica from arthrosis of the posterior vertebral joints
Putti's approach, gouge, splint
Putti-Chavany syndrome — unilateral sciatica with severe attacks of pain followed by foot paralysis
Putti-Platt director
Puusepp's operation — splitting of the central canal of the spinal cord for treatment of syringomyelia
Puusepp's reflex
Pyle's disease — familial metaphyseal dysplasia
Pynchon's applicator, speculum, tube
Pynchon-Lillie tongue depressor

Quaglino's operation — sclerotomy
Quain's ambiguous nucleus, degeneration, fatty heart, triangular fascia
Quant's sign
Quaranfil virus
Quarelli's syndrome — striatopallidal syndrome with parkinsonian tremor, seen in carbon disulfide poisoning
Quatrefages' angle

Queckenstedt's phenomenon, sign, test
Queckenstedt-Stookey test
Queensland fever, tick typhus
Quénu-Mayo operation — excision of the rectum and lymph glands for cancer
Quénu-Muret sign
Quervain's disease — same as *de Quervain's disease*
Quervain's forceps, fracture

Quervain-Sauerbruch retractor
Quesada's method
Quetelet's rule
Quevedo's forceps
Quevenne's iron
Queyrat's erythroplasia
Quick's method, test, tourniquet test
Quincke's disease — angioneurotic edema
Quincke's edema, meningitis, pulse, puncture, sign

Quincke-Tirmann-Schmelzer method
Quinlan's test
Quinquaud's disease — papular or pustular inflammation of the hair follicles of the scalp, with hair loss and scarring
Quinquaud's sign
Quinton's tube
Quisling's hammer

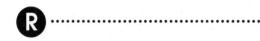

Raabe's test
Rabe-Salomon syndrome — congenital afibrinogenemia
Rabuteau's test
Racine's syndrome — swelling of the salivary glands and breasts four or five days premenstrually
Rademacher's disease — diminished immunity resulting in frequent infections, associated with hypogammaglobulinemia
Rademacher's system
Radford's nomogram
Radovici's sign
Raeder's paratrigeminal syndrome — a form of Bernard-Horner syndrome with cranial nerve disturbance caused by involvement of the carotid sympathetic plexus
Raimiste's sign
Rainey's corpuscles, tubes, tubules
Rainier's hemoglobin
Raiziss-Dubin method
Raji cell, cell radioimmune assay
Ralfe's test
Ralks' applicator, drill, forceps, magnet, mallet
Ralks-Davis mouth gag
Raman's effect, spectroscopy

Rambourg's stain
Ramdohr's sutures
Ramirez's dermatosis, shunt
Ramon's anatoxin, flocculation, flocculation test
Ramond's point, sign
Ramsay Hunt syndrome — same as Hunt's syndrome
Ramsay Hunt paralysis
Ramsbotham's hook, knife, sickle
Ramsden's eyepiece
Ramstedt's operation — same as Fredet-Ramstedt operation
Ramstedt's dilator, pyloromyotomy, pyloroplasty
Randall's curet, forceps, plaques, solution
Randolph's cannula, test
Raney's clip, drill, forceps, nickel, punch, retractor, rongeur
Raney-Crutchfield tongs
Raney Gigli-saw guide
Ranke's angle, complex, formula, stages
Rankin's clamp, forceps, retractor, tractor
Rankin-Crile forceps
Rankine's scale, thermometer
Ranson's pyridine silver stain
Rantzman's test

Ranvier's constrictions, crosses, internode, membrane, nodes, segment, tactile disks
Ranzewski's clamp
Raoult's law
Rapaport's dilator
Rapoport's test
Rapoport-Luebering cycle, shunt
Rappaport's classification
Raschkow's plexus
Rasin's sign
Rasmussen's aneurysm, nerve fibers, olivocochlear bundle
Rastelli's operation — to correct cardiac anomalies
Rathbun's syndrome — a congenital deficiency of alkaline phosphatase in the blood, marked by lack of calcification and abnormal cartilage maturation, with the cranial vault being nearly devoid of calcium
Rathke's columns, cysts, duct, folds, pocket, pouch, trabeculae, tumor
Ratliff-Blake forceps
Ratliff-Mayo forceps
Rau's apophysis, process
Rauber's layer, ligament, spinal crest
Rauchfuss' sling, triangle
Rauscher's leukemia virus
Ravich's cystoscope, lithotriptoscope
Ray's angulation method, curet, forceps, mania, speculum
Ray-Parsons-Sunday elevator
Rayer's disease — biliary xanthomatosis
Raygat's test
Rayleigh's light scatter
Raymond's apoplexy, type
Raymond-Céstan syndrome — same as *Céstan-Raymond syndrome*
Raynaud's disease(s) — idiopathic paroxysmal cyanosis of the digits, caused by arterial con-

Raynaud's disease(s) — *(continued)* traction from either cold or emotional disturbance; paralysis of the throat muscles following parotiditis
Raynaud's gangrene, phenomenon, sign
Rayner-Choyce eye implant
Read's formula
Réaumur's scale, thermometer
Reaves' punch
Rebuck's skin window technique, test
Recamier's curet
Rechcigl-Sidransky hepatoma
Recklinghausen's disease(s) — neurofibromatosis; osteitis with fibrous degeneration and formation of cysts and fibrous nodules on affected bones
Recklinghausen's canals, tonometer, tumor
Recklinghausen-Applebaum disease — hemochromatosis
Reclus' disease(s) — painless, cystic enlargement of the mammary glands; cellulitis with induration
Redlich's encephalitis
Redlich-Fisher miliary plaques
red Robinson catheter
Reed's cells
Reed-Hodgkin disease — same as *Hodgkin's disease*
Reed-Muench method
Reed-Sternberg cells
Reenstierna's antiserum
Rees' culture medium, test
Rees-Ecker diluting fluid, solution
Reese's syndrome — retinal dysplasia, congenital and always bilateral, usually associated with microphthalmia, cerebral agenesis and other abnormalities
Reese's dermatome, dysplasia, forceps, knife
Reese-Ecker fluid, method

Refetoff's syndrome — goiter and an elevated serum level of thyroid hormones but without true thyrotoxicosis

Refsum's disease — a hereditary disease of lipid metabolism, characterized by chronic polyneuritis, retinitis, cerebellar ataxia, and persistent elevation of protein in the cerebrospinal fluid

Regan's isoenzyme

Regan-Lowe agar

Regaud's fixative, fluid, tumor

Regnaud's residual body

Regnoli's operation — excision of the tongue

Rehberg's test

Rehfuss' method, test, tube

Reich-Nechtow clamp, dilator, forceps

Reichel's syndrome — osteochondromatosis marked by cartilaginous foreign bodies in the joint cavity or in the bursa of a tendon sheath

Reichel's cloacal duct

Reichert's syndrome — neuralgia of the glossopharyngeal nerve

Reichert's canal, cartilages, membrane, recess, scar, substance

Reichert-Meissl number

Reichl's test

Reichmann's disease/syndrome — excessive and continuous secretion of gastric juice

Reichmann's rod

Reichstein's substance

Reid's base line, index

Reid Hunt's reaction, test

Reifenstein's syndrome — a male form of pseudohermaphroditism, marked by ambiguous genitalia or hypospadias and by infertility due to sclerosis of the seminiferous tubules, sometimes accompanied by cryptorchidism and impotence

Reil's ansa, band, insula, island, limiting sulcus, ribbon, triangle, trigone

Reilly's bodies, granulations, phenomenon

Reimann's periodic disease — familial paroxysmal polyserositis

Reinecke's acid

Reiner's curet, D-xylose absorption test, knife, rongeur

Reiner-Beck snare

Reiner-Knight forceps

Reinhoff-Finochietto rib spreader

Reinke's crystalloids, crystals, edema

Reinsch's test

Reis-Bücklers disease — annular corneal dystrophy

Reisinger's forceps

Reisseisen's muscles

Reissner's fiber, membrane

Reiswig's reamer

Reiter's disease/syndrome — a triad of urethritis, iridocyclitis and arthritis

Reiter's protein complement-fixation

Reitland-Franklin unit

Rejchman's disease — same as *Reichmann's disease*

Rekoss' disk

Reliquet's lithotrite

Relton-Hall frame

Remak's band, fibers, ganglion, paralysis, plexus, reflex, sign, symptom, type

Remont's test

Renaut's bodies

Rendu's tremor

Rendu-Osler-Weber disease/syndrome — hereditary hemorrhagic telangiectasia

Renikhet disease — an acute, febrile disease of fowl caused by a paramyxovirus, marked by respiratory and nervous system symptoms. It is transmissi-

Renikhet disease — *(continued)* ble to humans, causing severe but transient conjunctivitis

Rénon-Delille syndrome — thyroovarian insufficiency, hypophyseal hyperfunction and acromegaly, associated with hypotension, tachycardia, hyperhidrosis, oliguria, insomnia, and intolerance to heat

Renpenning's syndrome — familial X-linked mental retardation

Renshaw's cells

Renver's funnel

Replogle's tube

Retan's treatment

Rett's syndrome — a progressive disorder present from birth in females, affecting the gray matter of the brain. It is marked by autism, ataxia, dementia, and seizures

Retter's needle

Retzius' body, cavity, fibers, foramen, gyrus, lines, space, striae, stripes, veins

Reuber's hepatoma

Reuss' color charts, formula, tables, test

Reuter's button, tube

Reverdin's operation — transplanting an epidermic graft to a defect

Reverdin's graft, method, needle

Revilliod's sign

Revol's disease — same as *Mortensen's disease*

Rey-Ostreich complex figure test

Reye's syndrome — sudden loss of consciousness in children following a premonitory, severe infection, marked by cerebral edema and fatty change in the liver, often followed by death

Reye-Johnson syndrome — same as *Reye's syndrome*

Reynold's clamp, number, scissors, test, tube

Rezek's forceps

Rhein's picks

Rheinberg's microscope

Rheinhard's myocarditis

Rheinstaedter's curet

Rhese's method

Rhinelander's clamp

Rhodesian trypanosomiasis

Rhoton's punch

Riba's meatotome

Ribas-Torres disease — a mild form of smallpox

Ribbert's theory, thrombosis

Ribbing's syndrome — hereditary multiple diaphyseal sclerosis

Ribble's bandage

Ribes' ganglion

Ricard's amputation

Ricco's law

Richard's forceps

Richards' clamp, nail, prosthesis, screw

Richards-Rundle syndrome — a congenital nervous system disorder marked by progressive sensorineural hearing loss, ataxia, muscle wasting, nystagmus, mental retardation, and failure to develop secondary sexual characteristics

Richardson's elevator, retractor, sign, sutures

Richardson-Eastman retractor

Richet's aneurysm, bandage, fascia

Richner-Hanhart syndrome — a familial syndrome consisting of keratosis of the palms and soles, growth retardation and mental retardation, transmitted as a recessive trait

Richter's syndrome — histiocytic lymphoma developing in chronic lymphocytic leukemia

Richter's forceps, hernia, sutures

Richter-Monro line

Rickett's organism

Rickham's reservoir

Ricord's treatment

Riddoch's syndrome — visual dis-orientation resulting from uni-lateral lesions of the parietal lobe

Riddoch's mass reflex

Rideal-Walker coefficient, method

Ridell's operation — excision of the anterior and posterior walls of the frontal sinus for treatment of malignant tu-mors

Ridgway's osteogenic sarcoma

Ridley's sinus

Ridlon's knife

Ridpath's curet

Rieckenberg's test

Riecker's bronchoscope

Riedel's disease — a rare, fibrous in-duration of the thyroid, with adhesion to adjacent struc-tures that may cause tracheal compression

Riedel's lobe, struma, thyroiditis

Rieder's cell, cell leukemia, lym-phocyte, paralysis

Riegel's pulse, symptoms, test

Rieger's syndrome — hypodontia, anal stenosis, mental defi-ciency, and absence of facial bones

Rieger's anomaly, malformation, phenomenon

Riegler's test

Riehl's melanosis

Rienhoff's dissector, forceps

Riesman's pneumonia, sign

Rietti-Greppi-Micheli syndrome — hemolytic jaundice, with in-creased red cell fragility

Rieux's hernia

Rifkind's sign

Rift Valley fever virus

Riga's aphthae, papilloma

Riga-Fede disease — granuloma of the lingual frenum in chil-dren that occurs after abra-sion by the lower central inci-sors

Rigal's sutures

Rigaud's operation — a plastic op-eration for urethral fistula

Rigby's retractor

Riggs' disease — compound peri-odontitis

Rigler's sign

Riley's needle

Riley-Day syndrome — familial dysfunction of the autonomic nervous system

Riley-Shwachman syndrome — osseous changes and hyper-reflexia, with a peculiar gait marked by stiff legs, ankle clo-nus, and calcaneal limp

Riley-Smith syndrome — macro-cephaly without hydrocepha-lus

Rimbaud-Passouant-Vallat syn-drome — febrile encephalitis with coma, convulsions, hemi-plegia, headache, vertigo, Cheyne-Stokes respiration, and deglutition disorders

Rimini's test

Rindfleisch's cells, folds

Ringenberg's electrode

Ringer's injection, irrigation, lac-tate, mixture, solution

Rinne's test

Rio-Hortega method

Riolan's anastomosis, arch, bone, muscle, nosegay, ossicles

Ripault's sign

Risdon's approach, incision, wire

Rish's chisel, knife

Risley's prism

Ritchie's formalin–ethyl acetate procedure, tenaculum

Ritgen's maneuver, method

Ritisch's sutures

Ritter's disease — exfoliative der-matitis supervening in bullous impetigo of the neonate; also called *staphylococcal scalded skin syndrome*

Ritter's dermatitis, dilator, fiber, for-ceps, law, rasp, sound, tetanus

Ritter-Oleson technique

Ritter-Rollet phenomenon, sign

Ritter-Valli law

Riva-Rocci sphygmomanometer

Rivalta's reaction, test

Riverius' alum curd, draft

Rivers' cocktail

Rivière's potion

Riviere's sign

Rivinus' canals, ducts, foramen, gland, incisure, notch, segment

Rizzo's retractor

Rizzoli's osteoclast

Rizzuti's lens expressor, retractor

Rizzuti-McGuire scissors

Roaf's syndrome — a nonhereditary craniofacial-skeletal disorder marked by early retinal detachment, cataracts, myopia, shortened long bones, and mental retardation

Roaf's method

Robb's cannula, forceps, syringe

Robert's syndrome — a hereditary syndrome marked by defective development of the long bones and cleft palate and other anomalies

Robert's ligament, pelvis

Robert Jones dressing

Roberts' applicator, esophagoscope, forceps, laryngoscope, speculum, test

Roberts-Nelson rib shears, tourniquet

Robertson's syndrome — a symptom of neurosyphilis, especially tabes dorsalis, and of other diseases of the central nervous system

Robertson's culture medium, pupil, sign

Robin's syndrome — same as *Pierre Robin syndrome*

Robin's spaces

Robinow's syndrome — dwarfism associated with malaligned

Robinow's syndrome — *(continued)* teeth, bulging forehead, depressed nasal bridge and short limbs; called also *Robinow's dwarfism*

Robinson's disease — cystic neoplasms of the sweat glands occurring on the face in the region of the eyes

Robinson's catheter, circle, stone basket

Robinson-Cohen slide

Robinson-Kepler test

Robinson-Kepler-Power water test

Robison's ester, ester degeneration, ester dehydrogenase

Robles' disease — infestation by worms of the genus *Onchocerca*

Robles' fever

Robson's line, point, position, staging system

Roch's lipomatosis

Roche's cutoff, sign

Rochester's awl, forceps, syringe, tube

Rochester-Carmalt forceps

Rochester-Ewald forceps

Rochester-Ferguson retractor, scissors

Rochester-Harrington forceps

Rochester-Mixter forceps

Rochester-Ochsner forceps

Rochester-Péan forceps

Rochester-Rankin forceps

Rochet's procedure

Rochon-Duvigneaud's syndrome — orbital and unilateral frontal headache with third, fourth, and sixth cranial nerve palsies, oculomotor paralysis, decrease of the field of vision, and other ocular changes

Rockey's cannula, endoscope, forceps, probe

Rockley's sign

Rocky-Davis incision

Rocky Mountain spotted fever

Rodman's incision
Rodrigues' aneurysm
Rodriguez-Alvarez catheter
Roe's clamp, solution
Roeder's clamp, forceps, treatment
Roemheld's syndrome — cardiac and gastrointestinal symptoms in excitable persons, most frequently in patients with thyroid disorders
Roffo's test
Roger's syndrome — continuous excessive secretion of saliva as a result of esophageal carcinoma
Roger's disease — ventricular septal defect
Roger's amputation, antigen, bruit, dissector, murmur, reaction, reflex, symptom, test
Roger Anderson apparatus
Roger-Josué test
Roger's sphygmomanometer
Rogor-Foot modification of Bielschowsky technique
Röhl's marginal corpuscles
Rohon-Beard cells
Rohr's agranulocytosis, layer, stria
Röhrer's index
Roida's tube
Rokitansky's disease — acute yellow atrophy of the liver
Rokitansky's acute yellow atrophy, diverticulum, hernia, kidney, pelvis
Rokitansky-Aschoff ducts, sinuses
Rokitansky-Cushing ulcers
Rokitansky-Küster-Hauser syndrome — same as *Mayer-Rokitansky-Küster-Hauser syndrome*
Rolando's angle, area, cells, column, fasciculus, fibers, fissure, funiculus, line, point, substance, tubercle, zone
Rolf's forceps, lance
Roller's nucleus
Rolleston's rule
Rollet's syndrome — sensorimotor ophthalmoplegia and optic at-

Rollet's syndrome — *(continued)* rophy, produced by lesions of the apex of the orbit involving the third, fourth, and sixth cranial nerves
Rollet's chancre, incision, irrigator, retractor, stroma
Rollier's formula, radiation, treatment
Romaña's sign
Romano-Ward syndrome — prolonged Q-R interval (atrial activity) in children subject to attacks of unconsciousness resulting from Adams-Stokes seizures and ventricular fibrillation
Romanovsky's (Romanowsky's) method, stain
Romberg's disease/syndrome — facial hemiatrophy
Romberg's hemiatrophy, sign, spasm, station, test, trophoneurosis
Romberg-Howship sign, symptom
Römer's reaction, test
Rommel-Hildreth cautery
Rommelaere's sign
Romney Marsh disease — hemorrhagic enterotoxemia of young calves, lambs, and piglets caused by *Clostridium perfringens* type C, which is usually fatal
Ronchese's test
Rönne's nasal step
Roos' osteotome, retractor
Ropes' test
Roper's cannula
Roques' syndrome — parallel sclerosis of the heart and lungs in chronic cor pulmonale in aged patients
Rorschach test
Rosa's law
Rose's operation — removal of the trigeminal ganglion
Rose's position, test, tetanus

Rose-Bradford kidney

Rose-Thompson cleft lip repair

Rose-Waaler test

Rosen's curet, incision, neuralgia, probe, tube

Rosen-Castleman-Liebow syndrome — pulmonary proteinosis

Rosenbach's syndrome — association of paroxysmal tachycardia with cardiac, gastric, and respiratory disturbances

Rosenbach's disease — a skin disease affecting persons coming in contact with meat or dead animals

Rosenbach's reaction, sign, test, tuberculin

Rosenbach-Gmelin test

Rosenberg-Bergstrom syndrome — an autosomal recessive syndrome marked by excessive uric acid in the urine, renal insufficiency, ataxia, and deafness

Rosenberg-Chutorian syndrome — a rare X-linked hereditary syndrome marked by optic atrophy, neural deafness, and polyneuropathy

Rosenfield's nomenclature, system

Rosenheim-Drummond's method, test

Rosenmüller's body, cavity, fossa, gland, node, organ, recess, valve

Rosenow's veal brain broth

Rosenthal's syndrome(s) — hereditary tendency to hemorrhage, resembling hemophilia but caused by plasma thromboplastin deficiency; paralysis on awakening, with inability to move although fully conscious

Rosenthal's canal, degeneration, fibers, test, vein

Rosenthal-Kloepfer syndrome — corneal opacities and acro-

Rosenthal-Kloepfer syndrome — (continued) megaloid appearance, with enlargement and thickening of the skin of the scalp so that it lies in folds

Rosenthaler's reagent

Rosenthaler-Turk reaction

Roser's line, mouth gag, sign

Roser-Braun sign

Rosewater's syndrome — a mild form of male familial hypogonadism

Rosi's prosthesis

Rosin's test

Ross' black spores, bodies, catheter, cycle, retractor

Ross-Jones test

Rossbach's disease — secretion of hydrochloric acid by the stomach cells

Rossel's test

Rosser's hook

Rössle-Urbach-Wiethe lipoproteinosis

Rossolimo's reflex, sign

Rostan's asthma, shunt

Rot's disease — same as *Rot-Bernhardt disease*

Rot's meralgia

Rot-Bernhardt disease — a condition marked by paresthesia, pain, and numbness of the thigh in the region supplied by the lateral femoral cutaneous nerve

Rot-Bielschowsky syndrome — paralysis of the conjugate gaze in one direction

Rotch's sign

Roth's disease — same as *Rot-Bernhardt disease*

Roth's spots

Roth-Bernhardt disease — same as *Rot-Bernhardt disease*

Rothera's nitroprusside test

Rothmann-Makai syndrome — idiopathic circumscribed pan-

Rothmann-Makai syndrome —
(*continued*)
niculitis with fat cell necrosis,
fatty granuloma, and cyst formation
Rothmund's syndrome — congenital cutaneous dystrophy
Rothmund's dystrophy
Rothmund-Thomson syndrome —
a hereditary syndrome marked
by poikiloderma and telangiectasia, associated with cataracts, bone defects, and hypogonadism
Rothschild's sign
Rotor's syndrome — chronic familial nonhemolytic jaundice
Rotter's nodes, test
Rotter-Erb syndrome — deformities
of the bones, joints, and tendons, marked by dwarfism,
multiple epiphyseal lesions,
multiple dislocations, bilateral
clubfoot, vertebral deformities, and cleft palate
Rouget's bulb, cells, muscle, pericyte
Roughton-Scholander apparatus,
syringe
Rougnon-Heberden disease —
angina pectoris
Rourke-Ernstein sedimentation
rate
Rous-associated virus (RAV)
Rous' sarcoma, sarcoma virus, test,
tumor
Roussel's law, sign
Rousselot's caustic
Roussin's test
Roussy-Cornil syndrome — progressive hypertrophic neuritis
Roussy-Dejerine syndrome — same
as *Dejerine-Roussy syndrome*
Roussy-Lévy syndrome — same as
Lévy-Roussy syndrome
Roussy-Lévy disease — familial
ataxia marked by disorders of
gait, clubfoot, and lack of ten-
don reflexes

Routier's operation — for
Dupuytren's contracture
Routte's operation — suturing the
saphenous vein so it will
open into the peritoneal cavity in order to drain the cavity in cases of ascites with cirrhosis of the liver
Rouviere's node
Roux's anastomosis, serum, stain
Roux-en-Y anastomosis, incision,
limb
Rovighi's sign
Rovsing's syndrome — horseshoe
kidney with nausea, abdominal discomfort, and pain
Rovsing's sign
Rowland's forceps, keratome, osteotome
Rowley-Rosenberg syndrome —
growth retardation, renal aminoaciduria, cor pulmonale,
and muscular hypoplasia, associated with alveolar hypoventilation, atelectasis, and right
ventricular hypertrophy — a
familial disorder that has
been observed in the children
of consanguineous parents
Rowntree-Geraghty test
Royce's knife, perforator
Royer's syndrome — association of
diabetes mellitus with hypo-
genital dystrophy
Rubin's test
Rubin-Brandborg tube
Rubin-Holth punch
Rubino's reaction, test
Rubins' cannula, needle, test, tube
Rubinstein's syndrome — a congenital syndrome marked by
mental and motor retarda-
tion, short stature, characteristic facies, various ocular
anomalies, pulmonary stenosis, keloid formation, and abnormalities of the vertebrae
and sternum
Rubinstein-Taybi syndrome —
same as *Rubinstein's syndrome*

Rubner's lactose test, law
Rubovits' clamp
Ruck's watery extract tuberculin
Rud's syndrome — a hereditary syndrome transmitted as an autosomal trait, marked by mental deficiency, epilepsy, infantilism, and congenital ichthyosis
Ruffini's brushes, corpuscles, cylinders, ending, organ
Rugby's forceps
Ruge's solution
Ruge-Phillipp test
Ruggeri's reflex, sign
Ruhemann's test, uricometer, uricometer method
Ruhr's rheumatism
Rukavina's syndrome — Indiana-type familial amyloid polyneuropathy
Rulf's convulsions
Rumel's clamp, forceps, splint, tourniquet
Rumel-Belmont tourniquet
Rummo's disease — downward displacement of the heart
Rumpel-Leede phenomenon, sign, test
Rumpf's sign, symptom, traumatic reaction
Rundles-Falls syndrome — familial hypochromic microcytic anemia with erythrocyte abnormalities, splenomegaly, and sometimes hepatomegaly, affecting only males
Runeberg's anemia, formula, type
Runyon's classification, group
Rusch's catheter, laryngoscope
Rusch-Foley catheter
Ruschelit's bougie, catheter
Rusconi's anus
Rush's clamp, extractor, mallet, nail, rod
Rushkin's balloon
Ruskin's forceps, rongeur, trocar
Ruskin-Liston forceps
Russe's incision
Russell's syndrome(s) — congenital dwarfism with short stature,

Russell's syndrome(s) —
  (continued)
disproportionately short arms, cryptorchidism, and other abnormalities; emaciation in infancy and childhood, caused by a diencephalic tumor and associated with initial growth acceleration, locomotor hyperactivity, euphoria, and pallor
Russell's bodies, double sugar agar, dwarf, effect, traction, unit, viper, viper venom
Russell-Buck tractor
Russell-Crooke cell
Russell-Silver syndrome — same as *Russell's syndrome*
Russian spring-summer encephalitis virus
Russo's reaction, test
Rust's disease — tuberculous spondylitis of the cervical vertebrae
Rust's syndrome — stiff neck and head with necessity for holding the head with both hands in lying down or rising up—a disorder occurring in tuberculosis, cancer, fracture of the spine, rheumatic or arthritic disease, or syphilitic periostitis
Rust's phenomenon, sign
Rustitskii's disease — same as *Kahler's disease*
Rutherford's atom, method, scattering
Rutherfurd's syndrome — a familial oculodental disorder of corneal dystrophy, gingival hypertrophy, and failure of tooth eruption
Ruttan-Hardisty test
Ruvalcaba's syndrome — abnormal shortness of the metacarpal or metatarsal bones, decreased gonadal function, and retardation characterized by skeletal abnormalities

Ruysch's disease — same as
  Hirschsprung's disease
Ruysch's glomeruli, membrane,
  muscle, tube, tunic, veins

Rye's classification
Ryerson's tenotome
Ryle's tube
Rytz's test

 S ....

Saalfield's extractor
Saathoff's test
Sabhi agar
Sabin's megaloblast, vaccine
Sabin-Feldman syndrome —
  chorioretinitis and cerebral
  calcifications—symptoms like
  those of toxoplasmosis but
  with negative tests for toxo-
  plasmosis
Sabin-Feldman dye test
Sabouraud's syndrome — a heredi-
  tary, congenital disease caus-
  ing beadlike enlargement and
  brittleness of hair
Sabouraud's agar, pastille
Sachs' disease — same as *Tay-Sachs
  disease*
Sachs' antigen, bur, spatula, tube
Sachs-Georgi reaction, test
Sachs-Vine tube
Sachs-Witebsky reaction, test
Sachsse's test
Saemisch's operation — transfixion
  of the cornea for cure of accu-
  mulation of pus in the eye
Saemisch's section, ulcer
Saenger's macula, reflex, sign, su-
  tures
Saethre-Chotzen syndrome — same
  as *Chotzen's syndrome*
Safar's bronchoscope
Sage's snare
Sagnac's rays
Sahli's method, reaction, reagent,
  test
Sahli-Nencki test
St. Agatha's disease — mastitis

St. Anthony's disease — chorea
St. Anthony's dance, fire
St. Appolonia's disease — tooth-
  ache
St. Avertin's disease — epilepsy
St. Avidus' disease — deafness
St. Blasius' disease — peritonsillar
  abscess
St. Clair-Thompson curet, forceps
St. Dymphna's disease — insanity
St. Erasmus' disease — colic
St. Fiacre's disease — hemorrhoids
St. Francis' fire
St. Gervasius' disease — rheuma-
  tism
St. Gotthard's tunnel disease —
  hookworm
St. Guy's dance
St. Hubert's disease — rabies
St. Job's disease — syphilis
St. John's dance, evil
St. Jude valve prosthesis
St. Louis encephalitis
St. Luke's retractor, rongeur
St. Main's evil
St. Mark's incision
St. Martin's evil
St. Mathurin's disease — idiocy
St. Modestus' disease — chorea
St. Roch's disease — plague
St. Sement's disease — syphilis
St. Valentine's disease — epilepsy
St. Vitus' dance
St. Zachary's disease — mutism
Saint's triad
Sakaguchi's reaction, test
Sakamoto's disease — infantile di-
  arrhea marked by explosive

Sakamoto's disease — *(continued)*
vomiting, milky stools, and
mild respiratory symptoms, occurring in epidemic form in
Japan

Sakati-Nyhan syndrome — acro-
cephalopoly/syndactyly, type
III

Sala's cells

Salah's needle

Salem's sump, tube

Salibi's clamp

Salisbury common cold virus

Salisbury-Melvin sign

Salk's vaccine

Salkowski's method, test

Salkowski-Arnstein method

Salkowski-Autenrieth-Barth
method

Salkowski-Ludwig test

Salkowski-Schipper test

Salmon's catheter

Salomon's test

Salter's incremental lines

Saltzman's method

Salus' arch

Salvatore-Maloney tracheotome

Salvioli's syndrome — a familial
syndrome involving the autonomic nervous system, bones,
endocrine glands, and phosphorus metabolism, causing
tremor, chorea, mental disorders, gynecomastia, hypergeni-
talism, and muscular atrophy

Salzmann's nodular corneal dystrophy

Sam Roberts esophagoscope, forceps, laryngoscope

Sampson's cyst, nail, prosthesis

Samuel's position

San Joaquin Valley disease — a
primary form of fungous
disease caused by infection
with *Coccidioides immitis;* the
secondary form is a virulent,
chronic, progressive

San Joaquin Valley disease —
(continued)
granulomatous disease
involving cutaneous and
subcutaneous tissues, viscera,
cerebral nervous system, and
lungs

San Joaquin Valley fever

Sanarelli's serum

Sanarelli-Shwartzman phenomenon

Sanchez Salorio's syndrome —
retinal pigmentary dystrophy
and cataract, with mental and
physical retardation

Sander's disease — a form of paranoia

Sanders' disease — epidemic keratoconjunctivitis

Sanders' bed, forceps, incision, laryngoscope

Sanders-Brown-Shaw needle

Sanderson's polsters

Sandhoff's disease — a form of
Tay-Sachs disease marked by
a more rapid course

Sandifer's syndrome — an unnatu-
ral position of the head occurring in children as a symptom of reflux esophagitis or
hiatal hernia

Sandström's bodies, glands

Sandwith's bald tongue

Sanfilippo's syndrome — a form of
mucopolysaccharidosis re-
sembling *Hurler's syndrome*
but with less severe effects

Sanford's test

Sanger's reagent

Sanger-Brown ataxia

Sansom's sign

Sanson's images

Sansregret modification of Chaussé
III method

Santavuori's syndrome — same as
Santavuori-Haltia syndrome

Santavuori-Haltia syndrome —
juvenile-type amaurotic famil-

Santavuori-Haltia syndrome —
   (*continued*)
   ial idiocy with symptoms present from birth
Santorini's canal, cartilage, caruncle, duct, fissure, ligament,
   muscle, papilla, parietal vein,
   plexus, tubercle
Santulli's clamp
Santy's forceps
Sanyal's conjunctivitis
Sappey's fibers, ligament, nucleus,
   subareolar plexus, veins
Sarbo's sign
Sarmiento's cast
Sarnoff's clamp
Sarns' saw
Sarot's clamp, forceps, thoraco-
   scope
Sarrouy's disease — anemia associ-
   ated with retarded growth,
   hepatosplenomegaly, hepa-
   tosplenic hematopoiesis, bone
   marrow hypoplasia and, usu-
   ally, terminal marasmus
Satinsky's clamp, forceps, scissors
Sato's knife
Satterlee's saw
Satterthwaite's method
Sattler's layer, veil
Satvioni's cryptoscope
Sauer's debrider, forceps, tonsillec-
   tome, vaccine
Sauer-Sluder tonsillectome
Sauerbruch's cabinet, prosthesis
Sauerbruch-Coryllos rib shears
Sauerbruch-Lebsche rongeur
Sauerbruch-Zukschwerdt retractor
Saundby's test
Saunders' disease — a dangerous
   condition of infants with di-
   gestive disturbances caused by
   excessive intake of carbohy-
   drates; it is marked by vom-
   iting, cerebral symptoms, and
   depression of circulation
Saunders' sign
Saunders-Paparella hook, needle,
   rasp

Saunders-Sutton syndrome —
   delirium tremens
Saussure's hygrometer
Sauvage's graft, prosthesis
Savill's disease — an acute, infec-
   tious disease of unknown
   cause, marked by vesicular
   dermatitis followed by desqua-
   mation and bodily symptoms
   of varying severity
Sawtell's applicator, forceps, retrac-
   tor
Sawtell-Davis forceps, hemostat
Sawyer's retractor
Saxtorph's maneuver
Sayre's operation — application of
   a plaster-of-Paris jacket for
   treatment of spondylitis and
   Pott's disease
Sayre's apparatus, bandage, jacket,
   splint
Sbarbaro's prosthesis
Scanlon's mastectomy
Scanzoni's operation — forceps ro-
   tation of the fetal head in the
   posterior position of the occi-
   put
Scanzoni's maneuver
Scardino's ureteropelvioplasty
Scarpa's operation — ligation of
   the femoral artery in Scarpa's
   triangle
Scarpa's fascia, fluid, foramen,
   fossa, ganglion, hiatus, liga-
   ment, liquor, membrane,
   nerve, sheath, shoe, staphy-
   loma, triangle
Scatchard's equation, plot
Sceleth's treatment
Schacher's ganglion
Schachowa's spiral tubes
Schaedler's blood agar, medium
Schaeffer's curet
Schaeffer-Fulton stain
Schaer's reagent
Schäfer's syndrome — a rare, hered-
   itary, congenital disorder
   marked by gross thickening of

Schäfer's syndrome — *(continued)* the nails, hyperkeratosis of the palms, soles, and knees; leukoplakia of the oral mucosa; and mental and physical retardation. Called also *Jadassohn-Lewandowsky syndrome*

Schäfer's dumbbell, method

Schäffer's reflex, test

Schales and Schales method

Schalfijew's test

Schall's tube

Schällibaum's solution

Schalm's test

Schamberg's disease — progressive pigmentary dermatosis in adolescent males

Schamberg's dermatitis, extractor

Schanz's syndrome — weakness of the spinal musculature, marked by fatigue, pain on pressure, and a tendency to curvature of the spine

Schanz's disease — traumatic inflammation of Achilles tendon

Schanz's brace

Schardinger's enzyme, reaction

Schatz's maneuver

Schatzki's ring

Schaudinn's fixative, fluid

Schaumann's disease/syndrome — sarcoidosis

Schaumann's benign lymphogranuloma, bodies, sarcoid, sarcoidosis

Schauta's operation — vaginal hysterectomy for cancer of the cervix uteri

Schauta-Wertheim operation — same as *Wertheim-Schauta operation*

Schede's operation(s) — resection of the thorax for empyema; for varicose veins of leg; excision of the necrosed part of a bone

Schede's clot, method, resection, treatment

Scheffe's test

Scheibe's deafness

Scheibler's reagent

Scheie's syndrome — a rare, hereditary mucopolysaccharidosis similar to *Hurler's syndrome* but without mental retardation

Scheie's disease — an autosomal recessive condition associated with normal or slightly reduced intellect and stature, with marked hirsutism, broad mouth, retinitis pigmentosa, corneal clouding, and joint stiffness

Scheie's operation(s) — scleral cauterization with iridectomy for glaucoma; a technique for needling and aspiration of cataract

Scheiner's experiment

Scheinmann's forceps

Schellong-Strisower phenomenon

Schemm's diet

Schenck's disease — sporotrichosis

Schepelmann's sign

Scherer's method, test

Scheuermann's disease — osteochondrosis of the vertebral epiphyses in youth

Scheuermann's kyphosis

Scheuthauer-Marie-Sainton syndrome — hereditary cleidocranial dysostosis

Schick's reaction, sign, test

Schiefferdecker's disks, symbiosis, theory

Schiemann's selective agar

Schiff's base, biliary cycle, reaction, reagent, test

Schilder's disease — a subacute or chronic form of leukoencephalopathy of children and adolescents; symptoms include blindness, deafness, and progressive mental deterioration

Schilder's encephalitis

Schilder-Foix disease — intracerebral symmetrical centrolobar sclerosis

Schiller's iodine, test

Schiller-Duval bodies

Schilling's blood count, index, leukemia, test

Schimmelbusch's disease — cystic disease of the breast

Schindler's esophagoscope, gastroscope

Schiøtz's tonometer

Schirmer's syndrome — an incomplete form of *Sturge-Kalischer-Weber syndrome*, consisting of angiomas of the face and choroid only, with early appearance of glaucoma

Schirmer's test

Schlange's sign

Schlatter's disease — same as *Osgood-Schlatter disease*

Schlatter's operation — total excision of the stomach for cancer

Schlatter's sprain

Schlatter-Osgood disease — same as *Osgood-Schlatter disease*

Schlein's arthroplasty

Schlemm's canal, ligaments

Schlesinger's phenomenon, sign, test

Schlichting's dystrophy

Schlichter's test

Schloffer's tumor

Schlösser's injection, method, treatment

Schlossmann's method

Schmalz's operation — introducing a thread into the lacrimal duct for cure of stricture

Schmeden's punch, scissors

Schmid-Fraccaro syndrome — congenital clefts of the iris, anal atresia, and other malformations; called also *cat's eye syndrome*

Schmidel's anastomosis

Schmidt's syndrome(s) — unilateral paralysis affecting the vocal cords, the trapezius, and the sternocleidomastoid muscles; an association of thyroid and adrenocortical insufficiency

Schmidt's diet, fibrinoplastin, keratitis, node, test

Schmidt-Lantermann clefts, incisures, segment

Schmidt-Strassburger diet

Schmiedel's ganglion

Schmieden's disease — prolapse of the gastric mucosa into the duodenum

Schmincke's tumor

Schmitt's disease — a lesion of the spinous process of the first thoracic vertebra, with displacement of the apophysis, caused by overstraining

Schmitz's bacillus

Schmorl's disease — herniation of the nucleus pulposus into an adjacent ventral body

Schmorl's bacillus, body, jaundice, method, nodes, nodule, reaction, stain

Schmutz pyorrhea

Schnabel's atrophy, caverns

Schneider's disease — a viral infection that occurs in spring and fall, marked by sudden high fever, chills, nasopharyngitis, arthralgia, malaise, vomiting, and headache, often followed by involvement of the central nervous system

Schneider's carmine, indicator, nail, rod

Schnidt's forceps

Schnyder's dystrophy

Schobinger's incision

Schöbl's scleritis

Schoemaker's anastomosis, clamp, gastrectomy, gastroenterostomy, line

Schoenberg's forceps

Schoenheimer-Sperry method
Scholl's knife, solution
Scholz's disease — a familial leu-
    koencephalopathy marked by
    demyelination of the cerebral
    white matter, sensory aphasia,
    cortical blindness, deafness,
    spasticity, paralysis, and de-
    mentia
Schön's theory
Schönbein's operation — staphylo-
    plasty that results in shutting
    off the nose from the mouth
Schönbein's reaction, test
Schönenberg's syndrome — dwarf-
    ism, congenital blepharop-
    tosis, congenital heart defects,
    and mental retardation
Schönlein's disease — same as
    Schönlein-Henoch disease
Schönlein's purpura
Schönlein-Henoch disease — a
    form of purpura, occurring
    chiefly in children, due to a
    vasculitis of unknown cause
    and marked by urticaria, ery-
    thema, arthropathy, and renal
    disturbance
Schönlein-Henoch purpura
Schopfer's test
Schott's bath, treatment
Schottmüller's disease — a general
    term used for infections
    caused by Salmonella of all
    groups except S. typhosa
Schramm's phenomenon
Schreger's bands, lines, striae
Schreiber's maneuver
Schridde's disease — congenital,
    generalized dropsy
Schridde's cancer hairs, granules
Schroeder's syndrome — high
    blood pressure, with notable
    gain in weight, from overacti-
    vity of the adrenal glands
Schroeder's disease — a condition
    probably caused by deficiency
    of gonadotropic hormone,

Schroeder's disease — (continued)
    marked by hypertrophic endo-
    metrium and excessive uter-
    ine bleeding
Schroeder's curet, forceps, scissors,
    test
Schroeder-Braun forceps
Schroeder van der Kolk's law
Schroetter's chorea
Schrön's granule
Schrön-Much granules
Schroth's treatment
Schrötter's catheter, chorea
Schubert's forceps, punch
Schubert-Dannmeyer test
Schuchardt's incision
Schüffner's dots, granules, puncta-
    tion, stippling
Schuknecht's chisel, excavator,
    gouge, prosthesis, scissors,
    speculum
Schüle's sign
Schüller's disease — same as Hand-
    Schüller-Christian disease
Schüller's ducts, glands, method,
    phenomenon, position
Schüller-Christian disease — same
    as Hand-Schüller-Christian dis-
    ease
Schulte's test, valve
Schultz's syndrome — malignant
    leukopenia
Schultz's disease/syndrome — drug-
    allergic agranulocytosis
Schultz's angina, method, reaction,
    stain, triad
Schültz-Charlton phenomenon, re-
    action, test
Schultz-Dale reaction
Schultze's acroparesthesia, bundle,
    cells, fasciculus, fold, phenom-
    enon, placenta, sign, test,
    tract, type
Schultze-Chvostek's sign
Schumann's rays
Schumm's test
Schürmann's test
Schütz's bundle, law, micrococcus,
    rule

Schütz-Borissov law, rule
Schwab and England scale
Schwabach's test
Schwalbe's amygdaloid tubercle, corpuscles, foramen, fissure, line, nucleus, ring, sheath, space
Schwann's cell, cell tumor, membrane, myelin, neurilemma, nucleus, sheath, substance
Schwartz's syndrome — a congenital hereditary disorder marked by myotonic myopathy, dystrophy of epiphyseal cartilage, joint contracture, and decrease in the palpebral aperture
Schwartz's leukemia virus, test
Schwartz-Bartter syndrome — inappropriate secretion of antidiuretic hormone
Schwartz-Jampel syndrome — same as *Schwartz-Jampel-Aberfeld* syndrome
Schwartz-Jampel-Aberfeld syndrome — a hereditary disorder marked by myotonic myopathy, dwarfism, blepharophimosis, joint contractures, and flat facies
Schwartz-Kerrison rongeur
Schwartz-McNeil test
Schwarz's activator, test
Schwediauer's disease — same as *Swediaur's disease*
Schweigger's forceps
Schweigger-Seidel sheath
Schweitzer's reagent
Schweizer's forceps
Schweninger's method
Schweninger-Buzzi anetoderma, macular atrophy
Scianna antigen, blood group system
Scivoletto's test
Sclavo's serum
Scobee-Allis forceps
Scott's cannula, resectoscope, splint, tube

Scott's tapwater substitute
Scott-Wilson method, reagent
Scoville's curet, forceps, needle, trephine
Scoville-Greenwood forceps
Scoville-Lewis clip
Scribner's shunt
Scriver-Goldbloom-Roy syndrome — a disorder of amino acid metabolism arising from disturbance of renal tubular transport
Scudder's clamp, forceps
Scully's tumor
Scultetus' bandage, binder, dressing, position
Searcy's erysiphake, forceps, tonsillectome, trephine
Seattle classification
Sebileau's bands, hollow
Sechenoff's (Setchenow's) centers, nuclei
Seckel's syndrome — dwarfism marked by small head, narrow birdlike face with a beaklike nose, large eyes, and receding lower jaw
Seckel's bird-headed dwarf
Secretan's disease — post-traumatic hard edema of the dorsum of the hand or foot resulting in restriction of digital flexion
Sédillot's syndrome — changes in the genitalia associated with psychoneurotic disturbances thought to arise from contraception or masturbation
Sédillot's operation(s) — correction of a midline cleft in the uvula and soft palate; flap operation for restoring the upper lip
Sédillot's elevator, raspatory
Sedlinger's needle
Seeligmüller's neuralgia, sign
Seessel's pocket, pouch
Séglas' type
Segond's forceps, spatula
Séguin's sign, signal symptom
Sehrt's clamp, compressor

Seibert's tuberculin

Seidel's scotoma, sign, test

Seidelin's bodies

Seidlitz's powder test, powders

Seidlmayer's syndrome — postinfectious purpura of infancy and childhood, marked by elevated lesions

Seifert's reaction

Seiffert's forceps, punch

Seignette's salt

Seiler's knife, scissors

Seitelberger's disease — infantile neuroaxonal dystrophy

Seitz's filter, metamorphosing respiration, sign

Selas' filter

Seldinger's needle, technique

Seletz's cannula, catheter, forceps, punch

Seletz-Gelpi retractor

Selivanoff's (Seliwanow's) reaction, reagent, test

Selker's reservoir

Sellard's test

Seller's stain

Sellick's maneuver

Sellor's clamp, knife, valvulotome

Selman's clamp, forceps

Selter's disease — acrodynia

Selter's tuberculin

Selverstone's clamp, hook, rongeur

Selye's syndrome — the aggregate of all systemic reactions of the body to long-continued exposure to stress; called also *general adaptation syndrome*

Semb's operation — causing the apex of the lung to collapse for pulmonary tuberculosis

Semb's forceps, retractor, shears

Semb-Sauerbruch rongeur

Semken's forceps

Semliki Forest virus

Semon's law, sign

Semon-Hering hypothesis, theory

Semon-Rosenbach law

Semple's treatment, vaccine

Semunya virus

Sen's syndrome — infantile cirrhosis of the liver

Sendai virus

Senear-Usher syndrome — an eruption of scaling erythematous macules, involving the scalp, face, and trunk, suggesting the coexistence of lupus erythematosus and pemphigus

Sengstaken's balloon, tube

Sengstaken-Blakemore tube

Senn's operation — intestinal anastomosis

Senn's bone plates

Senn-Dingman retractor

Senning's operation — surgical creation of two interatrial channels for crossing systemic and pulmonary venous circulations in transposition of the great vessels

Senning's clamp

Senter's syndrome — a rare disorder of ichthyosis, hyperkeratosis, and sensorineural deafness

Senturia's forceps, retractor, speculum

Serature's clip

Sereny's test

Sergent's white adrenal line

Serre's operation — correction of skin contractures that distort the angle of the mouth, which involves switching of a skin and subcutaneous tissue flap from one lip to another

Serres' angle, glands

Sertoli-cell-only syndrome — congenital absence of the germinal epithelium of the testes, the seminiferous tubes, marked by smaller than normal testes, and absence of spermatozoa in the semen

Sertoli's cell tumor, cells, column

Sertoli-Leydig cell tumor

Setchenow's (Sechenoff's) centers, nuclei

Settegast's method
Seutin's bandage
Sever's disease — inflammation of
    the cartilage of the heel
Sewall's cannula, forceps, trocar
Sexton's knife
Seyderhelm's solution
Sézary's syndrome — generalized
    exfoliative erythroderma
    caused by cutaneous infiltra-
    tion by reticular lymphocytes
Sézary's cell, erythroderma,
    lymphoma, reticulosis
Sézary-Lutzner cells
Sforzini's syndrome — a hereditary
    familial form of exophthalmos
    not associated with metabolic
    or endocrine disorders
Shaaf's forceps
Shaeffer's spore stain
Shäfer's syndrome — congenital
    dyskeratosis
Shaffer's method
Shaffer-Hartmann method
Shaffer-Marriott method
Shaldon's tube
Shallcross' forceps, hemostat
Shambaugh's adenotome, elevator,
    incision, retractor
Shambaugh-Derlacki chisel, eleva-
    tor, microscope
Shambaugh-Lempert knife
Shantz's osteotomy
Shapiro-Wilks test
Shapleigh's curet
Sharpey's fibers
Shattock's disease — granuloma
    caused by foreign-body reac-
    tion to implanted silica parti-
    cles
Shaver's syndrome — bauxite
    worker's disease, causing inter-
    stitial pulmonary fibrosis ac-
    companied by emphysema
    and pneumothorax
Shay's leukemia, ulcer
Shea's bur, drill, incision, stapedec-
    tomy, tube

Shea-Anthony antral balloon
Shear's test
Shearer's forceps, retractor, rongeur
Sheehan's syndrome — postpartum
    pituitary necrosis
Sheehan's chisel, osteotome, retrac-
    tor
Sheehy's syndrome — rapidly ad-
    vancing sensorineural hearing
    loss in children
Sheehy's forceps, knife, tube
Sheehy-House prosthesis
Shekelton's aneurysm
Sheldon's necrotic purpura
Sheldon-Pudenz dissector, tube
Sheldon-Spatz needle
Sheldon-Swann needle
Shenton's arch, line
Shepard's tube
Shepherd's fracture
Sherman's plate, unit
Sherman-Bourquin unit of vitamin
    B_2
Sherman-Munsell unit of vitamin
    A
Sherrington's law, phenomenon
Shibley's sign
Shichito disease — scrub typhus
Shier's prosthesis
Shiga's bacillus, toxin
Shiga-Kruse disease — bacillary
    dysentery
Shihabi-Bishop method
Shiley's shunt, tube
Shiley-Bjork tube
Shimoda's blood group system
Shimpo's syndrome — same as
    Crow-Fukase syndrome
Shine-Dalgarno sequence
Shiner's tube
Shinowara-Jones-Reinhard unit
Shirodkar's operation — for incom-
    petent cervix when cervical
    os is closed
Shirodkar's cerclage, needle, proce-
    dure
Shirodkar-Page cerclage
Shoemaker's clamp, shears

Shoepinger's incision

Shohl's solution

Shohl-Pedley method

Shone's syndrome — diversion of the tendinous cords of the atrioventricular valves into one papillary muscle instead of two

Shope's fibroma, papilloma

Shorr's stain

Shortbent's scissors

Shprintzen's syndrome — hereditary cardiac defects and craniofacial abnormalities, often associated with abnormalities of chromosome 22

Shrady's saw

Shrapnell's membrane

Shubich-Spatz Bismarck brown stain

Shulman's syndrome — inflammation of fasciae of the extremities with eosinophilia, edema, and swelling, frequently occurring after strenuous exercise

Shurly's retractor

Shuster's forceps

Shwachman's syndrome — primary pancreatic insufficiency with bone-marrow failure

Shwachman-Diamond syndrome — same as *Shwachman's syndrome*

Shwartzman's phenomenon, reaction

Shy-Drager syndrome — a progressive encephalomyelopathy involving the autonomic nervous system, marked by atrophy of the iris, incontinence, impotence, tremor, and wasting of muscle

Shy-Magee disease — a benign, congenital disease of muscle marked by intramuscular rodlike structures

Sia test

Sibley-Lehninger unit

Sibson's aponeurosis, fascia, furrow, groove, notch, vestibule

Sicar's sign

Sicard's syndrome — same as *Collet-Sicard syndrome*

Sicard-Cantelouble test

Sichel's disease — a type of pseudoptosis, with a fold of skin hanging from the upper lid margin

Sichel's ptosis

Sidler-Huguenin's endothelioma

Siebold's operation — surgical separation of the pubic bone lateral to the median line

Siebold-Bradbury test

Siegert's sign

Siegle's otoscope

Siegrist's spots, streaks

Siegrist-Hutchinson syndrome — post-traumatic chorioretinopathy marked by extreme dilation of the pupil, macular disorders, choroid rupture, or atrophy of the optic nerve

Siemens' syndrome — a familial type of keratosis involving the face, neck, forearms, and backs of the hands

Siemens' dermatosis

Siemens-Bloch pigmented dermatosis

Siemens-Halske cell

Siemerling's nucleus

Sierra-Sheldon tracheotome

Sieur's sign, test

Siffert's method

Siggaard-Andersen alignment nomogram

Sigmund's glands

Signorelli's sign

Sigualt's symphysiotomy

Siker's laryngoscope

Silex's sign

Silver's syndrome — a congenital syndrome marked by low birth weight, short stature,

Silver's syndrome — *(continued)* lateral asymmetry, syndactyly, triangular face, and precocious puberty

Silver's operation — surgical resection for repair of hallux valgus

Silver's bunionectomy, dwarf, osteotome, procedure

Silver-Russell syndrome — same as *Silver's syndrome*

Silverman's disease — an abnormality of the sternum, marked by pigeon breast

Silverman's needle

Silverskiöld's syndrome — a form of osteochondrodystrophy with slight vertebral changes but curved long bones of the extremities

Silvester's method

Silvestrini-Corda syndrome — failure of the liver to inactivate estrogens, marked by eunuchoid body, atrophy of the testes, defective libido, and sterility

Silvestroni-Bianco syndrome — constitutional microcytic anemia

Simbu hepatitis, virus

Simmerlin's dystrophy, type

Simmonds' disease — panhypopituitarism

Simmonds' cachexia

Simmons' citrate agar

Simon's dermatome, foci, incision, position, septic factor, sign, speculum, sutures, symptom

Simonart's bands, thread

Simonelli's test

Simons' disease — progressive disappearance of subcutaneous fat above the pelvis, facial emaciation, and abnormal deposition of fat about the thighs and buttocks. Also called *lipodystrophy*

Simonsen's phenomenon

Simpson's syndrome — adipose gynandrism affecting either sex

Simpson's forceps, lamp, light, splint

Simpson-Luikart forceps

Sims' position, speculum, suture, test

Sims-Huhner test

Sindbis virus

Sinding-Larsen-Johansson disease — same as *Larsen-Johansson disease*

Singer's node

Singer-Blom stoma valve

Singleton's incision

Singley's clamp, forceps

Sinkler's phenomenon

Sipple's syndrome — a hereditary association of pheochromocytoma with medullary thyroid carcinoma

Sippy's diet, method, powder, treatment

Sisto's sign

Sistrunk's operation — removal of thyroglossal cysts and sinuses

Sistrunk's retractor, scissors

Sivash's prosthesis

Sjögren's syndrome — a symptom complex of unknown cause occurring chiefly in older women, marked by keratoconjunctivitis and enlargement of the parotid gland. It is often associated with rheumatoid arthritis and sometimes with systemic lupus erythematosus. Called also *Gougerot-Nulock-Houwer syndrome*

Sjögren's antibodies

Sjögren-Larsson syndrome — congenital erythroderma in association with mental deficiency and spastic disorders

Sjöqvist's method

Skeele's curet

Skeer's sign, symptom

Skene's catheter, ducts, glands, tubules

Skevas-Zerfus disease — a condition occurring principally among sponge divers who come in contact with the stinging tentacles of sea anemones that are often attached to the base of sponges

Skillern's cannula, forceps, fracture

Skillman's forceps

Skinner's box, line

Skirrow's medium

Sklar-Schiøtz tonometer

Sklowsky's symptom

Skoda's sign, tympany

Slaughter's saw

Slavianski's membrane

Sloan's dissector, incision

Slocum's splint

Slocumb's syndrome — acute disseminated rheumatoid arthritis

Sluder's disease/syndrome — neuralgia of the sphenopalatine ganglia, causing burning maxillary pain with radiation into the neck and shoulder

Sluder's operation — removal of the tonsil and its capsule

Sluder's guillotine, method, neuralgia, tonsillectome, tonsillectomy

Sluder-Ballenger tonsillectome

Sluder-Demarest tonsillectome

Sluder-Jensen mouth gag

Sluder-Sauer guillotine, tonsillectome

Sly's syndrome — a lysosomal storage disease marked by skeletal manifestations, prominent sternum, organomegaly, cardiac murmur, short stature, and mental retardation

Small-Carrion prosthesis

Smart's forceps, scissors

Smead-Jones closure, sutures

Smedberg's drill

Smee's cell

Smellie's method, scissors

Smeloff-Cutter prosthesis, valve

Smiley-Williams needle

Smillie's meniscotome, retractor

Smith's disease(s) — acute infectious lymphocytosis; mucous colitis

Smith's operation — extraction of an immature cataract with an intact capsule

Smith's dislocation, fracture, pessary, phenomenon, reaction, sign, test

Smith-Dietrich method

Smith-Fisher knife, spatula

Smith-Hodge pessary

Smith-Lemli-Opitz syndrome — a hereditary syndrome marked by multiple congenital anomalies, including microcephaly, mental retardation, defective development of male genitalia, syndactyly, and others

Smith-Peterson nail, osteotome, pin, prosthesis

Smith-Robinson technique

Smith-Strang disease — a defect in methionine absorption, marked by malodorous urine, white hair, mental retardation, and convulsions

Smithwick's clamp, dissector, forceps

Smithwick-Hartmann forceps

Sneddon-Wilkinson disease — subcorneal pustular dermatosis

Snell's cell, law

Snellen's chart, reflex, reform eye, sign, test, test type

Snider's match test

Snitman's retractor

Snyder's agar, forceps, hemostat, Hemovac, test

Soave's operation — endorectal pull-through with normal

Soave's operation — (continued)
colon connected to the anus
for treatment of congenital
mega colon
Sobernheim's vaccine
Socin's operation — enucleation of
a goitrous or thyroidal tumor
from the healthy part of the
gland to avoid myxedema
Soemmering's crystalline swelling,
foramen, ganglion, gray sub-
stance, papilla, process, ring
cataract, spot, vein
Sohval-Soffer syndrome — a con-
genital syndrome marked by
male hypogonadism, multiple
skeletal abnormalities, and
mental retardation
Soldaini's reagent, test
Solera's test
Solow's sigmoidoscope
Somers' clamp, forceps
Somerset's bur
Somogyi effect, method, phenome-
non, unit
Sondergaard's cleft
Sondermann's canals
Sones' catheter
Sonne's dysentery
Sonne-Duval bacillus
Sonnenschein's test
Sörensen's buffer, method, reagent
Soresi's cannula
Soret's band, effect, phenomenon
Soriano's syndrome — hyperplastic,
osteogenic, recurrent osteoper-
iostitis with pseudotumoral de-
velopment
Sorondo-Ferre amputation
Sorsby's syndrome — a congenital
disorder consisting of retinal
macular defects, dystrophy of
the extremities, and abnormal
shortness of fingers and toes
Sorsby's disease — dystrophy of the
fundus beginning in the fifth
decade, causing unilateral
blurring of central vision and

Sorsby's disease — (continued)
followed by a similar disorder
in the other eye
Sorsby's macular degeneration
Sorval Porter–Blum ultramicro-
tome
Soto-Hall sign
Sotos' syndrome — cerebral gigan-
tism
Sottas' disease — progressive hyper-
trophic interstitial neuropathy
Souligoux-Morestin method
Souques' phenomenon, sign
Souques-Charcot geroderma
Sourdille's keratoplasty
South African–type porphyria
South American blastomycosis,
hemorrhagic fever
Southey's cannula, trocar, tube
Southey-Leech trocar, tube
Southgate's modification of
Mayer's stain
Southwick's clamp, osteotomy
Southworth's symptom complex
Souttar's cautery, tube
Soxhlet's apparatus
Soyka's milk-rice culture medium
Spalding's sign
Spallanzani's law
Spanish psyllium
Spanlang-Tappeiner syndrome —
congenital zonular corneal
opacity associated with hyper-
keratosis of the palms and
soles
Spearman's rank correlation coef-
ficient
Spee's curve, embryo
Speed's prosthesis
Spemann's induction
Spence's tail
Spence-Adson forceps
Spencer's disease — a form of epi-
demic gastroenteritis
Spencer's cannula, forceps, probe,
scissors
Spencer-Parker vaccine
Spencer-Wells forceps

Spengler's fragments, immune bodies, tuberculin

Spens' syndrome — same as *Adams-Stokes syndrome*

Speransky-Richen-Siegmund syndrome — necrotizing perforation of the hard palate into the maxillary sinus

Spero's forceps

Spicer's iron diamine method

Spiegelberg's sign

Spieghel's line

Spiegler's reagent, test, tumor

Spiegler-Fendt pseudolymphoma, sarcoid, sarcomatosis

Spielmeyer-Stock disease — retinal atrophy in amaurotic familial idiocy

Spielmeyer-Vogt disease — a late juvenile form of cerebral sphingolipidosis

Spies' punch

Spigelius' line

Spiller's syndrome — epidural ascending spinal paralysis

Spinelli's operation — reversing the prolapsed inverted uterus and restoring it to the correct position

Spira's disease — hypoplasia of the dental enamel caused by drinking water with high fluorine content

Spiro's test

Spitz's nevus

Spitzer's theory

Spitzka's nucleus, tract

Spitzka-Lissauer column, tract

Spivack's operation — cystostomy

Splendore-Hoeppli phenomenon

Spöndel's foramen

Spondweni virus

Spratt's curet, rasp

Sprengel's deformity

Sprinz-Dubin syndrome — same as *Dubin-Johnson syndrome*

Sprinz-Nelson syndrome — same as *Dubin-Johnson syndrome*

Spritz's bottle

Sprong's sutures

Spurling's forceps, rongeur, sign

Spurling-Kerrison forceps, punch, rongeur

Spurway's syndrome — an inherited condition in which bones are abnormally brittle and subject to fracture

Sputnik-Federov lens

Squire's catheter, sign

Srb's syndrome — aplasia and synostosis of the first two ribs, with a hornlike, bony protrusion of the cranial portion of the sternum

Ssabanejew-Frank operation — same as *Frank's operation*

Stacke's operation — removal of the mastoid and the contents of the tympanum

Stader's splint

Staderini's nucleus

Staehelin's test

Stafne's cyst, mandibular defect

Stahl's ear, No. 1, No. 2

Stähli's line

Stahr's gland

Stallard's sutures

Stamey test

Stamm's gastrostomy, tube

Stammer's method

Stammler's reaction

Stanbury-Hedge defect

Stanford's protocol, test

Stanley bacillus

Stanley Kent bundle

Stannius' follicle

Stanton's disease — an infectious disease of rodents transmissible to humans, caused by *Pseudomonas pseudomallei*

Stanton's clamp

Starck's dilator

Stargardt's disease — hereditary degeneration of the retinal macula

Starkey's soap

Starling's curve, hypothesis, law, mechanism

Starlinger's dilator

Starr-Edwards pacemaker, prosthesis, valve

Stas-Otto method

State's operation — end-to-end anastomosis of the colon for treatment of Hirschsprung's disease

Staub-Traugott effect, phenomenon, test

Staude-Moore forceps, tenaculum

Staunig's method

Staunton's sphygmomanometer

Stearns' alcoholic amentia

Stecher's method

Stedman's aspirator, pump, tube

Steele's dilator, elevator

Steele-Richardson-Olszewski syndrome — a progressive neurological disorder occurring in the sixth decade of life, marked by paralysis of the downward gaze, stumbling gait, dystonic rigidity of the trunk and neck, and dementia

Steell's murmur

Steenbock's unit of vitamin D

Steer's replicating device

Stefan-Boltzmann law

Stehle's method

Stein's operation — reconstruction of the lower lip with flaps taken from the upper lip

Stein's antigen, test

Stein-Abbe lip flap

Stein-Kazanjian flap

Stein-Leventhal syndrome — sclerocystic disease of the ovary marked by hirsutism, obesity, menstrual disturbances, infertility, and enlarged ovaries, probably due to excessive androgen secretion; called also *polycystic ovary disease* or *syndrome*

Steinach's operation — ligation of the vas deferens with resection of a portion of the vas

Steinach's method

Steinbrocker's syndrome — a disorder of the upper extremity marked by shoulder pain and stiffness and by swelling and pain in the hand, sometimes occurring after myocardial infarction or injury to the neck

Steindler's operation — surgical correction of clubfoot

Steindler's posterior syndrome — low back pain

Steindler's arthrodesis

Steiner's syndrome — hypertrophy of one side of the entire body; called also *Curtius' syndrome*

Steiner's tumor

Steiner-Vörner syndrome — multiple, symmetric, red, punctiform angiomas of the skin and mucous membranes with a variety of systemic disorders

Steinert's disease — myotonic dystrophy

Steinle-Kahlenberg test

Steinmann's extension, pin

Steinthol's groupings

Stellwag's brawny edema, sign, symptom

Stender's dish

Stenger's test

Stensen's canal, duct, experiment, foramen, plexus, veins

Stent's graft, mass

Stenvers' method, position, view

Stenzel's prosthesis, rod

Stephen's spots

Stepita's clamp

Sterles' sign

Sterling-Okuniewski sign

Stern's position, test

Stern-McCarthy electrotome, panendoscope, resectoscope

Sternberg's disease — same as *Hodgkin's disease*

Sternberg's giant cells, sign
Sternberg-Reed cells
Sternheimer-Malbin stain
Stevens' forceps, hook, scissors
Stevens-Johnson syndrome — same
as *Johnson-Stevens disease*
Stevenson's clamp, forceps,
scissors
Stewart's purple, test
Stewart-Holmes sign
Stewart-Morel syndrome — same
as *Morgagni's syndrome*
Stewart-Treves syndrome—
lymphangiosarcoma occurring
in upper extremities affected
by postmastectomy lymph-
edema
Sticker's disease — a mildly contagious disease of children
marked by a rose-colored, lace-
like macular rash
Sticker's sarcoma
Stickler's syndrome — a hereditary
syndrome marked by progressive myopia and by abnormal
epiphyseal development in
the vertebrae and long bones
Stieda's disease — same as *Pellegrini-Stieda disease*
Stieda's fracture, process
Stieda-Pellegrini syndrome —
traumatic calcification of the
collateral tibial ligament
Stierlin's sign, symptom
Stifel's figure
Still's syndrome — juvenile rheumatoid arthritis
Still's disease — a form of chronic
arthritis affecting children,
marked by enlargement of
lymph nodes and intermittent
fever
Still's murmur
Still-Chauffard syndrome — same
as *Chauffard's syndrome*
Stille's clamp, forceps, gouge, osteo-
tome, shears, trephine
Stille-Adson forceps
Stille-Bjork forceps
Stille-Horsley forceps

Stille-Leksell rongeur
Stille-Liston forceps
Still-Luer forceps, rongeur
Stiller's asthenia, rib, sign
Stilling's syndrome — same as
Duane's syndrome
Stilling's canal, column, fibers,
fleece, nucleus
Stilling-Turk-Duane syndrome —
same as *Duane's syndrome*
Stimson's sign
Stinson's method
Stintzing's tables
Stirling's modification of Gram's
stain
Stitt's catheter
Stock's test
Stock-Spielmeyer-Vogt syndrome —
juvenile amaurotic familial id-
iocy
Stocker's line, sign
Stockholm-Koch method
Stockman's clamp
Stoerck's loop
Stoerk's blennorrhea
Stoker's treatment
Stokes' syndrome — same as *Mor-
gagni-Adams-Stokes syndrome*
Stokes' operation — same as
Gritti's operation
Stokes' amputation, collar, expec-
torant, law, reagent, shift,
sign, test
Stokes-Adams syndrome — same
as *Morgagni-Adams-Stokes syndrome*
Stokvis' disease — a syndrome
caused by absorption of nitrates and sulfides from the intestine, marked by excessive
methemoglobin in the circulating blood associated with
cyanosis and by severe enteritis, dyspnea, syncope, anemia,
and occasionally by digital
clubbing
Stokvis' test
Stokvis-Talma syndrome — same
as *Stokvis' disease*

Stoll's test
Stoltz's pubiotomy
Stone's eye implant
Stone-Holcombe clamp
Stoneman's forceps
Stookey's reflex
Storck's test
Storey's forceps
Storm Van Leeuwen chamber
Stormer's viscosimeter
Storz's bronchoscope, telescope
Storz-Beck snare
Storz-Iglesias resectoscope
Stout's wiring
Stovall-Black method
Strachan's syndrome — same as *Strachan-Scott syndrome*
Strachan-Scott syndrome — nutritional deficiencies, particularly of vitamin B_2, with pain, numbness, and paresthesia of the palms, soles, joints, and shoulders; dimmed vision; deafness; and emaciation
Strange's test
Stransky-Regala syndrome — chronic familial hemolytic anemia, marked by erythroblastosis of the bone marrow with a profusion of immature erythroblasts
Strasburger's cell plate
Strassburg's test
Stratte's clamp, forceps
Straus' biological test, phenomenon, reaction
Strauss' cannula; needle, sign, test
Strayer's knife
Street's pin
Streeter's horizons
Stroganoff's (Stroganov's) treatment
Stroll's dilution egg count technique
Strombeck's operation — plastic reconstruction of the breast to augment or reduce its size
Strombeck's incision

Stromeyer's cephalhematocele, splint
Strong's bacillus
Struempel's forceps, rongeur
Strully's curet, hook, scissors
Strully-Kerrison rongeur
Strümpell's disease(s) — a hereditary form of lateral sclerosis in which spasticity is limited to the legs; polioencephalomyelitis
Strümpell's phenomenon, reflex, sign, type
Strümpell-Leichtenstern disease — hemorrhagic encephalitis
Strümpell-Lorrain disease — spinocerebellar degeneration
Strümpell-Marie disease — ankylosing spondylitis
Strümpell-Westphal disease — the cerebral changes of hepatolenticular degeneration
Strümpell-Westphal pseudosclerosis
Strunsky's sign
Struve's test
Struyken's forceps, punch
Stryker's dermabrader, dermatome, frame, saw
Stryker-Halbeisen syndrome — a scaling, macular eruption on the face and upper trunk from vitamin B complex deficiency, associated with macrocytic anemia
Stuart's broth, factor, transport medium
Stuart-Bras disease — veno-occlusive disease of the liver
Stuart-Prower factor
Stubbs' curet
Stühmer's disease — atrophy of the glans penis, resulting in stricture of the urethral meatus
Sturge's syndrome — same as *Sturge-Kalischer-Weber syndrome*
Sturge's disease — same as *Sturge-Kalischer-Weber syndrome*

Sturge-Kalischer-Weber syndrome — a congenital syndrome consisting of angiomas of the face, leptomeninges, and choroid and glaucoma — often associated with intracranial calcification, mental retardation, hemiplegia, and epilepsy. Called also *Dimitri's disease*

Sturge-Weber syndrome — same as *Sturge-Kalischer-Weber syndrome*

Sturge-Weber-Dimitri disease — same as *Sturge-Kalischer-Weber syndrome*

Sturm's conoid, interval

Sturmdorf's operation — excision of diseased endocervix

Stutsman's snare

Stuttgart's disease — canine typhus

Stypven time test

Sucquet-Hoyer anastomosis, canal

Sudan black B stain

Sudeck's disease — post-traumatic osteoporosis

Sudeck's atrophy, critical point, porosis

Sudeck-Leriche syndrome — post-traumatic osteoporosis with vasospasm

Sugg's catheter

Suker's sign

Sulkowitch's reagent, test

Sullivan's test

Sulzberger-Chase phenomenon

Sulzberger-Garbe syndrome — an exudative lichenoid dermatitis associated with other cutaneous and systemic manifestations

Sumner's method, reagent, sign

Sundt's clip

Suranyi's test

Surgaloy's sutures

Sutter's blood groups

Sutton's disease — a severe form of disease of the oral mucosa,

Sutton's disease — (*continued*) marked by ulcerative lesions surrounded by a red border, caused by local injury, allergic reaction, endocrine imbalance, and emotional stress

Sutton's nevus, ulcer

Sutton-Gull disease — arteriocapillary fibrosis

Suzanne's gland

Švec's leukemia

Svedberg's unit

Swan's syndrome — blind spot syndrome

Swan-Ganz catheter

Swank-Davenport method

Swann's antigen

Swanson's implant, prosthesis

Swediaur's (Schwediauer's) disease — inflammation of the calcaneal bursa

Sweeney's retractor, speculum

Sweet's syndrome — a rare disease predominant in women, marked by sudden onset of plaquelike lesions of the face, neck, and upper extremities accompanied by conjunctivitis, fever, malaise, and arthralgia

Sweet's forceps, method, punch, scissors

Swenson's operation — removal of the rectum and the aganglionic segment of the bowel for Hirschsprung's disease

Swenson's procedure

Swift's disease — same as *Swift-Feer disease*

Swift-Feer disease — acrodynia

Swyer-James syndrome — chronic obstructive pseudoemphysema; also called *Macleod's syndrome*

Sydenham's disease — an acute, toxic, infective disorder of the nervous system, usually associated with acute rheumatic fever in young persons,

Sydenham's disease—(*continued*) marked by involuntary, jerky movements of the face, neck, and limbs

Sydenham's chorea, cough

Sydney crease, line

Sylva's irrigator

Sylvest's disease — epidemic pleurodynia

Sylvest's syndrome — an acute, infectious disease caused by the Coxsackie B virus, marked by sudden onset of fever and severe pain in the muscles of the lower chest or abdomen

Sylvius' angle, aqueduct, cistern, fissure, fossa, iter, valve, ventricle

Syme's operation(s) — amputation of the foot at the ankle joint, with removal of both malleoli; external urethrotomy

Syme's amputation

Symington's body

Symmers' disease — giant follicular lymphoma

Symmer's clay pipestem fibrosis

Syms' tractor

Syrian ulcer

Szabo's test

Szent-Györgyi reaction

Sztehlo's clamp

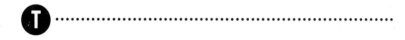

Tabb's curet, knife

Taenzer's disease — a skin disorder marked by redness and roughness of the eyebrows and spreading to the face and scalp

Taenzer's stain

Taenzer-Unna stain

Tahyna virus

Taillefer's valve

Taiwan acute respiratory strain

Takahara's syndrome — a congenital deficiency of blood catalase, with malignant alveolar pyorrhea and gangrene, seen in Japan and Switzerland

Takahara's disease — a rare disease occurring principally in Japan, caused by congenital absence of the enzyme catalase. It is marked by recurrent infections of the gingiva, but more often than not no symptoms are present

Takahashi's forceps

Takata's reagent

Takata-Ara test

Takatsuki's syndrome — same as *Crow-Fukase syndrome*

Takayama's stain

Takayasu's disease/syndrome — pulseless disease, same as *Martorell's syndrome*

Takayasu's arteritis

Talbot's law

Talfan disease — infectious porcine encephalomyelitis

Tallerman's apparatus, treatment

Tallqvist's scale

Talma's disease — delayed relaxation of muscle following contraction, from either injury or disease

Talma's operation — surgical production of artificial adhesions between the liver and spleen and the omentum and abdominal wall for ascites from cirrhosis of the liver

Tamm-Horsfall mucoprotein, protein

Tamura-Takahashi disease — hereditary black blood disease

Tangier disease — a disorder of lipoprotein and lipid metabolism

Tanner's operation — procedure in which the left and short gastric veins are divided and the stomach is bisected and resutured, for bleeding esophageal varices

Tanner's method, stage

Tanner-Roux procedure

Tanret's reaction, reagent, test

Tansini's operation(s) — amputation of the breast; removing a cyst of the liver; gastric resection

Tapia's syndrome — unilateral paralysis of the larynx and tongue, with atrophy of the tongue

Tar's symptom

Tardieu's ecchymoses, petechiae, spots, test

Targowla's reaction, test

Tarin's fascia, foramen, fossa, space

Tarini's recess

Tarinus' band, valve, velum

Tarlov's cyst

Tarnier's forceps

Tarrant's method

Tarui's disease — a hereditary disorder caused by deficiency of the muscle isozyme 6-phosphofructokinase

Tashkent ulcer

Tatum's clamp

Tauber's catheter, speculum

Taussig-Bing syndrome — complete transposition of the aorta, with ventricular septal defect, right ventricular hypertrophy, anterior situation of the aorta, and posterior situation of the pulmonary artery

Taussig-Bing complex, heart, malformation

Taussig-Snellen-Albers syndrome — drainage of the pulmonary vein into the inferior vena cava, associated with septal defects

Tawara's node

Tay's disease — degeneration of the choroid seen late in life, thought to be from an atheromatous condition of arteries

Tay's choroiditis, sign, spot

Tay-Sachs disease — the infantile form of cerebral sphingolipidosis, marked by degeneration of brain cells leading eventually to dementia, blindness, paralysis, and death

Taybi's syndrome — bone dysplasia, dwarfism, cleft palate, peculiar facies, deafness, and mental retardation

Taylor's syndrome — hyperemia of the ovary

Taylor's apparatus, curet, diet, method, speculum, splint, sutures, test

Taylor-Hulton method

Teale's operation — amputation that preserves a long, rectangular flap of muscle and integument on one side of the limb and a short, rectangular flap on the other

Teale's amputation, forceps

Teevan's law

Teichmann's crystals, test

Tellais' sign

Tellyesniczky's fluid, mixture

Temple-Fay retractor

Tenckhoff's catheter

Tenner's cannula

Tenney's changes

Tenon's capsule, fascia, membrane, space

Terry's syndrome — retrolental fibroplasia

Terson's disease — cerebral aneurysms, subarachnoid hemorrhage, ocular venous stenosis and venous saccular dilation of the eye

Terson's forceps, speculum

Teschen's disease — infectious porcine encephalomyelitis

Teschen's virus

Tesla's current

Testivin's sign

Teufel's method

Teutleben's ligaments

Teutschländer's syndrome — dystrophic metalipoid calcinosis

Textor's operation — removal of thin, split-thickness skin grafts by razor, knife, or dermatome

Thamm's tuberculin

Thane's method

Thatcher's nail

Thayer-Doisy unit

Thayer-Martin agar medium, test

Thaysen's syndrome — attacks of severe pain in the region of the anorectal ring and the internal and sphincter

Thaysen's disease — nontropical sprue, or celiac disease

Thebesius' veins

Theden's bandage

Theile's canal, glands

Theiler's mouse encephalomyelitis, virus

Theimich's lip sign

Theis' retractor

Theobald's probe

Theobald Smith's phenomenon

Thévenard's disease — same as *Hicks' syndrome*

Thézac-Porsmeur method

Thibierge-Weissenbach syndrome — calcinosis

Thiele's syndrome — pain and tenderness in the lower portion of the sacrum and coccyx and in contiguous tissues

Thiemann's disease — familial necrosis of the phalangeal epiphysis, resulting in deformity of the interphalangeal joints

Thiersch's operation — removal of skin grafts with a razor

Thiersch's canaliculus, graft, sutures, wire

Thiersch-Duplay urethroplasty

Thiry's fistula

Thiry-Vella fistula

Thoma's ampulla, counting chamber, fixative

Thoma-Zeiss counting cell, counting chamber

Thomas' syndrome(s) — a combination of disorders of equilibrium, adiadochokinesia, halting speech, ataxia, reflex and sensitivity disorders, and often cerebral catalepsy; hypothyroidism, with secondary hypertrophic osteoarthropathy and exophthalmos following partial thyroidectomy

Thomas' cryoextractor, heel, keratome, pessary, sign, splint, test

Thomas-Binetti test

Thomas-Warren incision

Thomayer's sign

Thompson's syndrome — congenital optic atrophy

Thompson's catheter, line, lithotrite, prosthesis, resectoscope, test

Thompson, F. R., hip prosthesis, rasp

Thoms' forceps, method, pelvimeter, tenaculum

Thoms-Allis forceps

Thoms-Gaylor forceps, punch

Thomsen's disease — a congenital, hereditary disease marked by tonic spasm and rigidity of muscles upon movement after rest

Thomsen's phenomenon

Thomsen-Friedenreich antigen

Thomson's disease — a hereditary developmental disease marked by hyperkeratotic lesions and xerodermatous changes

Thomson's clamp, sign

Thoraeus' filter

Thorek's aspirator, scissors

Thorek-Feldman scissors

Thorek-Mixter forceps

Thorel's bundle

Thormählen's test

Thorn's syndrome — a rare disorder caused by renal tubular damage of unknown origin, resulting in loss of sodium chloride, acidosis, dehydration, and vascular collapse

Thorn test

Thornton's nail, screw, sign

Thornwald's irrigator, perforator

Thornwaldt's (Tornwaldt's) disease — chronic inflammation of the pharyngeal bursa, accompanied by formation of pustular cyst and nasopharyngeal stenosis

Thornwaldt's (Tornwaldt's) abscess, bursa, bursitis, cyst

Thorpe's curet, forceps, scissors

Thorpe-Castroviejo scissors

Thorpe-Westcott scissors

Throckmorton's reflex

Thudichum's test

Thunberg's tube

Thygeson's disease — epithelial punctate keratitis associated with viral conjunctivitis

Tidy's test

Tiedemann's nerve

Tiemann's catheter

Tietz-Fiereck method

Tietze's syndrome — idiopathic, painful, nonsuppurative swellings of the costal cartilages; albinism, deaf-mutism, and hypoplasia of the eyebrows

Tillaux's disease — mastitis with multiple tumors of the breast

Tillaux-Phocas disease — same as *Cheatle's disease*

Timberlake's evacuator, obturator, resectoscope

Timbrall-Fisher incision

Timme's syndrome — ovarian and adrenal insufficiency

Timofeew's apparatus, corpuscles

Tindale's medium

Tinel's sign

Tischler's forceps, punch

Tisdall's method

Tiselius' apparatus

Titterington's method, position

Tizzoni's stain, test

Tobey's rongeur

Tobey-Ayer maneuver, test

Tobie, von Brand, and Mehlman's diphasic medium

Tobold's apparatus, forceps

Tobold-Fauvel forceps

Todd's bodies, button, cautery, cirrhosis, needle, palsy, paralysis, process, units

Todd-Hewitt broth

Toison's fluid, solution, stain

Tollens' test

Tollens, Neuberg, and Schwket test

Tolosa-Hunt syndrome — unilateral paralysis of the eye muscles

Tom Jones sutures

Toma's sign

Tomes' fibers, fibrils, granular layer, process

Tommaselli's disease — pyrexia and hematuria associated with excessive intake of quinine

Tommasi's sign

Tooke's knife, spatula

Toomey's evacuator, syringe, tube

Tooth's disease — progressive neuropathic muscular atrophy

Tooth's atrophy, type

Töpfer's test

Topinard's angle, line

Torek's operation(s) — for undescended testicle; for excision

Torek's operation(s) — (*continued*) of the thoracic part of the esophagus

Torkildsen's operation — ventriculocisternostomy

Tornwardt's (Thornwaldt's) abscess, cyst

Tornwaldt's (Thornwaldt's) disease — chronic inflammation of the pharyngeal bursa, accompanied by formation of pustular cyst and nasopharyngeal stenosis

Tornwaldt's (Thornwaldt's) abscess, cyst

Torquay's test

Torre's syndrome — multiple tumors of the sebaceous glands associated with visceral malignancy

Torres-Teixeira bodies

Torsten-Sjögren's syndrome — same as *Marinesco-Garland syndrome*

Toti's operation — dacryocystorhinostomy

Touraine's syndrome — angioid streaks in cardiovascular disorders

Touraine-Solente-Golé syndrome — thickening of the skin of the face and scalp, thickening of the bones of the limbs, and clubbing of the fingers

Tourette's disease — same as *Gilles de la Tourette's syndrome*

Tournay's sign

Tourtual's canal

Touton's giant cells

Tower's forceps, retractor

Towne's projection roentgenogram

Townes' syndrome — anomalies of the ears and limbs and digits, anal defects, and renal deficiency

Townley's forceps, prosthesis

Townsend's ionization

Toyama's disease — pityriasis

Toynbee's corpuscles, experiment, law, ligament, maneuver, otoscope

Tracy-Welker method

Trambusti's reaction, test

Trantas' dots

Trapp's coefficient, factor, formula

Trapp-Häser formula

Traquair's scotoma

Trattner's catheter

Traube's corpuscles, curves, double tone, dyspnea, heart, membrane, murmur, plugs, resonance theory, semilunar space, sign

Traube-Hering curves, waves

Trautmann's triangle

Treacher Collins syndrome — defective mandibulofacial bone formation

Treacher Collins–Franceschetti syndrome — same as *Treacher Collins syndrome*

Treitz's angle, arch, fossa, hernia, ligament, muscle

Trélat's speculum

Trendelenburg's operation(s) — excision of varicose veins; ligation of the great saphenous vein for varicose veins; synchondroseotomy; pulmonary embolectomy for the treatment of postoperative embolism

Trendelenburg's cannula, gait, position, sign, symptom, tampon, test

Trendelenburg-Crafoord clamp

Tresilian's sign

Tretop's test

Treves' operation — opening of abscess through the loin, irrigating and curetting the sac, and scraping away dead bone for Pott's disease

Treves' fold

Trevor's disease — a rare condition characterized by swellings of

Trevor's disease — (*continued*)
the extremities constituted by epiphyseal cartilage, resulting in limitation of joint movement

Triboulet's reagent, test

Trillat's method

Trimadeau's sign

Tripier's amputation

Troell-Junet syndrome — a combination of acromegaly, toxic goiter, diabetes mellitus, and hyperostosis of the cranial vault

Troeltsch's speculum

Troisier's syndrome — severe debility associated with diabetes

Troisier's ganglion, node, sign

Troisier-Hanot-Chauffard syndrome — diabetes mellitus, with hypertrophic cirrhosis of the liver and dark-brown skin pigmentation

Trolard's net, plexus, vein

Tröltsch's corpuscles, pouch, recesses, spaces

Trommer's test

Trömner's sign

Trotter's syndrome — unilateral neuralgia in the region of the mandible, tongue, and ear

Trousseau's syndrome — slowly advancing thrombophlebitis associated with visceral malignancy

Trousseau's apophysiary points, dilator, forceps, phenomenon, sign, spot, test, twitching

Trousseau-Jackson dilator

Trousseau-Lallemand bodies

Troutman's eye implant, forceps, gouge, scissors

Truant's stain

Trudeau's medium

Trueta's method, technique, treatment

Trümmerfeld line

Trusler's clamp

Tschernogowbou's test

Tschmarke's treatment

Tsuchiya's test

Tswett's method

Tubbs' dilator

Tucker's bronchoscope, esophagoscope, laryngoscope, telescope, tube

Tucker-McLean forceps

Tudor-Edwards costotome

Tuffier's ligament, method, test

Tuffier-Raney retractor

Tuffnell's bandage, treatment

Tullio's phenomenon

Tulpius' valve

Tuohy's catheter, needle

Türck's bundle, cell, column, degeneration, fasciculus, trachoma

Turck's zone

Turcot's syndrome — a hereditary syndrome marked by development of polyps of the brain and colon

Turek's spreader

Turell's forceps, proctoscope, sigmoidoscope

Türk's cell, irritation leukocyte, lymphomatosis

Turkel's trephine, tube

Turkestan ulcer

Turlington's balsam

Turnbull's blue reaction

Turner's syndrome — a hereditary chromosomal anomaly marked by gonadal dysgenesis, short stature, neck webbing, elbow deformity, and cardiac defects

Turner's cerate, dilator, hypoplasia, marginal gyrus, prosthesis, sign, sulcus, tooth

Turner-Warwick urethroplasty

Turpin's syndrome — congenital bronchiectasis, megaesophagus, tracheoesophageal fistula,

Turpin's syndrome — *(continued)* vertebral deformities, rib malformations, and heterotopic ductus thoracicus

Turyn's sign

Tuttle's forceps, proctoscope, sigmoidoscope, test

Twining's method

Twort-d'Herelle phenomenon

Tycos' sphygmomanometer

Tydings' forceps, knife, tonsillectome

Tydings-Lakeside forceps

Tyndall's cone, effect, light, phenomenon

Tyrode's solution

Tyrrell's fascia, hook

Tyson's crypts, glands, test

Tyzzer's disease — necrosis of the liver and intestine caused by *Bacillus piliformis*, occurring in many mammals and occasionally in humans

Tzanck's cell, preparation, test

U

Uchida's incision, technique

Uden's syndrome — coronary disorders resulting from high position of the diaphragm

Udránszky's test

Uebe's applicator

Uehlinger's syndrome — thickening of the skin of the face, scalp, and extremities; clubbing of the fingers; and deformity of the long bones

Uffelmann's reagent, test

Uganda S virus

Uhl's anomaly

Uhlenhuth's test

Uhthoff's sign

Ullmann's line

Ullrich's syndrome — congenital, atonic, sclerotic muscular dystrophy

Ullrich's retractor

Ullrich-Feichtiger syndrome — micrognathia, occurrence of an extra finger or toe, genital abnormalities, and other defects

Ullrich and Fremerey-Dohna syndrome — same as *Hallermann-Streiff syndrome*

Ullrich-Turner syndrome — same as *Noonan's syndrome*

Ulrich's test

Ultzmann's test

Umber's test

Underwood's disease — a disorder of lipid metabolism usually present at birth or shortly after, characterized by hardening of subcutaneous fat and development of multiple, firm nodules on the buttocks, trunk, thighs, cheeks, arms, and feet

Undritz's anomaly

Unna's disease — a chronic inflammatory disease of the skin marked by yellowish patches; greasy, moist, or dry scales; and itching

Unna's syndrome — an inherited, familial form of hypotrichosis, with eyelashes and eyebrows often missing at birth

Unna's alkaline methylene blue stain, boot, cell, dermatosis, layer, mark, nevus, paste, vesicle, wrap

Unna-Pappenheim stain

Unna-Taenzer disease — same as *Taenzer's disease*

Unna-Taenzer stain

Unna-Thost disease/syndrome — a congenital disease marked by symmetrical thickening of the epidermal horny layers of the palms and soles, often extending to the dorsal surfaces of the knuckles

Unschuld's sign

Unverricht's disease — progressive familial myoclonic epilepsy

Unverricht-Lundborg disease — same as *Unverricht's disease*

Updegraff's needle

Uppsala virus

Urbach's lipoproteinosis

Urbach-Oppenheim disease — a dermatosis occurring in diabetes, marked by necrosis of the elastic and connective tissue of the skin with degeneration of collagen

Urbach-Wiethe disease/syndrome — a rare familial and congenital lipid storage dis-

Urbach-Wiethe disease/syndrome — (*continued*) ease characterized by multiple lipoid infiltrations that produce waxiness and thickening of the skin and mucous membranes of the mouth, pharynx, larynx, and hypopharynx, resulting in hoarseness

Urbantschitsch's bougie

Uriolla's sign, test

Urov's disease — same as *Kashin-Bek disease*

Uruma virus

Uschinsky's culture medium

Usher's syndrome — congenital nerve deafness and retinitis pigmentosa, often ending in blindness

Uskow's pillars

Ussing's equation

Uyemura's syndrome — a combination of night blindess, epithelial xerosis, multiple white spots on the retina, and faulty dark adaptation

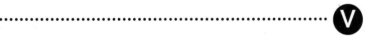

Vahlquist-Gasser syndrome — a chronic, benign form of granulocytopenia of children without systemic manifestations

Vail's syndrome — neuralgic pain in the nose, face, eye, ear, head, neck, and shoulder, usually unilateral, often nocturnal, associated with symptoms of nasal sinusitis

Valdini's method

Valenta's test

Valentin's corpuscles, ganglion, pseudoganglion

Valentine's position, splint, test tube

Valleix's points

Vallery-Radot and Blamoutier lipomatosis

Vallet's mass

Valli-Ritter law

Valsalva's experiment, ligaments, maneuver, sinus, test, zone

Valsuani's disease — progressive pernicious anemia in puerperal women

Van Allen's syndrome — Iowa-type familial amyloid polyneuropathy

Van Alyea's cannula, tube

van Bogaert's encephalitis, sclerosing leukoencephalitis

van Bogaert–Bertrand syndrome — same as *Canavan's disease*

van Bogaert–Divry syndrome — hereditary, diffuse, corticomeningeal venous angiomatosis, characterized by mental deficiency, epilepsy, pyramidal and extrapyramidal disorders, hemianopsia, pigmentation disorders, and telangiectasia

van Bogaert–Hozay syndrome — sudden arrest of growth of the extremities, followed by decalcification and osteolysis of various bones of the hands and feet

van Bogaert–Nyssen syndrome — same as *Nyssen–van Bogaert syndrome;* also called *van Bogaert–Nyssen-Peiffer syndrome*

van Bogaert–Scherer-Epstein syndrome–familial hypercholesterolemia

van Buchem's syndrome — a hereditary disorder marked by osteosclerosis of the skull, mandible, clavicles, ribs, and long bones, associated with elevated blood alkaline phosphatase and sometimes leading to optic atrophy and deafness

van Buren's disease — same as *Peyronie's disease*

van Buren's forceps

van Deen's test

Van de Graaff's generator

van de Kamer test

van den Bergh's disease — cyanosis arising from the foregut or originating within the small intestine

van den Bergh's test, technique

van den Velden's test

van der Hoeve's syndrome — a hereditary syndrome consisting

van der Hoeve's syndrome — (*continued*) of blue scleras, osteogenesis imperfecta, and otosclerotic deafness, usually transmitted as an autosomal dominant trait; also called *Adair-Dighton syndrome* and *Dighton-Adair syndrome*

van der Kolk's law

van der Waals bond, equation, forces, radius

van der Woude's syndrome — a hereditary syndrome marked by cleft lip or cleft palate occurring in association with cysts of the lower lip

Van Doren's forceps

van Gehuchten's cells, method

van Gieson's stain

van Helmont's mirror

van Hook's operation — ureteroureterostomy

Van Hoorn's maneuver

van Hoorne's canal

Van Lint's akinesia, block

Van Lint and Atkinson akinesia, block

Van Neck's disease — nonspecific ischiopubic osteochondritis in children of both sexes

Van Neck–Odelberg syndrome — same as *Van Neck's disease*

van Ness' rotation

Van Osdel's guillotine

Van Slyke's formula, method, amino acid procedure, test

Van Slyke-Cullen method, test

Van Slyke-Fitz method

Van Slyke-Meyer method

Van Slyke-Palmer method

Van Struycken forceps, punch

Vanderbilt's clamp, forceps

Vanghetti's prosthesis

Vannas' knife, scissors

van't Hoff's law, rule

Vanzetti's sign

Vaquez's disease — same as *Vaquez-Osler disease*

Vaquez-Osler disease — polycythemia vera

Varolius' bridge, valve

Vasconcelos-Baretto clamp

Vasiliev's disease — leptospiral jaundice

Vater's ampulla, corpuscles, duct, papilla

Vater-Pacini corpuscles

Vaudremer's tuberculin

Vaughan's disease — anemia characterized by immature leukocytes and nucleated red cells, usually observed in metastatic carcinoma of the bone marrow

Vaughan's split products

Vaughan-Novy test

Veau's elevator, palatoplasty

Vedder's agar, culture medium, sign

Veeneklaas' syndrome — chronic bronchitis associated with dental caries

Veenema's retractor

Veenema-Gusberg needle, punch

Veillon's tube

Vella's fistula

Velpeau's bandage, deformity, hernia

Venable's plate

Venable-Stuck nail

Venning Browne test

Venus' girdle

Veraguth's fold

Verbiest's syndrome — narrowing of the lumbar vertebral canal, characterized by symptoms of compression of the caudal nerve roots

Verbrugge's clamp

Verbrycke's syndrome — cholecystohepatic flexure adhesions

Verdan's syndrome — limited action of flexor activity of the uninvolved fingers in adhesive tenosynovitis

Verga's lacrimal groove, ventricle

Verheyen's stars

Verhoeff's operation — posterior sclerotomy followed by electrolytic punctures

Verhoeff's elastic method, forceps, scissors, stain, sutures

Verhoeff–van Gieson stain

Vermale's operation — amputation by double-flap transfixion

Verner-Morrison syndrome — diarrhea, hypokalemia, and achlorhydria, associated with secretion of a toxin by a pancreatic islet-cell tumor

Vernes' test

Vernet's syndrome — paralysis of the motor components of glossopharyngeal, vagal, and accessory cranial nerves, occurring most frequently as a result of head injury

Verneuil's disease — syphilitic disease of the bursa

Verneuil's canals, neuroma

Vernier's dial

Vernon's tube

Vernon-David proctoscope, sigmoidoscope

Verocay's bodies

Verres' needle, trocar

Verril's sign

Verse's disease — deposit of calcium in one or more intervertebral disks

Verstraeten's bruit

Vesalius' foramen, ligament

Vesely-Street nail

Vezien's scissors

Viamonte-Hobbs electrosurgical unit

Viamonte-Jutzy electrosurgical unit

Vickers' hyperbaric bed

Vicq d'Azyr's band, body, bundle, fasciculus, foramen, stripe, tract

Vidal's disease — a skin disease of psychogenic origin, marked by a confluent lichen and papular eruption

Vidal's operation — subcutaneous ligation of the veins for varicocele

Vierordt-Mesh formula

Vierra's sign

Viers' erysiphake

Vieth-Müller horopter

Vieussens' annulus, ansa, foramen, isthmus, limbus, loop, ring, valve, veins, ventricle

Vignal's cells

Vigouroux's sign

Vilanova-Cañadell syndrome — a combination of a papular, dry skin eruption, hypothyroidism, and vitamin A deficiency

Vilanova–Piñol Aguadé syndrome — a dermatological disorder characterized by pea-sized, subcutaneous nodules of the legs

Villard's button

Villaret's syndrome — unilateral paralysis of the ninth, tenth, eleventh, and twelfth cranial nerves, producing paralysis or anesthesia of the pharynx, soft palate, larynx, and vocal cords

Villemin's theory

Vim's needle

Vim-Silverman needle

Vincent's disease — necrotizing ulcerative gingivostomatitis

Vincent's angina, gingivitis, infection, organism, spirillium, stomatitis, tonsillitis

Vineberg's operation — to establish a collateral blood supply to the heart in which an internal mammary artery is implanted into the myocardium

Vinke's tongs, tractor

Vinson's syndrome — same as *Plummer-Vinson syndrome*

Vinson-Plummer syndrome — same as *Plummer-Vinson syndrome*

Virchow's disease — acute congenital encephalitis

Virchow's angle, cells, corpuscle, crystals, degeneration, gland, granulations, hydatid, law, line, nociceptor, node, viremia

Virchow-Robin spaces

Virchow-Seckel dwarfism

Virden's catheter

Vischer's lumboiliac incision

Visscher-Bowman test

Vitali's test

Vladimiroff's operation — removal of the heels, os calcis, and astragalus, and excision of the articular surfaces of the tibia, fibula, cuboid, and scaphoid

Vladimiroff's tarsectomy

Vleminckx's solution

Voegtlin's unit

Voelcker-Joseph test

Vogel's curet

Vogel-Lee test

Voges-Proskauer broth, reaction, test

Vogt's syndrome — a condition associated with birth trauma, marked by involuntary hand movements, difficulty in walking, outbursts of laughter or tears, speech disorders, and sometimes mental deficiency

Vogt's disease — a form of corneal dystrophy characterized by glints of a golden hue under indirect light

Vogt's angle, bone-free projection, cataract, cephalodactyly, cornea, degeneration, point, white limbal girdle

Vogt-Hueter point

Vogt-Koyanagi syndrome — uveomeningitis marked by exudative inflammation of the iris and choroid, associated with patchy depigmentation of the skin and hair and some-

Vogt-Koyanagi syndrome —
(*continued*)
times with retinal detachment
and deafness

Vogt-Koyanagi-Harada syndrome —
bilateral uveitis with exudative inflammation of the iris,
choroid meningism, and retinal detachment, occurring in
association with alopecia, vitiligo, poliosis, headache, vomiting, deafness, and vertigo or
glaucoma

Vogt-Spielmeyer disease —
amaurotic idiocy

Vohwinkel's syndrome — a mutilating disease characterized by
hyperkeratosis and keratotic
lesions on the dorsal surfaces
of the hands and feet, knees
and elbows, and by con-
stricted digits

Voigt's boundary lines

Voillemier's point

Voit's nucleus

Volavsek's syndrome — keratosis of
the palms, with involvement
of the periarticular areas of
the fingers

Volhard's nephritis, test

Volhard-Arnold method

Volhard-Harvey method

Volkmann's syndrome — post-traumatic muscular hypertonia
and degenerative neuritis;
also known as *Volkmann's contracture*

Volkmann's disease — congenital
deformity of the foot, caused
by tibiotarsal dislocation

Volkmann's operation — incision
of the tunica vaginalis for hydrocele

Volkmann's canals, cheilitis, contracture, deformity, ischemic
paralysis, membrane, retractor, splint, spoon, subluxation

Volkovitsch's sign

Vollmer's test

Voltolini's disease — acute, purulent inflammation of the inner ear with severe pain, followed by involvement of the
meninges with fever, delirium,
and unconsciousness

Voltolini's sign, tube

von Aldor's test

Von Apathy's gum syrup medium

von Bardeleben's prefrontal bone

von Behring's fluid

Von Bergmann's hernia

von Bezold's abscess

von Brun's flap

von Economo's disease — lethargic
encephalitis

von Economo's encephalitis

von Eichen's cannula

von Fürth–Charnass method

von Gierke's disease — glycogen
storage disease, accompanied
by enlargement of the liver
and heart with progressive
muscular degeneration

von Gies joint

von Graefe's cautery, forceps, sign,
speculum

von Haberer's gastroenterostomy

von Haberer-Aguirre gastrectomy

von Haberer-Finney gastrectomy,
gastroenterostomy

von Hansemann cells

von Hippel's disease — hemangiomatosis confined to the retina; with cerebral involvement it is known as *Hippel-
Lindau disease* or *von Hippel–
Lindau disease*

von Hippel–Lindau disease —
hereditary phakomatosis, characterized by congenital angiomatosis of the retina and cerebellum

von Jaksch's disease — an anemia
of young children accompanied by poikilocytosis, peripheral red blood cell immaturity,

von Jaksch's disease — *(continued)* leukocytosis, and hepatosplenomegaly

von Jaksch's anemia, test

von Kossa's method, stain

von Kupffer's cells

von Langenbeck's bipedicle mucoperiosteal flap

von Leber's atrophy

von Maschke's test

von Mering's reflex

von Meyenburg's disease — a degenerative disease of cartilage producing many and bizarre forms of arthritis

von Meyenburg's complex

von Monakow's fibers

von Mondak's forceps

von Petz's clamp

von Pirquet's cutireaction, reaction, test

von Recklinghausen's disease — same as *Recklinghausen's disease*

von Recklinghausen's neurofibromatosis, test

von Saal's pin

von Weber's triangle

von Willebrand's disease/syndrome — a congenital hereditary tendency to hemorrhage, marked by prolonged bleeding time and deficiency of Hageman coagulation factor

von Willebrand's antigen, factor

von Zeynek and Mencki test

von Zumbusch's psoriasis

Voorhees' bag, needle

Voorhoeve's disease — linear striation in the metaphyses of long and flat bones

Voorhoeve's dyschondroplasia

Vörner's heloderma

Voronoff's operation — transplantation into a man of the testes of an anthropoid ape in an effort to rejuvenate the recipient

Vossius' keratitis, lenticular ring

Vrolik's disease/syndrome — an inherited condition in which the bones are brittle and subject to fracture, sometimes accompanied by otosclerotic deafness; also called *osteogenesis imperfecta (type II)*

Vulpian's atrophy, law, test

W. Dean McDonald clamp

Waaler-Rose test

Waardenburg's syndrome(s) — a hereditary disorder marked by abnormal width of the nasal bridge, pigmentary disturbances, leukoderma, and sometimes cochlear deafness; a hereditary disorder marked by acrocephaly, orbital and facial deformities, syndactyly, cleft palate, muscular contraction, and cardiac malformation

Waardenburg-Jonkers disease — progressive corneal dystrophy of young infants, characterized by the appearance of minute dots on the parenchyma occupying the entire surface of the cornea

Wachendorf's membrane

Wachenheim-Reder sign
Wachsberger's bur
Wachstein-Meissel stain
Wachtenfeldt's clip, forceps
Wada's prosthesis, test
Wade's balsam, staining method
Wade-Fite staining method
Wade-Fite-Faraco staining method
Wadsworth-Todd cautery
Waelsch's urethritis
Wagener's retinitis
Wagner's disease — a familial form of retinal dystrophy characterized by progressive myopia associated with sclerosis and atrophy of the vessels of the choroid, macular degeneration, and patches of retinal detachment
Wagner's operation — osteoplastic resection of the skull
Wagner's corpuscles, hammer, line, osteogenic sarcoma, polymyositis, punch, resection, spot, test, theory
Wagner-Jauregg treatment
Wagner-Unverricht syndrome — an association of myositis with dermatitis, characterized by erythema of the face and eyelids and muscular pain and weakness
Wagstaffe's fracture
Wahl's sign
Walcher's position
Walcheren fever
Waldeau's forceps
Waldenberg's apparatus
Waldenström's syndrome — same as *Calvé-Legg-Perthes syndrome*
Waldenström's disease(s) — an acute form of thyrotoxicosis with muscular and cerebral complications; osteochondrosis of the capital femoral epiphysis
Waldenström's hepatitis, macroglobulinemia, purpura, test, uveoparotitis

Waldeyer's colon, fluid, fossa, gland, layer, ligament, ring, sulcus
Wales' bougie, dilator
Walker's carcinoma, carcinosarcoma, forceps, method, retractor, scissors, trephine
Walker-Apple scissors
Walker-Atkinson scissors
Walker-Warburg syndrome — a congenital disorder, usually fatal before the age of 1 year, marked by hydrocephalus, retinal dysplasia, and corneal opacity
Wallace-Diamond method
Walldius' prosthesis
Wallenberg's syndrome — a condition due to occlusion of the posterior inferior cerebellar artery, marked by loss of pain sensation in the face and extremities and muscular incoordination
Waller's law
Wallgren's disease — obstruction of the splenic vein, with venous stasis of the spleen, resultant splenomegaly, and development of collateral circulation
Wallhauser-Whitehead method
Walpole's sodium acetate buffer
Walsh's average, curet
Walsh-Ogura orbital decompression
Walsham's forceps
Walter's bromide test, forceps, spud
Walter-Bohmann syndrome — tachycardia, hypothermia, polypnea, pallor, and cold sweat following cholecystectomy or cholecystoduodenostomy
Walter-Deaver retractor
Walthard's cell rests, inclusions, islets

Walther's clamp, dilator, ducts, forceps, ganglion, oblique ligament, sound

Walther-Crenshaw clamp

Walton's forceps, knife, law, rongeur, scissors

Walton-Schubert forceps, punch

Wang's test

Wangensteen's apparatus, clamp, colostomy, drainage, forceps, suction, tube

Wanner's symptom

Wanscher's mask

Wappler's cystoscope, electrode

Warburg's syndrome — same as *Walker-Warburg syndrome*

Warburg's apparatus, coenzyme, ferment, theory

Ward's syndrome — multiple, nevoid, basal cell carcinomata associated with dyskeratosis palmaris et plantaris

Ward's triangle

Ward-French needle

Ward-Romano syndrome — same as *Romano-Ward syndrome*

Wardill four-flap method, palatoplasty

Wardrop's disease — acute inflammation of the matrix of the nails, occurring spontaneously in debilitated states or as the result of an injury

Waring's method, system

Warren's fat columns, incision, test

Wartenberg's disease — neuritis of the superficial ramus of the radial nerve

Wartenberg's sign, symptom

Warthen's clamp

Warthin's tumor

Warthin-Finkeldey cells

Warthin-Starry silver stain

Warthin-Starry-Faulkner method

Washio's flap

Wasko's probe

Wassén's test

Wassermann's antigen, reaction, test

Wassermann-positive pneumonia, pulmonary infiltrations

Wassilieff's disease — leptospiral jaundice

Watanabe heritable hyperlipidemic rabbetting

Waterhouse's urethroplasty

Waterhouse-Friderichsen syndrome — a rapidly fulminating meningococcal septicemia marked by massive purpura, bilateral adrenal hemorrhage, and shock

Waterman's bronchoscope

Waters' operation — a form of extraperitoneal cesarean section

Waters' position, view roentgenogram

Waterston's operation — anastomosis between the ascending aorta and right pulmonary artery

Waterston's anastomosis

Waters-Waldron position

Watkins' operation — for prolapse and procidentia uteri, in which the bladder is separated from the anterior wall of the uterus

Watson's forceps, method, speculum

Watson-Cheyne dissector

Watson-Crick helix

Watson-Jones gouge, incision

Watson-Schwartz test

Watson-Williams forceps, needle, rasp, rongeur

Watts' clamp, tenaculum

Wayson's stain

Weary's hook, spatula

Weaver's clamp

Webb's bolt, retractor, stripper

Weber's syndrome — paralysis of the oculomotor nerve, producing ptosis, strabismus, and loss of light reflex; also called *Weber's paralysis*

Weber's disease — same as *Sturge-Kalischer-Weber syndrome*

Weber's catheter, circle, corpuscle, douche, gland, implant, insufflator, law, method, organ, paradox, paralysis, retractor, scissors, sign, symptom, test, tubercle, zone

Weber-Christian syndrome — subcutaneous nodules and plaques resulting in atrophy of the subcutaneous fatty layer of the skin

Weber-Christian disease — relapsing, febrile, nodular, nonsuppurative panniculitis

Weber-Christian panniculitis

Weber-Cockayne syndrome — a form of epidermolysis in which large vesicles and erosions appear on the hands and feet in response to very slight injury

Weber-Dimitri syndrome — same as *Sturge-Kalischer-Weber syndrome*

Weber-Dimitri disease — same as *Sturge-Kalischer-Weber syndrome*

Weber-Fechner law

Weber-Fergusson incision

Weber-Fergusson-Longmire incision

Weber-Gubler syndrome — same as *Weber's syndrome*

Weber-Leyden syndrome — same as *Weber's syndrome* and *Leyden's paralysis*

Webril's bandage

Webster's operation — for retrodisplacement of the uterus

Webster's knife, retractor, technique, test, tube

Wechsler Adult Intelligence Scale, Intelligence Scale for Children

Weck's clamp, shears, tube

Wecker's spatula

Wedensky's facilitation, inhibition, phenomenon

Weder's retractor

Weder-Solenberger retractor

Wedl's cells

Weech's syndrome — same as *Christ-Siemens syndrome*

Weeks' bacillus, needle, speculum

Wegener's syndrome — a progressive disease marked by granulomatous lesions of the respiratory tract and, finally, by widespread inflammation of all organs of the body

Wegener's granulomatosis

Wegierko's coma

Wegner's disease — osteochondrotic separation of epiphyses in hereditary syphilis

Wegner's line, osteochondritis, sign

Weibel-Palade bodies

Weichardt's antikenotoxin, reagent

Weichbrodt's reaction, test

Weichselbaum's diplococcus

Weidel's reaction, test

Weigert's fibrin stain, iron hematoxylin stain, law, method, myelin sheath staining method, neuroglia fiber stain, resorcin-fuchsin stain

Weigert-Gram stain

Weigert-Pal technique

Weigl's vaccine

Weil's disease — leptospiral jaundice

Weil's syndrome(s) — same as *Larrey-Weil disease*; leptospiral jaundice

Weil's basal layer, forceps, icterus, rongeur, splint, stain, test, zone

Weil-Felix agglutinins, reaction, test

Weill's syndrome — same as *Adie's syndrome*

Weill's sign

Weill-Marchesani syndrome — a congenital disorder of connective tissues, transmitted as an

Weill-Marchesani syndrome — (*continued*) autosomal dominant or recessive trait and marked by short stature and brachydactyly

Weill-Reys syndrome — same as *Adie's syndrome*

Weill-Reys-Adie syndrome — same as *Adie's syndrome*

Weinberg's reaction, retractor, rule, spreader, test

Weinberg-Himelfarb syndrome — fetal endocardial fibroelastosis

Weiner's method

Weingarten's syndrome — tropical pulmonary eosinophilia

Weingartner's forceps, rongeur

Weinman's medium

Weir Mitchell's disease — bilateral vasodilatation of the extremities, with burning pain and increased skin temperature

Weir Mitchell's treatment

Weir's operation — appendicostomy

Weis' forceps

Weisbach's angle

Weisenbach's forceps

Weisman's forceps, tenaculum

Weisman-Graves speculum

Weismann's theory

Weismann-Netter's syndrome — congenital, familial anteroposterior curvature and thickening of the tibia and fibula of both legs

Weismann-Netter's dysostosis

Weismann-Netter and Stuhl syndrome — same as *Weismann-Netter's syndrome*

Weiss' reflex, sign, test

Weiss-Baker syndrome — same as *Charcot-Weiss-Baker syndrome*

Weissmann's bundle, fibers

Weitbrecht's cartilage, cord, foramen, ligament, retinaculum

Weitlaner's retractor

Welander's syndrome — late distal hereditary myopathy

Welch's abscess, bacillus

Welch Allyn forceps, laryngoscope, otoscope, proctoscope, retinoscope, sigmoidoscope, transilluminatory tube

Welcher's angle

Welcker's method

Welin's technique

Welker's method

Welker-Marsh method

Wellaminski's perforator

Welland's test

Wells' clamp, forceps, tractor

Wenckebach's disease — downward displacement of the heart

Wenckebach's block, heart block, period, phenomenon

Wender's test

Wenzell's test

Weppen's test

Werdnig-Hoffmann disease/syndrome — a hereditary, progressive, infantile form of muscular atrophy resulting from degeneration of the anterior horn cells of the spinal cord

Werdnig's disease — same as *Werdnig-Hoffmann syndrome*

Werdnig-Hoffmann atrophy, paralysis, type

Werlhof's disease — idiopathic thrombocytopenic purpura

Werlhof-Wichmann syndrome — same as *Werlhof's disease*

Wermer's syndrome — polyendocrine neoplasia

Werner's syndrome — premature senility of adults, marked by cataracts, hyperkeratinization, and sclerodermatous changes in the skin

Werner's disease — a rare hereditary condition marked by premature aging

Werner's test

Werner-His disease — an infection caused by *Rickettsia quinana*

Werner-His disease — *(continued)* transmitted by lice and marked by attacks of headache, hyperesthesia, and intermittent fever; called also *trench fever*

Werner-Schultz disease — agranulocytosis

Wernicke's syndrome — a mental condition, usually of old age, marked by defective memory, loss of sense of location, confusion, and bewilderment

Wernicke's disease — an inflammatory, hemorrhagic encephalopathy with lesions of the hypothalamus and periventricular region

Wernicke's aphasia, area, center, cramp, dementia, encephalopathy, field, fissure, reaction, sign, symptom, test, triangle, zone

Wernicke-Korsakoff syndrome — the coexistence of *Wernicke's syndrome* with *Korsakoff's disease*

Wernicke-Mann hemiplegia, type

Wertheim's operation — radical hysterectomy; removal of the uterus, tubes, and parametrium

Wertheim's clamp, forceps, hysterectomy, ointment, splint

Wertheim-Cullen clamp, forceps

Wertheim-Navratil needle

Wertheim-Reverdin clamp

Wertheim-Schauta operation — for cystocele, with interposition of the uterus between the base of the bladder and the anterior vaginal wall

Wesenberg-Hamazaki body

Wesolowski's prosthesis

Wesselsbron's disease — a mosquito-borne, fatal disease of lambs, transmissible to humans, in whom it causes a mild, febrile illness

Wesselsbron's virus

Wesson's mouth gag, retractor

West Nile fever

West's syndrome — an encephalopathy of infants causing spasms and arrest of psychomotor development

West's chisel, gouge

Westberg's space

Westcott's scissors

Wester's clamp, scissors

Westergren's method, sedimentation rate

Westermark's sign

Westgard multirule technique

Westphal's syndrome — familial paroxysmal paralysis

Westphal's disease — same as *Strümpell-Westphal disease*

Westphal's ataxia, neurosis, nucleus, phenomenon, pupillary reflex, sign, symptom, zone

Westphal-Leyden syndrome — an acute form of ataxia of unknown origin

Westphal-Piltz phenomenon, reflex

Westphal-Strümpell disease — same as *Wilson's disease*

Westphal-Strümpell pseudosclerosis

Wetzel's grid, test

Wever-Bray phenomenon

Weyers' syndrome(s) — congenital gastrointestinal atresia of parts of the gastrointestinal system, with obstruction of the adjoining vessels; iridodental dysplasia

Weyers' oligodactyly syndrome — a congenital syndrome consisting of deficiency of the ulna and ulnar rays, abnormal membrane in the interpalpebral fissure, malformations of the kidney and spleen, and cleft palate

Weyers-Fulling syndrome — multiple oculodentofacial abnor-

Weyers-Fulling syndrome —
(*continued*)
malities, including hypoplasia
of the dental root and early
loss of teeth, cataract, microphthalmia, glaucoma, and
peculiar facies

Weyers-Thier syndrome — a congenital syndrome consisting of
abnormal smallness of eyes,
twisted face due to maxillary
dysplasia, malocclusion of
teeth, and vertebral malformations

Weyl's test

Wharton's duct, gelatin, jelly

Whatman's filter paper

Wheatley Trichrome stain

Wheatstone's bridge

Wheeler's eye implant, knife, spatula

Wheeler-Johnson test

Wheelhouse's operation — perineal
section for impermeable stricture of the urethra

Whipple's disease/syndrome — a
malabsorption syndrome
marked by diarrhea, steatorrhea, arthritis, lymphadenopathy, and central nervous system lesions

Whipple's operation — radical pancreatoduodenectomy

Whipple's incision, intestinal lipodystrophy, method, pancreatoduodenectomy, resection, test,
triad

Whitcomb-Kerrison punch

White's disease — a familial eruption, beginning in childhood,
in which keratotic papules of
the trunk, face, scalp, and ax-
illae become crusted with
wartlike elevations

White's operation — castration for
hypertrophy of the prostate

White's chisel, forceps, mallet, scissors

White-Lillie forceps

White-Oslay forceps

White-Proud retractor

White-Smith forceps

Whitehead's operation(s) —
excision of hemorrhoids; removal of the tongue with scissors

Whitehorn's method

Whiteside's test

Whitfield's ointment

Whiting's rongeur, tonsillectome

Whitman's operation(s) — arthroplasty of the hip; a method of
astragalectomy

Whitman's frame

Whitmore's disease — an infectious disease of animals transmissible to humans, in whom
it causes either a chronic granulomatous pneumonia or a ful-
minant septicemia with high
mortality

Whitmore's bacillus, bag, fever,
staging system

Whitnall's ligament, tubercle

Whitten's effect

Whitver's clamp

Whytt's disease — tuberculous
meningitis causing acute
hydrocephalus

Wichmann's asthma

Wickersheimer's fluid, medium

Wickham's striae

Widal's disease/syndrome — same
as *Hayem-Widal syndrome*

Widal's reaction, test

Widal-Abrami syndrome — same
as *Hayem-Widal syndrome*

Widal-Abrami disease — acquired
hemolytic anemia

Wideroe's test

Widmark's conjunctivitis, test

Widowitz's sign

Wiechowski-Handorsky method

Wiedemann's syndrome — thalido-
mide embryopathy

Wiener's breast reduction, genetic
theory, keratome, speculum,
system

Wiener-Pierce rasp, trocar

Wigand's maneuver, version

Wigby-Taylor method

Wigmore's saw

Wijs' test

Wilbrand's prism test

Wilbur-Addis test

Wilcoxon rank sum statistic

Wildbolz reaction, test

Wilde's cords, forceps, incision, punch

Wilde-Blakesley forceps

Wilde-Bruening snare

Wilder's cystotome, diet, dilator, law, sign, stain, trephine

Wildemuth's ear

Wildervanck's syndrome — a hereditary familial syndrome marked by deaf-mutism, short neck, and paralysis of the external ocular muscles

Wildervanck-Waardenburg-Franceschetti-Klein syndrome — same as *Wildervanck's syndrome*

Wildgen-Reck locator, magnet

Wilke's brace

Wilkerson's bur, point system

Wilkie's disease — partial or complete block of the third segment of the duodenum

Wilkins' disease — congenital adrenal hyperplasia

Wilkins-Chilgren agar

Wilkinson's anemia

Wilkinson-Peter test

Wilks' disease — a form of cutaneous tuberculosis marked by verrucous lesions of the fingers

Willan's lepra

Willan-Plumbe syndrome — same as *Willan's lepra*

Willauer's raspatory, scissors

Willebrand's syndrome — same as *Willebrand-Jurgens syndrome* and *von Willebrand's disease*

Willebrand-Jurgens syndrome — hemorrhagic diathesis inher-

Willebrand-Jurgens syndrome — *(continued)* ited as a simple dominant trait, characterized by prolonged bleeding time and associated with epistaxis and bleeding from the gastrointestinal tract, gums, and uterus and at the sites of surgical operations

Willett's clamp, forceps

Williams' syndrome — a congenital disorder characterized by physical and mental deficiency, elfin facies, aortic stenosis and occasionally, elevated blood calcium; may be associated with hypersensitivity to vitamin D

Williams' colpopoiesis, craniotome, method, phenomenon, position, probe, sign, speculum, stain, tracheal tone

Williams-Campbell syndrome — congenital deficiency in the cartilaginous wall of the trachea or of a bronchus, leading to either obstructive emphysema or bronchiectasis

Williamson's blood test, sign

Willis' disease — diabetes mellitus

Willis' antrum, circle, cords, nerve, pancreas, paracusis, pouch, valve

Willner's spots

Willock's respiratory jacket

Willowbrook virus

Wills' anemia, factor

Willy Meyer incision, radical mastectomy

Wilman's clamp

Wilmer's chisel, retractor, scissors

Wilms' nephroblastoma, tumor

Wilson's syndrome — hepatolenticular degeneration

Wilson's disease — a rare, progressive disease due to a defect in the metabolism with

Wilson's disease — (continued) accumulation of copper in the liver, brain, kidney, and cornea; characterized by cirrhosis of the liver and degenerative changes in the brain

Wilson's awl, clamp, degeneration, leads, modification of Bowie's stain, muscle, spreader, trocar, wrench

Wilson-Blair culture medium

Wilson-Mikity syndrome — a rare and often fatal form of pulmonary insufficiency in low-birth-weight infants, marked by abnormal respiratory action and cyanosis

Wiltberger's spreader

Wimberger's sign

Wimshurst's machine

Winckel's disease — a fatal disease of newborn infants, marked by jaundice, hemoglobinuria, hemorrhage, cyanosis, convulsions, and collapse

Winckler's test

Wincor's scissors

Windscheid's disease — neurologic symptoms of arteriosclerosis

Winer's catheter

Winiwarter's operation — cholecystoenterostomy

Winiwarter-Buerger disease/syndrome — thromboangiitis obliterans (same as Buerger's disease)

Winkelstein's alkalinized milk drip

Winkler's disease — a painful disorder of the ear, marked by hard nodules involving the skin and cartilage

Winkler's body

Winkler-Waldeyer closing ring

Winogradsky's culture medium

Winslow's collateral fibers, epiploic foramen, hiatus, ligament, pancreas, star, test

Winter's syndrome — a congenital syndrome consisting of renal hypoplasia, anomalies of the genitalia, especially vaginal atresia, and abnormalities of the middle-ear ossicles

Winterbottom's sign, symptom

Winternitz's sound

Wintersteiner's compound

Winton's disease — same as Pictou's disease

Wintrich's sign

Wintrobe's hematocrit, macromethod, method, tube

Wintrobe-Landsberg method

Wirsung's canal, duct

Wis-Foregger layrngoscope

Wis-Hipple laryngoscope

Wisconsin medium

Wise's disease — same as Mucha-Habermann syndrome

Wise-Rein disease — same as Kaposi's disease (1)

Wiseman-Doan syndrome — primary splenic neutropenia

Wishard's catheter

Wishart's disease — tumors of the spinal nerve roots and auditory nerves

Wishart's test

Wiskott-Aldrich syndrome — a rare and usually fatal hereditary syndrome, transmitted as an X-linked recessive trait and characterized by chronic eczema, chronic suppurative otitis media, anemia, and thrombocytopenic purpura

Wiskott-Aldrich-Huntley syndrome — same as Wiskott-Aldrich syndrome

Wissler-Fanconi syndrome — high intermittent fever, exanthemata, arthralgia, carditis, pleurisy, neutrophil leukocytosis, and increased sedimentation rate

Wistar's pyramid

Witkop's disease — hereditary benign premature keratinization in individual cells of the epithelium

Witkop–Von Sallmann syndrome — a hereditary congenital disease of the oral mucosa and bulbar conjunctiva, characterized by gelatinous plaques of the conjunctiva and thickening of the oral mucosa

Witkop–Von Sallmann disease — same as *Witkop's disease*

Wittmaack-Ekbom syndrome — same as *Ekbom's syndrome*

Wittner's forceps

Witts' anemia

Witz's test

Witzel's operation — gastrostomy

Wladimiroff's operation — same as *Vladimiroff's operation*

Woakes' saw

Wohlfart-Kugelberg-Welander disease — progressive muscular dystrophy with fibrillary twitching

Wohlgemuth's unit

Wohlwill–Corino Andrade syndrome — same as *Andrade's syndrome*

Woillez's disease — acute idiopathic pulmonary congestion

Woldman's test

Wolf's syndrome — an association of multiple anomalies caused by partial deletion of the short arm of a chromosome of the B group

Wolf's catheter, method

Wolf-Hirschhorn syndrome — chromosomal abnormality marked by microcephaly, a vertical skin fold on either side of the nose, cleft palate, micrognathia, cryptorchidism, and hypospadias

Wolf-Orton body

Wolf-Schindler gastroscope

Wolfe's forceps, graft

Wolfe-Krause graft

Wolfenden's position

Wolff's duct, law, reagent

Wolff-Calmette reaction

Wolff-Chaikoff effect

Wolff-Eisner reaction, test

Wolff-Junghans test

Wolff-Parkinson-White syndrome — paroxysmal tachycardia, shown in an electrocardiographic pattern of short P-R interval (atrial activity) and prolonged QRS complex (ventricular activity)

Wölfler's operation — anterior gastrojejunostomy for pyloric obstruction

Wölfler's sign, sutures

Wolfram's syndrome — a hereditary association of diabetes mellitus, diabetes insipidus, optic atrophy, and neural deafness

Wolfring's glands

Wolfson's clamp, retractor

Wolkowitsch's sign

Wollaston's doublet

Wolman's disease — primary familial xanthomatosis in infants, usually leading to early death

Wolman's xanthomatosis

Wolter's method

Wolters' nevus

Wong's method

Wood's filter, glass, lamp, light, metal, sign, test

Woodbridge's sutures, treatment

Woodbury's test

Woodruff's catheter

Woods-Fildes hypothesis, theory

Woodson's elevator, spoon

Woodward's forceps, sound

Wookey's skin flap

Woolner's tip

Woringer's disease — a manifestation of faulty fat assimilation

Woringer's disease — (*continued*) occurring in children fed fat-rich food, characterized by hepatomegaly with colicky pain, headache, vomiting, nausea, fatigability, and pallor

Woringer-Kolopp disease/syndrome — a form of reticulosis, with multiple cutaneous tumors

Worm-Müller's test

Wormley's test

Worth's chisel, forceps

Woulfe's bottle

Wratten's filter

Wreden's sign

Wright's syndrome — a neurovascular syndrome caused by occlusion of the subclavian artery, resulting from malposition of the arm

Wright's antigen, method, plate, stain, version

Wright blood group system, respirometer

Wrisberg's cartilage, ganglion, ligament, line, nerve, staff, tubercle

Wuhrmann's disease — myocardial fibrosis

Wullen's stone dislodger

Wullstein's forceps, knife, retractor, scissors, tympanoplasty

Wullstein-House forceps

Wunderlich's syndrome — hemorrhage surrounding the kidney

Wunderlich's curve

Wundt's tetanus

Wundt-Lamansky law

Wurd's catheter

Wurster's test

Wurth's vein stripper

Wützer's operation — for the radical cure of inguinal hernia

Wutzler's scissors

Wyatt's disease — a systemic disorder of the neonatal period, from infection with a cytomegalovirus acquired before birth

Wyburn-Mason's syndrome — arteriovenous aneurysm of the midbrain, with retinal, facial, and mental changes

Wyeth's operation — amputation at the hip joint

Wylie's drain, forceps, pessary

Wynn's method

Wysler's sutures

Yankauer's operation — curettement of the bony end of the eustachian tube

Yankauer's bronchoscope, esophagoscope, forceps, nasopharyngoscope, tube

Yankauer-Little forceps

Yasargil's forceps, raspatory, scissors, technique

Yazujian's bur

Yellen's clamp

Yemen ulcer

Yeo's treatment

Yeomans' forceps, proctoscope, sigmoidoscope

Yerkes discrimination box

Yerkes-Bridges test

Yersin's serum

Yokogawa's fluke

Yorke's autolytic reaction

Yoshida's dissector, sarcoma, tumor

Youdon's plot

Young's syndrome — absence of spermatozoa in the semen and chronic infection of the sinuses and lungs

Young's operation(s) — partial prostatectomy; total excision of seminal vesicles and partial excision of ejaculatory ducts

Young's clamp, dilator, forceps, retractor, rule, test

Young-Dees-Leadbetter procedure

Young-Helmholtz theory

Young-Millin needle holder

Youssef's syndrome — a rare syndrome combining urinary incontinence and menstrual hematuria, caused by a vesicouterine fistula appearing after lower segment cesarean section

Yvon's coefficient, test

Zachary–Cope DeMartel clamp

Zahn's infarct, lines, pockets, ribs

Zahorsky's syndrome — an acute infectious disease of childhood caused by Coxsackie A viruses, characterized by sudden high fever and vesicular ulcerative lesions of the soft palate and faucial areas

Zahorsky's disease — an acute mild viral disease of young children, marked by fever and followed by rash

Zak's reaction

Zaleski's test

Zambesi ulcer

Zander's apparatus, cells

Zanelli's method

Zang's space

Zange-Kindler syndrome — block of the cerebrospinal fluid in the cisterna magna, from space-occupying lesions of the posterior cranial fossa

Zangemeister's test

Zanoli-Vecchi syndrome — convulsions with apnea and loss of consciousness, appearing suddenly two to three hours after surgery

Zappacosta's test

Zappert's syndrome — a cerebellar disorder characterized by ataxia of station and gait, intention tremor, nystagmus, and slurred speech; the onset is sudden in normal children or in children recovering from infectious diseases

Zappert's counting chamber

Zaufal's sign

Zeeman's correction method, effect

Zeis' glands

Zeisel's test

Zeissel's layer

Zellballen's pattern

Zeller's test

Zellweger's syndrome — a rare syndrome marked by muscular hypotonia, incomplete myelinization of nerve tissues, craniofacial malformations, and glomerular cysts of the kidney

Zener's breakdown, diode

Zenker's crystals, degeneration, diverticulum, dysplasia, fixative, fluid, necrosis, pouch, solution

Zero family

Zeune's law

Ziegler's operation — V-shaped iridectomy

Ziegler's cautery, forceps, speculum

Ziegler-Furniss clamp

Ziehen's test

Ziehen-Oppenheim disease — a progressive disorder of children marked by muscular contractions producing bizarre distortions of the spine and hips

Ziehl's carbolfuchsin stain, solution

Ziehl-Neelsen method, stain

Ziemann's dots, stippling

Ziemssen's motor points

Zieve's syndrome — hypercholesterolemia, hepatosplenomegaly, fatty infiltration of the liver, hemolytic anemia, and hypertriglyceridemia following the intake of large amounts of alcohol

Ziffern's test

Zika virus

Zimaloy's prosthesis

Zimany's bilobed flap

Zimmer's clamp, prosthesis, splint

Zimmerlin's atrophy, type

Zimmermann's arch, corpuscle, decoction, elementary particles, granule, pericyte, reaction, test, virus

Zinn's annulus, aponeurosis, artery, cap, circle, corona, ligament, membrane, ring, tendon, zone, zonule

Zinsser's inconsistency

Zinsser-Cole-Engman syndrome — a congenital syndrome characterized by dyskeratosis, pigmentation of the skin, nail dystrophy, aplastic anemia, hypersplenism, acrocyanosis, hyperhidrosis of the palms and soles, and leukoplakia of the tongue and hard palate

Zipser's clamp

Zittmann's decoction

Zoellner's needle, raspatory, scissors

Zoepffel's edema

Zoll's pacemaker

Zollinger-Ellison syndrome — a complex of symptoms consisting of intractable, fulminating peptic ulcer, severe gastric hyperacidity, and islet-cell tumors of the pancreas that may be benign or malignant

Zollinger-Ellison tumor

Zöllner's figures, lines

Zondek-Aschheim test

Zondek-Bromberg-Rozin syndrome — galactorrhea and hyperthyroidism

Zoon's balanitis, erythroplasia

Zouchlos' test

Zsigmondy's gold number method, test

Zuckerkandl's bodies, convolution, dehiscences, gland, organs

Zuelzer's syndrome — eosinophilia, leukocytosis, and hypergammaglobulinemia in infants and young children, with manifestations that include hepatomegaly, pulmonary infiltrations, asthma, joint lesions, urticaria, and convulsions

Zuelzer's awl, plate

Zuelzer-Kaplan syndrome(s) — a congenital familial form of chronic hemolytic anemia, characterized by jaundice, hepatosplenomegaly, osseous changes, and a tendency to-

Zuelzer-Kaplan syndrome(s) — (continued) ward development of mongoloid facies; a severe, chronic hypochromic microcytic anemia attributed to the interaction of the hemoglobin C gene with the thalassemia gene

Zuelzer-Ogden syndrome — a combination of hematopoietic disorders, characterized by progressive macrocytic anemia, leukopenia, and thrombocytopenia

Zuntz's theory

Zurich hemoglobin

Zutt's clamp

Zwahlen's syndrome — same as Franceschetti's syndrome

Zwanck's pessary

Zweifel–De Lee cranioclast

Zwenger's test

Appendices

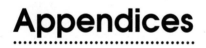

Appendix 1
Anticancer Drug Combinations

PROTOCOL	COMPONENT DRUGS (abbreviation key at end of table)
ABC	Adriamycin, BCNU, cyclophosphamide
ABCD	Adriamycin, bleomycin, CCNU, dacarbazine
ABCM	Adriamycin, bleomycin, cyclophosphamide, mitomycin C
ABDV	Adriamycin, bleomycin, DTIC, vinblastine
ABP	Adriamycin, bleomycin, prednisone
ABV	actinomycin D, bleomycin, vincristine
ABVD	Adriamycin, bleomycin, vinblastine, dacarbazine
AC	Adriamycin, CCNU
AC	Adriamycin, cyclophosphamide
ACe	Adriamycin, cyclophosphamide
ACE	Adriamycin, cyclophosphamide, etoposide
ACM	Adriamycin, cyclophosphamide, methotrexate
ACOP	Adriamycin, cyclophosphamide, Oncovin, prednisone
ACOPP	Adriamycin, cyclophosphamide, Oncovin, prednisone, procarbazine
ADBC	Adriamycin, DTIC, bleomycin, CCNU
ADIC	Adriamycin, dacarbazine (DTIC)
ADOAP	Adriamycin, Oncovin, ara-C, prednisone
ADOP	Adriamycin, Oncovin, prednisone
Adria-L-PAM	Adriamycin, melphalan
AIM	L-asparaginase, ifosfamide, methotrexate
ALOMAD	Adriamycin, Leukeran, Oncovin, methotrexate, actinomycin D
APC	amsacrine, prednisone, chlorambucil
APO	Adriamycin, prednisone, Oncovin
AV	Adriamycin, vincristine
AVDP	asparaginase, vincristine, daunorubicin, prednisone
AVM	Adriamycin, vinblastine, methotrexate
AVP	actinomycin D, vincristine, Platinol
AVP	Adriamycin, vincristine, procarbazine
BACO	bleomycin, Adriamycin, CCNU, Oncovin

Appendix 1
Anticancer Drug Combinations (Continued)

PROTOCOL	COMPONENT DRUGS (abbreviation key at end of table)
BACOD	bleomycin, Adriamycin, Cytoxan, Oncovin, dexamethasone
BACON	bleomycin, Adriamycin, CCNU, Oncovin, nitrogen mustard
BACOP	bleomycin, Adriamycin, cyclophosphamide, Oncovin, prednisone
BACT	BCNU, ara-C, cyclophosphamide, 6-thioguanine
BACT	bleomycin, Adriamycin, Cytoxan, tamoxifen citrate
BAMON	bleomycin, Adriamycin, methotrexate, Oncovin, nitrogen mustard
BAP	bleomycin, Adriamycin, prednisone
BAVIP	bleomycin, Adriamycin, vinblastine, imidazole carboxamide, prednisone
BCAVe	bleomycin, CCNU, Adriamycin, Velban
BCD	bleomycin, cyclophosphamide, dactinomycin
BCNU	bis-chloroethyl-nitrosourea
BCOP	BCNU, cyclophosphamide, Oncovin, prednisone
BCP	BCNU, cyclophosphamide, prednisone
BCVP	BCNU, cyclophosphamide, vincristine, prednisone
BCVPP	BCNU, cyclophosphamide, vinblastine, procarbazine, prednisone
B-DOPA	bleomycin, DTIC, Oncovin, prednisone, Adriamycin
BEP	bleomycin, etoposide, Platinol
BHD	BCNU, hydroxyurea, dacarbazine
BHDV	BCNU, hydroxyurea, dacarbazine, vincristine
B-MOPP	bleomycin, nitrogen mustard, Oncovin, procarbazine, prednisone
BMP	BCNU, methotrexate, procarbazine
BOAP	bleomycin, Oncovin, Adriamycin, prednisone
BOLD	bleomycin, Oncovin, lomustine, dacarbazine
BONP	bleomycin, Oncovin, Natulan, prednisolone

Appendix continued on following page

Appendix 1
Anticancer Drug Combinations (Continued)

PROTOCOL	COMPONENT DRUGS (abbreviation key at end of table)
BOP	BCNU, Oncovin, prednisone
BOPAM	bleomycin, Oncovin, prednisone, Adriamycin, mechlorethamine, methotrexate
BOPP	BCNU, Oncovin, procarbazine, prednisone
BVAP	BCNU, vincristine, Adriamycin, prednisone
BVCPP	BCNU, vinblastine, cyclophosphamide, procarbazine, prednisone
BVD	BCNU, vincristine, dacarbazine
BVDS	bleomycin, Velban, doxorubicin, streptozocin
BVPP	BCNU, vincristine, procarbazine, prednisone
CABOP	Cytoxan, Adriamycin, bleomycin, Oncovin, prednisone
CABS	CCNU, Adriamycin, bleomycin, streptozocin
CAD	cyclophosphamide, Adriamycin, dacarbazine
CAD	cytosine arabinoside, daunorubicin
CADIC	cyclophosphamide, Adriamycin, DTIC
CAE	cyclophosphamide, Adriamycin, etoposide
CAF	cyclophosphamide, Adriamycin, 5-fluorouracil
CAFP	cyclophosphamide, Adriamycin, 5-fluorouracil, prednisone
CAFVP	cyclophosphamide, Adriamycin, 5-fluorouracil, vincristine, prednisone
CAM	cyclophosphamide, Adriamycin, methotrexate
CAMB	Cytoxan, Adriamycin, methotrexate, bleomycin
CAMEO	cyclophosphamide, Adriamycin, methotrexate, etoposide, Oncovin
CAMF	cyclophosphamide, Adriamycin, methotrexate, 5-fluorouracil
CAMLO	cytosine arabinoside, methotrexate, leucovorin, Oncovin
CAMP	Cytoxan, Adriamycin, methotrexate, procarbazine hydrochloride
CAO	cyclophosphamide, Adriamycin, Oncovin
CAP	cyclophosphamide, Adriamycin, Platinol
CAP	cyclophosphamide, Adriamycin, prednisone

Appendix 1
Anticancer Drug Combinations *(Continued)*

PROTOCOL	COMPONENT DRUGS (abbreviation key at end of table)
CAP-BOP	cyclophosphamide, Adriamycin, procarbazine, bleomycin, Oncovin, prednisone
CAT	cytosine arabinoside, Adriamycin, 6-thioguanine
CAV	cyclophosphamide, Adriamycin, vincristine
CAV	Cytoxan, Adriamycin, Velban
CAVe	CCNU, Adriamycin, Velban
CAVMP	cyclophosphamide, Adriamycin, VP-16, methotrexate prednisone
CAVP-16	cyclophosphamide, Adriamycin, VP-16-213
CBPPA	cyclophosphamide, bleomycin, procarbazine, prednisone, Adriamycin
CBV	cyclophosphamide, BCNU, VP-16-213
CBVD	CCNU, bleomycin, vinblastine, dexamethasone
CCAVV	CCNU, cyclophosphamide, Adriamycin, vincristine, VP-16
CCFE	cyclophosphamide, cisplatin, 5-fluorouracil, estramustine
CCM	cyclophosphamide, CCNU, methotrexate
CCMA	CCNU, cyclophosphamide, methotrexate, Adriamycin
CCNU-OP	CCNU, Oncovin, prednisone
CCOB	CCNU, cyclophosphamide, Oncovin, bleomycin
CCOP	CCNU, Oncovin, prednisone
CCV	CCNU, cyclophosphamide, vincristine
CCV-AV	CCNU, cyclophosphamide, vincristine, Adriamycin, vincristine
CCVB	CCNU, cyclophosphamide, vincristine, bleomycin
CCVPP	cyclophosphamide, CCNU, vinblastine, procarbazine, prednisone
CCVPP	CCNU, cyclophosphamide, Velban, procarbazine, prednisone
CD	cytarabine, daunorubicin
CDC	carboplatin, doxorubicin, cyclophosphamide
CDDP	*cis*-diamminedichloroplatinum
CeeNU	lomustine

Appendix continued on following page

Appendix 1
Anticancer Drug Combinations *(Continued)*

PROTOCOL	COMPONENT DRUGS (abbreviation key at end of table)
CEP	CCNU, etoposide, prednimustine
CEV	cyclophosphamide, etoposide, vincristine
CF	cisplatin, 5-fluorouracil
CFL	cisplatin, 5-fluorouracil, leucovorin calcium
CFP	cyclophosphamide, 5-fluorouracil, prednisone
CFPT	cyclophosphamide, 5-fluorouracil, prednisone, tamoxifen
CHAD	cyclophosphamide, hexamethylmelamine, Adriamycin, *cis*-diamminedichloroplatinum
CHAM-OCA	cyclophosphamide, hydroxyurea, actinomycin D, methotrexate, Oncovin, citrovorum factor, Adriamycin
CHEX-UP	cyclophosphamide, hexamethylmelamine, 5-fluorouracil, Platinol
CHF	cyclophosphamide, hexamethylmelamine, 5-fluorouracil
CHIP	*cis*-dichlorotranshydroxy-bis-isopropylamine platinum IV
ChlVPP	chlorambucil, vinblastine, procarbazine, prednisone
CHO	cyclophosphamide, hydroxydaunomycin, Oncovin
CHOB	cyclophosphamide, Adriamycin, Oncovin, bleomycin
CHOD	cyclophosphamide, doxorubicin, Oncovin, dexamethasone
CHOP	cyclophosphamide, hydroxydaunomycin, Oncovin, prednisone
CHOP-BLEO	cyclophosphamide, hydroxydaunomycin, Oncovin, prednisone, bleomycin
CHOR	cyclophosphamide, hydroxydaunorubicin, Oncovin, and radiation
CHVP	cyclophosphamide, hydroxydaunomycin, VM-26, prednisone
CIA	CCNU, isophosphamide, Adriamycin
CISCA	cisplatin, Cytoxan, Adriamycin
cis-DDP	*cis*-diamminedichloroplatinum

Appendix 1
Anticancer Drug Combinations (Continued)

PROTOCOL	COMPONENT DRUGS (abbreviation key at end of table)
CLVPP	chlorambucil, vinblastine, procarbazine, prednisone
CMC	cyclophosphamide, methotrexate, CCNU
CMC-VAP	cyclophosphamide, methotrexate, CCNU, vincristine, Adriamycin, procarbazine
CMF	Cytoxan, methotrexate, 5-fluorouracil
CMF-AV	cyclophosphamide, methotrexate, 5-fluorouracil, Adriamycin, vincristine
CMFAVP	cyclophosphamide, methotrexate, 5-fluorouracil, Adriamycin, vincristine, prednisone
CMF-BLEO	cyclophosphamide, methotrexate, 5-fluorouracil, bleomycin
CMF-FLU	cyclophosphamide, methotrexate, 5-fluorouracil, fluoxymesterone
CMFH	cyclophosphamide, methotrexate, 5-fluorouracil, hydroxyurea
CMFP	cyclophosphamide, methotrexate, 5-fluorouracil, prednisone
CMFP-VA	cyclophosphamide, methotrexate, 5-fluorouracil, prednisone, vincristine, Adriamycin
CMFT	cyclophosphamide, methotrexate, 5-fluorouracil, tamoxifen
CMF-TAM	cyclophosphamide, methotrexate, 5-fluorouracil, tamoxifen
CMFV	cyclophosphamide, methotrexate, 5-fluorouracil, vincristine
CMFVAT	cyclophosphamide, methotrexate, 5-fluorouracil, vincristine, Adriamycin, testosterone
CMFVP	Cytoxan, methotrexate, 5-fluorouracil, vincristine, prednisone
C-MOPP	cyclophosphamide, mechlorethamine, Oncovin, procarbazine, prednisone
CMP	CCNU, methotrexate, procarbazine
CMPF	cyclophosphamide, methotrexate, prednisone, 5-fluorouracil
CMV	cisplatin, methotrexate, vinblastine
CNF	cyclophosphamide, Novantrone, 5-fluorouracil

Appendix continued on following page

Appendix 1
Anticancer Drug Combinations *(Continued)*

PROTOCOL	COMPONENT DRUGS (abbreviation key at end of table)
COAP	cyclophosphamide, Oncovin, ara-C, prednisone
COAP-BLEO	cyclophosphamide, Oncovin, ara-C, prednisone, bleomycin
COB	cisplatin, Oncovin, bleomycin
COBMAM	cyclophosphamide, Oncovin, bleomycin, methotrexate, Adriamycin, MeCCNU
COM	cyclophosphamide, Oncovin, MeCCNU
COM	cyclophosphamide, Oncovin, methotrexate
COMA-A	cyclophosphamide, Oncovin, methotrexate, Adriamycin, Ara-C
COMB	cyclophosphamide, Oncovin, MeCCNU, bleomycin
COMB	cyclophosphamide, Oncovin, methotrexate, bleomycin
COMBAP	Cytoxan, Oncovin, methotrexate, bleomycin, Adriamycin, prednisone
COMe	Cytoxan, Oncovin, methotrexate
COMET-A	cyclophosphamide, vincristine, methotrexate, leucovorin, etoposide, cytarabine
COMF	cyclophosphamide, Oncovin, methotrexate, 5-fluorouracil
COMLA	cyclophosphamide, Oncovin, methotrexate, leucovorin, ara-C
COMP	cyclophosphamide, Oncovin, methotrexate, prednisone
COP	cyclophosphamide, Oncovin, prednisone
COPA	cyclophosphamide, Oncovin, prednisone, Adriamycin
COPAC	CCNU, Oncovin, prednisone, Adriamycin, cyclophosphamide
COPB	cyclophosphamide, Oncovin, prednisone, bleomycin
COP-BLAM	cyclophosphamide, Oncovin, prednisone, bleomycin, Adriamycin, Matulane
COP-BLEO	cyclophosphamide, Oncovin, prednisone, bleomycin
COPP	CCNU, Oncovin, procarbazine, prednisone

Appendix 1
Anticancer Drug Combinations (Continued)

PROTOCOL	COMPONENT DRUGS (abbreviation key at end of table)
COPP	cyclophosphamide, Oncovin, procarbazine, prednisone
CPDD	*cis*-platinum diamminedichloride
CPM	chloroethyl cyclohexylnitrosourea, procarbazine, methotrexate
CPOB	cyclophosphamide, prednisone, Oncovin, bleomycin
CROP	cyclophosphamide, rubidazone, Oncovin, prednisone
CROPAM	cyclophosphamide, rubidazone, Oncovin, prednisone, L-asparaginase, methotrexate
CTX-Plat	cyclophosphamide, cisplatin
CV	cyclophosphamide, VP-16
CVA	cyclophosphamide, vincristine, Adriamycin
CVA-BMP	cyclophosphamide, vincristine, Adriamycin, BCNU, methotrexate, procarbazine
CVB	CCNU, vinblastine, bleomycin
CVEB	cisplatin, vinblastine, etoposide, bleomycin
CVM	cyclophosphamide, vincristine, methotrexate
CVP	cyclophosphamide, vincristine, prednisone
CVP-B	cyclophosphamide, vincristine, prednisone, bleomycin
CVP-BLEO	cyclophosphamide, vincristine, prednisone, bleomycin
CVPP	CCNU, vinblastine, prednisone, procarbazine
CVPP	cyclophosphamide, Velban, procarbazine, prednisone
CVPP-CCNU	cyclophosphamide, vinblastine, procarbazine, prednisone, CCNU
CyVADACT	cyclophosphamide, vincristine, Adriamycin, dactinomycin
CyVADTIC	cyclophosphamide, vincristine, Adriamycin, DTIC
CyVMAD	cyclophosphamide, vincristine, methotrexate, Adriamycin, DTIC
DA	daunomycin, cytosine, arabinoside

Appendix continued on following page

Appendix 1
Anticancer Drug Combinations *(Continued)*

PROTOCOL	COMPONENT DRUGS (abbreviation key at end of table)
DAT	daunomycin, ara-C, 6-thioguanine
DAVH	dibromodulcitol, Adriamycin, vincristine, Halotestin
DBH	dacarbazine, BCNU, hydroxyurea
DBV	dacarbazine, BCNU, vincristine
DCCMP	daunorubicin, cyclocytidine, 6-mercaptopurine, prednisone
DCMP	daunorubicin, cytarabine, 6-mercaptopurine, prednisone
DCPM	daunorubicin, cytarabine, prednisone, mercaptopurine
DCT	daunorubicin, cytarabine, thioguanine
DCV	dacarbazine, CCNU, vincristine
DMC	dactinomycin, methotrexate, cyclophosphamide
DOAP	daunorubicin, Oncovin, ara-C, prednisone
DTIC	diethyl-triazeno-imidazole, carboxamide
DVB	*cis*-diamminedichloroplatinum, vindesine, bleomycin
DVLP	daunomycin, vincristine, L-asparaginase, prednisone
DVPA	daunorubicin, vincristine, prednisone, L-asparaginase
DZAPO	daunorubicin, azacitidine, ara-C, prednisone, Oncovin
ECHO	etoposide, cyclophosphamide, hydroxydaunomycin, Oncovin
EMA	etoposide, methotrexate, actinomycin D
FA	5-fluorouracil, Adriamycin
FAC	5-fluorouracil, Adriamycin, cyclophosphamide
FAC-LEV	5-fluorouracil, Adriamycin, cyclophosphamide, levamisole
FACP	Ftorafur, Adriamycin, cyclophosphamide, Platinol
FACS	5-fluorouracil, Adriamycin, cyclophosphamide, streptozocin

Appendix 1
Anticancer Drug Combinations *(Continued)*

PROTOCOL	COMPONENT DRUGS (abbreviation key at end of table)
FACVP	5-fluorouracil, Adriamycin, cyclophosphamide, VP-16
FAM	5-fluorouracil, Adriamycin, mitomycin C
FAME	5-fluorouracil, Adriamycin, MeCCNU
FAMME	5-fluorouracil, Adriamycin, mitomycin C, MeCCNU
FAM-S	5-fluorouracil, Adriamycin, mitomycin C, streptozocin
FAP	5-fluorouracil, Adriamycin, cisplatin
5-FC	5-fluorocytosine
FCP	5-fluorouracil, cyclophosphamide, prednisone
FEC	5-fluorouracil, etoposide, cisplatin
FIME	5-fluorouracil, ICRF-159, MeCCNU
FMS	5-fluorouracil, mitomycin C, streptozocin
FMV	5-fluorouracil, MeCCNU, vincristine
FOAM	5-fluorouracil, Oncovin, Adriamycin, mitomycin C
FOMI	5-fluorouracil, Oncovin, mitomycin
FUDR	5-fluorouracil, deoxyribonucleoside
FUM	5-fluorouracil, methotrexate
FURAM	Ftorafur, Adriamycin, mitomycin C
FUTP	fluorouridine, triphosphate
HAC	hexamethylmelamine, Adriamycin, cyclophosphamide
HAD	hexamethylmelamine, Adriamycin, *cis*-diamminedichloroplatinum
HAM	hexamethylmelamine, Adriamycin, melphalan or methotrexate
HAMP	hexamethylmelamine, Adriamycin, methotrexate, Platinol
HCAP	hexamethylmelamine, cyclophosphamide, Adriamycin, Platinol
HCFU	hexylcarbamoyl, 5-fluorouracil
HOAP-BLEO	hydroxydaunomycin, Oncovin, ara-C, prednisone, bleomycin

Appendix continued on following page

Appendix 1
Anticancer Drug Combinations (Continued)

PROTOCOL	COMPONENT DRUGS (abbreviation key at end of table)
HOM	hexamethylmelamine, Oncovin, methotrexate
HOP	hydroxydaunomycin, Oncovin, prednisone
IMV	isophosphamide, methotrexate, vincristine
IMVP-16	isophosphamide, methotrexate, VP-16
IUDR	iododeoxyuridine
LAM	L-asparaginase, methotrexate
LAPOCA	L-asparaginase, prednisone, Oncovin, cytarabine, Adriamycin
LMF	Leukeran, methotrexate, 5-fluorouracil
LPAM	L-phenylalanine mustard
L-VAM	leuprolide acetate, vinblastine, Adriamycin, mitomycin
MA	mitomycin-C, Adriamycin
MABOP	Mustargen, Adriamycin, bleomycin, Oncovin, prednisone
MAC	methotrexate, Adriamycin, cyclophosphamide
MAC	mitomycin C, Adriamycin, cyclophosphamide
MACC	methotrexate, Adriamycin, cyclophosphamide, CCNU
MACOP-B	methotrexate, Adriamycin, cyclophosphamide, Oncovin, prednisone, bleomycin
MAD	MeCCNU and Adriamycin
MAP	L-phenylalanine mustard, Adriamycin, prednisone
M-BACOD	methotrexate, bleomycin, Adriamycin, cyclophosphamide, Oncovin, dexamethasone
MBC	methotrexate, bleomycin, cisplatin
MBD	methotrexate, bleomycin, diamminedichloroplatinum
MCA	megestrol, cyclosphosphamide, Adriamycin
MCBP	melphalan, cyclophosphamide, BCNU, prednisone
MCP	melphalan, cyclophosphamide, prednisone
MeCP	MeCCNU, cyclophosphamide, prednisone
MECY	methotrexate, cyclophosphamide

Appendix 1
Anticancer Drug Combinations *(Continued)*

PROTOCOL	COMPONENT DRUGS (abbreviation key at end of table)
MEFA	MeCCNU, 5-fluorouracil, Adriamycin
MF	mitomycin, 5-fluorouracil
MFP	melphalan, 5-fluorouracil, medroxyprogesterone acetate
MIFA	mitomycin C, 5-fluorouracil, Adriamycin
MM	mercaptopurine, methotrexate
MOAD	methotrexate, Oncovin, L-asparaginase, dexamethasone
MOB	mechlorethamine, Oncovin, bleomycin
MOB-III	mitomycin C, Oncovin, bleomycin, cisplatin
MOCA	methotrexate, Oncovin, cyclophosphamide, Adriamycin
MOF	MeCCNU, Oncovin, 5-fluorouracil
MOF-STREP	MeCCNU, Oncovin, 5-fluorouracil, streptozocin
MOMP	mechlorethamine, Oncovin, methotrexate, prednisone
MOP	methotrexate, Oncovin, prednisone
MOP-BAP	mechlorethamine, Oncovin, procarbazine, bleomycin, Adriamycin, prednisone
MOPP	mechlorethamine, Oncovin, procarbazine, prednisone
MOPP/ABV	methlorethamine, Oncovin, procarbazine, prednisone, Adriamycin, bleomycin, vinblastine
MPL + PRED	melphalan, prednisone
M-2 protocol	vincristine, carmustine, cyclophosphamide, melphalan, prednisone
MTX + MP + CTX	methotrexate, mercaptopurine, cyclophosphamide
M-VAC	methotrexate, vinblastine, Adriamycin, cisplatin
MVH	methotrexate, VP-16, hexamethylmelamine
MVP	mitomycin C, vinblastine, cisplatin
MVPP	mechlorethamine, vinblastine, procarbazine, prednisone
MVVPP	mechlorethamine, vincristine, vinblastine, procarbazine, prednisone

Appendix continued on following page

Appendix 1
Anticancer Drug Combinations *(Continued)*

PROTOCOL	COMPONENT DRUGS (abbreviation key at end of table)
NAC	nitrogen mustard, Adriamycin, CCNU
OAP	Oncovin, ara-C, prednisone
OAP-BLEO	Oncovin, ara-C, prednisone, bleomycin
OCA	Oncovin, cyclophosphamide, Adriamycin
O-DAP	Oncovin, dianhydrogalactitol, Adriamycin, Platinol
OMAD	Oncovin, methotrexate, Adriamycin, dactinomycin
OPAL	Oncovin, prednisone, L-asparaginase
OPP	Oncovin, procarbazine, prednisone
OPPA	Oncovin, procarbazine, prednisone, Adriamycin
PAC	Platinol, Adriamycin, cyclophosphamide
PATCO	prednisone, ara-C, thioguanine, cyclophosphamide, Oncovin
PAVE	procarbazine, Alkeran, Velban
PBV	Platinol, bleomycin, vinblastine
PCV	procarbazine, CCNU, vincristine
PE	Platinol, etoposide
PEB	Platinol, etoposide, bleomycin
PEP	Procytox, epipodophyllotoxin derivative, prednisolone
PFT	phenylalanine mustard, fluorouracil, tamoxifen
POC	procarbazine, Oncovin, CCNU
POCA	prednisone, Oncovin, cytarabine, Adriamycin
POCC	procarbazine, Oncovin, cyclophosphamide, CCNU
POMP	prednisone, Oncovin, methotrexate, Purinethol
PRIME	procarbazine, isophosphamide, methotrexate
ProMACE	prednisone, methotrexate, Adriamycin, cyclophosphamide, etoposide
ProMACE Cyta BOM	prednisone, methotrexate, Adriamycin, cyclophosphamide, etoposide, cytarabine, bleomycin, Oncovin, methotrexate
ProMACE MOPP	procarbazine, methotrexate, Adriamycin, Cytoxan, etoposide, Mustargen, Oncovin, procarbazine, prednisone

Appendix 1
Anticancer Drug Combinations (Continued)

PROTOCOL	COMPONENT DRUGS (abbreviation key at end of table)
PVB	Platinol, vinblastine, bleomycin
ROAP	rubidazone, Oncovin, ara-C, prednisone
SAM	streptozocin, Adriamycin, MeCCNU
SCAB	streptozocin, CCNU, Adriamycin, bleomycin
SMF	streptozocin, mitomycin C, 5-fluorouracil
TAD	6-thioguanine, Ara-C, daunomycin
T-CAP-III	triazinate, cyclophosphamide, Adriamycin, Platinol
T-MOP	6-thioguanine, methotrexate, Oncovin, prednisone
TOAP	thioguanine, Oncovin, cytosine arabinoside, prednisone
TRAP	thioguanine, rubidomycin, ara-C, prednisone
VA	vincristine, Adriamycin
VAB I	vinblastine, actinomycin D, bleomycin
VAB II	vinblastine, actinomycin D, bleomycin, cisplatin
VAB III	vinblastine, actinomycin D, bleomycin, cisplatin, chlorambucil, cyclophosphamide
VAB IV	vinblastine, actinomycin D, bleomycin, cisplastin, cyclophosphamide
VABCD	vincristine, Adriamycin, bleomycin, CCNU, DTIC
VAC	vincristine, actinomycin D, cyclophosphamide
VAD	vincristine, Adriamycin, dexamethasone
VADA	vincristine, Adriamycin, dexamethasone, actinomycin D
VAFAC	vincristine, Adriamycin, 5-fluorouracil, amethopterin, cyclophosphamide
VAFAC	vinblastine, amethopterin, 5-fluorouracil, Adriamycin, cyclophosphamide
VAM	VP-16-213, Adriamycin, methotrexate
VAMP	vincristine, amethopterin, 6-mercaptopurine, prednisone
VAP	vinblastine, actinomycin D, Platinol
VATD	vincristine, ara-C, 6-thioguanine, daunorubicin
VATH	vinblastine, Adriamycin, thiotepa, Halotestin

Appendix continued on following page

Appendix 1
Anticancer Drug Combinations (Continued)

PROTOCOL	COMPONENT DRUGS (abbreviation key at end of table)
VAV	VP-16-213, Adriamycin, vincristine
VB	vinblastine, bleomycin
VBA	vincristine, BCNU, Adriamycin
VBAP	vincristine, BCNU, Adriamycin, prednisone
VBC	vincristine, bleomycin, cisplatin
VBD	vinblastine, bleomycin, cis-diamminedichloroplatinum
VBM	vincristine, bleomycin, methotrexate
VBMCP	vincristine, BCNU, melphalan, cyclophosphamide, prednisone
VBP	vinblastine, bleomycin, Platinol
VC	VP-16, carboplatin
VCAP	vincristine, cyclophosphamide, Adriamycin, prednisone
V-CAP III	VP-16-213, cyclophosphamide, Adriamycin, Platinol
VCF	vincristine, cyclophosphamide, 5-fluorouracil
VCMP	vincristine, cyclophosphamide, melphalan, prednisone
VCP	vincristine, cyclophosphamide, prednisone
VDP	vincristine, daunorubicin, prednisone
VEMP	vincristine, Endoxan, mercaptopurine, prednisone
VENP	vincristine, Endoxan, Natulan, prednisone
VFAM	vincristine, 5-fluorouracil, Adriamycin, mitomycin C
VLP	vincristine, L-asparaginase, prednisone
VMAD	vincristine, methotrexate, Adriamycin, actinomycin D
VMCP	vincristine, melphalan, cyclophosphamide, prednisone
VMV	vincristine, methotrexate, VP-16
VOCAP	VP-16-213, Oncovin, cyclophosphamide, Adriamycin, Platinol

Appendix 1
Anticancer Drug Combinations (Continued)

PROTOCOL	COMPONENT DRUGS
VP	vincristine, prednisone
VP-16 + DDP	etoposide, cisplatin
VPB	vinblastine, Platinol, bleomycin
VPCMF	vincristine, prednisone, cyclophosphamide, methotrexate, 5-fluorouracil
VP-L-asparaginase	vincristine, prednisone, L-asparaginase
VPVCP	vincristine, prednisone, vinblastine, chlorambucil, procarbazine

Note:

actinomycin D (dactinomycin)
Adriamycin (doxorubicin)
Alkeran (melphalan)
AMSA (amsacrine)
Ara-C (cytarabine)
BCNU (carmustine)
BCNU (bis-chloroethyl-nitrosourea)
Blenoxane (bleomycin)
BLEO (bleomycin)
CCNU (lomustine)
CDDP (cisplatin)
CPM (cyclophosphamide)
CTX (cyclophosphamide)
Cytosar-U (cytarabine)
Cytoxan (cyclophosphamide)
DACT (dactinomycin)
DDP (cisplatin)
DOX (doxorubicin)
DTIC (dacarbazine)
Ftorafur (tegarfur)
5-FU (5-fluorouracil)
FUDR (floxuridine)

ICRF-159 (razoxane)
IUDR (iododeoxyuridine)
levamisole (imidazole)
L-PAM (melphalan)
MeCCNU (semustine)
methyl-CCNU
MITO (mitomycin)
MTX (methotrexate)
Mutamycin (mitomycin)
nitrogen mustard (mechlorethamine)
Oncovin (vincristine)
PCB (procarbazine)
Platinol (cisplatin)
PRDL (prednisolone)
PRED (prednisone)
TMX (tamoxifen)
VBL (vinblastine)
VCR (vincristine)
VDS (vindesine)
Velban (vinblastine)
VePesid (etoposide)
VP-16 (etoposide)

Appendices
Table of Elements

Name	Symbol	At. No.	At. Wt.*	Name	Symbol	At. No.	At. Wt.*
Actinium	Ac	89	227.028	Mendelevium	Md	101	(258)
Aluminum	Al	13	26.982	Mercury	Hg	80	200.59
Americium	Am	95	(243)	Molybdenum	Mo	42	95.94
Antimony	Sb	51	121.75	Neodymium	Nd	60	144.24
Argon	Ar	18	39.948	Neon	Ne	10	20.179
Arsenic	As	33	74.922	Neptunium	Np	93	237.0482
Astatine	At	85	(210)	Nickel	Ni	28	58.69
Barium	Ba	56	137.33	Niobium	Nb	41	92.906
Berkelium	Bk	97	(247)	Nitrogen	N	7	14.007
Beryllium	Be	4	9.012	Nobelium	No	102	259
Bismuth	Bi	83	208.980	Osmium	Os	76	190.2
Boron	B	5	10.811	Oxygen	O	8	15.999
Bromine	Br	35	79.904	Palladium	Pd	46	106.42
Cadmium	Cd	48	112.41	Phosphorus	P	15	30.974
Calcium	Ca	20	40.08	Platinum	Pt	78	195.08
Californium	Cf	98	(251)	Plutonium	Pu	94	(244)
Carbon	C	6	12.011	Polonium	Po	84	(209)
Cerium	Ce	58	140.12	Potassium	K	19	39.098
Cesium	Cs	55	132.905	Praseodymium	Pr	59	140.908
Chlorine	Cl	17	35.453	Promethium	Pm	61	(145)
Chromium	Cr	24	51.996	Protactinium	Pa	91	231.036
Cobalt	Co	27	58.933	Radium	Ra	88	226.025
Copper	Cu	29	63.546	Radon	Rn	86	(222)
Curium	Cm	96	(247)	Rhenium	Re	75	186.207
Dysprosium	Dy	66	162.50	Rhodium	Rh	45	102.906
Einsteinium	Es	99	(252)	Rubidium	Rb	37	85.468
Element 106		106	(263)	Ruthenium	Ru	44	101.07
Erbium	Er	68	167.26	Rutherfordium	Rf	104	(261)
Europium	Eu	63	151.96	Samarium	Sm	62	150.36
Fermium	Fm	100	(257)	Scandium	Sc	21	44.956
Fluorine	F	9	18.998	Selenium	Se	34	78.96
Francium	Fr	87	(223)	Silicon	Si	14	28.086
Gadolinium	Gd	64	157.25	Silver	Ag	47	107.868
Gallium	Ga	31	69.72	Sodium	Na	11	22.990
Germanium	Ge	32	72.59	Strontium	Sr	38	87.62
Gold	Au	79	196.967	Sulfur	S	16	32.064
Hafnium	Hf	72	178.49	Tantalum	Ta	73	180.948
Hahnium	Ha	105	(261)	Technetium	Tc	43	(98)
Helium	He	2	4.003	Tellurium	Te	52	127.60
Holmium	Ho	67	164.930	Terbium	Tb	65	158.925
Hydrogen	H	1	1.008	Thallium	Tl	81	204.383
Indium	In	49	114.82	Thorium	Th	90	232.038
Iodine	I	53	126.905	Thulium	Tm	69	168.934
Iridium	Ir	77	192.22	Tin	Sn	50	118.69
Iron	Fe	26	55.847	Titanium	Ti	22	47.88
Krypton	Kr	36	83.80	Tungsten	W	74	183.85
Lanthanum	La	57	138.906	Uranium	U	92	238.029
Lawrencium	Lw	103	(260)	Vanadium	V	23	50.942
Lead	Pb	82	207.2	Xenon	Xe	54	131.29
Lithium	Li	3	6.941	Ytterbium	Yb	70	173.04
Lutetium	Lu	71	174.967	Yttrium	Y	39	88.906
Magnesium	Mg	12	24.312	Zinc	Zn	30	65.38
Manganese	Mn	25	54.938	Zirconium	Zr	40	91.22

*Atomic weights are corrected to conform with the 1979 values of the International Union of Pure and Applied Chemistry, expressed to the fourth decimal point, rounded off to the nearest thousandth. The numbers in parentheses are the mass numbers of the most stable or most common isotope.

Appendix 3
Symbols

Symbols consisting of letters of the alphabet appear in Abbreviations.

Ⓛ	left	←	is due to
Ⓡ	right, trademark	⇌	reversible reaction
Ⓜ	murmur	⊖	normal
⊙	start of operation	√c̄	check with
⊗	end of operation	φ	none
□	male	∨	systolic blood pressure
○	female	∧	diastolic blood pressure
♂	male	#	gauge, number, weight,
♀	female		pound(s)
*	birth	℞	recipe, take
†	death	°	degree
∝	is proportional to	24°	24 hours
Δ	prism diopter	1°	primary
Δt	time interval	2°	secondary
ΔA	change in absorbance	2d	second
ΔpH	change in pH	2ndry	secondary
Ω	ohm	1×	once
π	3.1416—ratio of circumference	2×	twice
	of a circle to its diameter	×2	twice
σ	1/100 of a second, standard	′	foot, minute, primary accent,
	deviation		univalent
χ^2	chi square (test)	″	inch, second, secondary accent,
τ	life (time)		bivalent
τ½	half-life (time)	ii̅	two
?	question of, questionable,	/	of, per
	possible	:	ratio (is to)
>	greater than	::	equality between ratios, "as"
≯	not greater than	∴	therefore
≧	greater than or equal to	+	plus, positive, present
<	less than	−	minus, negative, absent
≮	not less than	÷	divided by
≦	less than or equal to	=	equals
∼	approximate	≠	does not equal, not equal to
≃	approximately equal to	≅	approximately equals
±	not definite, plus/minus	%	per cent
(+)	significant	θ	angle (measuring divergence of
(−)	insignificant		two intersecting lines or planes)
(±)	possibly significant	℥	ounce
↓	decreased, depression	f℥	fluid ounce
↑	elevation, increased	℈	scruple
⇧	up	♏	minim
↑V	increase due to *in vivo* effect	ʒ	drachm, dram
↓V	decrease due to *in vivo* effect	fʒ	fluidrachm, fluidram
↑C	increase due to chemical	√	root, square root, radical
	interference during the assay	²√	square root
↓C	decrease due to chemical	³√	cube root
	interference during the assay	∞	infinity
→	causes, no change, transfer to	◡	combined with

Appendix 4
Positions of Fetus

Cephalic Presentation

1. Vertex—occiput, the point of direction

Left occipitoanterior	L.O.A.
Left occipitotransverse	L.O.T.
Right occipitoposterior	R.O.P.
Right occipitotransverse	R.O.T.
Right occipitoanterior	R.O.A.
Left occipitoposterior	L.O.P.

2. Face—chin, the point of direction

Right mentoposterior	R.M.P.
Left mentoanterior	L.M.A.
Right mentotransverse	R.M.T.
Right mentoanterior	R.M.A.
Left mentotransverse	L.M.T.
Left mentoposterior	L.M.P.

3. Brow—the point of direction

Right frontoposterior	R.F.P.
Left frontoanterior	L.F.A.
Right frontotransverse	R.F.T.
Right frontoanterior	R.F.A.
Left frontotransverse	L.F.T.
Left frontoposterior	L.F.P.

Breech or Pelvic Presentation

1. Complete breech—sacrum, the point of direction (feet crossed and thighs flexed on abdomen)

Left sacroanterior	L.S.A.
Left sacrotransverse	L.S.T.
Right sacroposterior	R.S.P.
Right sacroanterior	R.S.A.
Right sacrotransverse	R.S.T.
Left sacroposterior	L.S.P.

2. Incomplete breech—sacrum, the point of direction
Same designations as above, adding the qualifications footling, knee, etc.

Transverse Lie or Shoulder Presentation

Shoulder—scapula, the point of direction

Left scapuloanterior	L.Sc.A.	Back anterior positions
Right scapuloanterior	R.Sc.A.	
Right scapuloposterior	R.Sc.P.	Back posterior positions
Left scapuloposterior	L.Sc.P.	

Appendix 5
Greek Alphabet

The Greek alphabet has 24 letters

Name	Lowercase	Uppercase	Transcription
alpha	α	A	a
beta	β	B	b
gamma	γ	Γ	g
delta	δ	Δ	d
epsilon	ε	E	e
zeta	ζ	Z	z
eta	η	H	ē
theta	θ	Θ	th
iota	ι	I	i
kappa	κ	K	c, k
lambda	λ	Λ	l
mu	μ	M	m
nu	ν	N	n
xi	ξ	Ξ	x
omicron	o	O	o
pi	π	Π	p
rho	ρ	P	r
sigma	σ	Σ	s
tau	τ	T	t
upsilon	υ	Υ	y
phi	φ	Φ	ph
chi	χ	X	ch
psi	ψ	Ψ	ps
omega	ω	Ω	ō

VANDERBILT UNIVERSITY

3 0081 024 680 021